TAKING SIDES

Clashing Views in

Drugs and Society

EIGHTH EDITION

TAKING SIDES

Clashing Views in

Drugs and Society

EIGHTH EDITION

Selected, Edited, and with Introductions by

Raymond Goldberg
State University of New York College at Cortland

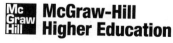

McGraw-Hill
Higher Education

Boston   Burr Ridge, IL   Dubuque, IA   New York   San Francisco   St. Louis
Bangkok   Bogotá   Caracas   Kuala Lumpur   Lisbon   London   Madrid   Mexico City
Milan   Montreal   New Delhi   Santiago   Seoul   Singapore   Sydney   Taipei   Toronto

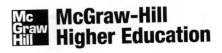

The **McGraw·Hill** Companies

McGraw-Hill
Higher Education

TAKING SIDES: CLASHING VIEWS IN DRUGS AND SOCIETY,
EIGHTH EDITION

Published by McGraw-Hill, a business unit of The McGraw-Hill Companies, Inc., 1221 Avenue of
the Americas, New York, NY 10020. Copyright © 2008 by The McGraw-Hill Companies, Inc. All
rights reserved. Previous edition(s) 1993–2006. No part of this publication may be reproduced or
distributed in any form or by any means, or stored in a database or retrieval system, without the
prior written consent of The McGraw-Hill Companies, Inc., including, but not limited to, in any
network or other electronic storage or transmission, or broadcast for distance learning.

Some ancillaries, including electronic and print components, may not be available to customers
outside the United States.

Taking Sides® is a registered trademark of the McGraw-Hill Companies, Inc.
Taking Sides is published by the **Contemporary Learning Series** group within the McGraw-Hill
Higher Education division.

 This book is printed on recycled, acid-free paper containing
10% postconsumer waste.

1 2 3 4 5 6 7 8 9 0 DOC/DOC 0 9 8 7

MHID: 0-07-351511-6
ISBN: 978-0-07-351511-3
ISSN: 1094-7566

Managing Editor: *Larry Loeppke*
Production Manager: *Faye Schilling*
Senior Developmental Editor: *Jill Peter*
Editorial Assistant: *Nancy Meissner*
Production Service Assistant: *Rita Hingtgen*
Permissions Coordinator: *Lori Church*
Senior Marketing Manager: *Julie Keck*
Marketing Communications Specialist: *Mary Klein*
Marketing Coordinator: *Alice Link*
Project Manager: *Jane Mohr*
Design Specialist: *Tara McDermott*
Senior Administrative Assistant: *DeAnna Dausener*
Senior Operations Manager: *Pat Koch Krieger*
Cover Graphics: *Maggie Lytle*

Compositor: ICC Macmillan Inc.
Cover Image: © Brand X Pictures/Punchstock

Library of Congress Cataloging-in-Publication Data

Main entry under title:
   Taking sides: clashing views in drugs and society/selected, edited, and with introductions by
   Raymond Goldberg.—8th ed.
Includes bibliographical references.
1. Drug abuse—Social aspects. I. Goldberg, Raymond, *comp.*
                                      362.29

www.mhhe.com

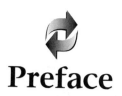

Preface

One of the hallmarks of a democratic society is the freedom of its citizens to disagree. This is no more evident than on the topic of drugs. The purpose of this eighth edition of *Taking Sides: Clashing Views in Drugs and Society* is to introduce drug-related issues that (1) are pertinent to the reader and (2) have no clear resolution. In the area of drug abuse, there is much difference of opinion regarding drug prevention, causation, and treatment. For example, should drug abuse be prevented by increasing enforcement of drug laws or by making young people more aware of the potential dangers of drugs? Is drug abuse caused by heredity, personality characteristics, or environment? Is drug abuse a medical, legal, or social problem? Are the dangers of some drugs such as Ecstasy, caffeine, and steroids overexaggerated? Should there be more stringent enforcement of marijuana use and underage drinking?

There are many implications to how the preceding questions are answered. If addiction to drugs is viewed as hereditary rather than as the result of flaws in one's character or personality, then a biological rather than a psychosocial approach to treatment may be pursued. If the consensus is that the prevention of drug abuse can be achieved by eliminating the availability of drugs, then more money and effort will be allocated for interdiction and law enforcement than education. If drug abuse is viewed as a legal problem, then prosecution and incarceration will be the goal. If drug abuse is identified as a medical problem, then abusers will be given treatment. However, if drug abuse is deemed a social problem, then energy will be directed at underlying social factors, such as poverty, unemployment, health care, and education. Not all of the issues have clear answers. One may favor increasing penalties for drug violations *and* improving treatment services. And it is possible to view drug abuse as a medical *and* social *and* legal problem.

The issues debated in this volume deal with both legal and illegal drugs. Although society seems most interested in illegal drugs, it is quite pertinent to address issues related to legal drugs because they cause more deaths and disabilities. No one is untouched by drugs, and everybody is affected by drug use and abuse. Billions of tax dollars are channeled into the war on drugs. Thousands of people are treated for drug abuse, often at public expense. The drug trade spawns crime and violence. Medical treatment for illnesses and injuries resulting from drug use and abuse creates additional burdens to an already extended health care system. Babies born to mothers who used drugs while pregnant are entering schools, and teachers are expected to meet the educational needs of these children. Ritalin is prescribed to several million students to deal with their lack of attention in the classroom. Drug use by secondary students is rampant. The issues debated here are not whether drug abuse is a problem, but what should be done to rectify this problem.

Many of these issues have an immediate impact on the reader. For example, Issue 3, "Are Drinking Age Laws Effective?" has an impact on anyone under age twenty-one who imbibes alcohol. Issue 14, "Does Secondhand Smoke Endanger the Health of Nonsmokers?" is relevant to smokers and nonsmokers because restrictions on smoking are discussed. Issue 10, "Are Psychotherapeutic Drugs Overprescribed for Treating Mental Illness?" is important because millions of people have been diagnosed with depression or some other type of mental illness. And the question "Should Laws Prohibiting Marijuana Use Be Relaxed?" (Issue 9) is relevant to the millions of people who smoke marijuana.

Plan of the book   In this eighth edition of *Taking Sides: Clashing Views in Drugs and Society*, there are 38 selections dealing with 19 issues. Each issue is preceded by an introduction and followed by a postscript. The purpose of the introduction is to provide some background information and to set the stage for the debate as it is argued in the "yes" and "no" selections. The postscript summarizes the debate and challenges some of the ideas brought out in the two selections, which can enable the reader to see the issue in other ways. Included in the postscripts are additional suggested readings on the issue. Also, Internet site addresses (URLs) have been provided at the beginning of each unit, which should prove useful as starting points for further research. The issues, introductions, and postscripts are designed to stimulate readers to think about and achieve an informed view of some of the critical issues facing society today. At the back of the book is a list of all the contributors to this volume, which gives information on the physicians, professors, authors, and policymakers whose views are debated here.

Taking Sides: Clashing Views in Drugs and Society is a tool to encourage critical thinking. In reading an issue and forming your own opinion, you should not feel confined to adopt one or the other of the positions presented. Some readers may see important points on both sides of an issue and may construct for themselves a new and creative approach. Such an approach might incorporate the best of both sides, or it might provide an entirely new vantage point for understanding.

Changes to this edition   This eighth edition represents a significant revision. Eight of the 19 issues are new: Should Drug Laws Against Drug Use Remain Restrictive? (Issue 1); Are Drinking Age Laws Effective? (Issue 3); Are the Dangers of Ecstasy (MDMA) Overstated? (Issue 4); Should the Federal Government Play a Larger Role in Regulating Steroid Use? (Issue 7); Are Psychotherapeutic Drugs Overprescribed for Treating Mental Illness? (Issue 10); Does Secondhand Smoke Endanger the Health of Nonsmokers? (Issue 14); Should Marijuana Be Approved for Medical Use? (Issue 16); and Is Abstinence an Effective Strategy for Drug Education? (Issue 19). For eight of the remaining eleven issues from the previous edition, one or both selections were replaced to reflect more current points of view.

A word to the instructor   To facilitate the use of *Taking Sides*, an *Instructor's Resource Guide with Test Questions* (multiple choice and essay) and a general guidebook called *Using Taking Sides in the Classroom*, which discusses methods and techniques for implementing the pro-con approach into any classroom setting, can be obtained from the publisher. An online version of *Using Taking Sides in the Classroom* and a correspondence service for *Taking Sides* adopters can be found at http://www.mhcls.com/usingts/. For students, we offer a field guide to analyzing argumentative essays called *Analyzing Controversy: An Introductory Guide,* with exercises and techniques to help them to decipher genuine controversies.

Taking Sides: Clashing Views in Drugs and Society is only one title in the *Taking Sides* series. If you are interested in seeing the table of contents for any of the other titles, please visit the *Taking Sides* Web site at http://www.mhcls.com/takingsides/.

Acknowledgments   A number of people have been most helpful in putting together this eighth edition. I would like to thank those professors who adopted the seventh edition of this book and took the time to make suggestions for this subsequent edition:

Donald Brodeur
Sacred Heart University

Owen Cater
California State University, Sacramento

Mark Kaelin
Montclair State University

I am also grateful to my students and colleagues, who did not hesitate to share their perceptions and to let me know what they liked and disliked about the seventh edition. Without the editorial staff at McGraw-Hill Contemporary Learning Series, this book would not exist. The insight and professional contributions have been most valuable. Their thoughtful perceptions and encouragement were most appreciated. In no small way can my family be thanked. I am grateful for their patience and support.

Raymond Goldberg
State University of New York at Cortland

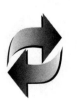

Contents in Brief

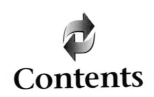

Contents

Judith McMullen, a law professor at Marquette University, argues that laws prohibiting underage drinking have been ineffective. Young adults between the ages of 18 and 21 who do not live at home have opportunities to drink alcohol without parental interference. In addition, this same age group has other legal rights, such as the right to marry, drive a car, or join the military. Enforcement of underage drinking laws, says McMullen, is destined for failure. The United States Department of Health and Human Services maintains that underage drinking is fraught with numerous problems ranging from motor vehicle crashes to homicide and suicide. Also, underage drinking is related to unhealthy risk-taking behaviors and poor academic performance. Rather than tolerate underage drinking, more effort should be placed on enforcing underage drinking laws.

Issue 4.   Are the Dangers of Ecstasy (MDMA) Overstated?   97

Jacob Sullum, a senior editor at *Reason* magazine, contends that the effects of drugs such as Ecstasy, particularly in regard to sexual behavior, are exaggerated. Sullum refers to the history of marijuana and how it was deemed a drug that would make people engage in behaviors that they would not typically engage in. Sullum feels that the public's reaction is unjustified. Club drugs such as Ecstasy allow partygoers to dance and remain active for long periods of time according to the National Institute on Drug Abuse (NIDA). However, Ecstasy may produce a number of adverse effects such as high blood pressure, panic attacks, loss of consciousness, seizures, and death. Moreover, Ecstasy can produce negative effects on the brain, resulting in confusion, depression, memory impairment, and attention difficulties.

Issue 5.   Should Pregnant Drug Users Be Prosecuted?   120

Paul A. Logli, an Illinois prosecuting attorney, argues that it is the government's duty to enforce every child's right to begin life with a healthy, drug-free mind and body. Logli maintains that pregnant women who use drugs should be prosecuted because they harm the life of their unborn children. He feels that it is the state's responsibility to ensure that every baby is born as healthy as possible. Carolyn Carter, a social work professor at Howard University, argues that the stigma of drug use during pregnancy has resulted in the avoidance of treatment. Carter asserts that the prosecution of pregnant drug users is unfair because

Robert A. Levy, a senior fellow at the Cato Institute, and Rosalind B. Marimont, a mathematician and scientist who retired from the National Institute of Standards and Technology, claim that the government distorts and exaggerates the dangers associated with cigarette smoking. Levy and Marimont state that factors such as poor nutrition and obesity are overlooked as causes of death among smokers. They note that cigarette smoking is harmful, but the misapplication of statistics should be regarded as "junk science." The 2004 Surgeon General's report on smoking states that the evidence pointing to the dangers of smoking is overwhelming. The report clearly links cigarette smoking to various forms of cancer, cardiovascular diseases, respiratory diseases, reproductive problems, and a host of other medical conditions.

Issue 9.   Should Laws Prohibiting Marijuana Use Be Relaxed?   211

Ethan Nadelmann, founder and executive director of the Drug Policy Foundation, argues that law enforcement officials are overzealous in prosecuting individuals for marijuana possession. Eighty-seven percent of marijuana arrests are for possession of small amounts of the drug. The cost of marijuana enforcement to U.S. taxpayers ranges from $10–15 billion. In addition, punishments are unjust in that they vary greatly. The Office of National Drug Control Policy (ONDCP) contends that marijuana is not a harmless drug. Besides causing physical problems, marijuana affects academic performance and emotional adjustment. Moreover, dealers who grow and sell marijuana may become violent to protect their commodity.

Issue 10.   Are Psychotherapeutic Drugs Overprescribed for Treating Mental Illness?   236

Professor Leemon McHenry, a professor with the Philosophy Department at the California State University at Northridge, questions the effectiveness of psychiatric drugs, especially antidepressant drugs known as selective serotonin reuptake inhibitors (SSRIs). McHenry maintains that the increase in the prescribing of antidepressant drugs results from their promotion by the pharmaceutical industry. McHenry also argues that pharmaceutical companies should be more forthright in the efficacy of these drugs. Medical doctor Bruce M. Cohen maintains that psychiatric medicines are very beneficial in enabling individuals with a variety of illnesses to return to normal aspects of consciousness. Cohen points out that people with conditions such as anxiety, depression, and psychosis respond very well to medications. These types of drugs have been utilized successfully for hundreds of years.

James Thornton from *Men's Health* describes caffeine as an addictive substance that results in withdrawal symptoms. The stimulating effects of caffeine are muted by tolerance that develops to the drug. One downside to caffeine is that it impedes one's ability to get to sleep. The lack of sleep may result in jitteriness and arrhythmias in adults. In large amounts caffeine can cause anxiety and panic attacks. According to medical doctor Sally Satel, caffeine may have addictive qualities but its dangers are overstated. Caffeine's addictive qualities are modest. Most caffeine users are able to moderate their consumption of caffeine. Headaches are one by-product of caffeine cessation. Very few people consume caffeine compulsively. Moreover, individuals who have difficulty moderating their caffeine use often have other psychiatric problems.

Writer Michael Fumento disputes the idea that Ritalin is over prescribed. He notes that there are many myths associated with Ritalin. It does not lead to abuse and addiction. Fumento argues that Ritalin is an excellent medication for ADHD. One reason it is not as accepted is because it has been demonized by various groups. It is possible that the drug is underutilized. Fumento contends that more students would benefit from Ritalin and other stimulants. Pediatrician and family therapist Lawrence Diller contends that Ritalin is overused because diagnosing ADHD is imprecise. Symptoms such as distractibility, inattention, and impulsivity are typical behaviors of many children. Moreover, it is unclear whether the use of Ritalin and other stimulants carry over to long-term academic success. Diller argues that the proliferation in the use of Ritalin stems from its promotion by the pharmaceutical industry.

Merrill Matthews, a health policy advisor with the American Legislative Exchange Council, argues that the advertising of prescription drugs directly to consumers will result in better-informed consumers. Additionally, communication between doctors and patients may improve because patients will be more knowledgeable about drugs. Writers Robert Langreth and Matthew Herper contend that the pharmaceutical industry spends much more money promoting drugs that are similar to existing drugs rather than researching how to develop new and better drugs. The top ten pharmaceutical companies spend twice as much money on marketing and administration as on research. Too often, claim Langreth and Herper, the excessive marketing of drugs creates demand even when the demand is not present.

According to the Surgeon General's report on secondhand smoke, in 2005 more than 3,000 adult nonsmokers died from lung cancer, 46,000 from coronary heart disease, and about 430 newborns from sudden infant death syndrome. In addition, children exposed to secondhand smoke have an increased risk of acute respiratory infections, ear problems, and severe asthma. Simply separating smokers from nonsmokers or having separately ventilated areas for smoking is ineffective. Statisticians J. B. Copas and J. Q. Shi argue that research demonstrating that secondhand smoke is harmful is biased. They contend that many journals are more likely to publish articles if secondhand smoke is shown to be deleterious and that the findings of many studies exaggerate the adverse effects of secondhand smoke.

The National Institute on Alcohol Abuse and Alcoholism (NIAAA) contends that heredity plays a large role in the development of alcoholism. Family environment may play a role in whether one becomes an alcoholic but individuals inherit characteristics that increase the possibility of developing alcoholism. The NIAAA notes that identical twins are twice as likely to become alcoholic as fraternal twins. Grazyna Zajdow, a lecturer in sociology at Deakin University, maintains that the concept of alcoholism results from a social construct of what it means to be alcoholic. Because alcoholism is a social stigma, it is viewed as a disease rather than as a condition caused by personal and existential pain. Environmental conditions, especially consumerism, says Zajdow, are the root cause of alcoholism.

Sherwood O. Cole, a professor emeritus of psychology at Rutgers University, argues in favor of allowing marijuana for medicinal purposes despite the fact that it has some adverse effects, especially on cognition and mental health and on the respiratory and cardiovascular systems. Some of the potential medical uses of marijuana include reducing fluid pressure in the eyes of glaucoma patients, reducing nausea associated with cancer treatment, stimulating appetite in AIDS patients, and reducing convulsions of epileptic patients. The Drug Enforcement Administration (DEA) states that marijuana has not been proven to have medical utility. The DEA cites the positions of the American Medical Association, the American Cancer Society, the American Academy of Pediatrics, and the National Multiple Sclerosis Society to support its position. The DEA feels that any benefits of medicinal marijuana are outweighed by its drawbacks.

The Office of National Drug Control Policy (ONDCP), an agency of the federal government, maintains that it is important to test students for illicit drugs because testing reduces drug use and improves the learning environment in schools. The ONDCP purports that the majority of students support drug testing. In addition, drug testing does not decrease participation in extracurricular activities. Jennifer Kern and associates maintain that drug testing is ineffective and that the threat of drug testing may dissuade students from participating in extracurricular activities. Moreover, drug testing is costly, it may make schools susceptible to litigation, and it undermines relationships of trust between students and teachers. Drug testing, according to Kern, does not effectively identify students who may have serious drug problems.

Author Susan L. Ettner and associates maintain that not only do people in substance abuse treatment benefit, but that taxpayers also benefit. They estimate that about seven dollars is saved for every dollar spent on treatment. Individuals in treatment are less likely to engage in criminal activity and they are more likely to be employed. The report from the United Nations Office on Drugs and Crime argues that drug abuse treatment does not cure drug abuse. Most people who go through drug treatment relapse. Drug abuse treatment does not get at the root causes of drug abuse: crime, family disruption, loss of economic productivity, and social decay. At best, treatment may minimize drug abuse.

Issue 19.   Is Abstinence an Effective Strategy for Drug Education?   441

Tracy J. Evans-Whipp, of the Murdoch Children's Research Institute in Melbourne, Australia, and her colleagues maintain that an abstinence message coupled with harsh penalties is more effective at reducing drug use than a message aimed at minimizing the harms of drugs. They contend that an abstinence message is clear and that a harm reduction message may give a mixed message. Drug researcher Marsha Rosenbaum states that because many teens experiment with drugs, a message to reduce the harms associated with drugs is necessary. Rosenbaum believes that scare tactics and misinformation about drugs increases the likelihood that teens may have problems if or when they experiment with drugs. Also, a problem with the abstinence-only message is that teens have no one to turn to if they experience problems with drugs.

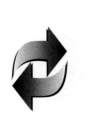

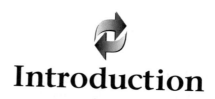

Introduction

Drugs: Divergent Views

An Overview of the Problem

The topic of drugs remains a controversial topic in today's society. Very few topics generate as much debate and concern as drugs. Drug use, either directly or indirectly, affects everyone. Drugs and issues related to drugs are evident in every aspect of life. There is much dismay that drug use and abuse cause many of the problems that plague society. Individuals, families, and communities are adversely affected by drug abuse, and many people wonder if the very fabric of society will continue to experience decay because of the abuse of drugs. The news media are replete with horrific stories about people under the influence of drugs committing crimes or perpetrating violence against others; of people who die senselessly; of men, women, and children who compromise themselves for drugs; and of women who deliver babies that are addicted or impaired by drugs. In some countries drug cartels have a major impact on government. Clearly, one does not need to be a drug user to experience its deleterious effects.

From conception until death, almost everyone is touched by drug use. For example, stimulants such as Ritalin are prescribed for children so that they can learn or behave better in school. Some college students take stimulants so that they can stay up late to write a term paper or lose a few pounds. Moreover, college students who use Ritalin are more likely to use illegal drugs (Teter, Esteban, Boyd, and Guthrie, 2003). Many teenagers take drugs to cope with daily stresses and increasing responsibilities or because they want to be accepted by their friends. For many people, young and old, the elixir for relaxation may be sipped, swallowed, smoked, or sniffed. Some people who live under poverty-stricken conditions anesthetize themselves with drugs as a way to escape consciously from their unpleasant environment. On the other hand, some individuals who seem to have everything immerse themselves in drugs, possibly out of boredom, emptiness in their lives, or simply to find the next thrill. To contend with the ailments that accompany getting older, the elderly often rely on drugs. Many people use drugs to confront their pains, problems, frustrations, and disappointments. Others take drugs simply because they like their effects or they take drugs due to curiosity. Some people just want to experience more happiness in their lives. Others use drugs to deal with issues of mental health. This last concern is debated in Issue 10, which examines whether or not psychotherapeutic drugs are overprescribed for treating mental illness.

Background on Drugs

Despite one's feelings about drug use, legal and illegal drugs are an integral part of society. The popularity of various drugs rises and falls with the times. For example, according to annual surveys of eighth-, tenth-, and twelfth-grade students in the United States, the use of marijuana and cocaine increased from the early 1990s to the late 1990s and then decreased from 2000 to the present (Johnston, O'Malley, Bachman, and Schulenberg, 2005). Especially alarming is the fact that approximately one of every six eighth-grade students has tried marijuana. One particular drug that increased significantly in the latter 1990s was MDMA (Ecstasy). MDMA spiked in 2001 and decreased since then. Nevertheless, Ecstasy and other club drugs remain popular with many young people. However, in the year 2002 many types of drugs have declined in use. Nevertheless, Ecstasy and other "club drugs" such as ketamine (Special K) and GHB remain popular with many young people. Issue 4 looks at whether or not the dangers of Ecstasy are overstated.

Understanding the history and role of drugs in society is critical to our ability to address drug-related problems. Drugs have been used throughout human history. Alcohol played a significant role in the early history of the United States. According to Lee (1963), for example, the Pilgrims landed at Plymouth Rock because they ran out of beer. Marijuana use dates back nearly 5,000 years, when the Chinese Emperor Shen Nung prescribed it for medical ailments like malaria, gout, rheumatism, and gas pains. Ironically, 5000 years after marijuana was first used medicinally, its medical benefits remain a matter of contention. Some issues simply refuse to go away. Hallucinogens have existed since the beginning of humankind and have been used for a variety of reasons. For example, hallucinogens were used to enhance beauty or to cast spells on enemies. About 150 of the estimated 500,000 different plant species have been used for hallucinogenic purposes (Schultes and Hofmann, 1979).

Opium, from which narcotics are derived, was written about extensively by the ancient Greeks and Romans; opium is even referred to in Homer's *Odyssey* (circa 1000 B.C.). In the Arab world opium and hashish were widely used (primarily because alcohol was forbidden). The Arabs were introduced to opium through their trading in India and China. Arab physician Avicenna (A.D. 1000) wrote an extremely complete medical textbook in which he describes the benefits of opium. Ironically, Avicenna died from an overdose of opium and wine. Eventually, opium played a central role in a war between China and the British government.

Caffeine remains the most commonly consumed drug throughout the world. It is estimated that more than 9 out of every 10 Americans drink beverages that include caffeine. Coffee dates back to A.D. 900, when, to stay awake during lengthy religious vigils, Muslims in Arabia consumed coffee. However, coffee was later condemned because the Koran, the holy book of Islam, described coffee as an intoxicant (Brecher, 1972). Drinking coffee became a popular activity in Europe, although it was banned for a short time. In the mid-1600s, coffeehouses were prime locations for men to converse, relax, and conduct business. Medical benefits were associated with coffee, although England's

King Charles II and English physicians tried to prohibit its use. Many claims have been made regarding the safety of caffeine. A study involving 15,000 people found no relationship between caffeine and cancer (*Men's Health*, 2004). Issue 11 discusses whether or not the consequences of caffeine outweigh its benefits.

Coffeehouses served as places of learning. For a one-cent cup of coffee, one could listen to well-known literary and political leaders (Meyer, 1954). Lloyd's of London, the famous insurance company, started around 1700 from Edward Lloyd's coffeehouse. However, not everyone was pleased with these "penny universities," as they were called. In 1674, in response to the countless hours men spent at the coffeehouses, a group of women published a pamphlet titled *The Women's Petition Against Coffee*, which criticized coffee use. Despite the protestations against coffee, its use proliferated. Today, more than 300 years later, coffeehouses are still flourishing as centers for relaxation and conversation.

Coca leaves, from which cocaine is derived, have been chewed since before recorded history. Drawings found on South American pottery illustrate that coca chewing was practiced before the rise of the Incan Empire. The coca plant was held in high regard: Considered a present from the gods, it was used in religious rituals and burial ceremonies. When the Spaniards arrived in South America, they tried to regulate coca chewing by the natives but were unsuccessful. Cocaine was later included in the popular soft drink Coca-Cola. Another stimulant, amphetamine, was developed in the 1920s and was originally used to treat narcolepsy. It was later prescribed for treating asthma and for weight loss. Today, the stimulant Ritalin, and similar variations are given to approximately six million school-age children annually in the United States to address attention deficit disorders. Some people claim that too many children are receiving Ritalin, while others assert that not enough students are receiving the drug. The question of whether or not Ritalin and other stimulants should be used for treating attention deficit disorder is debated in Issue 12.

Minor tranquilizers, also called "antianxiety drugs," were first marketed in the early 1950s. The sales of these drugs were astronomical. Drugs to reduce anxiety were in high demand. Another group of antianxiety drugs are benzodiazepines. Two well-known benzodiazepines are Librium and Valium; the latter ranks as the most widely prescribed drug in the history of American medicine. Xanax, which has replaced Valium as the minor tranquilizer of choice, is one of the five most prescribed drugs in the United States today. Minor tranquilizers are noteworthy because they are legally prescribed to alter one's consciousness. Mind-altering drugs existed prior to minor tranquilizers, but they were not prescribed for that purpose. In many instances, consumers request prescribed drugs from their physicians after seeing them advertised in the media. It is estimated that one-third of all prescriptions are written at the request of the patient. Pharmaceutical companies spend more than $2.5 billion on advertising drugs to consumers (Roth, 2003). Is it a good practice for patients to encourage their physicians to prescribe drugs that they saw advertised? Whether or not there should be more regulation on advertising prescription drugs directly to consumers is examined in Issue 13.

Combating Drug Problems

The debates in *Taking Sides: Clashing Views in Drugs and Society* confront many important drug-related issues. For example, what is the most effective way to reduce drug abuse? Should laws preventing drug use and abuse be more strongly enforced, or should drug laws be less punitive? How can the needs of individuals be met while serving the greater good of society? Should drug abuse be seen as a public health problem or a legal problem? Are drugs an American problem or an international problem? The debate whether the drug problem should be fought nationally or internationally is addressed in Issue 2. Many people argue that America would benefit most by focusing its attention on stopping the proliferation of drugs in other countries. Others feel that reducing the demand for drugs should be the primary focus. If federal funding is limited, should those funds focus on reducing the demand for drugs or stopping their importation?

One of the oldest debates concerns whether or not drug use should be decriminalized. In recent years this debate has become more intense because well-known individuals such as political analyst William F. Buckley, Jr., and economist Milton Friedman have come out in support of changing drug laws. For many people the issue is not whether drug use is good or bad, but whether people should be punished for taking drugs. Is it worth the time and expense for law enforcement officials to arrest nonviolent drug offenders? One question that is basic to this debate is whether drug decriminalization causes more or less damage than keeping drugs illegal. Issue 1 addresses the question of whether restrictive drug laws are effective at reducing drug use and abuse.

In a related matter, should potentially harmful drugs be restricted even if they may be of medical benefit? Some people are concerned that drugs used for medical reasons may be illegally diverted. Yet most people agree that patients should have access to the best medicine available. In referenda in numerous states, U.S. voters have approved the medical use of marijuana. Is the federal government consistent in allowing potentially harmful drugs to be used for medical purposes? For example, narcotics are often prescribed for pain relief. Is there a chance that patients who are given narcotics will become addicted? Issue 9 debates whether or not laws prohibiting marijuana should be relaxed. Regardless whether one feels that marijuana laws should be relaxed, the fact remains that over 25 million people have used marijuana in the previous year (Pacula, 2004/2005).

Addiction to drugs is a major problem in society. Yet, most people who stop their addiction to drugs do so on their own (Parmar, Salagubang, and Smith, 2004). Issue 6 looks at the issue of drug addiction and whether addiction is based on heredity or whether it is a choice that people make. In other words, is drug abuse a disease or is it a matter of poor decisions?

A major emphasis in society today is on competition, especially athletic competition. With a win-at-all-cost mentality, many athletes try to get the upper edge. One way to achieve this is through the use of performance-enhancing drugs. A particularly alarming point is that many athletes use anabolic steroids at extremely high dosage levels (*Business Week,* 2004). The issue of whether or not the federal government should play a larger role in regulating steroid use is discussed in Issue 7.

Many of the issues discussed in this book deal with drug prevention. As with most controversial issues, there is a lack of consensus on how to prevent drug-related problems. For example, Issue 5 debates whether or not prosecuting women who use drugs during pregnancy will affect drug use by other women who become pregnant. On the other hand, will pregnant women avoid prenatal care because they fear prosecution? Will newborns be better served if pregnant women who use drugs are charged with child abuse? Are these laws discriminatory, because most cases that are prosecuted involve poor women?

Some people contend that drug laws discriminate not only according to social class, but also according to age and ethnicity. Many drug laws in the United States were initiated because of their association with different ethnic groups: Opium smoking, for example, was made illegal after it was associated with Chinese immigrants. Cocaine became illegal after it was linked with blacks. And marijuana was outlawed after it was linked with Hispanics.

Drug-related issues are not limited to illegal drugs. Tobacco and alcohol are two pervasive legal drugs that generate much debate. For example, are the adverse effects of smoking exaggerated (Issue 8)? At a congressional hearing, executives at the largest tobacco companies swore tobacco is not addictive (Godrej, 2004). Should nonsmokers be concerned about the effects of second-hand smoke on their health (Issue 14)? With regard to alcoholism, a debate is whether alcoholism is caused by one's heredity or whether it is caused by environmental factors (Issue 15). A fourth issue relating to legal drugs deals with whether or not underage drinkers should be taught how to drink responsibly (Issue 3).

Gateway Drugs

Drugs like inhalants, tobacco, and alcohol are considered "gateway" drugs. These are drugs that are often used as a prelude to other, usually illegal, drugs. Inhalants are composed of numerous products, ranging from paints and solvents to glues, aerosol sprays, petroleum products, cleaning supplies, and nitrous oxide (laughing gas). Inhalant abuse, also known as "huffing," is a relatively new phenomenon in the United States. It seems that until the media started reporting on the dangers of inhalant abuse, its use was not particularly common (Brecher, 1972). Increasingly, movies depict smoking behavior. Celebrities are shown smoking cigarettes in movies (Dalton et al., 2003).

Advertisements are an integral part of the media, and their influence can be seen in the growing popularity of cigarette smoking among adolescents. In the 1880s cigarette smoking escalated in the United States. One of the most important factors contributing to cigarettes' popularity at that time was the development of the cigarette-rolling machine (previously, cigarettes could be rolled at a rate of only four per minute). Also, cigarette smoking, which was considered an activity reserved for men, began to be seen as an option for women. As cigarettes began to be marketed toward women, cigarette smoking became more widespread. As is evident from this introduction, numerous factors affect drug use. One argument is that if young people were better educated about the hazards of drugs and were taught how to understand the role of the media, then limits on advertising would not be necessary.

Drug Prevention and Treatment

Some people maintain that educating young people about drugs is one way to prevent drug use and abuse. Studies show that by delaying the onset of drug use, the likelihood of drug abuse is reduced. In the past, however, drug education had little impact on drug-taking behavior (Goldberg, 2005). Another strategy being adopted in many schools is to drug test students. The belief is that the threat of drug testing will reduce drug use. However, one needs to balance the possible benefits against the costs. The expense of drug testing ranges from $14 to $30 per test, except in the case of anabolic steroids, which costs $100 per test (Yamaguchi, Johnston, and O'Malley, 2003). Issue 17 examines whether or not drug testing of students serves as an effective deterrent to drug use.

Another way to reduce drug abuse that has been heavily promoted is drug abuse treatment. However, is drug abuse treatment effective? Does it prevent recurring drug abuse, reduce criminal activity and violence, and halt the spread of drug-related disease? Issue 18 examines whether or not drug abuse treatment affects these outcomes. The results of drug treatment are contradictory. A European study found that the majority of people in drug treatment drop out (*The Economist,* 2004). Other studies show that drug abuse treatment may have some benefits. But do the benefits outweigh the costs of the treatment? If society feels that treatment is a better alternative to other solutions, such as incarceration, it is imperative to know if treatment works.

Some illegal drugs may produce beneficial effects. For example, marijuana is claimed to help individuals deal with the side effects of chemotherapy. Others believe that marijuana helps people with glaucoma and multiple sclerosis as well as with many other ailments. However, because marijuana is illegal, should it be considered for medicinal use? Can medicinal use of marijuana turn into excessive, unhealthy use? Should marijuana use be encouraged for individuals who have a history of drug abuse in their families? Issue 16 discusses whether or not marijuana should be approved for medical use.

A logical place to address drug use is in schools because schools are able to reach the greatest number of potential drug users. Schools have employed various strategies to reduce drug use by students. One strategy that has been adopted is that of abstinence. Yet, is the abstinence approach the best vehicle for reducing or stopping young people from using drugs? Issue 19 focuses on whether or not the abstinence approach is an effective strategy for drug education.

Distinguishing Between Drug Use, Misuse, and Abuse

Although the terms *drug, drug misuse,* and *drug abuse* are commonly used, they have different meanings to different people. Defining these terms may seem simple at first, but many factors affect how they are defined. Should a definition for a drug be based on its behavioral effects, its effects on society, its pharmacological properties, or its chemical composition? One simple, concise definition of a drug is "any substance that produces an effect on the mind, body, or both." One could also define a drug by how it is used. For example, if watching television and listening to music are forms of escape from daily problems, then they may be considered drugs.

Legal drugs cause far more death and disability than illegal drugs, but society appears to be most concerned with the use of illegal drugs. The potential harms of legal drugs tend to be minimized. By viewing drugs as illicit substances only, people can fail to recognize that commonly used substances such as caffeine, tobacco, alcohol, and over-the-counter preparations are drugs. If these substances are not perceived as drugs, then people might not acknowledge that they can be misused or abused.

Definitions for misuse and abuse are not affected by a drug's legal status. Drug misuse refers to the inappropriate or unintentional use of drugs. Someone who smokes marijuana to improve his or her study skills is misusing marijuana because the drug impairs short-term memory. Drug abuse alludes to physical, emotional, financial, intellectual, or social consequences arising from chronic drug use. Under this definition, can a person abuse food, aspirin, soft drinks, or chocolate? Also, should people be free to make potentially unhealthy choices?

The Cost of the War on Drugs

The United States government spends billions of dollars each year to curb the rise in drug use. A major portion of that money goes toward law enforcement. Vast sums of money are used by the military to intercept drug shipments, while foreign governments are given money to help them with their own wars on drugs. A smaller portion of the funds is used for treating and preventing drug abuse.

The expense of drug abuse to industries is staggering: Experts estimate that about 14 percent of full-time construction workers in the United States between the ages of 18 and 49 use illicit drugs while at work (Gerber and Yacoubian, 2002). The cost of drug abuse to employers is approximately $171 billion each year (Kesselring and Pittman, 2002). Compared to nonaddicted employees, drug-dependent employees are absent from their jobs more often, and drug users are less likely to maintain stable job histories than nonusers. In its report *America's Habit: Drug Abuse, Drug Trafficking and Organized Crime*, the President's Commission on Organized Crime supported testing all federal workers for drugs. It further recommended that federal contracts be withheld from private employers who do not implement drug-testing procedures. Students who use drugs on a regular basis perform more poorly academically than students who do not use drugs.

A prerequisite to being hired by many companies is passing a drug test. Drug testing may be having a positive effect. From 1987 to 1994 the number of workers testing positive declined 57 percent (Center for Substance Abuse Prevention, 1995). Many companies have reported a decrease in accidents and injuries after the initiation of drug testing. However, most Americans consider drug testing degrading and dehumanizing. An important question is, What is the purpose of drug testing? Drug testing raises three other important questions: (1) Does drug testing prevent drug use? (2) Is the point of drug testing to help employees with drug problems or to get rid of employees who use drugs? and (3) How can the civil rights of employees be balanced against the rights of companies?

How serious is the drug problem? Is it real, or is there simply an unreasonable hysteria regarding drugs? In the United States there has been a growing intolerance toward drug use. Drugs are a problem for many people. Drugs can affect one's physical, social, intellectual, and emotional health. Ironically, some people take drugs because they produce these effects. Individuals who take drugs receive some kind of reward from the drug; the reward may come from being associated with others who use drugs or from the feelings derived from the drug. Many people use illegal drugs or legal drugs like tobacco and alcohol as forms of self-medication. If people did not receive rewards from their use of drugs, then people would likely cease using drugs.

The disadvantages of drugs are numerous: They interfere with career aspirations, educational achievement, athletic performance, and individual maturation. Drugs have also been associated with violent behavior; addiction; discord among siblings, children, parents, spouses, and friends; work-related problems; financial troubles; problems in school; legal predicaments; accidents; injuries; and death. Yet are drugs the cause or the symptom of the problems that people have? Perhaps drugs are one aspect of a larger scenario in which society is experiencing much change and in which drug use is merely another thread in the social fabric.

References

E. M. Brecher, *Licit and Illicit Drugs.* Little, Brown, 1972.

Business Week, "Can Drug-Busters Beat New Steroids? It's Scientist vs. Scientist as the Athens Olympics Approach," June 14, 2004, p. 82.

Center for Substance Abuse Prevention, Substance Abuse and Mental Health Services Administration, *Drug-Free for a New Century,* 1995.

M. A. Dalton, J. D. Sragent, M. L. Beach, L. Titus-Ernstoff, J. J. Gibson, M. B. Ahrens, J. J. Tickle, and T. F. Heatherton, "Effects of Viewing Smoking in Movies on Adolescent Smoking Initiation: A Cohort Study," *The Lancet,* July 26, 2003, pp. 281–290.

The Economist, "Coming Clean; Drug Treatment," October 16, 2004, p. 34.

J. K. Gerber and G. S. Yacoubian, "An Assessment of Drug Testing Within the Construction Industry," *Journal of Drug Education,* vol. 32, no. 1, 2002, pp. 53–68.

D. Godrej, "Smoke Gets In Your Eyes," *New International,* July 2004, pp. 9–12.

R. Goldberg, *Drugs Across the Spectrum.* Wadsworth Publishing, 2005.

L. D. Johnston, P. O. O'Malley, J. G. Bachman, and J. Schulenberg, *Monitoring the Future.* National Institute on Drug Abuse, 2005.

R. G. Kesselring and J. P. Pittman, "Drug Testing Laws and Employment Injuries," *Journal of Labor Research,* vol. 32, no. 2, 2002, pp. 293–302.

H. Lee, *How Dry We Were: Prohibition Revisited.* Prentice Hall, 1963.

Men's Health, "Start Me Up," October 2004, pp. 172–175.

H. Meyer, *Old English Coffee Houses.* Rodale Press, 1954.

R. L. Pacula, "Marijuana Use and Policy: What We Know and Have Yet to Learn," *NBER Reporter* Winter, 2004/2005, pp. 22–24.

N. Parmar, J. Salagubang, and S. A. Smith, "The Surprising Truth About Addiction," *Psychology Today,* May/June, 2004, pp. 43–46.

M. S. Roth, "Media and Message Effects on DTC Prescription Drug Print Advertising Awareness," *Journal of Advertising Research,* June, 2003, pp. 180–193.

R. E. Schultes and A. Hofmann, *Plants of the Gods: Origins of Hallucinogenic Use.* McGraw-Hill, 1979.

C. Teter, S. Esteban, C. Boyd, and S. Guthrie, "Illicit Methylphenidate Use in an Undergraduate Student Sample: Prevalence and Risk Factors," *Pharmacotherapy,* 2003, pp. 609–617.

R. Yamaguchi, L. D. Johnston, and P. M. O'Malley, "Relationship Between Student Illicit Drug Use and School Drug-testing Policies," *Journal of School Health,* April 2003, pp. 159–165.

Internet References . . .

Drug Policy Alliance

Formerly the Drug Policy Foundation, this site is an excellent source of information dealing with legal issues as they relate to drugs.

http://www.drugpolicyfoundation.org

Office of National Drug Control Policy (ONDCP)

This site provides information regarding the government's position on many drug-related topics. Funding allocations by the federal government to deal with drug problems is included also.

http://www.whitehousedrugpolicy.gov

National Institute on Drug Abuse—Club Drugs

Current information regarding club drugs such as Ecstasy, Rohypnol, ketamine, methamphetamines, and LSD can be accessed through this site.

http://www.clubdrugs.org

National Institute on Drug Abuse (NIDA)

Health risks associated with anabolic steroids and strategies for preventing steroid abuse can be obtained at this location.

http://www.steroidabuse.org

Drugs and Public Policy

*D*rug abuse causes a myriad of problems for society: The psychological and physical effects of drug abuse can be devastating; many drugs are addictive; wreak havoc on families; disability and death result from drug overdoses; and drugs frequently are implicated in crimes, especially violent crimes. Identifying drug-related problems is not difficult. What is unclear is the best course of action to take when dealing with these problems.

Three scenarios exist for dealing with drugs: policies can be made more restrictive, they can be made less restrictive, or they can remain the same. The position one takes depends on whether drug use and abuse are seen as legal, social, or medical problems. Perhaps the issue is not whether drugs are good or bad, but how to minimize the harm of drugs. The debates in this section explore these issues.

- Should Laws Against Drug Use Remain Restrictive?

- Should the United States Put More Emphasis on Stopping the Importation of Drugs?

- Are Drinking Age Laws Effective?

- Are the Dangers of Ecstasy (MDMA) Overstated?

- Should Pregnant Drug Users Be Prosecuted?

- Should Drug Addiction Be Considered a Disease?

- Should the Federal Government Play a Larger Role in Regulating Steroid Use?

ISSUE 1

Should Laws Against Drug Use Remain Restrictive?

YES: **Herbert Kleber and Joseph A. Califano Jr.**, from "Legalization: Panacea or Pandora's Box?" *World and I* (January 2006)

NO: **Peter Gorman**, from "Veteran Cops Against the Drug War," *The World and I* (January 2006)

ISSUE SUMMARY

YES: Herbert Kleber, the executive vice president of the Center on Addiction and Substance Abuse (CASA), and Joseph Califano, founder of CASA, maintain that drug laws should remain restrictive because legalization would result in increased use, especially by children. Kleber and Califano contend that drug legalization would not eliminate drug-related violence and harm caused by drugs.

NO: Author Peter Gorman states that restrictive drug laws have been ineffective. He notes that drug use and drug addiction have increased since drug laws became more stringent. Despite the crackdown on drug use, the availability of drugs has increased while the cost of drugs has decreased. In addition, restrictive drug laws, says Gorman, are racist and endanger civil liberties.

In 2008 the federal government allocated nearly $13 billion to control drug use and to enforce laws that are designed to protect society from the perils created by drug use. Some people believe that the government's war on drugs could be more effective but that governmental agencies and communities are not fighting hard enough to stop drug use. They also hold that laws to halt drug use are too few and too lenient. Others contend that the war against drugs is unnecessary; that, in fact, society has already lost the war on drugs. These individuals feel that the best way to remedy drug problems is to end the fight altogether by ending the current restrictive policies regarding drug use.

There are conflicting views among both liberals and conservatives on whether legislation has had the intended result of curtailing the problems of drug use. Many argue that legislation and the criminalization of drugs have been counterproductive in controlling drug problems. Some suggest that the criminalization of drugs has actually contributed to and worsened the social ills associated with drugs. Proponents of drug legalization maintain that the war on drugs, not drugs themselves, is damaging to American society. They do not advocate drug use; they argue only that laws against drugs exacerbate problems related to drugs.

Proponents of drug decriminalization argue that the strict enforcement of drug laws damages American society because it drives people to violence and crime and that the drug laws have a racist element associated with them. People arrested for drug offenses overburden the court system, thus rendering it ineffective. Moreover, proponents contend that the criminalization of drugs fuels organized crime, allows children to be pulled into the drug business, and makes illegal drugs more dangerous because they are manufactured without government standards or regulations. Hence, drugs may be adulterated or of unidentified potency. Decriminalization advocates also argue that decriminalization would take the profits out of drug sales, thereby decreasing the value of and demand for drugs. In addition, the costs resulting from law enforcement are far greater to society than the benefits of criminalization.

Some decriminalization advocates argue that the federal government's prohibition stance on drugs is an immoral and impossible objective. To achieve a "drug-free society" is self-defeating and a misnomer because drugs have always been a part of human culture. Furthermore, prohibition efforts indicate a disregard for the private freedom of individuals because they assume that individuals are incapable of making their own choices. Drug proponents assert that their personal sovereignty should be respected over any government agenda, including the war on drugs. Less restrictive laws, they argue, would take the emphasis off of law enforcement policies and allow more effort to be put toward education, prevention, and treatment. Also, it is felt that most of the negative implications of drug prohibition would disappear.

Opponents of this view maintain that less restrictive drug laws are not the solution to drug problems and that it is a very dangerous idea. Less restrictive laws, they assert, will drastically increase drug use. This upsurge in drug use will come at an incredibly high price: American society will be overrun with drug-related accidents, loss in worker productivity, and hospital emergency rooms filled with drug-related emergencies. Drug treatment efforts would be futile because users would have no legal incentive to stop taking drugs. Also, users may prefer drugs rather than rehabilitation, and education programs may be ineffective in dissuading children from using drugs.

Advocates of less restrictive laws maintain that drug abuse is a "victimless crime" in which the only person being hurt is the drug user. Opponents argue that this notion is ludicrous and dangerous because drug use has dire repercussions for all of society. Drugs can destroy the minds and bodies of many people. Also, regulations to control drug use have a legitimate social aim to protect society and its citizens from the harm of drugs.

In the following selections, Henry Kleber and Joseph Califano explain why they feel drugs should remain illegal, whereas Peter Gorman describes the detrimental effects that he believes occur as a result of the restrictive laws associated with drugs.

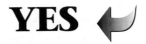

YES

Herbert Kleber and
Joseph A. Califano Jr.

Legalization:
Panacea or Pandora's Box

Introduction

Legalization of drugs has recently received some attention as a policy option for the United States. Proponents of such a radical change in policy argue that the "war on drugs" has been lost; drug prohibition, as opposed to illegal drugs themselves, spawns increasing violence and crime; drugs are available to anyone who wants them, even under present restrictions; drug abuse and addiction would not increase after legalization; individuals have a right to use whatever drugs they wish; and foreign experiments with legalization work and should be adopted in the United States.

In this, its first White Paper, the Center on Addiction and Substance Abuse at Columbia University (CASA) examines these propositions; recent trends in drug use; the probable consequences of legalization for children and drug-related violence; lessons to be learned from America's legal drugs, alcohol and tobacco; the question of civil liberties; and the experiences of foreign countries. On the basis of its review, CASA concludes that while legalization might temporarily take some burden off the criminal justice system, such a policy would impose heavy additional costs on the health care system, schools, and workplace, severely impair the ability of millions of young Americans to develop their talents, and in the long term overburden the criminal justice system.

Drugs like heroin and cocaine are not dangerous because they are illegal; they are illegal because they are dangerous. Such drugs are not a threat to American society because they are illegal; they are illegal because they are a threat to American society.

Any relaxation in standards of illegality poses a clear and present danger to the nation's children and their ability to learn and grow into productive citizens. Individuals who reach age 21 without using illegal drugs are virtually certain never to do so. Viewed from this perspective, substance abuse and addiction is a disease acquired during childhood and adolescence. Thus, legalization of drugs such as heroin, cocaine, and marijuana would threaten a pediatric pandemic in the United States.

From The National Center on Addiction and Substance Abuse at Columbia University, September 1995 Copyright © 2006 by The National Center on Addiction and Substance Abuse at Columbia University. Reprinted by permission.

While current prohibitions on the import, manufacture, distribution, and possession of marijuana, cocaine, heroin, and other drugs should remain, America's drug policies do need a fix. More resources and energy should be devoted to prevention and treatment, and each citizen and institution should take responsibility to combat drug abuse and addiction in America. . . .

Legalization, Decriminalization, Medicalization, Harm Reduction: What's the Difference?

The term "legalization" encompasses a wide variety of policy options from the legal use of marijuana in private to free markets for all drugs. Four terms are commonly used: legalization, decriminalization, medicalization, and harm reduction—with much variation in each.

Legalization usually implies the most radical departure from current policy. Legalization proposals vary from making marijuana cigarettes as available as tobacco cigarettes to establishing an open and free market for drugs. Variations on legalization include: making drugs legal for the adult population, but illegal for minors; having only the government produce and sell drugs; and/or allowing a private market in drugs, but with restrictions on advertising, dosage, and place of consumption. Few proponents put forth detailed visions of a legalized market.

Decriminalization proposals retain most drug laws that forbid manufacture, importation, and sale of illegal drugs, but remove criminal sanctions for possession of small amounts of drugs for personal use. Such proposals suggest that possession of drugs for personal use be legal or subject only to civil penalties such as fines. Decriminalization is most commonly advocated for marijuana.

Medicalization refers to the prescription of currently illegal drugs by physicians to addicts already dependent on such drugs. The most frequently mentioned variation is heroin maintenance. Proponents argue that providing addicts with drugs prevents them from having to commit crimes to finance their habit and insures that drugs they ingest are pure.

Harm reduction generally implies that government policies should concentrate on lowering the harm associated with drugs both for users and society, rather than on eradicating drug use and imprisoning users. Beginning with the proposition that drug use is inevitable, harm reduction proposals can include the prescription of heroin and other drugs to addicts; removal of penalties for personal use of marijuana; needle-exchange programs for injection drug users to prevent the spread of AIDS and other diseases that result from needle sharing among addicts; and making drugs available at low or no cost to eliminate the harm caused by users who commit crimes to support a drug habit.

Variations on these options are infinite. Some do not require any change in the illegal status of drugs. The government could, for instance, allow needle exchanges while maintaining current laws banning heroin, the most commonly injected drug. Others, however, represent a major shift from the current role of government and the goal of its policies with regard to drug use and availability. Some advocates use the term "harm reduction" as a politically attractive cover for legalization.

Where We Are

Most arguments for legalization in all its different forms start with the contention that the "war on drugs" has been lost and that prevailing criminal justice and social policies with respect to drug use have been a failure. To support the claim that current drug policies have failed, legalization advocates point to the 80 million Americans who have tried drugs during their lifetime. Since so many individuals have broken drug laws, these advocates argue, the laws are futile and lead to widespread disrespect for the law. A liberal democracy, they contend, should not ban what so many people do.[1]

The 80 million Americans include everyone who has ever smoked even a single joint. The majority of these individuals have used only marijuana, and for many their use was brief experimentation. In fact, the size of this number reflects the large number of young people who tried marijuana and hallucinogenic drugs during the late 1960s and the 1970s when drug use was widely tolerated. During this time, drug use was so commonly accepted that the 1972 Shafer Commission, established during the Nixon Administration, and later, President Jimmy Carter called for decriminalization of marijuana.[2]

Since then, concerned public health and government leaders have mounted energetic efforts to de-normalize drug use, including First Lady Nancy Reagan's "Just Say No" campaign. As a result, current* users of any illicit drugs, as measured by the National Household Survey on Drug Abuse, decreased from 24.8 million in 1979 to 13 million in 1994, a nearly 50 percent drop. Over the same time period, current marijuana users dropped from 23 million to 10 million and cocaine users from 4.4 million to 1.4 million.[3] The drug-using segment of the population is also aging. In 1979, 10 percent of current drug users were older than 34; today almost 30 percent are.[4]

With these results and only 6 percent of the population over age 12 currently using drugs,[5] it is difficult to say that drug reduction efforts have failed. This sharp decline in drug use occurred during a period of strict drug laws, societal disapproval, and increasing knowledge and awareness of the dangers and costs of illegal drug use.

Several factors, however, lead many to conclude that we have not made progress against drugs. This feeling of despair stems from the uneven nature of the success. While casual drug use and experimentation have declined substantially, certain neighborhoods and areas of the country remain infested with drugs and drug-related crime, and these continuing trouble spots draw media attention. At the same time, the number of drug addicts has not dropped significantly and the spread of HIV among addicts has added a deadly new dimension to the problem. The number of hardcore** cocaine users (as estimated by the Office of National Drug Control Policy based on a number of surveys including the Household Survey, Drug Use Forecasting, and Drug

---

*Throughout this paper, "current" drug users refers to individuals who have used drugs within the past month, the definition used in most drug use surveys.

**Throughout this paper, "hardcore" users refers to individuals who use drugs at least weekly.

Abuse Warning Network) has remained steady at roughly 2 million.[6] The overall number of illicit drug addicts has hovered around 6 million, a situation that many experts attribute both to a lack of treatment facilities[7] and the large numbers of drug-using individuals already in the pipeline to addiction, even though overall casual use has dropped.

Teenage drug use has been creeping up in the past three years. In the face of the enormous decline in the number of users, however, it is difficult to conclude that current policies have so failed that a change as radical as legalization is warranted. While strict drug laws and criminal sanctions are not likely to deter hardcore addicts, increased resources can be dedicated to treatment without legalizing drugs. Indeed, the criminal justice system can be used to place addicted offenders into treatment. In short, though substantial problems remain, we have made significant progress in our struggle against drug abuse.

Will Legalization Increase Drug Use?

Proponents of drug legalization claim that making drugs legally available would not increase the number of addicts. They argue that drugs are already available to those who want them and that a policy of legalization could be combined with education and prevention programs to discourage drug use.[8] Some contend that legalization might even reduce the number of users, arguing that there would be no pushers to lure new users and drugs would lose the "forbidden fruit" allure of illegality, which can be seductive to children.[9] Proponents of legalization also play down the consequences of drug use, saying that most drug users can function normally.[10] Some legalization advocates assert that a certain level of drug addiction is inevitable and will not vary, regardless of government policies; thus, they claim, even if legalization increased the number of users, it would have little effect on the numbers of users who become addicts.[11]

The effects of legalization on the numbers of users and addicts is an important question because the answer in large part determines whether legalization will reduce crime, improve public health, and lower economic, social, and health care costs. The presumed benefits of legalization evaporate if the number of users and addicts, particularly among children, increases significantly.

Availability

An examination of this question begins with the issue of availability, which has three components:

- **Physical,** how convenient is access to drugs.
- **Psychological,** the moral and social acceptability and perceived consequences of drug use.
- **Economic,** the affordability of drugs.

Physical

Despite assertions to the contrary, the evidence indicates that presently drugs are not accessible to all. Fewer than 50 percent of high school seniors and young adults under 22 believed they could obtain cocaine "fairly easily" or "very easily.[12] Only 39 percent of the adult population reported they could get cocaine; and only 25 percent reported that they could obtain heroin, PCP, and LSD.[13] Thus, only one-quarter to one-half of people can easily get illegal drugs (other than marijuana). After legalization, drugs would be more widely and easily available. Currently, only 11 percent of individuals reported seeing drugs available in the area where they lived;[14] after legalization, there could be a place to purchase drugs in every neighborhood. Under such circumstances, it is logical to conclude that more individuals would use drugs.

Psychological

In arguing that legalization would not result in increased use, proponents of legalization often cite public opinion polls which indicate that the vast majority of Americans would not try drugs even if they were legally available.[15] They fail to take into account, however, that this strong public antagonism towards drugs has been formed during a period of strict prohibition when government and institutions at every level have made clear the health and criminal justice consequences of drug use. Furthermore, even if only 15 percent of population would use drugs after legalization, this would be triple the current level of 5.6 percent.

Laws define what is acceptable conduct in a society, express the will of its citizens, and represent a commitment on the part of the Congress, the President, state legislatures, and governors. Drug laws not only create a criminal sanction, they also serve as educational and normative statements that shape public attitudes.[16] Criminal laws constitute a far stronger statement than civil laws, but even the latter can discourage individual consumption. Laws regulating smoking in public and workplaces, prohibiting certain types of tobacco advertising, and mandating warning labels are in part responsible for the decline in smoking prevalence among adults.

The challenge of reducing drug abuse and addiction would be decidedly more difficult if society passed laws indicating that these substances are not sufficiently harmful to prohibit their use. Any move toward legalization would decrease the perception of risks and costs of drug use, which would lead to wider use.[17] During the late 1960s and the 1970s, as society, laws, and law enforcement became more permissive about drug use, the number of individuals smoking marijuana and using heroin, hallucinogens, and other drugs rose sharply. During the 1980s, as society's attitude became more restrictive and anti-drug laws stricter and more vigorously enforced, the perceived harmfulness of marijuana and other illicit drugs increased and use decreased.

Some legalization advocates point to the campaign against smoking as proof that reducing use is possible while substances are legally available.[18] But it has taken smoking more than 30 years to decline as much as illegal drug use did in 10.[19] Moreover, reducing use of legal drugs among the young has proven especially difficult. While use of illegal drugs by high school seniors dropped 50 percent from 1979 to 1993, tobacco use remained virtually constant.[20]

Economic

By all of the laws of economics, reducing the price of drugs will increase consumption.[21] Though interdiction and law enforcement have had limited success in reducing supply (seizing only 25 percent to 30 percent of cocaine imports, for example)[22] the illegality of drugs has increased their price.[23] Prices of illegal drugs are roughly 10 times what they would cost to produce legally. Cocaine, for example, sells at $80 a gram today, but would cost only $10 a gram legally to produce and distribute. That would set the price of a dose at 50 cents, well within the reach of a school child's lunch money.[24]

Until the mid-1980s, cocaine was the drug of the middle and upper classes. Regular use was limited to those who had the money to purchase it or got the money through white collar crime or selling such assets as their car, house, or children's college funds. In the mid-1980s, the $5 crack cocaine vial made the drug inexpensive and available to all regardless of income. Use spread. Cocaine-exposed babies began to fill hospital neonatal wards, cocaine-related emergency room visits increased sharply, and cocaine-related crime and violence jumped.[25]

Efforts to increase the price of legal drugs by taxing them heavily in order to discourage consumption, if successful, would encourage the black market, crime, violence, and corruption associated with the illegal drug trade. Heroin addicts, who gradually build a tolerance to the drug, and cocaine addicts, who crave more of the drug as soon as its effects subside, would turn to a black market if an affordable and rising level of drugs were not made available to them legally.

Children

Drug use among children is of particular concern since almost all individuals who use drugs begin before they are 21. Furthermore, adolescents rate drugs as the number one problem they face.[26] Since we have been unable to keep legal drugs, like tobacco and alcohol, out of the hands of children, legalization of illegal drugs could cause a pediatric pandemic of drug abuse and addiction.

Most advocates of legalization support a regulated system in which access to presently illicit drugs would be illegal for minors.[27] Such regulations would retain for children the "forbidden fruit" allure that many argue legalization would eliminate. Furthermore any such distinction between adults and minors could make drugs, like beer and cigarettes today, an attractive badge of adulthood.

The American experience with laws restricting access by children and adolescents to tobacco and alcohol makes it clear that keeping legal drugs away from minors would be a formidable, probably impossible, task. Today, 62 percent of high school seniors have smoked, 30 percent in the past month.[28] Three million adolescents smoke cigarettes, an average of one-half a pack per day, a $1 billion a year market.[29] Twelve million underage Americans drink beer and other alcohol, a market approaching $10 billion a year. Although alcohol use is illegal for all those under the age of 21, 87 percent of high school seniors report using alcohol, more than half in the past month.[30] These rates of use persist despite school, community, and media activities that inform youths about the dangers of smoking and drinking and despite increasing public awareness of these risks. This record indicates that efforts to ban drug use among minors while allowing it for adults would face enormous difficulty.

Moreover, in contrast to these high rates of alcohol and tobacco use, only 18 percent of seniors use illicit drugs, which are illegal for the entire society.[31] It is no accident that those substances which are mostly easily obtainable—alcohol, tobacco, and inhalants such as those found in household cleaning fluids—are those most widely used by the youngest students.[32]

Supporters and opponents of legalization generally agree that education and prevention programs are an integral part of efforts to reduce drug use by children and adolescents. School programs, media campaigns such as those of the Partnership for a Drug-Free America (PDFA), and news reports on the dangers of illegal drugs have helped reduce use by changing attitudes towards drugs. In 1992, New York City school children were surveyed on their perceptions of illegal drugs before and after a PDFA campaign of anti-drug messages on television, in newspapers, and on billboards. The second survey showed that the percentage of children who said they might want to try drugs fell 29 points and those who said drugs would make them "cool" fell 17 points.[33] Another study found that 75 percent of students who saw anti-drug advertisements reported that the ads had a deterrent effect on their own actual or intended use.[34]

Along with such educational programs, however, the stigma of illegality is especially important in preventing use among adolescents. From 1978 to 1993, current marijuana use among high school seniors dropped twice as fast as alcohol use.[35] California started a $600 million anti-smoking campaign in 1989, and by 1995, the overall smoking rate had dropped 30 percent. But among teenagers, the smoking rate remained constant—even though almost one-quarter of the campaign targeted them.[36]

In separate studies, 60 to 70 percent of New Jersey and California students reported that fear of getting in trouble with the authorities was a major reason why they did not use drugs.[37] Another study found that the greater the perceived likelihood of apprehension and swift punishment for using marijuana, the less likely adolescents are to smoke it.[38] Because a legalized system would remove much, if not all of this deterrent, drug use among teenagers could be expected to rise. Since most teens begin using drugs because their peers do[39]—not because of pressure from pushers[40]—and most drugs users initially exhibit few ill effects, more teenagers would be likely to try drugs.[41]

As a result, legalization of marijuana, cocaine, and heroin for adults would mean that increased numbers of teenagers would smoke, snort, and inject these substances at a time when habits are formed and the social, academic, and physical skills needed for a satisfying and independent life are acquired.

Hard Core Addiction

A review of addiction in the past shows that the number of alcohol, heroin, and cocaine addicts, even when adjusted for changes in population, fluctuates widely over time, in response to changes in access, price, societal attitudes, and legal consequences. The fact that alcohol and tobacco, the most accepted and available legal drugs, are the most widely abused, demonstrates that behavior is influenced by opportunity, stigma, and price. Many soldiers who were regular heroin users in Vietnam stopped once they returned to the

United States where heroin was much more difficult and dangerous to get.[42] Studies have shown that even among chronic alcoholics, alcohol taxes lower consumption.[43]

Dr. Jack Homer of the University of Southern California and a founding member of the International System Dynamics Society estimates that without retail-level drug arrests and seizures—which reduce availability, increase the danger of arrest for the drug user, and stigmatize use—the number of compulsive cocaine users would rise to between 10 and 32 million, a level 5 to 16 times the present one.[44]

Not all new users become addicts. But few individuals foresee their addiction when they start using; most think they can control their consumption.[45] Among the new users created by legalization, many, including children, would find themselves unable to live without the drug, no longer able to work, go to school, or maintain personal relationships. In fact, as University of California at Los Angeles criminologist James Q. Wilson points out with regard to cocaine,[46] the percentage of drug triers who become abusers when the drugs are illegal, socially unacceptable, and generally hard to get, may be only a fraction of the users who become addicts when drugs are legal and easily available—physically, psychologically, and economically.

Harming Thy Neighbor and Thyself: Addiction and Casual Drug Use

To offset any increased use as a result of legalization, many proponents contend that money presently spent on criminal justice and law enforcement could be used for treatment of addicts and prevention.[47] In 1995, the federal government is spending $13.2 billion to fight drug abuse, nearly two-thirds of that amount on law enforcement; state and local governments are spending at least another $16 billion on drug control efforts, largely on law enforcement.[48] Legalization proponents argue that most of this money could be used to fund treatment on demand for all addicts who want it and extensive public health campaigns to discourage new use.

With legalization, the number of prisoners would initially decrease because many are currently there for drug law violations. But to the extent that legalization increases drug use, we can expect to see more of its familiar consequences. Costs would quickly rise in health care, schools, and businesses. In the long term, wider use and addiction would increase criminal activity related to the psychological and physical effects of drug use and criminal justice costs would rise again. The higher number of casual users and addicts would reduce worker productivity and students' ability and motivation to learn, cause more highway accidents and fatalities, and fill hospital beds with individuals suffering from ailments and injuries caused or aggravated by drug abuse.

Costs

It is doubtful whether legalization would produce any cost savings, over time even in the area of law enforcement. Indeed, the legal availability of alcohol has not eliminated law enforcement costs due to alcohol-related violence. A third of state prison inmates committed their crimes while under the influence of alcohol.[49] Despite intense educational campaigns, the highest number of arrests in 1993—1.5 million—was for driving while intoxicated.[50] Even if, as some legalization proponents propose, drug sales were taxed, revenues raised would be more than offset by erosion of the general tax base as abuse and addiction limited the ability of individuals to work.

Like advocates of legalization today, opponents of alcohol prohibition claimed that taxes on the legal sale of alcohol would dramatically increase revenues and even help erase the federal deficit.[51] The real-world result has been quite different. The approximately $20 billion in state and federal revenues from alcohol taxes in 1995[52] pay for only half the $40 billion that alcohol abuse imposes in direct health care costs,[53] much less the costs laid on federal entitlement programs and the legal and criminal justice systems, to say nothing of lost economic productivity. The nearly $13 billion in federal and state cigarette tax revenue[54] is one-sixth of the $75 billion in direct health care costs attributable to tobacco,[55] to say nothing of the other costs such as the $4.6 billion in social security disability payments to individuals disabled by cancer, heart disease, and respiratory ailments caused by smoking.[56]

Health care costs directly attributable to illegal drugs exceed $30 billion,[57] an amount that would increase significantly if use spread after legalization. Experience renders it unrealistic to expect that taxes could be imposed on newly legalized drugs sufficient to cover the costs of increased use and abuse.

Public Health

Legalization proponents contend that prohibition has negative public health consequences such as the spread of HIV from addicts who share dirty needles, accidental poisoning, and overdoses from impure drugs of variable potency. In 1994, more than one-third of new AIDS cases were among injection drug users who shared needles, cookers, cottons, rinse water, and other paraphernalia; many other individuals contracted AIDS by having sex, often while high, with infected injection drug users.[58]

Advocates of medicalization argue that while illicit drugs should not be freely available to all, doctors should be allowed to prescribe them (particularly heroin, but also cocaine) to addicts. They contend that giving addicts drugs assures purity and eliminates the need for addicts to steal in order to buy them.[59]

Giving addicts drugs like heroin, however, poses many problems. Providing them by prescription raises the danger of diversion for sale on the black market. The alternative—insisting that addicts take drugs on the prescriber's premises—entails at least two visits a day, thus interfering with the stated goal of many maintenance programs to enable addicts to hold jobs.

Heroin addicts require two to four shots each day in increasing doses as they build tolerance to its euphoric effect. On the other hand, methadone can be given at a constant dose since euphoria is not the objective. Addicts maintained on methadone need only a single dose each day and take it orally, eliminating the need for injection.[60] Because cocaine produces an intense, but short euphoria and an immediate desire for more,[61] addicts would have to be given the drug even more often than heroin in order to satisfy their craving sufficiently to prevent them from seeking additional cocaine on the street.

Other less radical harm reduction proposals also have serious flaws. Distributing free needles, for example, does not guarantee that addicts desperate for a high would refuse to share them. But to the extent that needle exchange programs are effective in reducing the spread of the AIDS virus and other diseases without increasing drug use, they can be adopted without legalizing drugs. Studies of whether needle exchange programs increase drug use have generally focused on periods of no longer than 12 months.[62] While use does not seem to increase in this period, data is lacking on the long-term effects of such programs and whether they prompt attitude shifts that in turn lead to increased drug use.

Some individuals do die as a result of drug impurities. But while drug purity could be assured in a government regulated system (though not for those drugs sold on the black market), careful use could not. The increased numbers of users would probably produce a rising number of overdose deaths, similar to those caused by alcohol poisoning today.

The deaths and costs due to unregulated drug quality pale in comparison to the negative impact that legalization would have on drug users, their families, and society. Casual drug use is dangerous, not simply because it can lead to addiction or accidental overdoses, but because it is harmful per se, producing worker accidents, highway fatalities, and children born with physical and mental handicaps. Each year, roughly 500,000 newborns are exposed to illegal drugs in the womb; many others are never born because of drug-induced spontaneous abortions.[63] Newborns already exposed to drugs are far more likely to need intensive care and suffer the physical and mental consequences of low birth weight and premature birth, including early death.[64] The additional costs just to raise drug-exposed babies would outweigh any potential savings of legalization in criminal justice expenditures.[65]

Substance abuse aggravates medical conditions. Medicaid patients with a secondary diagnosis of substance abuse remain in hospitals twice as long as patients with the same primary diagnosis but with no substance abuse problems. Girls and boys under age 15 remain in the hospital three and four times as long, respectively, when they have a secondary diagnosis of substance abuse.[66] One-third to one-half of individuals with psychiatric problems are also substance abusers.[67] Young people who use drugs are at higher risk of mental health problems including depression, suicide, and personality disorders.[68] Teenagers who use illegal drugs are more likely to have sex[69] and are less likely to use a condom than those who do not use drugs.[70] Such sexual behavior exposes these teens to increased risk of pregnancy as well as AIDS and other sexually transmitted diseases.

In schools and families, drug abuse is devastating. Students who use drugs not only limit their own ability to learn, they also disrupt classrooms, interfering with the education of other students. Drug users tear apart families by failing to provide economic support, spending money on drugs, neglecting the emotional support of the spouse and guidance of children, and putting their children at greater risk of becoming substance abusers themselves.[71] With the advent of crack cocaine in the mid-1980s, foster care cases soared over 50 percent nationwide in five years; more than 70 percent of these cases involved families in which at least one parent abused drugs.[72]

Decreased coordination and impaired motor skills that result from drug use are dangerous. A recent study in Tennessee found that 59 percent of reckless drivers who, having been stopped by the police, test negative for alcohol on the breathalyzer, test positive for marijuana and/or cocaine.[73] Twenty percent of New York City drivers who die in automobile accidents test positive for cocaine use.[74] The extent of driving while high on marijuana and other illegal drugs is still not well known because usually the police do not have the same capability for roadside drug testing as they do for alcohol testing. . . .

Crime and Violence

Legalization advocates contend that *drug-related* violence is really *drug-trade-related* violence. They argue that what we have today is not a drug problem but a drug prohibition problem, that anti-drug laws spawn more violence and crime than the drugs themselves. Because illegality creates high prices for drugs and huge profits for dealers, advocates of legalization point out that users commit crimes to support their habit; drug pushers fight over turf; gangs and organized crime thrive; and users become criminals by coming into contact with the underworld.[75]

Legalization proponents argue that repeal of current laws, which criminalize drug use and sales, and wider availability of drugs at lower prices will end this black market and thus reduce the violence, crime, and incarceration associated with drugs.

Researchers divide drug-related violence into three types: systemic, economically compulsive, and psychopharmacological:[76]

- **Systemic violence** is that intrinsic to involvement with illegal drugs, including murders over drug turf, retribution for selling "bad" drugs, and fighting among users over drugs or drug paraphernalia.
- **Economically compulsive violence** results from addicts who engage in violent crime in order to support their addiction.
- **Psychopharmacological violence** is caused by the short or long-term use of certain drugs which lead to excitability, irrationality and violence, such as a brutal murder committed under the influence of cocaine.

Legalization of the drug trade and lower prices might decrease the first two types of violence, but higher use and abuse would increase the third. Dr. Mitchell Rosenthal, President of the Phoenix House treatment centers warns, "What I and many other treatment professionals would expect to see in a drug-legalized America is a sharp rise in the amount of drug-related crime that is *not* committed for gain—homicide, assault, rape, and child abuse. Along with this, an increase in social disorder, due to rising levels of drug consumption and a growing number of drug abusers."[77]

In a study of 130 drug-related homicides, 60 percent resulted from the psychopharmacological effects of the drug; only 20 percent were found to be related to the drug trade; 3.1 percent were committed for economic reasons. (The remaining 17 percent either fell into more than one of these categories or were categorized as "other.")[78] U.S. Department of Justice statistics reveal that six times as many homicides, four times as many assaults, and almost one and a half times as many robberies are committed under the influence of drugs as are committed in order to get money to buy drugs.[79] Given these facts, any decreases in violent acts committed because of the current high cost of drugs would be more than offset by increases in psychopharmacological violence, such as that caused by cocaine psychosis.

The threat of rising violence is particularly serious in the case of cocaine, crack, methamphetamine, and PCP—drugs closely associated with violent behavior. Unlike marijuana or heroin, which depress activity, these drugs cause irritability and physical aggression. For instance, past increases in the New York City homicide rate have been tied to increases in cocaine use.[80]

Repeal of drug laws would not affect all addicts in the same way. Addicts engage in criminal behavior for different reasons. A small proportion of addicts is responsible for a disproportionately high number of drug-related crimes and arrests. Virtually all of these addicts committed crimes before abusing drugs and use crime to support themselves as well as their habits. Their criminal activity and drug use are symptomatic of chronic antisocial behavior and attitudes. Legally available drugs at lower prices would do little to discourage crime by this group. For a second group, criminal activity is associated with the high cost of illegal drugs. For these addicts, lower prices would decrease drug-related crimes. For a third group, legally available drugs would mean an opportunity to create illegal diversion markets, as some addicts currently do with methadone.[81]

Legalization advocates point to the exploding prison population and the failure of strict drug laws to lower crime rates.[82] Arrests for drug offenses doubled from 470,000 in 1980 to 1 million in 1993.[83] Some 60 percent of the 95,000 federal inmates are incarcerated for drug-law violations.[84]

Rising prison populations are generated in large part by stricter laws, tough enforcement, and mandatory minimum sentencing laws—policy choices of the public and Congress. But the growing number of prisoners is also a product of the high rate of recidivism—a phenomenon tied in good measure to the lack of treatment facilities, particularly in prison. Eighty percent of prisoners have prior convictions and 60 percent have served time before.[85] Despite the fact that more than 60 percent of all state inmates have used illegal drugs regularly and 30 percent were under the influence of drugs at the time they committed the crime for which they were incarcerated,[86] fewer than 20 percent of inmates with drug problems receive any treatment.[87] Many of these inmates also abuse alcohol, but there is little alcoholism treatment either for them or for those prisoners dependent only on alcohol.[88]

While strict laws and enforcement do not deter addicts from using drugs, the criminal justice system can be used to get them in treatment. Because of the nature of addiction, most drug abusers do not seek treatment voluntarily, but many respond to outside pressures including the threat of incarceration.[89] Where the criminal justice system is used to encourage participation in treatment, addicts are more likely to complete treatment and stay off drugs. . . .[90]

Notes

1. Kurt Schmoke, "Decriminalizing Drugs: It Just Might Work—And Nothing Else Does," in *Drug Legalization: For and Against*, ed. Rod Evans and Irwin Berent (Lasalle: Open Court Press, 1992), p. 216; Merrill Smith, "The Drug Problem: Is There an Answer?" in Evans and Berent, eds., p. 84; Steven Wisotsky, "Statement Before the Select Committee on Narcotics Abuse and Control," in Evans and Berent, eds., p. 189.

2. National Commission on Marijuana and Drug Abuse, *Marijuana: Signal of Misunderstanding* (Washington, DC: GPO, 1972); Musto, p. 267.

3. U.S. Department of Health and Human Services, *Preliminary Estimates from the 1994 National Household Survey on Drug Abuse* (September 1995), pp. 2, 58.

4. Dept. of Health and Human Services (1995), p. 11.

5. Dept. of Health and Human Services (1995), p. 2.

6. Office of National Drug Control Policy (ONDCP), *National Drug Control Strategy: Strengthening Communities' Response to Drugs and Crime* (February 1995), p. 139.

7. ONDCP, *Breaking the Cycle of Drug Abuse* (September 1993), pp. 6–9.

8. Todd Austin Brenner, "The Legalization of Drugs: Why Prolong the Inevitable," in Evans and Berent, eds., p. 173; Schmoke, in Evans and Berent, eds., p. 218; Smith, in Evans and Berent, eds., p. 85.

9. Smith, in Evans and Berent, eds., p. 83–86; Kevin Zeese, "Drug War Forever?" in *Searching for Alternatives: Drug-Control Policy in the United States,* eds. Melvyn Krauss and Edward Lazear (Stanford: Hoover Institute Press, 1992), p. 265.

10. Ethan Nadelmann, "The Case for Legalization," in *The Drug Legalization Debate,* ed. James Inciardi (Newbury Park: Sage Publications, 1991), pp. 39–40.

11. Michael Gazzaniga, "The Opium of the People: Crack in Perspective," in Evans and Berent, eds., p. 236.

12. Lloyd Johnston, Patrick O'Malley, and Jerald Bachman, *National Survey Results on Drug Use from The Monitoring the Future Study, 1975–1993* (Rockville: 1994), Vol. 1, p. 191 and Vol. 2, p. 144; Center on Addiction and Substance Abuse at Columbia University, *National Survey of American Attitudes on Substance Abuse* (July 1995).

13. Dept. of Health and Human Services *Preliminary Estimates from the 1993 National Household Survey: Press Release* (July 1994), p. 4.

14. Dept. of Health and Human Services (July 1994), p. 4.

15. See for example, Lester Grinspoon and James Bakalar, "The War on Drugs—A Peace Proposal," *The New England Journal of Medicine,* 330(5) 1994, pp. 357–60; Arnold Trebach, "For Legalization of Drugs" in *Legalize It? Debating American Drug Policy,* Arnold Trebach and James Inciardi, eds., (Washington: American University Press, 1993), p. 108.

16. Mark Moore, "Drugs: Getting a Fix on the Problem and the Solution," in Evans and Berent, eds., p. 152.

17. Johnston, O'Malley and Bachman, Vol. 1, p. 206.

18. Schmoke, in Evans and Berent, eds., p. 218; Brenner, in Evans and Berent, eds., p. 171; Wisotsky in Evans and Berent, eds., p. 210.

19. ONDCP (1995), p. 139; Centers for Disease Control, *Morbidity and Mortality Weekly Report,* 34(SS-3) 1994, p. 8.

20. Johnston, O'Malley and Bachman, Vol. 1, p. 79.

21. Moore in Evans and Berent, eds., p. 148; and Mark Moore, "Supply Reduction and Law Enforcement" in *Drugs and Crime,* Michael Tonry and James Wilson, eds., Crime and Justice: A Review of Research, Volume 13 (Chicago: University of Chicago Press, 1990), pp. 109–158; Michael Grossman, Gary Becker and Kevin Murphy, "Rational Addiction and the Effect of Price on Consumption," in Krauss and Lazear, eds., p. 83.

22. ONDCP (1995), p. 146.

23. Michael Farrell, John Strang and Peter Reuter, "The Non-Case for Legalization" in *Winning the War on Drugs: To Legalize or Not* (Institute of Economic Affairs: London, 1994).

24. Herbert Kleber, "Our Current Approach to Drug Abuse—Progress, Problems, Proposals," *The New England Journal of Medicine* 330(5) 1994, pp. 362–363; for higher estimates of the differences between illegal and legal costs see Moore, in Evans and Berent, eds., p. 148 and Wisotsky, in Evans and Berent, eds., p. 190.

25. Moore, in Evans and Berent, eds., p. 129–130.

26. Center on Addiction and Substance Abuse at Columbia University, *National Survey of American Attitudes on Substance Abuse* (July 1995).

27. See for example, Wisotsky, in Evans and Berent, eds. p. 204.

28. Johnston, O'Malley and Bachman, Vol. 1, pp. 76–79.

29. K. Michael Cummings, Terry Pechacek and Donald Shopland, "The Illegal Sale of Cigarettes to US Minors: Estimates by State," *American Journal of Public Health,* 84(2) 1994, pp. 300–302.

30. Johnston, O'Malley and Bachman, Vol. 1, pp. 76–79.

31. Johnston, O'Malley and Bachman, Vol. 1, p. 79.

32. Lloyd Johnston, "A Synopsis of the Key Points in the 1994 Monitoring the Future Results" (December 1994), Table 1; Johnston, O'Malley and Bachman, Vol. 1, pp. 136–137.

33. Drug Strategies, *Keeping Score* (Washington, DC: 1995), p. 11.

34. Evelyn Cohen Reis et al, "The Impact of Anti-Drug Advertising: Perceptions of Middle and High School Students," *Archives of Pediatric and Adolescent Medicine,* 148, December 1994, p. 1262–1268.

35. Johnston, O'Malley and Bachman, Vol. 1, p. 79.

36. "Hooked on Tobacco: The Teen Epidemic," *Consumer Reports,* March 1995, pp. 142–148.

37. Rodney Skager and Gregory Austin, *Fourth Biennial Statewide Survey of Drug and Alcohol Use Among California Students in Grades 7, 9, and 11,* Office of the Attorney General, June 1993; Wayne Fisher, *Drug and Alcohol Use Among New Jersey High School Students,* New Jersey Department of Law and Public Safety, 1993.

38. David Peck, "Legal and Social Factors in the Deterrence of Adolescent Marijuana Use," *Journal of Alcohol and Drug Education,* 28(3) 1983, pp. 58–74.

39. Diedre Dupre, "Initiation and Progression of Alcohol, Marijuana and Cocaine Use Among Adolescent Abusers," *The American Journal on Addiction,* 4, 1995, pp. 43–48.

40. Ronald Simmons, Rand Conger and Leslie Whitbeck, "A Multistage Learning Model of the Influences of Family and Peers Upon Adolescent Substance Abuse," *Journal of Drur Issues* 18(3) 1988, pp. 293–315.

41. Simmons, Conger and Whitbeck, p. 304; Mark Moore, "Drugs: Getting a Fix on the Problem and the Solution," in Evans and Berent, eds., p. 143.

42. Musto, p. 258–259.

43. Philip Cook, "The Effect of Liquor Taxes on Drinking, Cirrhosis, and Auto Accidents" in *Alcohol and Public Policy: Beyond the Shadow of Prohibition,* Mark Moore and Dean Gerstein, eds. (Washington, DC: National Academy Press, 1981), p. 256.

44. Jack Homer, "Projecting the Impact of Law Enforcement on Cocaine Prevalence: A System Dynamics Approach," *Journal of Drug Issues* 23(2) 1993, p. 281–295.

45. Kleber, p. 361.

46. James Q. Wilson, "Against the Legalization of Drugs," *Commentary* (February 1990), pp. 21–28.

47. See for example, Schmoke in Evans and Berent, eds., p. 218.

48. ONDCP (1995), p. 138.

49. Bureau of Justice Statistics, *Survey of State Prison Inmates, 1991* (Washington, DC: 1993), p. 26.

50. Bureau of Justice Statistics, *Prisoners in 1994* (Washington, DC: 1995), p. 13.

51. Paul Aaron and David Musto, "Temperance and Prohibition in America: A Historical Overview," in Moore and Gerstein, eds., p. 172.

52. Drug Enforcement Administration (DEA), *How to Hold Your Own in a Drug Legalization Debate* (Washington, DC, 1994), p. 26, adjusted to 1995.

53. Center on Addiction and Substance Abuse at Columbia University (CASA), *The Cost of Substance Abuse to America's Health Care System, Final Report* (To be issued, 1995).

54. The Tobacco Institute (1994), adjusted to 1995.

55. CASA (To be issued, 1995).

56. Center on Addiction and Substance Abuse at Columbia University, *Substance Abuse and Federal Entitlement Programs* (February 1995).

57. CASA (To be issued, 1995).

58. Centers for Disease Control, National AIDS Clearinghouse (1994).

59. See for example, "Prescribing to Addicts Appears to Work in Britain: Interview with Dr. John Marks," *Psychiatric News,* December 17, 1993, pp. 8, 14.

60. Joyce Lowinson et al, "Methadone Maintenance, "pp. 550–561; Jerome Jaffe, "Opiates: Clinical Aspects," pp. 186–194; and Eric Simon, "Opiates: Neurobiology," pp. 195–204 in *Substance Abuse: A Comprehensive Textbook,* 2nd ed., Joyce Lowinson, Pedro Ruiz and Robert Millman, eds. (Baltimore: Williams and Wilkins, 1992).

61. Mark Gold, "Cocaine (and Crack): Clinical Aspects," in Lowinson, Ruiz and Millman, eds., pp. 205–221.

62. Peter Lurie, Arthur Reingold et al, *The Public Health Impact of Needle Exchange Programs in the United States and Abroad,* 2 vols., (University of California, 1993).

63. Dept. of Justice (1992), p. 12; Paul Taubman, "Externalities and Decriminalization of Drugs," in Krauss and Lazear, eds., p. 99.

64. Dept. of Justice (1992), p. 12; Joel Hay, "The Harm They Do to Others," in Krauss and Lazear, eds., p. 204–213.

65. Hay, in Krauss and Lazear, eds., p. 208.

66. Center on Addiction and Substance Abuse at Columbia University (CASA), *The Cost of Substance Abuse to America's Health Care System, Report 1: Medicaid Hospital Costs,* (July 1993), p. 38–46.

67. Ronald Kessler et al, "Lifetime and 12-month prevalence of DSM-III-R psychiatric disorders in the United States: Results from the National Comorbidity Study," *Archives of General Psychiatry,* 51(1) 1994, pp. 8–19.

68. Dept. of Justice (1992), p. 11.

69. Centers for Disease Control, "Youth Risk Behavior Survey, 1991."

70. M. Lynne Cooper, Robert Pierce, and Rebecca Farmer Huselid, "Substance Abuse and Sexual Risk taking Among Black Adolescents and White Adolescents," *Health Psychology* 13(3) 1994, pp. 251–262.

71. Dept. of Justice (1992), p. 9.

72. General Accounting Office, *Foster Care: Parental Drug Abuse Has Alarming Impact on Young Children* (Washington, DC: 1994).

73. Daniel Brookoff et al, "Testing Reckless Drivers for Cocaine and Marijuana" *The New England Journal of Medicine* 331(8) 1994, pp. 518–522.

74. Peter Marzuk, Kenneth Tardiff, et al, "Prevalence of Recent Cocaine Use among Motor Vehicle Fatalities in New York City," *Journal of the American Medical Association* 1990; 263, pp. 250–256.

75. See for example, Nadelmann, in Inciardi (1991), ed., p. 31–32; Brenner, in Evans and Berent, eds., p. 174; Ira Glasser, "Drug Prohibition: An Engine for Crime," in Krauss and Lazear, eds., p. 271–283; Milton Friedman, "The War We are Losing," in Krauss and Lazear, eds., p. 53–57.

76. Paul J. Goldstein, "The Drugs/Violence Nexus: A Tripartite Conceptual Framework," *Journal of Drug Issues* (Fall 1985) pp. 493–516.

77. Mitchell Rosenthal, "Panacea or Chaos: The Legalization of Drugs in America," *Journal of Substance Abuse Treatment* 11(1) 1994, pp. 3–7.

78. Henry Brownstein and Paul J. Goldstein, "A Typology of Drug-Related Homicides" in *Drugs, Crime and the Criminal Justice System,* Ralph Weisheit, ed., (Cincinnati, OH: Anderson Publishing Co., 1990), pp. 171–191.

79. Bureau of Justice Statistics (1993), p. 22.

80. Kenneth Tardiff et al, "Homicide in New York City: Cocaine Use and Firearms," *Journal of the American Medical Association,* 272(1) 1994, p. 43–46.

81. Jon Chaiken and Marcia Chaiken, "Varieties of Criminal Behavior," (Santa Monica: Rand, 1982); HK Wexler and George De Leon, "Criminals as Drug Abusers and Drug Abusers Who Are Criminals" Paper presented to the Annual Convention of the American Psychological Association, Washington, DC, 1980; cited in George De Leon, "Some Problems with the Anti-Prohibitionist Position on Legalization of Drugs," *Journal of Addictive Diseases,* 13(2) 1994, p. 38.

82. See for example, New York City Bar Association, "A Wiser Course: Ending Drug Prohibition," *The Record* 49(5) 1994, pp. 525–534.

83. Bureau of Justice Statistics (1995), p. 13.

84. Bureau of Justice Statistics (1995), pp. 1, 10.

85. Bureau of Justice Statistics (1993), p. 11.

86. Bureau of Justice Statistics (1993), p. 21.

87. General Accounting Office, *Drug Treatment: State Prisons Face Challenges in Providing Services* (Washington, DC: 1991).

88. Bureau of Justice Statistics (1993), p. 26.

89. De Leon, p. 38.

90. M. Douglas Anglin. "The Efficacy of Civil Commitment in Treating Narcotic Addiction" in *Compulsory Treatment of Drug Abuse: Research and Clinical Practice,* NIDA Research Monograph 86, 1988, pp. 8–34; Robert Hubbard et al, *Drug Abuse Treatment: A National Study of Effectiveness* (Chapel Hill: University of North Carolina Press, 1989).

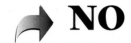

Veteran Cops Against the Drug War

Howard Woolridge is outside of Utica, New York, heading east on horseback on a beautiful late summer day. He's wearing a T-shirt with the slogan "Cops Say Legalize Drugs. Ask Me Why." For the last 3,000 miles, he's been switching off between his two horses, Misty and Sam. But the T-shirt slogan had stayed the same.

The rangy, good-looking guy is also talking on the cell phone to a reporter back in North Texas. But he interrupts that conversation to speak to someone who pulls up next to him in a car. "That's right—cops say legalize," he tells the newcomer in a deep voice. "Why? Because if we do, we just might be able to keep drugs out of the hands of your 14-year-old."

"Right on!" the motorist shouts, and drives off.

Woolridge is not a lunatic and he's not been out in the sun too long, even if he did cross the United States on horseback in the summer heat. He's a retired law enforcement officer with 18 years on the job who finally decided that the war on drugs was more of a problem than the illicit drugs it was purporting to fight.

He's also a serious long-distance horseman, on the road this time since March 4, when he left Los Angeles for the 3,400-mile ride to New York Harbor. It's the second time Woolridge has crossed the United States to publicize the campaign to repeal most of the drug laws in this country. In 2003 he rode from Georgia to Oregon. When he finished this trip on October 5, looking out at the Statue of Liberty, he was honored by the Long Riders' Guild as only the second person known to have ridden horseback all the way across the country in both directions. And he'll still be wearing one of his "Ask Me Why" T-shirts, the same shirts he's been wearing for six years.

"When I first started wearing it," he says, "people in Texas thought I was crazy. They thought my idea would destroy Texas and America. They believed the government propaganda that millions of people would pick up heroin or meth-amphetamines and become junkies overnight if you legalized it." But in the last two to three years, he's seen a sea change in the attitude of the American public regarding the war on drugs.

Jailed Over Medicinal Marijuana

"At any given Arby's, McDonald's, Rotary Club or veterans hall," he says, "people are overwhelmingly in favor of calling a halt to drug prohibition. Overwhelmingly."

Many of the houses Woolridge is riding past carry plaques attesting to the Utica area's involvement in the Underground Railroad that once funneled runaway slaves from the south up to Canada. It makes him think about Bernie Ellis, a fellow soldier in the war against the drug war, who has lost his own freedom.

"For 10 years he provided free medical marijuana to three oncologists in the Nashville, Tennessee, area for their patients undergoing chemotherapy. He never once met the doctors, of course; it was all cloak-and-dagger. He'd bring the marijuana to an office worker who'd get it to the patient.

"Well, he finally got busted last year. Now he's looking at five years mandatory federal prison time, though that might go up to 10 because he had a shotgun on his farm when he got busted. And of course his million-dollar farm has been forfeited because he grew the medical marijuana there."

The phone goes quiet for a minute, and there's the sound of a strangled sob. "Sorry. Got a little choked up for a second," he says. He pauses to explain his T-shirt to a motorist, then he's back on the phone talking about Bernie. "This is a guy who broke the law to help people and is now facing the consequences of that. Poor son of a bitch. Next time I see him he'll be in prison."

Woolridge is not a lone ranger in the fight to legalize drugs. He's a founding member of an organization called Law Enforcement Against Prohibition or LEAP, an organization made up entirely of current or former members of law enforcement who feel the drug war's a failure and believe legalization and regulation are preferable to the incarceration of drug users and control of the drug market by organized crime.

Founded in March 2002 by five police officers, LEAP now counts about 3,000 members, from the ranks of policemen, prison guards, Drug Enforcement Administration (DEA) agents, judges and even prosecutors in 48 states and 45 foreign countries. The idea behind LEAP is that, as with the Vietnam Veterans Against the War, the call for an end to the drug war carries more weight when it comes from folks who were in the trenches.

"We're the ones who fought the war," said Jack Cole, LEAP's executive director, who retired from the New Jersey state police as a detective lieutenant after 26 years, including 14 in their Narcotics Bureau, mostly undercover. "And I bear witness to the abject failure of the U.S. war on drugs and to the horrors these prohibitionist policies have produced."

The LEAP Web site provides the statistical backup for that argument. "After nearly four decades of fueling the U.S. policy of a war on drugs with over half a trillion tax dollars and increasingly punitive policies, our confined population has quadrupled," it says. "More than 2.2 million of our citizens are currently incarcerated and every year we arrest an additional 1.6 million for nonviolent drug offenses—more per capita than any country in the world. . . . Meanwhile, people continue dying in our streets while drug barons and terrorists continue to grow richer."

To get that message out, LEAP members have given nearly 1,500 speeches since 2003. And they don't preach to the choir. "We don't do hemp rallies or Million Man Marijuana Marches," said Woolridge. "We do Kiwanis Clubs and PTA meetings and cop conventions. That's where the people we've got to reach go."

To parents and teachers and Rotarians and other cops, LEAP members tell their own stories, about their work and about how they came to feel the drug war was not the answer.

Woolridge, for instance, was a street cop in Michigan for 15 of his 18 years of service, before moving up to the rank of detective. "I didn't work directly with the drug war, in that I wasn't in narcotics," he said. "Still, as a detective I was constantly working with felonies that touched on the drug war. Eight of 10 burglary suspects I dealt with were on crack at the time. They were stealing for drug money."

The burglary victims "were all in real pain," he said. "And I got so fed up with it I began saying, 'Why not let these guys have all the crack they want until they die?' Now I'd say, 'Have all you want for a dollar.' That makes it their choice to live or die. Either way, you don't have people breaking into houses for drug money anymore."

"Dehumanizing" Drug Users

To Cole, who did work directly in narcotics, the whole concept of the war on drugs is wrong. "You declare war, you need soldiers. You have soldiers, they need an enemy. So we've effectively taken a peacekeeping force—the police—and turned them into soldiers whose enemies are the 110 million people who have tried illegal substances in the U.S."

To be an effective soldier, you've got to dehumanize your enemy. "When I started out in narcotics I believed everything they told me," said Cole, a no-BS kind of guy. "Drugs were bad. The people who did them were less than human. I was all for locking them up."

Worse, he said, he and others often applied what they called a little "street justice" to the people they were arresting. "In our training we were taught to believe that drug users were the worst people in the world and whatever we did to them to try to stop their drug use was justified."

What they did was kick in home or apartment doors and have every man woman and child inside lie on the floor. If people didn't cooperate immediately, they were thrown to the floor. Then the place was ransacked. "When we searched for drugs we pretty much did as much damage as possible. We'd break bureaus, turn over beds, smash mirrors, throw things on the floor. Didn't matter, because the people there weren't humans, right? And then, if we did find any drugs, we'd arrest everyone in the house: parents, sisters, brothers. And since we'd already kicked the door down when we came in, it would be left open and anyone who wanted to enter could steal what they wanted. We never cared about that."

Street justice didn't stop there, said Cole. In court, he said officers routinely changed testimony to insure convictions—times, locations, amounts of drug, "anything that couldn't be checked to catch the officer in a lie."

It didn't take long for Cole to reach the conclusion that the drug war and its street justice weren't for him. He was mostly going after small-timers, and his job, he came to feel, was to insert himself into voluntary, private business transactions. "To do that, I had to become someone's confidant, their best friend. And once I was, I would bust them."

But he, too, got hooked—on the adrenaline high of the game. "By the time I came to my senses, I was working on big-timers, and pitting your mind against theirs was a great rush," he said. "Also, it was hard to quit because we were considered by the public and our peers as heroes. And then, given that I'd worked with a lot of cops who applied bad street justice, I let myself believe that at least if I was the one catching [the dopers] they'd be legally caught, and I'd tell the truth and justice would prevail."

He laughed. "Know what was the worst? When I realized that I liked and respected a lot of the bad guys much more than I liked or respected the guys I was working with."

Prohibition: Has It Worked by Its Own Standards?

The stated goals of the war on drugs are to lower drug consumption, reduce addiction and dependence, and decrease the quality and quantity of illegal drugs available on American streets. Those have been the goals since President Richard Nixon first declared the war as part of his attempt to look tough on crime during the presidential election in 1968.

Since then, the strategy of prohibition has been ramped up by every succeeding administration. Few people in this country—or anywhere—have escaped the effects of the U.S. drug war, from the toll of burglaries and car thefts committed to pay for drugs, to the tax bills for prisons to hold the increasing percentages of citizens locked up for nonviolent drug-related crimes, to the millions of kids who've grown up without one or both parents as a result of drug convictions and drug addictions. Drug-related murders reach into the tens of thousands in this country, and the toll is much higher in drug-producing and—shipping nations, from Colombia to Afghanistan to Jamaica. Thousands of peace officers have died fighting the drug war. Whole countries have found themselves under the boot of the illegal drug industry, their governments controlled or intimidated by drug cartels, their politicians and police forces infiltrated, and honest public servants assassinated.

The assumption in American drug policy has always been that those are the impacts of illegal drugs themselves. But LEAP members have come to believe those are the wages, not of drugs, but of the war on drugs. And they want the rest of the country to look closely at the costs of that strategy and what they see as its failures.

Despite the billions of dollars spent on the fight in nearly 40 years, LEAP members point out, the drug war has failed on every one of its own stated goals.

Drug consumption, for instance, shows little sign of dropping. Whereas in 1965, according to the Drug Enforcement Administration, fewer than 4 million Americans had ever tried an illegal drug, the figure is now more than 110 million. In 2000, the federal government estimated that there were about 33 million people in this country who had used cocaine at least once—a more than 700 percent increase over the total number of people 35 years before who had used any illegal drug.

Dependence and addiction? According to the Office of National Drug Control Policy (ONDCP), the federal agency that sets and administers U.S. drug policy, in 2002 more than 7 million Americans were either dependent on or abusing illegal substances—nearly double the number of people who had even tried such drugs when Nixon declared his war. Heroin addicts have jumped from a few hundred thousand in the 1960s to between 750,000 and one million today according to the ONDCP.

Attempts to decrease the quality of available drugs also have failed. In 1970, average street heroin in this country had a potency of 1 to 2 percent. In 2000, according to the DEA, that purity figure was 36.8 percent—although U.S. drug czar John Walters did praise anti-drug forces recently for reducing the strength of street heroin coming from South America to 32.1 percent. Similarly, street cocaine was roughly 2 to 4 percent pure in 1968—and a whopping 56 percent in 2001, according to the ONDCP. The average strength of the active ingredient (THC) in marijuana sold in this country more than doubled between the late 1970s and 2001.

Nor is there much good news on drug quantities and availability, at least not judging by the numbers of users and the prices on the street. The ONDCP estimates that Americans' use of cocaine and crack has dropped from 447 tons in 1990 to 259 tons in 2000. But the price of cocaine has dropped from $100 per gram in 1970 to $25 to $50 per gram in 2002—for cocaine that was many times stronger. At the wholesale level, a kilogram of cocaine (2.2 pounds at roughly 25 percent purity) cost $45,000 in New York City in 1970. Today, in any large city in the U.S., it costs less than $15,000 and it's about 65 percent pure.

Only marijuana showed a price increase. In 1970, a bag of Mexican ditchweed (roughly an ounce) cost $20. In 2005, that same bag costs nearly $50. But most Americans who can afford it don't smoke Mexican ditchweed. They smoke U.S.-grown sinsemilla, which runs up to $400 per ounce.

With availability, price, and quality making drugs as attractive as ever, the only other barometer of the success of the drug war might be if it's stopped anyone from trying drugs—an area where programs like DARE, a huge effort targeted at schoolkids—have had a noted lack of success. "It didn't stop George Bush, Bill Clinton, Al Gore or me from smoking pot," said Woolridge. "I don't think it probably ever stopped anyone."

Collateral Damage

The cops and prosecutors and judges who belong to LEAP think the bad results of the drug war go beyond its policy failures, even beyond the lives lost to drug violence and incarceration.

"Let's be honest," Cole said. "The war on drugs has taken an incredible toll in terms of the loss of our civil liberties, particularly in terms of the Fourth Amendment, from property forfeiture laws that fund law enforcement agencies to warrantless searches. It's promoted institutionalized racism, and it's created a systemic level of corruption among law enforcement unheard of prior to its initiation."

Law enforcement veterans like Cole and Woolridge believe the increase in institutional racism is one of the deepest wounds. They point out, for instance, that crack users (generally inner-city blacks) are subject to mandatory minimum sentences of five years for possession of five grams of crack, while powder cocaine users (generally middle-class whites) have to be caught with 500 grams to get the same mandatory sentence.

While ONDCP statistics show that whites use more than 70 percent of all illegal drugs, blacks are sentenced to prison for drug crimes seven times more often than whites.

"Imagine," said Cole, "one of the most racist places in the world: South Africa, 1993. At that time, the South African government was incarcerating black males at the rate of 859 per 100,000 population." And yet in 2004 in the United States—with more people and a higher percent of its population in prison than any country in the world—the incarceration rate for black males was 4,919 per 100,000 (compared to 726 overall).

He pointed to an FBI estimate that one in three black male babies born in the U.S. in 2004 have an expectation of going to prison during their lifetime. "That just blows my mind," he said.

LEAP members believe that a large percentage of the corruption found in U.S. police agencies is tied to drugs. In Texas, recent drug-related scandals included the Dallas fake-drugs operation, in which a snitch was paid more than $200,000 over a two-year period to provide local cops with drug dealers. The "dealers" turned out to be nearly all illegal immigrants; their "drugs" turned out to be crushed sheetrock and pool chalk.

And then there was Tulia, in the Texas Panhandle, in which a multi-county drug task force hired a corrupt deputy sheriff to rid the town of its drug problem; when it turned out there wasn't one, the deputy created one, and more than 40 people wound up arrested.

LEAP spokesmen see both of those high-profile Texas drug corruption cases as indicative of a much wider problem: officers cutting corners to get the arrest numbers that will keep the fuel line of federal and state anti-drug funding open. And those scandals don't begin to touch on the border patrol agents, police, and other law enforcement officials who have been corrupted because the drug money is so available.

More Law-Enforcement Corruption

Rusty White, another LEAP member, is a self-described redneck who grew up hard in east Texas and now, after many stops in other states and countries, lives just north of Fort Worth. At 13, he saw a friend shoot up black-tar heroin and decided he didn't like hard drugs. By 16, he'd been to juvenile detention five times and gotten kicked out of his high school "because I was traveling with an older crowd of bad-ass kids that I was trying to live up to."

In quick succession, he married, became a father, joined the Army and got divorced. After a second tour with the Army, he ended up in Florence, Arizona, where he went to work at the state penitentiary, which, he said, was "one of the most violent prisons in the United States at that time."

From 1973 to 1978, he worked as a guard on maximum security, death row, and administrative segregation cellblocks, dealing with horrors daily. "Life meant very little to those inside the walls," he said, noting that two prison guards were killed and mutilated by inmates in 1973. "And drugs were one of the biggest problems we had. They were the cause of most of the deaths and power struggles." And most of the drugs were brought in by family members of prison workers. "I got fed up with the corruption and left to go into the oil-drilling business in 1979," he said.

After working overseas for several years, White moved to Oklahoma. And there, he said, he got to see the war on drugs from a very different vantage point. "The county I lived in had a sheriff who controlled the drug market. And he did so with force. It was common knowledge that if you crossed him he could be—and had been—deadly."

But the same sheriff regularly flew around the county in National Guard helicopters, providing photo ops for news crews to show how tough he was on drugs. "The only thing he was getting rid of was the competition," said White disgustedly.

His only personal encounter with the sheriff and his machine occurred when White's brother-in-law, a small-time pot dealer, was busted. "He was poor, didn't have a car that ran, and was living off [government] commodities. Yet he was going to be played by the sheriff as a drug-dealing kingpin," the former prison guard said.

"Anyway, he's the father of three little ones, all younger than six, and when the police arrived, he offered to go with them willingly. But he asked that his kids be allowed to stay with an uncle who was there rather than dragging them down to the station. Well, you know how people feel about 'drug dealers.' The police said no, the kids were coming to the station to watch their father get busted, and then they'd be released to the uncle."

When the man's trial came up, White said, it turned out the district attorney didn't have any evidence against him as a big-time dealer. Nonetheless, he was offered a plea deal: Admit to being a big dealer and get a one- to three-year sentence. If he took it to trial, however, the prosecutor promised he'd ask for a full 10 years.

"He copped to the plea. But to see him struggle with having to lie in front of his kids and admit to something he hadn't done—well, I sort of snapped and screamed at the prosecutor and asked him if he'd thought he'd earned his money that day and why he was playing God, and he looked at me and answered, 'Because in this county, I am God.'"

A couple of years later, White said, the DA went back into private practice and shortly thereafter was arrested and convicted for dealing methamphetamines. "How the sheriff escaped that net, I don't know," White said. "But the thing to remember is that . . . this sort of thing is happening every day in the war on drugs, all over the country. And that abuse of trust and power is far more harmful to Americans than drugs could ever be."

No Place for "Anyone with a Conscience"

Shortly after his brother-in-law's conviction, White went back to work in the prison system, and became a drug-dog trainer and handler. It was the sort of work White said he was meant to do. "I tracked several escapees from the prison and even some cop killers using my track K-9s. We helped departments all over the state. I'd be sent to prisons to look for drugs—I had no problem with that. But the more we were used with other police organizations the more my conscience started to become a problem."

Two incidents stick in White's mind. Once while his partner was helping another officer, part of a joint was discovered in the ashtray of an old pickup belonging to an elderly man. The dogs were brought in, and in the camper shell on the back of the truck in which the old man lived the dogs sniffed out a brief-case with more than $9,000 in it. Because it was a drug dog that had alerted on it, the money was confiscated. "And they just stood around laughing as the old man begged them not to take his life savings. It just made me sick and ashamed. Heck, it's common knowledge that over 90 percent of the paper money in this country is tainted with a drug scent a dog can find. But using that to rob our people disgusts me. Heck, if you walk any K-9 into a bank vault the dog will mark on that money, too. How come that money isn't confiscated?"

The second incident occurred one night when White and his drug dog were called to help a local police department search a house for drugs. When he pulled up to the house, he asked to see the warrant. The officer told him it wasn't there yet but to go ahead and start the search, and it would be there shortly. "I told him that's just not how it works. I needed the warrant for the search to be legal. So I put my K-9 back into the truck and brought him back to the kennel. And then I got called on the carpet for refusing to assist."

White thought getting into trouble for following the law he'd sworn to uphold was just too much, so he quit. "Heck, there was so much corruption, even among K-9 handlers. If they didn't want someone with drugs caught they'd say the dog didn't mark. If they did, well, we heard of cases where guys went so far as to 'salt' the areas their dogs were searching to make sure someone got busted. It was so bad that, being honest, you couldn't do it. . . . I don't think anyone with a conscience can be part of law enforcement anymore."

Richard Watkins saw the same corruption inside prison that White did, but from a unique perspective. A decorated Vietnam veteran with a Ph.D. in education, Watkins worked at Texas' Huntsville prison for 20 years; the last several as warden of Holiday Unit, a 2,100-bed facility housing a range of criminals from nonviolent to violent/maximum security.

He was originally hired to revamp and professionalize the correctional officers training program—something the prison system was forced to do by federal mandate, and which Watkins said was badly needed. "It was just horrible. Corrupt, bad, just plain horrible," he said.

Watkins had always had reservations about the war on drugs. He figured the drug dealers wouldn't go away as long as there was a market. And looking at this country's experience with Prohibition, "and how that created mobsters and criminal gangs," he figured that legalizing drugs made more sense. When selling and drinking booze became legal in this country again, he said, "you had so much more control of it. You had supporting laws that managed the use of alcohol."

Watkins was first exposed to drugs in Vietnam. He didn't use them—he preferred alcohol—but he saw a lot of other guys getting high on marijuana and other drugs. Many of those men wound up in prison when they came home with addiction problems. "And in prison, you could always get whatever drugs you wanted. Heck, we arrested a mom one time who was putting a lip-lock on her son to pass him a balloon full of heroin. But most of the drugs came in through the guards. Drugs are packaged so small, it's almost impossible to keep them out. Think about that: If you can't keep drugs out of a maximum-security prison, you can't keep them out of schools or anywhere else."

Once drugs lands someone in prison in Texas, he said, life's prospects get a lot dimmer. "We've got these minor players put in with professional criminals. If they weren't criminals going in they damn sure are when they get out. Imagine a system where we put people into a society that's really a training ground for criminals, then don't provide them with either schooling or treatment, then put them back on the streets where they came from. Do you really expect them to be reformed? Life doesn't work that way."

He wishes people wouldn't make the decision to use drugs. "But if they did use them, I wouldn't put them in prison. I'd rather see the money we spend on prisons going to give these kids the tools they need to make better choices."

Voices Opposing LEAP's Perspective

You might imagine that it would be easy to find law enforcement agencies and personnel who oppose LEAP's call for legalization and regulation as an alternative to the war on drugs. But neither the FBI nor the DEA would discuss the subject.

"Our job is to stop the flow of illegal drugs both at home and abroad, as well as to stop our citizens from wanting to use them, through education and prevention methods," said an ONDCP representative. "We will not discuss legalization or any organization which thinks that would be a solution."

Jack Cole wasn't surprised. "They're good soldiers," he said. "They're not allowed to question their commands. Our job is to simply have their commanders change their marching orders."

Mike Smithson, who runs LEAP's speakers bureau, said he's made more than 100 attempts to get law enforcement and drug policy officials to come out and debate LEAP, "and we've only been taken up on it five times. Policymakers generally say that debating us will lend us credence. We think they're just afraid. How can they defend a policy that is already being defended by every major drug dealer, cartel and drug-producing government worldwide?"

Woolridge says that on his entire ride from Los Angeles he's talked to only two officers who disagreed with LEAP's point of view. "One guy thought we'd destroy America if we legalized drugs. He was so angry when he couldn't find anything to write me a ticket for that he gave me the finger as he drove away. And there was a state trooper with 22 years on the job who told me to take off my shirt because it said "Cops say legalize drugs," and he didn't agree with that. I told him go make up his own shirt."

One person did agree to discuss his opposition to LEAP's stand was Sheriff John Cooke of Wells County in Colorado. Cooke is a member of a Rotary Club at which Howard Woolridge spoke. He was so taken aback by the idea of legalizing drugs that he demanded equal time and recently spoke to the Rotary Club himself.

"In my opinion, there are several reasons not to legalize drugs," Cooke told Fort Worth Weekly. First of all, when people say you're going to eliminate the black market, does that mean you're going to sell drugs to 12- and 15-year olds? Because if you don't, someone will. Law enforcement surely hasn't done a good job at keeping alcohol and cigarettes out of the hands of kids, so what makes them think they'll do any better with drugs? And if you don't sell drugs to them, there will be a black market created to sell to them. So I don't buy the end of the black market theory.

"Secondly, we already have social ills from the legal use of alcohol and tobacco. Why on earth would we want to turn other addictive substances loose on the public?

"Thirdly, these LEAP folks want to throw in the towel, say we've lost the drug war. But the thing is that I think we're winning the war on drugs. I think drug use is down. I think if we keep at it, we will win.

"Then there's the question of use. Right now, I believe that the threat of the hammer of law enforcement is keeping a great many people from doing drugs. The threat of prison time is a big hammer. I think if we legalized you'd see the number of people doing drugs in this country skyrocket. I believe we'd have a drug-dependent society . . . and I don't want to see America as a drug-dependent country."

Michael Gilbert, director of the Department of Criminal Justice at the University of Texas at San Antonio, said he doubted that there would be any sizeable black market aimed at teens if drugs were legalized. Gilbert is a LEAP member who worked in prisons—including Leavenworth—and with Justice Department agencies for more than 20 years.

"The reason there's so much money in the black market is not because of the small portion of destabilized street addicts we have, or even kids experimenting with drugs. It's because you have long-time productive millions [of people] who regularly purchase small quantities of the drugs of their choice but they don't use them in a way that becomes destructive to their lives," he said. "They're working, paying their taxes and so forth. The real money is from the enormous number of middle-class people who use drugs. So while you might still have a small market of teens purchasing drugs, it wouldn't be large enough to fund criminal enterprises as it does today."

While few policy makers will discuss the benefits of drug prohibition, several well-known former policy makers have come out against it. Among them are Nobel Prize-winning economist Milton Friedman, a former member of President Reagan's Economic Advisory Board; former Secretary of State (under Ronald

Reagan) George P. Shultz; former governor of New Mexico Gary Johnson; former Baltimore Mayor Kurt Schmoke; and U.S. Rep. Dennis Kucinich of Ohio, a former presidential candidate.

Benefits of the LEAP Solution

None of the LEAP members interviewed for this article believes abusing drugs is a good choice. But that's different, they say, from the legal system further ruining people's lives because of that bad choice. They also figure that, like tattoos, hair color decisions, and bad marriages, drug use is a poor choice that society should only care about when it hurts other people. In town, running around in your yard naked and screaming at 4 a.m. breaks the social contract. On a ranch where no one else can see or hear, few people would care about it. Likewise, LEAP members figure, if you can do drugs and not break the social contract, go ahead. And in fact, the federal government figures that 72 percent of chronic drug users continue to function well in society, without harming others.

Even considering the harm that drugs can cause, however, LEAP members believe that the war on drugs is even more harmful. Legalizing drugs, on the other hand, would take profits out of the hands of criminals and hugely reduce the need for people to commit crime to pay for drugs, they say. Regulation would take drug manufacture out of the hands of bathtub chemists and put it into the hands of real chemists, eliminating many of the deaths from bad drugs—much like the end of Prohibition did for deaths from homemade booze. HIV and hepatitis C, rampant among needle-sharing junkies, could be significantly reduced with the availability of clean needles, reducing a major health-care burden for the country.

"Don't forget my favorite," Woolridge said. "If as Bush said, drug money funds terrorists, [then] legalizing drugs would take half a billion dollars a day out of Afghanistan alone, much of which is going to al Qaeda to buy weapons to be used to kill our boys. We could eliminate that overnight."

Legalization, in fact, would probably not increase drug use long-term, many believe—especially since nearly half the population has already tried it. "In all likelihood," Watkins said, "you would see a spike in use as we did with the end of alcohol prohibition. But that normalized pretty quickly, and would probably be the same with drugs. There would be a period of experimentation that would level out, and we'd be left with all the benefits and none of the negatives."

It was Sunday afternoon and Howard Woolridge and Misty were still in upstate New York, having made it from Utica to a ghetto in Schenectady. Woolridge was back on the phone again, when a woman approached him.

"What do you mean cops say legalize drugs?" she could be heard asking.

"Just that. Let's legalize drugs, take them off the street corner."

"What kind of drugs?"

"Heroin, crack, methamphetamine, anything you can think of."

"Are you crazy? I don't want my kids doing those drugs!"

"Neither do I," he told her. "They're no good. But that doesn't keep them from being sold on the corner in this very neighborhood, does it? I'd legalize them and get them into pharmacies. Keep your kids from being shot while walking down the street."

There was a pause and then she laughed. "I never thought of it that way before. You're making me think now."

POSTSCRIPT

Should Laws Against Drug Use Remain Restrictive?

Kleber and Califano assert that utilizing the criminal justice system to maintain the illegal nature of drugs is necessary to keep society free of the detrimental effects of drugs. Loosening drug laws is unwise and dangerous. They argue that international control efforts, interdiction, and domestic law enforcement are effective and that many problems associated with drug use are mitigated by drug regulation policies. They maintain that restrictive drug laws are a feasible and desirable means of dealing with the drug crisis.

Gorman charges that restrictive drug laws are highly destructive and discriminatory. He professes that if drug laws remain stringent, the result would be more drug users in prison and that drug abusers and addicts would engage in more criminal activity. Also, there is the possibility that more drug-related social problems would occur. Gorman concludes that society cannot afford to retain its intransigent position on drug legalization. The potential risks of the current federal policies on drug criminalization outweigh any potential benefits. Society suffers from harsh drug laws, says Gorman, by losing many of its civil liberties.

Proponents for less restrictive drug laws argue that such laws have not worked and that the drug battle has been lost. They believe that drug-related problems would diminish if more tolerant policies were implemented. Citing the legal drugs alcohol and tobacco as examples, legalization opponents argue that less restrictive drug laws would not decrease profits from the sale of drugs (the profits from cigarettes and alcohol are incredibly high). Moreover, opponents argue, relaxing drug laws does not make problems associated with drugs disappear (alcohol and tobacco have extremely high addiction rates as well as a myriad of other problems associated with their use).

Many European countries, such as the Netherlands and Switzerland, have a system of legalized drugs, and most have far fewer addiction rates and lower incidences of drug-related violence and crime than the United States. These countries make a distinction between soft drugs (those identified as less harmful) and hard drugs (those with serious consequences). However, would the outcomes of less restrictive laws in the United States be the same as in Europe? Relaxed drug laws in the United States could still be a tremendous risk because its drug problems could escalate and reimposing strict drug laws would be difficult. This was the case with Prohibition in the 1920s, which, in changing the status of alcohol from legal to illegal, produced numerous crime- and alcohol-related problems.

Many good articles debate the pros and cons of this issue. These include "Reorienting U.S. Drug Policy," by Jonathon Caulkins and Peter Reuter (*Issues in Science and Technology,* Fall 2006); "No Surrender: The Drug War Saves Lives," by

John Walters (*National Review,* September 27, 2004), the current director of the Office of National Drug Control Policy; "Lighting Up In Amsterdam," by John Tierney (*New York Times,* August 26, 2006); "What Drug Policies Cost. Estimating Government Drug Policy Expenditures," by Peter Reuter (*Addiction,* March 2006); "An Effective Drug Policy to Protect America's Youth and Communities," by Asa Hutchinson (*Fordham Urban Law Journal,* January 2003); and, "The War at Home: Our Jails Overflow with Nonviolent Drug Offenders. Have We Reached the Point Where the Drug War Causes More Harm Than the Drugs Themselves," by Sanho Tree (*Sojourners,* May–June 2003).

ISSUE 2

Should the United States Put More Emphasis on Stopping the Importation of Drugs?

YES: Office of National Drug Control Policy, from *The National Drug Control Strategy* (February 2007)

NO: Cathy Inouye, from "The DEA, CIA, DoD, & Narcotrafficking," *Z Magazine* (July/August 2004)

ISSUE SUMMARY

YES: The Office of National Drug Control Policy (ONDCP) argues that the importation of drugs must be stopped to reduce drug use and abuse. If the supply of drugs being trafficked across American borders is reduced, then there would be fewer drug-related problems. The ONDCP maintains that a coordinated international effort is needed to combat the increased production of heroin, cocaine, and marijuana.

NO: Cathy Inouye, a human rights volunteer for NGO SEDEM (Seguridad en Democracia), feels that the corroboration of numerous United States with leaders in foreign governments have resulted in continued human rights abuses and has enriched those leaders in countries where the drug trade is prominent. Inouye notes that the federal government should reexamine its role of cooperation with other governments, especially those involved in the drug trade.

$\mathbf{S}$ince the beginning of the 1990s, overall drug use in the United States has increased. Up to now, interdiction has not proven to be successful in slowing the flow of drugs into the United States. Drugs continue to cross U.S. borders at record levels. This point may signal a need for stepped-up international efforts to stop the production and trafficking of drugs. Conversely, it may illustrate the inadequacy of the current strategy. Should the position of the U.S. government be to improve and strengthen current measures or to try an entirely new approach?

Some people contend that rather than attempting to limit illegal drugs from coming into the United States, more effort should be directed at reducing the demand for drugs and improving treatment for drug abusers. Foreign countries would not produce and transport drugs like heroin and cocaine into the United States if there was no market for them. Drug policies, some people maintain, should be aimed at the social and economic conditions underlying domestic drug problems, not at interfering with foreign governments.

Many U.S. government officials believe that other countries should assist in stopping the flow of drugs across their borders. Diminishing the supply of drugs by intercepting them before they reach the user is another way to eliminate or curtail drug use. Critical elements in the lucrative drug trade are multinational crime syndicates. One premise is that if the drug production, transportation, distribution, and processing functions as well as the money laundering operations of these criminal organizations can be interrupted and eventually crippled, then the drug problem would abate.

In South American countries such as Peru, Colombia, and Bolivia, where coca—from which cocaine is processed—is cultivated, economic aid has been made available to help the governments of these countries fight the cocaine kingpins. An alleged problem is that a number of government officials in these countries are corrupt or fearful of the cocaine cartel leaders. One proposed solution is to go directly to the farmers and offer them money to plant crops other than coca. This tactic, however, failed in the mid-1970s, when the U.S. government gave money to farmers in Turkey to stop growing opium poppy crops. After one year the program was discontinued due to the enormous expense, and opium poppy crops were once again planted.

Drug problems are not limited to the Americas. Since the breakup of the Soviet Union, for example, there has been a tremendous increase in opium production in many of the former republics. These republics are in dire need of money, and one source of income is opium production. Moreover, there is lax enforcement by police officials in these republics.

There are many reasons why people are dissatisfied with the current state of the war on drugs. For example, in the war on drugs, the casual user is generally the primary focus of drug use deterrence. This is viewed by many people as a form of discrimination because the vast majority of drug users and sellers who are arrested and prosecuted are poor, members of minorities, homeless, unemployed, and/or disenfranchised. Also, international drug dealers who are arrested are usually not the drug bosses but lower-level people working for them. Finally, some argue that the war on drugs should be redirected away from interdiction and enforcement because they feel that the worst drug problems in society today are caused by legal drugs, primarily alcohol and tobacco.

The following selections address the issue of whether or not the war on drugs should be fought on an international level. The Office of National Drug Control Policy takes the view that international cooperation is absolutely necessary if we are to stem the flow of drugs and reduce drug-related problems in the United States. Cathy Inouye argues that an international approach to dealing with drugs has been ineffective because many of the foreign countries receiving U.S. financial aid profit from the drug trade and that many of these countries engage in numerous human rights violations.

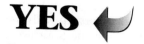
National Drug Control Strategy

Converging Threats on the Southwest Border

Securing our borders is a top priority for the U.S. Government. The Southwest Border poses an urgent challenge to national security. A recent study by DEA's El Paso Intelligence Center confirms that drug trafficking organizations collect fees to facilitate the movement of all types of contraband from Mexico into the United States. These "gatekeeper" organizations control the approaches to the Southwest Border and direct smuggling—of drugs, aliens, counterfeit goods, and potentially even terrorists into the United States. Power struggles between these organizations are responsible for widespread violence and corruption. By making headway against drug trafficking in partnership with the Mexican government, we can combat all of these serious threats to border security.

To coordinate Federal efforts to address the central position that the drug trade occupies among border threats, the Administration has developed a *National Southwest Border Counternarcotics Strategy* and an associated *Implementation Plan*. These two documents will help guide border control efforts and will increase the emphasis on disrupting the flow of drugs into the United States and the massive backflow of illicit cash into Mexico.

The counternarcotics capabilities supporting the *National Southwest Border Counternarcotics Strategy* will be enhanced by the Department of Homeland Security's (DHS) Secure Border Initiative (SBI), a comprehensive multiyear, multithreat, border security plan that will be implemented by U.S. Customs and Border Protection (CBP). SBI will increase the number of Border Patrol agents and expand associated physical infrastructure and technology. A critical component of SBI will leverage aerial surveillance and detection sensor technology to monitor border activity. A prototype of the new border control system will be deployed along the Southwest Border in the next several months.

Central to both the *National Southwest Border Counternarcotics Strategy* and SBI is a commitment by Federal agencies to substantially increase collaboration with State, local, and tribal agencies. One example of such collaboration is the DHS—led Border Enforcement Security Task Force, which combines personnel from different Federal agencies with key State and local law enforcement agencies to target violent criminal organizations along the Southwest Border. These efforts, through the Organized Crime Drug Enforcement Task Force

From the Office of National Drug Control Policy, February 2007, pp. 33–45.

(OCDETF), HIDTA program, EPIC, the DHS-supported State and Local Fusion Centers, and other entities, combined with a continued partnership with the Government of Mexico, will enhance our effectiveness along the Southwest Border against all threats.

Mexico

Across the Southwest Border in Mexico, drug trafficking and associated violence pose a grave threat not only to the health and safety of the Mexican people, but to the sovereignty of Mexico itself. Threats, intimidation, and attacks have instilled widespread fear, challenged Mexico's free press, and compromised the ability of municipalities, states, and even the national government to exercise authority. This lawlessness is fueled by Mexico's position as the primary transit corridor for most of the cocaine available on American streets, as well as a considerable share of the heroin, methamphetamine, and marijuana destined for the U.S. market. The threat to the security of Mexico, as well as its impact on the drug situation in the United States, has served to strengthen the resolve of both countries to take on this challenge together.

DEA and other U.S. law enforcement agencies have developed highly productive relationships with key Mexican counterparts that are yielding positive results. Anticorruption initiatives and institutional reforms by the Mexican government have increased DEA's ability to share information and conduct joint investigations. In 2006, Mexico extradited 63 criminals to the United States. Twenty-seven of these cases involved narcotics traffickers, including a member of the feared Tijuana-based Arellano-Felix Organization. The eradication of illicit crops remains a priority mission for the Mexican Army, which eradicated nearly 30,000 hectares of marijuana in 2006. Mexican authorities continue to seize significant amounts of drugs as they flow into Mexico and toward the United States.

President Felipe Calderon has demonstrated that his administration will continue to pursue the strong counterdrug commitment he inherited from his predecessor, former President Vicente Fox. Mexico's extradiction to the United States in early 2007 of 16 major drug traffickers is a concrete indication of Mexico's commitment to directly attack and disrupt major drug trafficking oganizations. The United States will continue to stand with Mexico and looks forward to increasing bilateral cooperation against the full array of cross-border drug threats.

Eradicating Domestic Marijuana Crops

Marijuana is the most widely used and readily available drug in the United States. DEA formed the Domestic Cannabis Eradication/Suppression Program (DCE/SP) to vigorously target, disrupt, and dismantle large-scale domestic marijuana growing operations. Working with ONDCP, DEA identified the top seven states for marijuana cultivation—California, Hawaii, Kentucky, Oregon, Tennessee, Washington, and West Virginia—and has shifted funding priorities to counter growing operations in these states. With these additional resources, the top seven states eradicated more than 5.5 million marijuana plants and the other states in the DCE/SP program accounted for the eradication of an additional 770,000 plants in 2006.

DEA's DCE/SP program has forced many traffickers to abandon large outdoor marijuana plots in favor of smaller, better concealed illicit gardens. Cultivators also have turned to sophisticated hydroponic technology to cultivate marijuana plants indoors, using high-nutrient solutions rather than conventional soil to increase the potency of their marijuana plants. The National Drug Intelligence Center's *National Drug Threat Assessment 2007* notes that several Asian criminal groups have moved their indoor marijuana cultivation networks from Canada to residential neighborhoods in the United States. In a recent example, 44 homes in a Sacramento, California suburb were found to be filled with marijuana plants under indoor cultivation, all managed by a single Asian drug organization.

Federal, State and local authorities will continue to focus on the disruption of both indoor and outdoor marijuana production, both to discourage its production and use and to prevent traffickers from benefiting from what remains the most lucrative crop in the drug trafficker's illegal product line.

Organizational Attack: Denying Drug Traffickers Their Profits

Money is the primary motivation of individuals involved in the drug trade at all levels and illicit funds are the lifeblood of drug trafficking organizations. Drug proceeds sustain production and trafficking operations and fuel corruption. By denying drug trafficking organizations their funds, law enforcement can inflict significant damage on their illicit business.

The *U.S. Money Laundering Threat Assessment*, published in December 2005, identifies the smuggling of bulk cash as a key money laundering threat. Most of the illicit money generated by drug sales in the United States is transported in cash across the Southwest Border into Mexico. Once the cash from drug sales in the United States is smuggled into Mexico, one of three things happens. First, the cash is converted into large denominations ($50s and $100s) and transported to drug source countries such as Colombia or wired to third-party countries. Second, the cash is kept in Mexico and used by Mexico-based trafficking organizations to support their operations. Third, the currency is repatriated to the United States through money service businesses (commonly referred to as "casas de cambio" or "centros cambiarios"), armored cars, or couriers, and then is deposited into U.S. financial institutions as "clean" money. Federal agencies are aggressively working to disrupt all of these movements of illicit funds.

DEA is actively targeting the illicit proceeds of drug traffickers in all of its investigations and is applying this heightened focus on financial matters to bulk currency movement, the Black Market Peso Exchange, and casas de cambio. DEA's *Money Trail Initiative* targets drug and money transportation organizations operating in the United States with the goal of connecting these organizations to sources of drug supply in Mexico. Since its inception in 2005, the *Money Trail Initiative* has resulted in the dismantling of six national drug and money transportation organizations as well as the identification and dismantling of the Chihuahua, Mexico based Arriola-Marquez drug trafficking organization. As a result of both concentrated and broad-based efforts to attack the financial structures of drug trafficking organizations, DEA denied drug trafficking and money laundering organizations $1.6 billion in revenue and seized a total of $341 million in U.S. currency in FY 2006.

ICE liaisons in Mexico, Ecuador, and Panama, in concert with special national law enforcement units located in each of these countries, are working on a bulk cash smuggling initiative known as *Operation Firewall*. This operation targets bulk cash smuggling by Mexican traffickers in the land, sea, air, passenger, and commercial transportation systems. As of October 2006, *Operation Firewall* has yielded more than 130 arrests and the seizure of more than $52 million in cash and financial instruments. This initiative will expand to additional partner nations in 2007.

The Treasury Department's Office of Foreign Assets Control (OFAC) has worked closely with both DEA and ICE to target the financial networks of Mexican drug trafficking organizations. Recent investigations resulted in the July 2006 identification (pursuant to the Foreign Narcotics Kingpin Designation Act) of a key Arellano Felix Organization money laundering cell that included several money service businesses and an armored car company. OFAC's actions effectively shut down this major illicit finance operation.

In an effort to combat the repatriation of illicit funds, the Treasury Department's Financial Crimes Enforcement Network (FinCEN) issued an advisory to U.S. financial institutions in April 2006 on the potential money laundering threat associated with the smuggling of bulk U.S. currency into Mexico and its subsequent return to the United States through the misuse of relationships with U.S. financial institutions by certain Mexican financial institutions, including Mexican casas de cambio. Law enforcement agencies are also increasing their focus on other Bank Secrecy Act (the principal U.S. regulatory regime targeting money laundering and terrorist financing) data and violations to help disrupt the flow of illegal funds into and through U.S. financial institutions.

Finally, Federal law enforcement agencies, along with their State and local law enforcement partners, are aggressively working to identify money laundering cells in the United States. The OCDETF Fusion Center and the National Seizure System (NSS) operated out of EPIC will support and enhance anti-money laundering intelligence and coordination. The information provided by the OCDETF Fusion Center and the NSS will allow law enforcement to identify disparate information and target organizational leaders for investigation and prosecution.

Colombia

During the past year, Colombia has continued to expand its aggressive efforts against drug trafficking. With U.S. assistance, Colombian forces were able to spray more than 160,000 hectares of coca. Another 40,000 hectares were manually eradicated. For the first time, manual and aerial spray eradication operations were conducted in key national parks and indigenous reserves that were once safe havens for the narco-terrorist group known as the Revolutionary Armed Forces of Colombia (FARC). Through aggressive eradication, the Colombian government also has effected a significant decrease in opium poppy cultivation over the last several years. In addition, Colombian and U.S. interdiction activities resulted in the seizure of more than 150 metric tons of seizures of cocaine and cocaine base in 2006, and the Colombian government completed several extraditions of key drug traffickers and FARC leaders for trial and conviction in U.S. courts.

Colombia also has worked to disarm and demobilize the two other major illegally armed groups that have been tied to drug trafficking. Through careful negotiation, more than 31,000 members of the United Self-Defense Forces of Colombia (AUC) have been demobilized, and talks that could lead to a demobilization process for members of the National Liberation Army (ELN) have begun as well. Demobilization reduces the options available to drug traffickers seeking protection from law enforcement forces in Colombia and has drastically reduced the level of violence and insecurity in the Colombian countryside.

The more secure climate that has resulted from Colombia's counterdrug efforts has enabled the increasing growth of legitimate business and industry. Prior to 2000, the Colombian economy was severely impacted by crime, violence and the ongoing conflict with the FARC; investment was low and national unemployment hovered near 16 percent. Since 2001, the Colombian gross domestic product (GDP) has grown an average of 4 percent a year, and reached a 6-percent growth rate by the end of 2006. Inflation has dropped from the decades-old rate of 20 percent to 4.5 percent and unemployment has fallen from 15.7 percent in 2000 to 10.4 percent in 2006. Private investment in Colombia has also recovered, rising from 10.9 percent of GDP in 1999 to 17.5 percent of GDP in 2005. Strong drug control policies have helped to spark a remarkable economic turnaround that is creating a brighter future for all Colombians.

Drug traffickers have started to respond to the success of eradication, interdiction, and law enforcement efforts in multiple ways. Coca cultivators have undermined the impact of aerial eradication by pruning or replanting their crops with seedlings. They also have begun planting smaller fields in more remote areas that are harder for spray aircraft and manual eradicators to reach. Traffickers also have taken advantage of neighboring countries to export drugs and to move precursors, money, and arms into Colombia. In addition, because drug trafficking organizations are now smaller, they have become less visible and less exposed to targeting by law enforcement officials.

Colombia and the United States are working to counter these challenges with efforts focused on improving the effectiveness of coca eradication programs. President Uribe has increased the pressure on coca cultivators by expanding the number of personnel focused on countering coca cultivation through a directive that makes coca eradication the responsibility of all public security forces in Colombia. The United States and Colombia also are investing

SUCCEEDING WITH PLAN COLOMBIA

Due to the bravery and dedication of Colombian authorities, and the assistance provided by the United States, remarkable progress has been made toward the accomplishment of Plan Colombia's many goals, as indicated below:

- *Create the conditions for peace in Colombia:* More than 31,000 members of the AUC have demobilized; more than 10,000 dissidents from illegally armed groups have deserted, including 5,500 members of the FARC; and negotiations with the ELN, if successful, could lead to an additional 3,500 demobilized personnel.
- *Strengthen institutional presence, efficiency, and effectiveness at national, regional, and local levels to improve governance in the nation and increase the citizens' confidence in the state:* Public services have been improved in 143 municipalities and 111 municipalities have been strengthened financially.
- *Initiate rapid steps in the South to facilitate the transition to legal activities and to generate socially, economically, and environmentally sustainable alternatives to drug trafficking and violence:* More than 81,000 families have benefited from alternative development and livelihood programs; more than 102,000 hectares of licit crops have been cultivated; and more than 23,000 hectares of illicit crops have been manually eradicated.
- *Provide humanitarian assistance to those segments of the population that have been victimized by violence, with special emphasis on the displaced population and the most vulnerable groups:* More than 2.7 million internally displaced persons have been assisted, and the number of internally displaced persons seeking assistance has dropped from more than 92,000 in 2002 to about 12,000 in 2006.
- *Prevent further deterioration of ecosystems and implement measures to conserve and recover their environmental functions and build sustainable development options:* A Forest Ranger program has been established with more than 20,000 participants protecting more than 168,000 hectares of national forests that are being threatened by coca cultivators.
- *Instill respect for human rights and promote compliance with international humanitarian law in Colombian society:* In the past 3 years, all members of the Colombian Security Forces have participated in at least two human rights training sessions. Human rights complaints against public security forces have dropped by 40 percent since 1995.
- *Promote citizen involvement as a means for developing participatory democracy:* More than 333 new citizen oversight committees have been formed and 400 existing ones have received support.
- *Increase the presence and effectiveness of the Justice System:* Forty-three houses of justice ("Casas de Justicia") have been established in Colombia, handling more than 4.8 million cases. Colombia is undergoing an historic transition from an inquisitory criminal justice system (proceedings that are conducted only by a judge who reviews evidence listed on paper) to an accusatory system (with an investigative stage separate from a trial phase in which witnesses testify in open court). The new system has demonstrated greater effectiveness and efficiency in the regions where it has been initiated and it is now gaining the public's confidence for the first time.
- *Establish the security conditions that permit the implementation of government programs:* Public Security Forces have grown by more than 32 percent since 2002, 56 companies of mobile rural police (Carabineros) with 8,600 men have been created, 598 platoons consisting of 24,000 citizen-soldiers have

been established throughout Colombia, and the Colombian National Police has established a presence in all 1,098 municipalities in Colombia for the first time in history.

- *Reduce the production, processing, trafficking, and corruptive influence of drug trafficking organizations:* Coca cultivation dropped more than 15 percent nationwide, including a 61 percent drop in the Putumayo; the purity of heroin seized at major U.S. ports of entry has sharply declined from 87 percent pure in 2000 to 68 percent pure in 2005, suggesting a decrease in Colombian heroin production; and more than 390 drug traffickers have been extradited to the United States over the past 4 years, undermining the drug trafficking organizations' ability to corrupt public officials.

- *Increased public safety:* The focus of Plan Colombia was to break the cycle of violence and reduce the impact of the FARC on farmers who wanted to begin cultivating licit products by increasing security throughout Colombia—a formidable task necessitating heavy investment. The improvements in security are remarkable.

in additional aircraft to increase overall aerial eradication capabilities. This will allow spray aircraft to continue to concentrate on aerial eradication in key cultivation zones while expanding efforts to identify and spray new coca crops more quickly in other areas of Colombia. Finally, the United States and Colombia are collaborating to acquire better data on coca cultivation and drug trafficking to assess and update the joint strategy as the drug trade in Colombia continues to evolve.

Andean Ridge Developments

Peru is the world's second leading producer of cocaine and President Alan Garcia has renewed Peru's commitment to counter illicit coca cultivation. Although the UN Office on Drugs and Crime estimates that Peruvian cocaine production dropped by 10 metric tons between 2004 and 2005, coca acreage in Peru increased from an estimated 27,500 hectares to some 38,000 hectares over the same period. To counter this increase, Peru employs a strong integrated counternarcotics strategy of eradication and alternative development. This nexus has led to the eradication of more than 12,000 hectares of coca in 2006, the development of infrastructure projects, and millions of dollars in sales of licit products in coca-growing regions through the assistance of the U.S. State Department's Bureau for International Narcotics and Law Enforcement Affairs (INL). With U.S. assistance, Peru is also advancing an aggressive container-screening program in its major ports which resulted in the seizure of nearly 12 metric tons of cocaine in its first year—a three fold increase over seizures during the previous year.

Bolivia, the world's third largest producer of cocaine, has unfortunately adopted several policies that have allowed the expansion of coca cultivation. As cocaine production rises in Bolivia, foreign drug traffickers are increasing their presence there. Yet, after a slow start, the Bolivian government met its stated goal of eradicating 5000 hectares of coca in 2006. The United States is strongly encouraging Bolivia to establish tight controls on the sale of licit coca leaf for traditional use and to increase controls on the precursor chemicals used to make cocaine. The United States also continues to advance development initiatives to assist Bolivian coca farmers in developing licit crops as alternatives to coca, increasing the competitiveness of licit enterprises, strengthening local democracy and state presence, and improving social services.

Ecuador and Venezuela have become major transit countries for drugs produced in the Andean Ridge. Northern Ecuador is a major transit point for cocaine, chemicals, and supplies for the FARC and other Colombian drug traffickers. Significant quantities of cocaine originating from Columbia or Peru and leaving South America by sea also depart from Ecuador. Cocaine seizures in Ecuador increased from 3 metric tons in FY 2004 to 34 metric tons in FY 2005, and more than 45 metric tons were seized in FY 2006. The volume of illicit drugs moving through Venezuela is also increasing, with the number of suspected drug flights traveling from Venezuela to Haiti, the Dominican Republic, and other points in the Caribbean more than doubling in 2006.

In September 2006, the U.S. Coast Guard and Ecuadorian authorities agreed on enhanced operational procedures for maritime counterdrug cooperation. The United States seeks to expand on that improved cooperation to reach a full maritime law enforcement agreement with Ecuador and will continue to seek opportunities for counterdrug cooperation with Venezuela.

Transit Zone Interdiction

Four consecutive record-setting years of illicit drug seizures in the transit zone have forced narcotics traffickers to adjust from well-established routes and methods to those they believe will be less susceptible to interdiction. Despite these shifts, the sum of transit zone cocaine seizures and high-confidence losses exceeded 288 metric tons in 2006.

Interdiction efforts in the transit zone over the past year have been bolstered by technological and procedural advances, along with a continuous flow of law enforcement intelligence. For example, the U.S. Coast Guard and Colombian counterparts are engaging in an effort that targets the fishing vessels that sail far out into the Eastern Pacific to serve as refuelers for go-fast speedboats. The U.S. Coast Guard has now been authorized to board Colombian-flagged fishing vessels that are operating outside of their officially documented purpose or beyond Colombian fishing zones. If the Coast Guard determines that these vessels are carrying excess fuel (presumably to refuel go-fast boats carrying drugs), they now have the means and the authority to render this fuel unusable.

Another example of such advances is the broad expansion of armed counterdrug helicopter capabilities used to disable fleeing vessels or to compel them to stop. The U.S. Coast Guard is cascading this capability beyond its special armed helicopter squadron into its HH-65C helicopter fleet. United Kingdom Royal Navy ships are now deploying with armed helicopters and U.S. Navy helicopters are now operating with Coast Guard gunners on board.

Highly successful initiatives like these contributed to an approximate 44 percent reduction in the number of confirmed and suspected go-fast smuggling events in 2006. U.S. efforts were greatly assisted by the cooperation of El Salvador as the site of a Cooperative Security Location.

A key element of this year's interdiction successes has been DEA's *Operation All Inclusive*. This bilateral, intelligence driven strategy is specifically designed to disrupt the flow of illicit drugs, money, and chemicals between source zones and the United States by attacking the drug organizations' vulnerabilities in their supply, transportation systems, and financial infrastructures. In 2005 and 2006, DEA implemented *Operation All Inclusive* throughout Central America, sharply boosting seizures of cocaine, marijuana, and precursor chemicals. As a result of these operations, drug trafficking organizations were forced to delay or suspend their drug operations, divert their routes, change their modes of transportation, and jettison loads. The success of these multi-agency and bilateral operations exemplified the cooperation among law enforcement entities throughout the United States, Latin America, and Central America.

The close cooperation of partner nations was also demonstrated in October 2006 when a Dutch Maritime Patrol Aircraft, operating out of its base in Curacao, detected a suspect fishing vessel in the Caribbean. The Belgian Navy Ship *WESTDIEP* and the British Royal Fleet Auxiliary *WAVE RULER*, both with embarked U.S. Coast Guard Law Enforcement Detachments, converged on the Honduran flagged fishing vessel. The existing U.S.-Honduran bilateral agreement was invoked and the vessel was boarded, leading to the seizure of nearly 3 metric tons of cocaine en route to Central America. Such seamless cooperation by partner nations has been critical in maintaining a strong interdiction presence across the transit zone. In addition, continued bilateral cooperation with Colombian Navy units will advance similar operations closer to the source zone, along the north and west coasts of Colombia.

Expanding the level of cooperation with partner nations across the transit zone will deny traffickers the freedom of movement they enjoy within the territorial waters of nations that do not have the means to interdict them. Building on the success of existing maritime bilateral agreements, similar arrangements are needed throughout the Eastern Pacific and Caribbean transit zones to further increase the risks associated with trafficking illicit drugs.

To ensure increased disruption of cocaine flow and continued disruption of trafficker means, methods and modes going forward, this Strategy is setting an aggressive 40 percent transit zone interdiction goal for 2007, as measured against the Consolidated Counterdrug Database (CCDB) estimate of cocaine movement. Specifically, the 40 percent metric will be applied to the CCDB all-confidence estimate of cocaine movement through the transit zone toward the United States from October 1, 2005 through September 30, 2006 (to ensure that all data being considered have been fully vetted by the time this Strategy is published). This flow estimate is conservative, because it measures only the cocaine movement that interagency operators and analysts are aware of; however, if this level of interdiction is achieved, it will constitute the largest transit zone disruption of the illicit cocaine market in history.

Intelligence-Driven Counterdrug Operations

Intelligence support to interdiction operations provides a model of cooperation among U.S. and cooperating nation military, law enforcement, and intelligence communities, demonstrating the tremendous increases in effectiveness and efficiency such creative collaboration can bring. *Operation Firewall and Operation Panama Express*, multiagency cocaine interdiction programs, combine investigative and intelligence resources to interdict cocaine from the northern coast of Colombia to the United States. Since the first year of *Operation Firewall* (July 2002 to June 2003), maritime cocaine seizures have nearly tripled—from 4.1 metric tons to approximately 11 metric tons. *Operation Panama Express*, a multiagency OCDETF program, collects and analyzes vital law enforcement data and disseminates this information to U.S. Southern Command's JIATF-South. JIATF-South is the key interdiction command and control facility with tactical control over interagency detection and monitoring forces. EPIC collects intelligence to support law enforcement information collected at JIATF-South; together this law enforcement information is fused with foreign intelligence to guide ongoing interdiction operations. This collaboration has been a key factor in the record transit zone drug seizures of the past several years. Since the implementation of *Operation Panama Express*, 443.5 metric tons of cocaine have been seized/scuttled and 1,272 individuals have been arrested. At the end of FY 2006, these combined operations have resulted in total seizures of 512.8 metric tons of cocaine.

The Administration is now attempting to improve intelligence coordination and support of counterdrug operations in the U.S. arrival zone. To enhance border intelligence, CBP and DEA are sharing border crossing and violator vehicle data relative to drug and currency smuggling at an unprecedented level. This change has revealed that approximately 300 vehicles of interest to ICE, DEA, and CBP are crossing our borders on a daily basis.

The counterdrug intelligence structure is evolving further along our Nation's borders to better meet the changing drug threat while applying lessons learned from our interdiction experience. To be successful, law enforcement and border agencies must develop intelligence structures and processes to extract information from open case files, disseminate this intelligence, and fuse it with other national data. The resulting fused intelligence should be used to drive counterdrug detection and monitoring, law enforcement, and interdiction operations.

Such exacting systemic requirements can only be met by establishing intelligence structures and protocols for the rapid sharing of critical information and the establishment of specialized interagency intelligence centers where this information can be integrated, analyzed, and further disseminated. Ongoing initiatives, described in the textbox below, will substantially improve our intelligence structure nationally, at our borders, and internationally.

Agencies are not only in the process of substantially improving their ability to collect, share, and use intelligence information, but are also working to expand their ability to marshal both intelligence and operational data to evaluate the effectiveness of drug enforcement initiatives by region. As part of this broader effort, DEA is developing the Significant Investigation Impact

Measurement System (SIIMS) and DrugSTAR. SIIMS has been used to assess such major investigations as *Operation Candy Box, Operation Cookie Dough,* and *Operation All-Inclusive.* DrugSTAR seeks to employ real-time statistical

SUCCESS IN THE TRANSIT ZONE—THE USS GETTYSBURG MAKES HER MARK

During a 6-month period beginning in late 2005, the USS Gettysburg, with a U.S. Navy helicopter detachment and a U.S. Coast Guard Law Enforcement Detachment (LEDET), severely impacted trafficker operations in the deep Eastern Pacific Ocean and the Caribbean Sea. Patrolling an area exceeding the entire width of the United States, this formidable mix of counterdrug assets, with U.S. interagency and partner nation support, disrupted the movement of more than 28 metric tons of cocaine and arrested 42 drug traffickers.

The hunt began in early October 2005. After receiving intelligence from Joint Interagency Task Force South (JIATF-South) and EPIC, a USS Gettysburg helicopter disrupted a drug trafficking speedboat operation near Honduran waters, where the traffickers rushed the boat ashore and fled into the countryside.

When a U.S. Customs and Border Protection P-3 maritime patrol aircraft located three suspect fishing vessels 1,100 miles from the nearest shoreline, JIATF-South directed the Gettysburg to move in. Once on scene, the U.S. Coast Guard LEDET boarded one of the vessels and seized 244 bales of contraband, resulting in the seizure of more than 9 metric tons (20,470 lbs.) of cocaine and the arrest of 7 drug traffickers.

Less than a week later, and more than 1,300 miles from the previous interdiction, the Gettysburg detected a go-fast operating well off the coast of Panama and U.S. maritime patrol aircraft were diverted to assist in tracking it down. A maritime patrol aircraft caught the suspect dumping contraband overboard and quickly guided the Gettysburg into position for the intercept. The Gettysburg recovered 48 bales (1.5 metric tons) of illicit drugs and detained another 4 suspects.

In late February 2006, maritime patrol aircraft cued by fused intelligence detected a suspect fishing vessel and a go-fast operating almost 1,000 miles west of the Galapagos Islands. The now-seasoned Gettysburg team intercepted the fishing vessel and the go-fast, adding to their seizure tally another 211 bales (5 metric tons) of contraband and detention of 8 drug traffickers.

The highly successful Gettysburg deployment highlights the importance of synchronized interagency action and the rapid fusion and dissemination of actionable intelligence in effectively detecting, interdicting, and apprehending drug smugglers on the high seas. Throughout the duration of her 6-month deployment, the USS Gettysburg repeatedly proved that with the right combination of end game capability, intelligence, and maritime patrol aircraft support, impressive interdiction successes can be achieved in the transit zone.

ENHANCED COUNTERDRUG INTELLIGENCE PROGRAMS

DEA's El Paso Intelligence Center

The DEA's El Paso Intelligence Center (EPIC) monitors the movement of drugs, weapons, and currency, and is dedicated to post-seizure analysis and the establishment of links between recent border law enforcement actions and ongoing investigations. This DEA-led multiagency intelligence center also coordinates training for State and local officers in the methods of highway drug and drug currency interdiction. As part of a revitalization effort, additional interagency staff has been added and EPIC's connectivity with State and local governments has been enhanced through its new Open Portal and National Seizure System, which also allows access to the Clandestine Laboratory Seizure System.

DHS Intelligence Integration

The Department of Homeland Security (DHS) is working to establish an intelligence organization that ensures integrated and coordinated departmentwide intelligence support. Key DHS intelligence initiatives include a Border Security Intelligence Campaign Plan that will provide coordinated intelligence collection, analysis, and dissemination; a National Border Intelligence Center concept to support all DHS missions; and CBP intelligence units to support field operations. DHS also has deployed a Homeland Intelligence Support Team to EPIC to develop a concept of operations for improving DHS intelligence support to border law enforcement across all threats.

Drug Terror Nexus Division

The Department of Homeland Security's Office of Counternarcotics Enforcement (CNE), through its Drug Terror Nexus Division, has been tasked with tracking and severing connections between illegal drug trafficking and terrorism. CNE works within the Joint Terrorism Task Force construct and brings together the collective knowledge of DHS's Office of Intelligence & Analysis and other components of DHS with information from the entire interagency to more clearly identify the links between drug trafficking and terrorism. CNE, along with the National Drug Intelligence Center, will assist in providing intelligence overviews and focused assessments on links between drugs and terrorism for specific regions, including the Southwest Border.

HIDTA Intelligence Centers

The National Guard Bureau is establishing a network of analysts on the Southwest Border as part of a larger project that has already linked 15 of the 32 HIDTA intelligence centers. The National Guard analysts, working out of the HIDTA intelligence centers are linked together via a classified Department of Defense communication system that provides a secure means to disseminate up-to-date intelligence and information. This intelligence network leverages military, law enforcement, and intelligence resources to provide greater interagency and State and local coordination, collaboration, and cooperation in counterdrug operations.

OCDETF Fusion Center

The OCDETF Fusion Center gathers, stores, and analyzes all-source drug and related financial investigative information and intelligence to support coordinated, multijurisdictional investigations focused on the disruption and dismantlement of the most significant drug trafficking and money laundering enterprises. The Fusion Center's "Compass System" is now being used by agents and analysts to develop leads and intelligence products for the field. To date, more than 640 analytical products have been produced that support a wide array of investigations targeting the highest levels of the transnational drug trade and their supporting financial infrastructure.

---

data to develop effective enforcement strategies and assess performance in a manner somewhat similar to that of the New York Police Department's CompStat program. Drug traffickers are constantly adjusting their tactics: the only way to stay ahead of them is to continuously improve U.S. intelligence capabilities and understand the impact our operations have on their illicit enterprise.

Evolution in Afghanistan's Drug Fight

Afghanistan continues to be a pivotal battleground in the Global War on Terror, a linchpin in our global struggle to preserve and expand democracy, and the key to reducing the global supply of illicit opiates. Efforts to fight drug trafficking in Afghanistan, combined with campaigns to counter terrorist elements and to consolidate democracy, are central to our Nation's *National Security Strategy.*

Although the Afghan people, supported by the United States and the international community, have made substantial progress in denying international terrorist elements the ability to operate in Afghanistan and establishing a legitimate, democratic government, many challenges remain. After a significant drop in 2005, opium poppy cultivation has rebounded and increased significantly in some areas of the country. The problem of narcotics production and trafficking may present the single greatest challenge to Afghanistan's future stability. The ultimate goal of the counternarcotics mission in Afghanistan is to eliminate the country's narco-economy while developing the legitimate economy and denying drug trafficking organizations the nearly $2.6 billion generated annually from this illicit trade.

Although the opium trade poses a threat to all of Afghanistan, the actual cultivation of opium poppy is largely concentrated in a few core provinces.

After the fall of the Taliban, the United Kingdom coordinated international efforts to build the capacity of the Afghan government to combat the narcotics cultivation and trafficking problem that the country has long faced. In 2004, the U.S. Government implemented a comprehensive five-pillar strategy, in cooperation with the British, to support Afghan government efforts to eliminate narcotics production and trafficking in the country. The five pillars include public information, alternative livelihoods programs, poppy elimination and eradication, interdiction, and law enforcement and justice reform.

The five-pillar counternarcotics strategy has made headway in every pillar, including, for the first time, the eradication pillar. Ultimate success will require consistent progress across all pillars. The U.S. Government is working to strengthen the political will of the government of Afghanistan across the board. The Department of State is working to improve Afghan elimination and eradication capacity by supporting provincial governors and improving the capacity of the Counternarcotics Ministry's eradication force. DEA, Department of Justice, Department of Defense, and Department of State programs are building the capacity of the counternarcotics police, border management forces, and the Afghan court system. The international community must also continue to pursue opportunities for cooperation in areas such as trade, border management, and regional infrastructure integration, which can help suppress the drug trade and promote the sustainable economic development that will lead to broader counternarcotics success in Afghanistan.

As part of its poppy elimination and eradication pillar, the United States has worked with the governments of the United Kingdom and Afghanistan to develop a Good Performer's Fund (GPF) for 2007 to provide incentives to provinces that reduce poppy cultivation and which have been and remain free of poppy cultivation. The goal of the fund is to encourage provincial and district administrations to reduce plantings and eradicate poppies while holding leadership accountable for their antidrug performance. A three-pronged approach has been developed to target strategic locations in Afghanistan. Specifically, the fund will be used to:

- Increase the number of poppy-free provinces from 6 to 14.
- Sustain poppy reduction in five successful provinces by setting specific targets.
- Reduce, through dissuasion and eradication, poppy production by at least 25 percent in Helmand Province.

Working in the law enforcement and interdiction pillars, DEA has taken on the mission to help the government of Afghanistan to target the command and control of the largest drug organizations in Afghanistan. DEA has done so by building Afghan institutions and by acting against Afghan narcotics trafficking networks directly. DEA operations in Afghanistan are an extension of *Operation Containment*, a DEA-led international effort that involves 19 countries and seeks to choke the flow of drugs and precursor chemicals into and out of Afghanistan. DEA's Afghanistan Foreign-deployed Advisory Support Teams (FAST) in Afghanistan have rapidly developed Afghan interdiction units and have improved the capacity of the Afghan Counternarcotics Police. At the same time DEA teams in Afghanistan have identified narcotics traffickers involved in targeting U.S. forces with improvised explosive devices. By providing critical information obtained from DEA human intelligence sources to U.S. Special Forces Teams, DEA has helped to protect the lives of our service members and our coalition partners.

The experience gained from comprehensive counternarcotics programs in other countries demonstrates that eliminating illicit crop cultivation is a long process that requires continued perseverance and dedication. The five pillar strategy in support of the Government of Afghanistan remains the best approach, but greater intensification of current initiatives and long-term resolve is needed. In doing so, the United States will refine its programs in each pillar based on lessons learned over the past year. In 2007, the United States will increasingly reap the benefits of past investments in the law enforcement and interdiction arena: the increasingly capable Afghan interdiction units, the counternarcotics courts and associated prosecutorial task force, and the greater understanding DEA has developed of Afghanistan's narcotics networks resulting from arrests, prosecutions, and convictions of senior traffickers operating in Afghanistan.

Cathy Inouye

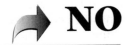

The DEA, CIA, DoD, & Narcotrafficking

The U.S. Military and the Drug Enforcement Administration (DEA) are at it again, this time in Guatemala. The State Department's recently released 2003 International Narcotics Control Strategy Report states that Guatemala has become "the preferred Central American staging point for cocaine shipments northwards to Mexico and the United States." That Guatemala is a major transport route for illegal drugs is nothing new and neither is the DEA's presence here. However, what is new and troubling is the U.S. government's recent overtures of military aid towards Guatemala and the reimplementation of Plan Mayan Jaguar, a joint DEA-Department of Defense project that sets no limit on the number of U.S. military and DEA personnel that could be deployed in Guatemala on joint anti-narcotrafficking operations. Add to this the familiar irony that many of the drug kingpins in the country benefited from previous trainings by either the DEA or the CIA and all the pieces are in place for more chaos and disaster in this latest chapter in the war on drugs.

Less than two years ago, Plan Mayan Jaguar was put on ice due to what the State Department termed "corruption in Guatemala's special counternarcotics force, within the National Civil Police and . . . threats against human rights workers." A month later, Otto Reich, assistant secretary of state for Latin American Affairs, further lambasted the government of Guatemala, pointedly stating, "Retired military officials, linked to violent organized crime, have significant influence within the armed forces, the police, the Executive powers, and the Judiciary." These criticisms are all the more pointed, given that Otto Reich, who directed the State Departments Office for Public Diplomacy during the height of the Iran-contra scandal, is no liberal-leaning diplomat. Reich also cited a report by Minugua, the United Nations presence in Guatemala, that referred to "growing indications" of links between the police, the Public Ministry, military intelligence, and clandestine groups that "operate with impunity" in the country.

Guatemalan human rights organizations and international analysts believe that these clandestine groups work at the behest of a hidden power structure, made up of former military, business leaders, drug tycoons, and politicians. According to a report by the Washington Office on Latin Affairs, this power structure uses the appearance of democracy within Guatemala as a façade behind which to order the intimidation and occasional execution of journalists,

From *Z Magazine*, July/August 2004, pp. 49–53. Copyright © 2004 by Institute for Social & Cultural Communication. Reprinted by permission.

activists, and other members of civil society. Amnesty International put it best when they referred to Guatemala as a Corporate Mafia State. Terrorizing activists and buying the judiciary accomplishes their goal of total impunity and allows this group of people to make a fortune while, according to the United Nations, over 80 percent of the population lives in poverty.

What role does the DEA and the U.S. military have to play in this debacle? During the 1980s, the U.S. military and the CIA played an active support role in Guatemala's transition from military to civilian rule. This transition was orchestrated by the Guatemalan military seeking to maintain power behind the scenes while creating a sense of legitimacy for the Guatemalan government through the appearance of democracy. The Guatemalan military was aided in this project by U.S. agencies whose main objective was not to do anything about the Guatemalan military's continuing human rights abuses, but rather to "professionalize" the force. This idea of creating an efficient, though not necessarily just, military apparatus and later police force, was taken up by the DEA in its attempts to control the flow of drugs through the country. This desire for efficiency led the DEA, the CIA, and the DoD to collaborate with the country's military intelligence, a move that proved to be the equivalent of striking a deal with the devil. The criminal element in the country's military intelligence—a Guatemalan institution that has excelled in the art of forced disappearance, torture, and assassination—used the support of these U.S. agencies to their own benefit, becoming heads of narcotrafficking cartels and key players in the hidden network that is the real power in Guatemala.

This power dynamic had become so entrenched and the government's relationship with narcotrafficking so obvious that at the beginning of 2003, the U.S. government decertified Guatemala as a country active in the fight against drug trafficking. Plan Mayan Jaguar appeared to be suspended indefinitely and even the continuation of a type of military aid known as Expanded IMET seemed to be in jeopardy. Guatemalan human rights activists cheered the move as a condemnation of the country's rampant corruption and deteriorating human rights situation. But the decertification lasted less than a year. By September 2003, Plan Mayan Jaguar was back on track. By February 2004, the Guatemalan Congress broadened the mandate of Plan Mayan Jaguar to allow more U.S. troops in Guatemala to conduct joint counternarcotraffic patrols with Guatemalan officials, a move that was opposed by some Guatemalan politicians who see the plan as a threat to Guatemalan sovereignty.

So what changed in Guatemala to drastically alter the U.S. government's official stance? Not much. Sure, there was an election that replaced pro-military President Portillo with pro-business President Berger. But this change is in many ways cosmetic, as the behind-the-scenes power structure in Guatemala remains in place. Also, Guatemala's re-certification and the re-implementation of Plan Mayan Jaguar happened before the Portillo regime left office. The explanation lies in Guatemala's strategic position in the larger war on drugs.

Plan Mayan Jaguar fits in the strategy of Operation Central Skies. Coupled with Plan Colombia, a billion dollar program designed to stop drug production "at the source" (i.e., in the South American Andes region), Operation Central Skies, with a smaller, though still significant, operating budget, is an attempt to stop the inflow of these same South American drugs through Central America, Mexico, and on into the United States. Operation Central Skies, administered by the U.S. Department of Defense, began in 1998 as a means to provide military aid, primarily in the form of helicopters and personnel, to various Central American governments for use in anti-narcotrafficking operations. Guatemala has participated in Operation Central Skies "deployments," as have security forces from Costa Rica, Belize, El Salvador, and Honduras. Several officers have been trained under the auspices of Operation Central Skies, many in the School of the Americas.

Guatemalan security forces have been denied full admission to the School of the Americas due to their atrocious human rights records and indices of corruption. This is highly ironic, as, during the Cold War, administrators of the School of the Americas trained the Guatemalan military intelligence in the polarizing "us-against-them" mind-set that served as a justification for Guatemala's notorious record of human rights abuse. However, Guatemalans can still attend partial U.S. military training through a program called Expanded International Military Education and Training program (E-IMET). Officials at the U.S. Department of Defense justifiy their actions by saying that these training courses will create a more professional military, thus strengthening Guatemala's democracy. This claim is doubtful.

The CIA was involved in attempts in the late 1980s and early 1990s to "professionalize" the military intelligence apparatus, which is believed to be responsible for the majority of human rights abuses throughout the civil war and up to the present day. CIA support enabled Guatemala to construct a new military intelligence academy in the capital and provide intelligence gathering technology to intelligence services. The goal of these attempts at professionalization was not to confront the atrocious human rights abuses and criminal mentality possessed by the military intelligence services, but to increase their efficiency. This was a dangerous policy, as, even at that time, Guatemalan Minister of Defense Gramajo acknowledged that the intelligence services were "out of control," operating with their own mandate often against the wishes of the military hierarchy or the civilian government.

Since that time, the situation has only grown worse, as key players in the intelligence services have allegedly become the heads of organized crime. One example is retired General Luis Francisco Ortega Menaldo, who has been described as "the most powerful man in Guatemala." Ortega Menaldo had an illustrious history in military intelligence during the Lucas regime in Guatemala (1978–1982). Working in a military intelligence office within the Ministry of Public Finance, Ortega Menaldo was responsible for detecting suspicious shipments likely meant for the left-wing guerrillas. In this capacity he allegedly held shipment containers hostage at the borders, forcing the owners to pay an informal "tax" to release their goods. By the time he was appointed as head of the elite military intelligence unit in the country, the Estado Mayor Presidencial (EMP) in 1991, he was already involved in narcotics trafficking and was in the center of a highly evolved criminal network. At this point in his career, he came into contact with the DEA, which was working closely with military intelligence officials to coordinate anti-narcotrafficking operations. According to Jose Reubén Zamora, a Guatemalan journalist, Ortega Menaldo and his associates were able to use this contact to their own benefit, expanding their criminal network with impunity.

Ortega Menaldo retired in 1996, when a close colleague of his, Alfredo Moreno Molina, long suspected of being involved in drug trafficking, was arrested for tax fraud, falsification of documents, and illicit enrichment. Ortega Menaldo was himself investigated for possible links to organized crime two weeks after the United States government suspended his visa in 2002 on the grounds of his suspected links to narcotics trafficking. Also under investigation for involvement in narcotics trafficking was retired Colonel Jacobo Esdras Salán Sanchez, another member of Guatemala's military intelligence and a graduate of the School of the Americas. Salán Sanchez also worked closely with the DEA, a relationship that ended badly when the DEA accused him of stealing confiscated drugs. Despite their now rocky relationship with the U.S. government, Ortega Menaldo and Salán Sanchez apparently continue to profit from their one-time patrons, the CIA and DEA. Guatemalan media reports speculate that much of the fancy gadgetry the CIA provided the Guatemalan military intelligence in the early 1990s has been used by Ortega Menaldo and his colleagues to spy on rival cartels and intimidate the judges and prosecutors who were charged with bringing them to justice.

Given the corrupt nature of the Guatemalan judiciary system, Moreno Molino, Salán Sanchez, and Ortega Menaldo have been cleared of any wrong doing. Moreno Molino was absolved by Judge Ruiz Wong of the Tenth Court of Appeals, who had himself been implicated in Moreno Molino's criminal network. The investigation of Ortega Menaldo was called a "clown show" by Iduvina Hernandez of the Guatemalan NGO SEDEM. She stated, "This trial seems like a show that will only put at risk whatever judge seeks to follow through on the case." After a year of haphazard investigation, during which the chief prosecutor was shot at by unknown assailants, Ortega Menaldo was also cleared of any links to organized crime. By the mid-1990s, the DEA must have realized that using Guatemala's military intelligence services to uphold the law was impossible. The DEA shifted its focus to developing an anti-narcotics squad within the National Civil Police. In a fact sheet prepared by the U.S. Embassy in Guatemala, the DEA is said to be training and financing Guatemala's anti-narcotics programs. The DEA "provided the impetus for the establishment of the elite counternarcotics force, the Department of Antinarcotics Operations (DOAN). Today (1996), the DOAN has various specialized counternarcotics units that are equipped and trained" by the DEA. Unfortunately, though not surprisingly, the DOAN had to be completely disbanded in 2002 due to rampant corruption and cooperation with the drug cartels they were supposed to be investigating.

Part of the blame for the continued miscalculation of the DEA, in concert with the DoD and the CIA, is a flawed oversight system and the overt optimistic, often misleading reports that these organizations make to themselves. In the 1999 International Narcotics Control Strategy Report, the State Department commends the government of Guatemala for "working, with USG (United States Government) assistance to develop effective integrated law enforcement and counternarcotics training programs to improve the quality of this small elite force (the DOAN)." The 2003 report skips over the complete failure of the DOAN and credits the formation of the Antinarcotics Information and Analysis Service (SAIS) as one of the greatest advances in the Guatemalan war on drugs. The report overlooks the fact that the SAIS is beset by the exact same corruption and abuse of authority problems as its predecessor. One of Guatemala's national newspapers, *Prensa Libre*, reports that in its one year of existence, the SAIA has been accused of torture, illegal detentions, robbery of drugs, and assassination.

The State Department isn't the only federal department analyzing Central America through rose-tinted glasses. In his 2000 testimony before the House Appropriations Committee, James Bodner, principal deputy undersecretary of defense for policy, makes the extraordinary claim that full IMET funding should be extended to Guatemala because of the "Guatemalan military's vigorous efforts to comply with the Peace Accords" and the "strong support" President Portillo had demonstrated for "respecting human rights." There aren't enough words in the English language to convey the utter falseness of these two claims. The Peace Accords were signed in 1996 between representatives of the Guatemalan government and leftist guerrilla groups. They were a comprehensive agreement outlining plans for everything from civilian control of the military to land reform to indigenous language rights. The Peace Accords remain unimplemented and human rights activists, international observers, and even representatives of the State Department lay the blame with certain members of the Guatemalan military. As for Bodner's analysis of the Portillo regime, perhaps he can be forgiven, since at the time of his testimony Portillo's government had not yet proven itself to be the most corrupt in the modern history of Guatemala, sponsoring a wave of political violence that would rip through the country in 2002 and 2003.

Despite these destructively optimistic reviews of the political reality in Guatemala, the United States does possess the correct intelligence on the area. In an interview with the Guatemalan press in 2002, Stephen MacFarland, business attaché to the U.S. Embassy in Guatemala, stated, "We (the United States) are preoccupied by the existence of parallel powers in this country and their links with narcotrafficking . . . we are preoccupied by the influence they can have in this country, especially over certain aspects of the armed forces." But it looks like the State Department analysis has once again fallen on deaf ears, as the Guatemalan government now courts the Bush Jr. administration for an end to the 1977 congressional embargo against military aid. The DEA, CIA, and DoD have been able to side step this prohibition through an accounting loophole, however, the Bush Jr. administration is contemplating renewing official military aid in June of this year. "During his visit to Washington, George W. Bush offered Guatemalan President Óscar Berger helicopters, planes, and communication equipment to modernize Guatemala's army," stated *Prensa Libre*. Berger told the press that "a team of experts will be coming here (at the end of May) to analyze what help the United States can give to modernize the Army."

Presumably, the current administration hopes that this latest round of "modernization" of arguably the most corrupt and brutal armed forces in

Latin America will lead to a victory in the Central American front of the "war on drugs." Likely the team of experts they are sending to Guatemala will gloss over the dense politics of this Central American country, equating a "professional" army with one that follows the rule of law and has an understanding of human rights. This is a dangerous assumption, given that past and continuing actions of the CIA, DEA, and DoD have only succeeded in the creation of an efficient criminal apparatus that masquerades as the forces of law and order. So it looks like we're in for another round of lunacy in the war on drugs. Operation Mayan Jaguar will be in effect for at least the next two years—during which time the DEA can expect to play a part in strengthening the drug network in Guatemala. Seminars on professionalism and a couple of CH-47 Chinook helicopters won't be able to change the economic and political realities that give rise to rampant corruption in Guatemala. Initiatives by U.S. agencies won't be able to tackle the legions of corrupt and underpaid police officers, the manipulative intelligence service that honed its criminal capacities with equipment and training by the CIA or the 80 percent of the population that lives in poverty and could use a few extra dollars by transporting drugs from one end of their country to the other. Even if Operation Central Skies does somehow manage to limit the flow of drugs through Central America, the victory would be questionable. The drugs aren't going to stay in South America. Another "preferred staging point" will be found, possibly a return to transporting cocaine through the Caribbean, as was the case in the 1980s.

Trying to decipher the purposes of all these code named anti-narcotrafficking joint operations has become impossible, especially from the perspective of the host country. But there is something telling about the attitudes of the DoD and the DEA blithely writing their optimistic annual country reports, asking for more money.

The war on drugs is not about drugs, but about self-justification. The more corrupt the security forces are in Guatemala, the more apparent the need to have some U.S. personnel down there, keeping an eye on things. The continuing failures to get the Guatemalan police to stop stealing cocaine from drug busts works fine for the DEA, as long as they get more funding to professionalize the force. Meanwhile, the U.S. military can maintain a presence, protecting any U.S. interests that need protecting. Daniel Lazare's analysis in the *NACLA Report on the Americas* is astute: "The goal (of the drug war) has not been to stamp out drugs per se, but to create a war-time atmosphere of hysteria in which the government would feel justified in using extraordinary measures to counter an extraordinary threat. Rather than eradication, the purpose of the drug war is . . . war itself." Using this analysis, Operation Central Skies makes perfect sense and the people in the DEA and the DoD are doing a fine job.

References

1. U.S. Department of State. *International Narcotics Control Strategy Report, 2003.* Released By the Bureau for International Narcotics and Law Enforcement Affairs. Washington DC. March 2004.
2. Pérez, Sonia D. (2002) Maya Jaguar sin apoyo de EEUU. *Prensa Libre.* September 12, 2002: 5.

3. Alvarado, H. and Jiménez, J. (2002) EE.UU. vincula al Gobierno con crimen organizado. *Siglo Veintiuno*. October 11, 2002: 4–5.

4. Peacock, Susan C. and Beltrán, A. (2003) *Hidden Powers in Post-Conflict Guatemala*. WOLA: Washington.

5. Schirmer, Jennifer. (1999) *Las Intimidades Del Proyecto Político de los Militares en Guatemala*. FLACSO: Guatemala. (Spanish Translation of *A Violence Called Democracy*)

6. Zamora, Jose Ruben. (2002) El Crimen Organizade, el Ejército, y el Futuro de los Guatemaltecos. *El Periodico*. November 12, 2002: 2–4.

7. ibid.

8. Pérez, Sonia D. (2002) Investigarán a Cinco Militares. *Prensa Libre*. October 24 2002: 3.

9. Narcotics Affairs Section—United States Embassy n Guatemala. *Fact Sheet: Counter-Narcotics Programs in Guatemala*. March 27, 1996.

10. U.S. Department of State. *International Narcotics Control Strategy Report, 1999*. Released By the Bureau for International Narcotics and Law Enforcement Affairs. Washington DC. March 2000.

11. U.S. Department of State. *International Narcotics Control Strategy Report, 2003*.

12. Presa Libre Staff. (2003) Saia repite los errores del Doan. *Prensa Libre*. October 24, 2003. p 12.

13. Mr. James Bodner, Principal Deputy Undersecretary of Defense for Policy. Testimony Before the House Appropriations Committee, Foreign Operations Subcommittee. April 6, 2000.

14. Paredes Diaz, Jennyffer. (2002) Fisk pide actuar contra corrupción y narcotráfico. *Prensa Libre*. November 13, 2002: 3.

15. Gonzaléz, Francisco. (2004) EE.UU. Analizará Dar Equipo al Ejecito. *Prensa Libre*. May 5, 2004.

16. Lazare, Daniel. (2001) A Battle Against Reason, Democracy and Drugs: The Drug War Deciphered. *NACLA Report on the Americas 35* (1): 13–17.

POSTSCRIPT

Should the United States Put More Emphasis on Stopping the Importation of Drugs?

The drug trade spawns violence: people die from using drugs or by dealing with people in the drug trade; families are ruined by the effects of drugs on family members; prisons are filled with tens of thousands of people who were and probably still are involved with illegal drugs; and drugs can devastate aspirations and careers. The adverse consequences of drugs can be seen everywhere in society. How should the government determine the best course of action to follow in remedying the negative effects of drugs? Would more people be helped by reducing the availability of drugs, or would more people benefit if they could be persuaded that drugs are harmful to them?

Two paths that are traditionally followed involve reducing either the supply of drugs or the demand for drugs. Four major agencies involved in the fight against drugs in the United States—the Drug Enforcement Administration (DEA), the Federal Bureau of Investigation (FBI), the U.S. Customs Service, and the U.S. Coast Guard—have seized thousands of pounds of marijuana, cocaine, and heroin during the past few years. Drug interdiction appears to be reducing the availability of drugs. But what effect does drug availability have on use? If a particular drug is not available, would other drugs be used in its place? Would the cost of drugs increase if there were a shortage of drugs? If costs increase, would violence due to drugs go up as well?

Annual surveys of 8th-, 10th-, and 12th-grade students indicate that availability is not a major factor in drug use. Throughout the 1980s drug use declined dramatically even though marijuana and cocaine could be easily obtained. According to the surveys, the perceived harm of these drugs, not their availability, is what affects students' drug use. As individuals' perceptions of drugs as harmful increase, usage decreases; as perceptions of harm decrease, usage increases. Generally, availability of drugs is a weak predictor of drug use.

Efforts to prevent drug use may prove fruitless if people have a natural desire to alter their consciousness. In his 1989 book *Intoxication: Life in the Pursuit of Artificial Paradise* (E. P. Dutton), Ronald Siegel contends that the urge to alter consciousness is as universal as the craving for food and sex.

A publication that examines trends in world drug markets is the *World Drug Report* (2006) by the United Nations Office on Drugs and Crime. Another publication that critically views current drug policies is *How Goes the War on Drugs? An Assessment of U.S. Drug Problems and Policy* by Jonathon Caulkins and associates (RAND Drug Policy Research Center, 2005). Articles that examine international efforts to deal with the issue of drugs include

"The New Opium War," by Matthew Quirk (*The Atlantic Monthly*, March 2005), "The Price of Powder" (*The Economist*, November 27, 2004), "U.S. Versus Them: Challenging America's War on Drugs—U.S. Policy," by Susan Taylor Martin (*St. Petersburg Times*, July 29, 2001); "Narcoterrorism as a Threat to International Security," by Stephen Blank (*World and I*, December 2001); and "Addicted to the Drug War," by Kenneth Sharp (*The Chronicle of Higher Education*, October 6, 2000).

ISSUE 3

Are Drinking Age Laws Effective?

YES: Judith G. McMullen, from "Underage Drinking: Does Current Policy Make Sense?" *Lewis & Clark Law Review* (Summer 2006)

NO: U.S. Department of Health & Human Services, from "Underage Drinking: Why Do Adolescents Drink, What Are the Risks, and How Can Underage Drinking Be Prevented?" *Alcohol Alert* (January 2006)

ISSUE SUMMARY

YES: Judith McMullen, a law professor at Marquette University, argues that laws prohibiting underage drinking have been ineffective. Young adults between the ages of 18 and 21 who do not live at home have opportunities to drink alcohol without parental interference. In addition, this same age group has other legal rights, such as the right to marry, drive a car, or join the military. Enforcement of underage drinking laws, says McMullen, is destined for failure.

NO: The United States Department of Health and Human Services maintains that underage drinking is fraught with numerous problems ranging from motor vehicle crashes to homicide and suicide. Also, underage drinking is related to unhealthy risk-taking behaviors and poor academic performance. Rather than tolerate underage drinking, more effort should be placed on enforcing underage drinking laws.

Over 90 percent of high school seniors consume alcohol and a significant percentage of those students engage in binge drinking. There is little doubt that many students drink to excess and that many young people drink alcohol irresponsibly. Regardless of the message that many underage drinkers receive, it is unhealthy, unlawful, and potentially dangerous for young people to drink alcohol, especially in excess. The question evolves around the best way to reduce the harms associated with alcohol use. Can young people be taught to consume alcohol so that the health risks and dangerous behaviors are minimized? Or, is it more prudent to simply say don't drink?

61

One important question is whether or not young people will respond to a message of responsible alcohol consumption. Because it is a recognized fact that the vast majority of people under age 21 drink alcohol, simply telling young people to not drink does not stop that behavior. However, does it make more sense to teach young people how to drink alcohol responsibly so they do not endanger themselves, their friends, or innocent bystanders? On the other hand, should someone under age 21 be taught how to drink responsibly if the very act of drinking alcohol while under age 21 is illegal? One could argue that instructing an underage person to drink responsibly is teaching that person to disregard the law. Is contempt or disregard for the law a good message?

Another relevant question deals with what is meant by "responsible alcohol consumption." One could argue that avoiding drunkenness is being responsible. Other examples of being responsible could entail being in control of oneself while drinking so that one does not engage in reckless behavior. For others, responsible alcohol use means not operating a motor vehicle after any amount of consumption. One could argue that calling a parent or taking a taxi-cab after drinking are examples of being responsible. If the responsible drink-ing message is favored, at what age should this be promoted? Should the responsible message be targeted to 14-year-olds, 16-year-olds, or 18-year-olds?

Whether or not a responsible drinking message is appropriate depends on one's goal for those individuals who are under age 21. If the goal is to prohibit all alcohol consumption for those under age 21, then the only acceptable mes-sage is do not drink. Yet, if the goal is to reduce the harm associated with underage drinking, then a message of responsibility may be more appropriate. It is also possible to provide the message that anyone under age 21 should not drink, but that underage drinkers should be responsible if they drink.

In 2007, the United States surgeon general published a paper with sugges-tions to reduce underage drinking. In this paper, the surgeon general outlined numerous goals. One goal focused on societal changes that would reduce underage drinking. Another goal attempted to get parents, caregivers, schools, communities, and all social systems to work together to address this problem. The surgeon general recommended improving surveillance of underage drinking as well as additional research on adolescent alcohol use.

In the following selections, Judith McMullen believes that our message of abstinence is ineffective as well as inconsistent with other behaviors that are allowed for individuals under age 21. The report from the U.S. Department of Health and Human Services advocates that underage drinking be prevented due to the damage it causes to the developing adolescent: intellectually, physically, and emotionally.

YES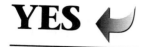

Judith G. McMullen

Underage Drinking: Does Current Policy Make Sense?

This Article examines the history of laws and policies regulating consumption of alcoholic beverages by young people in the United States, and examines youth drinking patterns that have emerged over time. Currently, all 50 states have a minimum drinking age of 21. Various rationales are offered for the 21 drinking age, such as the claim that earlier drinking hinders cognitive functions and the claim that earlier drinking increases the lifetime risk of becoming an alcoholic. While there is sufficient evidence to support the claim that it would be better for adolescents and young adults if they did not drink prior to age 21, research shows that vast numbers of underage persons consume alcoholic beverages, often in large quantities. The Article discusses the question of why underage drinking laws have not been able to effectively stop underage drinking.

Normally, discussions of underage drinking focus on persons under age 21 as one group. This Article breaks underage drinkers into two groups: minors (drinkers under the age of 18) and young adults (drinkers between the ages of 18 and 21). The Article goes on to separately analyze the two groups' drinking patterns and reasons for drinking. The Article concludes that prohibitions on drinking by minors could be made more effective because restrictions on activities by minors are expected and normally honored by parents, law, and society. The Article also concludes, however, that the enforcement of a drinking prohibition for young adults between the ages of 18 and 21 is doomed to remain largely ineffective because the drinking ban is wholly inconsistent with other legal policies aimed at that age group. The Article discusses three areas (health care decisions, educational decisions, and smoking) where persons over the age of 18 have virtually unfettered personal discretion, and applies the reasoning of those situations to the decision about whether to consume alcoholic beverages. The Article also compares the total drinking ban for young adults with the graduated privilege policies applied to drivers' licensing. The Article concludes that the total prohibition of alcohol consumption for young adults is inconsistent with other policies affecting young adults, and this inconsistency, coupled with harms that may come from the 21 drinking age, make the current policies ineffective and ill-advised for young adults between the age of 18 and 21.

From *Lewis and Clark Law Review*, Summer 2006. Copyright © 2006 by Judith G. McMullen. Reprinted by permission.

Introduction

On the surface, youth alcohol policy is simple and straightforward: the legal age for alcohol consumption is 21 in all states, and drinking before then is illegal. As it happens, though, these laws are not terribly effective. Huge numbers of youngsters age 12 and up (and probably younger) consume alcoholic beverages, despite the law.[1] The numbers of underage drinkers skyrocket once kids are over 18, and college campuses are known hotbeds of underage consumption.[2] According to researchers, large numbers of young people drink alcohol, many heavily, before they attain the legal drinking age.[3]

This Article addresses the question of why underage drinking laws have not been able to effectively stop underage drinking. It examines some of the classic reasons: ambivalence among adults as to the law, feelings of entitlement by young people, and glorification of alcohol consumption by society as a whole. The Article argues that alcohol consumption by adolescents under the age of 18 could be reduced by stricter and more consistent enforcement. However, the Article goes on to conclude that the prohibition of alcohol consumption cannot ever be effective for the 18 to 21 year old cohort, because it is wholly inconsistent with other legal policies aimed at that age group. Further, the Article argues that outlawing alcohol consumption for young adults[4] may cause harm because the policy may encourage unhealthy alcohol consumption patterns in young adults, and it carries the risk of engendering a lack of respect for the law in general.

Underage drinking laws need to be assessed in two parts. One policy is the prohibition of alcohol consumption for minors, i.e. persons under the age of 18. The second policy is prohibition of alcohol consumption for persons between the ages of 18 and 21. While similar justifications are offered for the restrictions on each of these groups, in fact, as we shall see, there are very different factors at play in terms of parental control, societal expectations, and overall consistency with other situations where the law asserts control over individual behaviors. Most articles on youth alcohol policy address whether the current policy is a good thing. This Article concedes that it might indeed be a good thing if persons under age 21 abstained from alcohol. However, the Article goes on to discuss how the youth alcohol policy fits—or does not fit—into the patchwork of laws and policies concerning state intervention into the lives of parents and their children.

This Article argues that banning alcohol consumption for the under-18 crowd is consistent with other child protective policies advanced by state laws, largely because the law does not accord many rights of self-determination to minors. Thus, the ban could be reasonably effective if enforcement were increased—perhaps with such measures as holding parents and other adults accountable for behaviors that facilitate illegal underage drinking. However, the Article also concludes that current alcohol policy for persons over age 18 is *not* consistent with analogous policies for persons who are legally adults: e.g., the right to refuse medical treatment or the right to smoke cigarettes. In fact, the alcohol laws governing young adults seem to substitute state policies for both parental judgment and the young person's self-determination on this single issue. Thus, the Article concludes that the policy cannot ever be widely effective with this group, and creates as many problems as it solves. This is despite the inarguable fact that alcohol consumption may well be harmful to persons in this disputed age group.

First, the Article gives an overview of drinking policies in the United States, from colonial times to the present.[5] Second, the Article discusses the current laws and the justifications offered for them.[6] Next, the Article examines the effectiveness of the laws and the drinking patterns among younger underage youths (up to age 18),[7] and older underage youths (ages 18 to 21).[8] The Article compares youth drinking policies with other policies affecting young adults and argues that the practical and philosophical differences between the drinking ban for 18 to 21 year-olds and other legal policies affecting that age group make the alcohol ban for young adults largely unenforceable.[9] The Article also discusses problems arguably caused by the prohibition of alcohol use by young adults and examines whether the drinking age law might have significant value despite its unenforceability.[10] Finally, the Article suggests that alcohol use by 18 to 21 year olds might be more appropriately addressed in a manner analogous to drivers' licensing policies for young drivers: by providing a combination of alcohol education and supervision to young adults who choose to drink.

Assessing Current Policies and Patterns

A. Structure of Current Laws

Currently, all fifty states have a minimum legal drinking age of 21.[11] Enforcement is aimed at both underage drinkers and their suppliers. Underage drinkers may be penalized with municipal or state citations or drivers' license suspensions.[12] Parents or other individual adults who supply alcohol to underage persons may be held criminally responsible, which might result in assessment of a fine or a jail sentence, although several states do not impose these penalties on parents who are serving alcoholic beverages to their *own* children.[13] Adults who provide alcohol to minors may also be exposed to civil liability in the event of harm caused by the underage drinker.[14] Bar owners or storeowners may be hit with fines or may lose their liquor licenses.[15] Penalties for underage driving while under the influence are effectively more severe for young adults than for adults over the age of 21, because the offense is typically committed if the young driver has *any* detectable alcohol in her blood.[16]

B. Policy Objectives

There are two stated justifications for enforcing a minimum drinking age: protection of young people, and protection of society. Numerous studies and statistics are offered to support each justification.

The first argument, that a 21 drinking age protects young people from harm, is supported by recent research that suggests alcohol can have an especially detrimental effect on the developing brain. The American Medical Association released a report in 2002 stating that drinking by adolescents and young adults could result in long-term brain damage, including diminishment of memory, reasoning, and learning abilities.[17] Experts think that memory and learning impairment is worse in adolescents, who may experience adverse effects after consuming only half as much alcohol as adults.[18] Human research at the University of Pittsburgh showed that heavy-drinking girls between the ages of 14 and 21 had smaller hippocampi than girls of the same age who were non-drinkers.[19] Admittedly, this research does not prove whether it is the heavy drinking that causes changes in the hippocampus, or the reduced size of the hippocampus that causes the urge to engage in heavy drinking.[20] Moreover, teenage hormonal changes, eating habits, or abuse of other substances like marijuana could also be causes of learning and memory impairment.[21] However, research with rats has shown similar bad effects from alcohol consumption on the rodents' learning and memory, even extending into adulthood.[22]

In addition, some researchers contend that alcohol abuse in the teenage years is more likely to lead to alcohol dependence later in life than if the drinking had begun at a later age. A study released in 1998 by the National Institute of Alcohol Abuse and Alcoholism concluded that "[c]hildren who begin drinking regularly by age 13 are more than four times as likely to become alcoholics as those who delay consuming alcohol until age 21 or older. . . ."[23] The study found that children who started drinking regularly at age 13 faced a 47% lifetime risk of becoming an alcoholic, compared with a 25% risk for youth who began drinking at age 17, and a 10% risk for people who began drinking at age 21.[24] However, it is not clear why some children are prone to such early and heavy drinking and others are not. It may be, for example, that children who begin drinking heavily at age 13 do so because of some biological characteristic that also causes them to have more of a lifetime risk for alcoholism.[25] In other words, rather than the early drinking causing the later alcoholism, it may be a symptom of the existing vulnerability to alcoholism.

It is also claimed that withholding drinking privileges until a later age protects young people by reducing the number of fatal automobile accidents involving teenagers. Indeed, "[t]he National Highway Traffic Safety Administration estimates that since the '70s, the age-21 policy has saved 20,970 teenage lives from serious car crashes alone."[26] For example, "[i]n 1982, a study by the National Highway Traffic Safety Administration found that 5,380 persons between the ages of 15 and 20 had died in drunken driving accidents that year. . . . [By 1995] the number had been reduced to 2,206 nationwide. . . ."[27] However, drunk driving enforcement in general has been taken more seriously since the drinking age was changed, and this might also account for some of the improvement.[28]

The second argument, that a 21 drinking age protects society from the bad effects of underage drinking, is partly supported by data on traffic fatalities that could be caused by young drunk drivers.[29] In addition, there is another claimed benefit to society in banning underage drinking: the possible reduction of crime perpetrated by persons under age 21. Alcohol has been shown to be a major contributing factor in teen deaths from accidents, homicide, and

suicide, and it has also been shown to increase the chances of juvenile delinquency and crime.[30] Alcohol abuse appears to increase the likelihood that young
people will engage in unprotected sex or acquaintance rape, suicide, and other
violent behavior.[31] Of course, alcohol is a known inhibition-reducer and is implicated in crimes for all age groups.[32] Moreover, both the drinking and other problem behaviors may be caused by the general turmoil of adolescence, which is
characterized by impulsiveness, sensation seeking, and unconventionality.[33]

There is no doubt that a significant number of young people consume
alcohol in violation of the minimum age laws. While state laws outlaw alcohol
purchase and consumption for all persons under age 21, there are in fact two
distinct groups of underage drinkers who present different issues. First of all
are the minors (high school and younger drinkers), and second are the young
adults or college age drinkers.[34]

C. Underage Drinking by Minors

Studies show that a significant minority of high school students consume
alcohol on a regular basis: "According to 2002 Monitoring the Future (MTF)
data, almost half (48.6 percent) of twelfth graders reported recent (within the
past 30 days) alcohol use."[35] Although younger teens report lower incidences
of alcohol use, "NHSDA[36] data indicate that the average age of self-reported
first use of alcohol among individuals of all ages reporting any alcohol use
decreased from 17.6 years to 15.9 years between 1965 and 1999."[37] Moreover,
underage drinkers are more likely than adults to be heavy drinkers.[38]

Even for those minors who are not regular drinkers, certain rites of passage
such as school dances, proms, and graduation can be the occasion of much
alcoholic excess. A notorious incident that occurred in Scarsdale, New York in
2002 provides an excellent example of the dynamics. In the fall of 2002, The
New York Times reported that the prestigious Scarsdale High School home-
coming dance and pre-dance parties included widespread binge drinking
"which left scores of students falling-down drunk, 27 with three-day school
suspensions and five hospitalized with acute alcohol poisoning. . . ."[39] When
the principal arrived at the dance shortly after its 8 pm start, he "found perhaps
a third of the 600 students there in a stupor from drinking screwdrivers they
had mixed at various homes. They had used vodka sneaked from their
parents['] liquor cabinets and disguised in Poland Spring water bottles."[40]

While major high school events have precipitated underage drinking for
generations, the New York Times cited differences noted by education and
mental health experts. First, "[t]he drinking starts younger. . . . The quantity
and speed of alcohol consumption are dangerously high and the goal seems to
be total oblivion."[41] Second, certain psychological factors are different: baby
boomer parents are less likely to be seen as authority figures by their children,
and the children in upscale communities are in a super-competitive atmosphere
with "enormous pressure to succeed."[42] If they don't meet parental expectations, they may drown their sorrows in drugs or alcohol. Finally, "[e]ducators
and mental health professionals also say that affluence breeds a sense of entitlement in children. 'They're told from the time they're young that they're the

prize of the community. . . . The conclusion an adolescent may draw is: "I'm special. I get to do what I want."'"[43]

The Scarsdale incident also illustrates another phenomenon that has become common: placing much of the blame for underage drinking on adults, especially parents. According to Geraldine Greene, executive director of the Scarsdale Family Counseling Service, underage drinking is "an adult failure. In every case, an adult has let a child down. Somewhere along the way they haven't exercised due care."[44] Although Greene's comments could be directed at a large variety of adults, including parents, vendors, and teachers, she is most critical of affluent parents who she feels do not take enough time to raise their teenagers properly.[45] Adolescent psychologist Dr. Alan Tepp said that while parents hold their adolescents to ever-higher achievement standards, "at the same time, we're putting less restraint on them, watching them less. We push them, and then allow them out."[46]

Studies provide some support for these opinions. Large amounts of time free from adult supervision, including after-school time without parent contact, has been related to higher alcohol consumption among teens.[47] "'Hanging out' with friends in unstructured, unsupervised contexts is generally related to negative outcomes, while spending time with others in adult-sanctioned, structured contexts is generally related to positive outcomes."[48]

There is, of course, a more direct way in which parents can be responsible for youth drinking: they may provide the liquor consumed by high school aged children. Some parents take the position that kids will drink anyway, and if the parents allow supervised drinking at home parties, this will reduce more dangerous binge drinking or drinking in cars, followed by driving while intoxicated.[49] For example, a 17-year-old graduate of Scarsdale High School said, "I know one of my friend's parents said, 'If you're staying in the house, then I don't have a problem with you drinking.' That's kind of promoting it. . . ."[50] Indeed, "having parents who sanction alcohol use (even in 'controlled' settings) is related to heavier drinking among adolescents."[51] A Westchester County District Attorney commented that the "number of kids getting drunk at home is on the increase, as is the frequency of alcohol being provided by an adult or older sibling. . . ."[52]

Herein lies part of the enforcement problem: some parents think drinking is a normal rite of passage for teenagers; others believe in zero-tolerance. A Scarsdale police detective, firmly in the latter camp, said, "Parents should send a clear message to their kids that this behavior will not be condoned. . . ."[53]

Yet even parents who might be willing to crack down are not always convinced that it will work. A principal in Chappaqua, New York quoted a parent who told him that "setting earlier curfews just makes the kids drink faster."[54] He added that since many parents feel powerless to stop their kids from drinking, they have adopted the view that "until society solves the problem, I want my kids alive."[55]

There are a number of different issues jumbled together here. First, we must consider whether it is reasonable for the state to prevent children under the age of 18 from consuming alcohol. Second, we must address whether we have consensus on this issue in this society. Finally, we must assess the reasonableness of the notion that parents can in large degree control the drinking behavior of their offspring.

Ever since *Prince v. Massachusetts*[56] upheld the state's right to protect a young Jehovah's Witness from the dangers of street preaching, it has been clear that a state can adopt reasonable policies to protect children, even over the heartfelt objections of their parents.[57] Unlike *Prince*, challenges to a state's protective alcohol policy do not rest on First Amendment free exercise claims; at best they depend upon arguments that reasonable parents might exercise their prerogative in favor of allowing their children to engage in moderate social drinking. A state's purposes of preventing traffic accidents, crime, and potential damage to a young imbiber's health or cognitive function would clearly survive any constitutional claim of infringement on parental authority. This is especially true in those few states that allow parents to serve alcohol to their own minor children while those children are in the parent's presence.[58] Even the most inconclusive of the scientific studies cited in Part III.B signals enough risk of harm that a state could reasonably prohibit alcohol consumption by minors.[59]

As to whether we have consensus about whether the absolute ban on consumption is a good thing, the answer is that we clearly do not. While a majority may favor the ban, a significant minority either thinks that it is counterproductive, or simply ineffective. These are the folks that may either look the other way or actually provide alcohol, on the theory that kids will drink anyway, and "I would rather know where they are."[60] In some national surveys, many parents admit to purchasing alcohol for their teenagers, in the hopes of providing a safe place for their kids to drink.[61] Ironically, these parents contribute to the fact that the ban is ineffective, and they make it ineffective not only for their own children, but for other people's children as well.

In fact, the combination of typical adolescent rebellion and readily available alcohol supplied by dissenting or indifferent adults makes it impossible for individual parents to completely control whether or not their children consume alcohol, unless the parents achieve round-the-clock supervision, amounting to lockdown, of their children.[62] Thus, penalizing parents for facilitating consumption, but not holding them accountable for the behavior of sneaky adolescent drinkers, makes good sense.

There are a myriad of situations where parents or the state effectively control situations involving persons under age 18. Parents are held responsible for the support and education of their minor children.[63] The law is generally structured to help parents in these endeavors, and to regulate parents who fall short. Thus, fit parents are generally entitled to custody of their minor children,[64] and deference is given to parental decisions about the incidents of that custody.[65] Laws that regulate minors' activities, such as truancy or curfew laws that may penalize errant children, are widely viewed as reinforcements to judicious parental controls.[66] Parents who stray from societal norms, such as parents who abuse their children or parents who are complicit in the truancy of their children, can be subjected to various penalties.[67]

Statutes and cases have attempted to strike a balance between parental prerogatives, children's rights, and societal interests in regulating minors' activities.[68] Where underage drinking is concerned, parents have an important role in restricting minors' access to alcohol.[69] Due to the fact that most minors live with at least one adult, greater adult consensus on the value of banning alcohol consumption by minors, as well as greater adult compliance with the laws, could combine to significantly reduce alcohol consumption by persons under age 18. Moreover, even if adolescent consumption is not reduced to zero, it could be reduced from current epidemic proportions, and abstinence from underage alcohol consumption could be internalized by minors as an important social norm.

D. Underage Drinking by Young Adults

Regulation of underage drinking becomes more problematic after a young person reaches the age of majority—usually 18—or moves away from home into a dorm or apartment. However imperfect parental supervision may have been before, it becomes nearly impossible at that time. Persons over the age of 18 are legally adults for any purpose *except* consuming alcohol. Even parents of economically dependent college students may not know whether their children are drinking, since schools have no obligation to notify parents when a young person violates underage drinking laws or school rules.[70]

Drinking in the 18 to 21 age group, however, is rampant. Young people in this age group who do not attend college drink less than those that do attend, but they are not teetotalers as a group.[71] And although not every child goes to college, these are the prime college age years for those that do, and college campuses are notorious for widespread alcohol consumption. According to one source, 44% of college students report binge drinking in the past two weeks, and 23% report frequent binge drinking.[72] Apparently, membership in fraternities and sororities greatly increases the likelihood of excessive drinking: a 2001 survey "showed that three-quarters of fraternity or sorority house residents (80 percent and 69 percent, respectively) are binge drinkers," an improvement over the 1993 figure of 83%.[73] Although binge drinking is typically defined as five or more drinks per occasion, the bingeing at many Greek organizations is reportedly far more extreme. One consultant stated:

> Our organization has worked extensively with Greek groups over the past twenty years and has found some chapters to report that more than 70 percent of their members consume thirteen or more drinks per occasion. We frequently hear from other professionals on campuses that fifteen to twenty drinks per occasion, though not the norm, is not uncommon among some groups of students.[74]

Theories abound as to why drinking is so extreme on college campuses. Researchers Wechsler and Wuethrich think one reason is that students "developed a sense of entitlement to alcohol" after the drinking age was lowered to 18 during the 1970s and then re-raised to 21.[75] They also point to the relaxation of dormitory supervision, the increasingly cultivated party images of fraternities and even schools themselves, and the rising importance of college sports as big business, with attendant alcohol industry sponsorships.[76] They also acknowledge alcohol's role in larger society as a factor.[77]

I believe that there is another important reason for widespread drinking among young adults: with the exception of alcohol, parental control over the young person's activities grinds to a halt after age 18, if not before then. Moreover, with the exception of alcohol, and to some extent drivers' licenses, state control of the activities of a person over 18 is no different for the 18 to 21 age group than for an adult of any age. Once a person attains age 18, he or she can legally marry without parental permission, join the military, enter contracts, smoke, make decisions concerning medical care, or drop out of school. These newfound freedoms occur at age 18, despite the fact that the young person may be immature or financially dependent on his parents, and despite the fact that he may have parents who disapprove of his decisions. It is this legal autonomy in other areas, I think, that makes enforcement of a 21 drinking age impossible.

For the sake of discussion, I will compare the 21 drinking age policy with policies aimed at the 18 to 21 age group in the areas of medical decision-making, decisions to forgo education, decisions about smoking, and regulations concerning driving. All of these represent adult privileges that can have serious consequences for the young person, and potentially for others around him. All also represent situations where a mistake in judgment, perhaps due to immaturity, can have dire consequences. Yet, unlike current alcohol policy, the policies in these areas defer to the judgment of the young person, for good or ill. If the main reason for forbidding alcohol consumption for persons under the age of 21 is protection from the adverse physical effects of youth drinking, such as greater likelihood of later alcoholism or greater damage to the brain, then the policy is entirely consistent with other policies for children under the age of 18. It is, however, completely unprecedented compared with other policies for young people in the 18 to 21 age group.

Problems Caused by the Prohibition of Alcohol Use by Young Adults

There are two potential problems that may result from the prohibition of alcohol use by young adults. The first problem is that the impossibility of enforcing the law will engender a lack of respect for the law in general among young adults. The second problem is that, for those who choose to violate the law, the necessity of sneaking around to drink may lead to more dangerous drinking patterns and may preclude access to avenues that might imbue healthier drinking habits.

A. The Difficulty of an Unenforceable Law

Laws that are difficult or impossible to enforce have always been problematic. Of course, no law is one hundred percent enforceable: history is replete with unsolved crimes and unpunished offenders of every sort.[78] However, laws may serve a useful symbolic or deterrent function despite sporadic enforcement. Indeed, "the effectiveness of symbolic laws depends on public affirmation rather than legal enforcement. 'People obey symbolic laws not for fear of legal sanction, but because they are backed by the consensus of society and the force of major social institutions.'"[79] As Lawrence Friedman has pointed out, even laws that are imperfectly enforced may reduce a given behavior by making it more costly: "[P]olicy choices are essentially selections among various techniques and means of encouraging or discouraging behavior, by making that behavior safer, cheaper, and more pleasant; or more expensive, more aversive."[80]

When we examine the 21 drinking age in this context, it can be argued that the current law reduces drinking by young adults and conveys important social values to all young adults, even those who violate the law. Advocates of the 21 drinking age claim that the law has resulted in more college-age students who abstain from alcohol use (and are willing to admit it), which thereby reduces alcohol-related problems of all sorts.[81] Not everyone credits the 21 drinking age with this progress, however. Richard Keeling, a physician and former director of health services at the University of Wisconsin-Madison, believes that enforcement methods such as crackdowns on house parties and increased fines for alcohol-related offenses are more likely reasons for changes in young adult behavior.[82]

The argument that a 21 drinking age conveys important societal values to teenagers and young adults is less persuasive in light of the fact, already discussed,[83] that the drinking ban for young adults does not seem to be backed by a broad consensus of society. As we have seen, many parents and other adults disagree with the law in principle.[84] These adults may view drinking as a rite of passage, or may believe that an earlier drinking age would be conducive to more moderate drinking habits later. Such adults may not only ignore violations of the drinking ban by young adults, but they may enable the young adults to commit the violations by supplying alcohol or hosting drinking parties.[85] In these circumstances, where the social consensus on youth drinking is divided at best, it is harder to claim that a strong moral message is being delivered to underage drinkers.

In addition, alcohol continues to be glorified in sports sponsorships and advertising, making it unclear exactly what social message teenagers and young adults are getting about alcohol. Research has shown that adolescents who are exposed to alcohol advertising are more likely to consume alcohol and to consume it in greater amounts.[86] It is clear that vast numbers of adolescents are in fact exposed to alcohol advertising. Voluntary conduct codes adopted in the late 1990s by the Distilled Spirits Council of the United States suggest that ads should only run in media outlets having no more than 30% of their audience under the age of 21.[87] However, 30% of a broadcast such as a sporting event can be a substantial number of underage viewers.

Sporting events often have alcohol companies as sponsors, such as the sponsorship of NASCAR driver Dale Earnhardt by Budweiser beer and the Busch beer sponsorship of the NASCAR Busch series.[88] Stadiums such as Miller Park in Wisconsin and Coors Field in Colorado associate their corporate sponsors with sports. College sports are no exception, with the NCAA allowing one minute per hour of alcohol ads during broadcast of NCAA events.[89] In a recent report, the Center for Science in the Public Interest argued that because the NCAA has many underage followers (including kids as young as 9 or 10), the NCAA is effectively helping brewers to recruit kids to beer drinking in general, as well as to particular brands of beer.[90] The American Medical Association recently joined the Center for Science in the Public Interest in urging the NCAA to ban alcohol advertising during events,[91] but the NCAA decided to retain its existing policy.[92]

B. Potential Harmful Effects of a 21-Year-Old Drinking Age

Mixed messages sent to young drinkers are only part of the problem. In addition, it is possible that the drinking ban for young adults may have harmful effects.[93] We have seen that even during Prohibition, commentators bemoaned the lack of respect for the law that came from the widely flaunted ban.[94] Some argue that Prohibition may have exacerbated alcohol abuse, at least for some consumers:

> It's the same pattern observed during Prohibition, when illicit stills would blow up, and there was a rise in deaths from alcohol poisoning. Far from instilling virtue in Americans, Prohibition caused them to switch from beer and wine to hard liquor. Overall consumption of alcohol might even have increased.[95]

In modern times, many parents and adults fear that banning alcohol outright leads rebellious young adults to drink in more dangerous ways: "The pattern for underage students is more dangerous. . . . Afraid of being caught, they drink a lot in a short period of time. They do it less often but more intensely."[96]

The legal ban on drinking before age 21 also eliminates the possibility of teaching responsible drinking behaviors to young adults who, because of relative economic dependence, are often accessible to parents, college administrators, and others. The president of Middlebury College in Vermont, John McCardell, believes that the lack of supervised drinking experience for young adults causes much of the problem.[97] He argues that colleges should play an active role in teaching students how to drink responsibly.[98] Says McCardell: "You have to give them some exposure. . . . That doesn't mean sending everybody out to get drunk. But if you're serious about teaching somebody biology, you're going to include a laboratory. College campuses could be little laboratories of progressiveness."[99]

Nor is McCardell alone in his views. A recent article in the student newspaper at Tufts University quoted several University administrators who expressed similar concerns. "It's very complicated when you're living in a country where the legal drinking age forces you to bury your head in the sand," said Margot Abels, Director of Drug and Alcohol Education Services.[100] Tufts Dean of Students, Bruce Reitman, regrets that the 21 drinking age makes it impossible for faculty members to "model responsible drinking," as they did when an 18 drinking age allowed Friday afternoon student-faculty sherry hours where alcohol was used in a civilized, non-abusive manner.[101] Nowadays, Reitman notes, it is "naïve" to tell freshmen that he expects them to never touch alcohol, especially in light of a recent survey of Tufts freshmen that indicated that more than 80% of respondents had tried alcohol before arriving at the University.[102]

The notion of allowing young adults to drink, at least in supervised settings such as college-sponsored parties, has some parallels with the grant of driving privileges to young drivers. Combining education and supervision with probationary privileges allows young drivers to acquire necessary skills. If they proceed through their probationary period without incident, they may obtain regular drivers' licenses. If they have violations, they may face delays or lose their licenses altogether.[103] Likewise, college campuses could sponsor parties where adult supervision is provided. Alcohol education could be incorporated into the mandatory curriculum. Nor are colleges the only institutions that could institute this approach. Churches, community centers, or other organizations frequented by young people could also provide much needed education and supervision to young adults who choose to drink. Otherwise, the furtive, excessive drinking patterns exhibited by a significant percentage of young adults may cause far greater problems than would come from lowering the drinking age.

Conclusion

This Article has attempted to show that prohibiting alcohol consumption by young adults aged 18 to 21 is a policy that is neither currently effective, nor likely to be effective in the future. This failure is partly due to the fact that parents, who are key players in the control of minors, no longer have legally enforceable control over offspring who have attained the age of majority. The failure of policy is also due to the fact that an outright ban on drinking by young adults is philosophically different from policies governing analogous decisions that may be made by adults in our society. Whereas adults may make questionable decisions in areas such as education, health, or smoking, decisions about alcohol are uniquely restricted. Due to this dichotomy, I believe that prohibition of alcohol use by young adults will never be widely effective, no matter how desirable a teetotaler young adult population might be.

Notes

1. *See, e.g.,* NAT'L RES. COUNCIL INST. OF MED., REDUCING UNDERAGE DRINKING: A COLLECTIVE RESPONSIBILITY 35–57 (Richard J. Bonnie & Mary Ellen O'Connel eds., 2004).

2. *Id.* at 43–48.

3. *Id.* at 40–42.

4. Throughout the Article, I will use the term "young adults" to denote persons in the 18 to 21 year-old age group.

5. *See infra* Part II.

6. *See infra* Part III.A–B.

7. *See infra* Part III.C.

8. *See infra* Part III.D.

9. *See infra* Part IV.

10. *See infra* Part V.

11. Shelley, *supra* note 19, at 709.

12. *See, e.g.*, MNOOKIN & WEISBERG, *supra* note 29, at 663; WIS. STAT. § 125.07(4) (2004).

13. One Maryland father was charged with maintaining a disorderly house, "a misdemeanor subject to a fine of up to $300 or a maximum jail sentence of six months." Other possible charges include "contributing to the delinquency of a minor" and "drinking in prohibited places." Veronica T. Jennings, *Md. Parents Cited in Teen Drinking Crackdown*, WASH. POST, June 14, 1988, at B1. Some states impose criminal liability on persons who provide alcohol to minors, where the minor later dies or suffers bodily harm as a consequence of the drinking. *See, e.g.*, WIS. STAT. § 125.075 (2004). However, some states, such as Wisconsin and Texas, allow drinking in the presence of a minor's own parent. MNOOKIN & WEISBERG, *supra* note 29, at 664.

14. *See, e.g.*, WIS. STAT. § 125.035 (2004); Congini v. Portersville Valve Co., 470 A.2d 515 (Pa. 1983) (holding that guardian had a cause of action against the minor ward's employer where the employer served alcohol at a party, minor became drunk, drove away from the party with the knowledge of employer's agent, and the minor was subsequently injured in an automobile accident.). *But see* Charles v. Seigfried, 651 N.E.2d 154, 165 (Ill.1995) (holding that there is no common law right of action against social hosts who serve alcohol to minors).

15. *See, e.g.*, MNOOKIN & WEISBERG, *supra* note 29, at 663–64; WIS. STAT. § 125.07.

16. *See* JAMES H. HEDLUND & ANNE T. MCCARTT, DRUNK DRIVING: SEEKING ADDITIONAL SOLUTIONS 8 (2002). . . .

17. Michael Stroh, *Younger Drinkers Risk Damaging Brain Cells*, BALTIMORE SUN, Dec. 10, 2002, at 1A.

18. Joseph A. Califano, Jr., Editorial, *Don't Make Teen Drinking Easier*, WASH. POST, May 11, 2003, at B7.

19. Stroh, *supra* note 51. The hippocampus is a part of the brain involved in memory and learning.

20. Id.

21. Id.

22. *Id.*; Kathleen Fackelmann, *Teen Drinking, Thinking Don't Mix; Alcohol Appears to Damage Young Brains, Early Research Finds*, USA TODAY, Oct. 18, 2000, at 1D (citing Aaron M. White et al., *Binge Pattern Ethanol Exposure in Adolescent and Adult Rats: Differential Impact on Subsequent Responsiveness to Ethanol*, 24 ALCOHOLISM: CLINICAL & EXPERIMENTAL RES. 1251 (2000)).

23. Sally Squires, *Early Drinking Said to Increase Alcoholism Risk*, WASH. POST, Jan. 20, 1998, at Z7 (These findings "are drawn from the National Longitudinal Alcohol Epidemiologic Survey, a national sample that included face-to-face interviews with nearly 28,000 current and former drinkers aged 18 years and older.").

24. *Id.* However, there were some gender and racial variations in these risk statistics: "Early drinking is especially risky for boys. Those who began drinking by age 13 had a 50 percent lifetime risk of alcoholism. For girls, the risk was 43 percent for those who began drinking at age 13. Among blacks, those who were drinking alcohol at age 13 had a 44 percent lifetime risk of alcoholism, while nonblack children the same age had a 48 percent lifetime risk." *Id.*

25. Id.

26. Alexander Wagenaar, Letter to the Editor, *Teenage Drinking: Rites and Wrongs*, WASH. POST, May 9, 2003, at A34.

27. Kevin Cullen & Karen Avenoso, *Deaths Show Backsliding on Alcohol; Teen-age Drinking May Undo Progress*, BOSTON GLOBE, Aug. 6, 1996, at B1.

28. *See* HEDLUND & MCCARTT, *supra* note 50, at 7–9 (citing several examples of improved public awareness and enforcement of drunk driving laws through-out the 1980s and 1990s, including mandatory driver's license suspension, mandatory jail time, administrative license revocation, widely used breath test equipment, training in field sobriety testing, sobriety checkpoints, special drunk driving saturation patrols, zero tolerance for youth, and lowering of BAC limits to 0.08 by many states). *See also* Glen Martin, *Holiday Sees Rise in DUI Arrests; 3,000 Officers Join Effort to Prevent Highway Deaths*, S.F. CHRON., May 31, 2005, at B1 (California Highway Patrol Officer Mike Wright said, "Each year we've been able to throw more and more resources at the problem, so we're getting more and more arrests. . . . Bigger is better. We have more people looking for drunks, so we're catching more drunks.").

29. Cullen & Avenoso, *supra* note 61.

30. Califano, Jr., *supra* note 52.

31. Cullen & Avenoso, *supra* note 61.

32. Nat'l Council on Alcoholism and Drug Dependence, FYI: Alcohol & Crime. . . .

33. Nat'l Inst. on Alcohol Abuse and Alcoholism, *Youth Drinking: Risk Factors and Consequences*, ALCOHOL ALERT NO. 37, July 1997. . . .

34. I am using the terms "college age" and "young adult" to refer to persons between the ages of 18 and 21. Of course, some kids are only 17 when they enter college, many young people in that age group do not attend college, and many people attending colleges and universities are over age 21. However, many studies and discussions of underage drinking concern college students and refer to drinking patterns among persons of "college age," perhaps because there is a significant drinking culture on many college campuses.

35. NAT'L RES. COUNCIL INST. OF MED., *supra* note 1, at 35.

36. *See id.* at 36 (now called the National Survey on Drug Use and Health).

37. *Id.* at 38.

38. *Id.* at 39 (This was true even among the 7% of 12–14–year-olds who reported drinking at all. "With increasing age, more youth drink and more drinkers are heavy drinkers.").

39. Jane Gross, *Teenagers' Binge Leads Scarsdale to Painful Self-Reflection*, N.Y. TIMES, Oct. 8, 2002, at B1.

40. Id.

41. Id.

42. Id.

43. Id.

44. Id.

45. Id.

46. *Scarsdale School Suspends 28 Students for Drunkenness*, N.Y. TIMES, Sept. 27, 2002, at B6.

47. NAT'L RES. COUNCIL INST. OF MED., *supra* note 1, at 82.

48. Id.

49. Id.

50. Elizabeth Nesoff, *A Prim Suburb Rallies to Curb Teen Drinking*, CHRISTIAN SCI. MONITOR, July 22, 2003, at 2.

51. NAT'L RES. COUNCIL INST. OF MED., *supra* note 1, at 82.

52. Corey Kilgannon, *Drinking Young*, N.Y. TIMES, Oct. 27, 2002, at WE1.

53. Nesoff, *supra* note 84.

54. Kilgannon, *supra* note 86.

55. *Id.*

56. 321 U.S. 158 (1944).

57. *Prince v. Massachusetts* was an appeal from convictions for violation of Massachusetts' child labor laws by Sarah Prince, who had allowed her 9-year-old niece to offer Jehovah's Witness literature for sale one evening, shortly before 9 pm. Mrs. Prince argued that her right to religious freedom coupled with her right to raise her children as she saw fit made the enforcement of the statute unconstitutional. However, the U.S. Supreme Court upheld the statute and the convictions, stating that the State's power to protect children from the dangers of street preaching was not foreclosed by the presence of parents, who could reduce, but not eliminate, the possible dangers. The Court famously proclaimed: "Parents may be free to become martyrs themselves. But it does not follow they are free, in identical circumstances, to make martyrs of their children before they have reached the age of full and legal discretion when they can make that choice for themselves." *Id.* at 170.

58. Several states allow parents to supply alcoholic beverages to their own children. *See* MNOOKIN & WEISBERG, *supra* note 29, at 664; WIS. STAT. § 125.07 (2004).

59. *See* NAT'L RES. COUNCIL INST. OF MED., *supra* note 1, at 64–65; Stroh, *supra* note 51; Fackelmann, *supra* note 56.

60. *See* NAT'L RES. COUNCIL INST. OF MED., *supra* note 1, at 82; Kilgannon, *supra* note 86.

61. Karina Bland, *Crackdown on Teen Keggers; Don't Buy Liquor, Parents Warned*, ARIZ. REPUBLIC, May 26, 2004, at A1.

62. In another context, I have noted that advocates of such an extreme form of parental supervision are few. *See* Judith G. McMullen, *"You Can't Make Me!": How Expectations of Parental Control over Adolescents Influence the Law*, 35 LOY. U. CHI. L.J. 603 (2003) [hereinafter McMullen, *"You Can't Make Me!"*]. In his 1995 book, *Parent in Control*, author Gregory Bodenhamer advises close monitoring of difficult children and teens, including following them, accompanying them on every outing, and physically forcing or restraining actions. GREGORY BODENHAMER, PARENT IN CONTROL 102–07 (1995). I could find no other authors who advocate such an extreme hands-on approach, although most parenting experts advocate discipline, persuasion, and communication.

63. *See* MNOOKIN & WEISBERG, *supra* note 29, at 144–46 (quoting WILLIAM BLACKSTONE, 2 COMMENTARIES *446, *446–51).

64. *See* MICHAEL GROSSBERG, GOVERNING THE HEARTH: LAW AND THE FAMILY IN NINETEENTH-CENTURY AMERICA 234–59 (1985) (discussing the historical evolution of parental fitness as the basis of custody).

65. Troxel v. Granville, 530 U.S. 57, 65–66 (2000).

66. *See* Ginsberg v. New York, 390 U.S. 629, 639 (1968) (stating that the "legislature could properly conclude that parents and others, teachers for example, who have this primary responsibility for children's well-being are entitled to the support of laws designed to aid discharge of that responsibility"). *Ginsberg* upheld a New York statute that restricted access of minors to sexually suggestive publications, in this case "girlie magazines." *Id.* at 631–33.

67. McMullen, *"You Can't Make Me!"*, *supra* note 96, at 622–25.

68. *See Ginsberg*, 390 U.S. at 639 (The Court balanced parental prerogatives in allowing children access to pornographic literature with the State's interest in limiting such access. The Court concluded that the State had an interest in restricting minor's access to sexually suggestive publications, but noted that the New York statute, which forbade the *sale* of such literature to persons under the age of 17, did not preclude a parent from allowing his own child to view such literature purchased by the parent.). *See also* Wisconsin v. Yoder, 406 U.S. 205, 214, 234 (1972) (The Court balanced the social interest in an educated citizenry with the right of parents to bring up children according to the parents' own religious beliefs. Here, the Court found that the state interest did not justify enforcing compulsory education rules requiring formal education until 16 against Amish parents whose religious convictions required them to remove their children from school after the eighth grade.).

69. *See* NAT'L RES. COUNCIL INST. OF MED., *supra* note 1, at 82 (stating that "both agesegregation and lack of adult supervision have been related to . . . greater alcohol consumption").

70. *Id.* at 204 (In the Higher Education Amendments of 1998, "Section 952 clarified that institutions of higher education are allowed (but not required) to notify parents if a student under the age of 21 at the time of notification commits a disciplinary violation involving alcohol or a controlled substance.").

71. *Id.* at 45 (The 2000 National Household Survey of Drug Abuse (NHSDA) reported that "41 percent of full-time college students aged 18 to 22 engaged in heavy drinking, compared with 36 percent of young adults who were attending college part time or not at all.").

72. *Providing Substance Abuse Prevention and Treatment Services to Adolescents: Hearing Before the Subcomm. on Substance Abuse and Mental Health Services of the Comm. on Health Education, Labor, and Pensions*, 108th Cong. 19 (2004) (prepared statement of Sandra A. Brown, Professor of Psychology and Psychiatry, Univ. of Cal.-San Diego).

73. WECHSLER & WUETHRICH, *supra* note 26, at 35.

74. *Id.* at 38 (quoting Mark Nason, prevention consultant with Prevention Research Institute, "a nonprofit organization that develops curricula to reduce the risk of alcohol and drug problems").

75. *Id.* at 30.

76. *Id.* at 30–31.

77. *Id.* at 31–32.

78. "Small" crimes, such as purse-snatching or low-level speeding while driving are examples of laws that often go unpunished because of the difficulty of apprehending every suspect. However, serious crimes sometimes go unpunished as well. The infamous and unsolved case of Jack the Ripper is but one example. L. PERRY CURTIS, JR., JACK THE RIPPER & THE LONDON PRESS 1 (2001).

79. Elizabeth A. Heaney, *Pennsylvania's Doctrine of Necessities: An Anachronism Demanding Abolishment*, 101 DICK. L. REV. 233, 259 (1996) (quoting Note, *The Unnecessary Doctrine of Necessaries*, 82 MICH. L. REV. 1767, 1798 (1984)).

80. Lawrence M. Friedman, *Two Faces of Law*, 1984 WIS. L. REV. 13, 14 (1984).

81. *See* Rutledge, *supra* note 158 (citing comments of Susan Crowley, director of PACE (Policy, Alternatives, Community and Education), a "10-year, $1.2 million program aimed at curtailing underage drinking" funded by the Robert Wood Johnson Foundation).

82. *Id.*

83. *See supra* Part III.C.

84. *See id.*

85. *See id.*

86. CTR. FOR SCI. IN THE PUBLIC INTEREST, TAKE A KID TO A BEER: HOW THE NCAA RECRUITS KIDS FOR THE BEER MARKET 10 (2005) . . . Alan W. Stacy et al., *Exposure to Televised Alcohol Ads and Subsequent Adolescent Alcohol Use*, 28 AM. J. OF HEALTH BEHAV. 498, 507–08 (2004); Susan E. Martin et al., *Alcohol Advertising and Youth*, 26 ALCOHOLISM: CLINICAL & EXPERIMENTAL RES. 900, 905 (2002).

87. Melanie Warner, *A Liquor Maker Keeps a Close Watch on Its Ads*, N.Y. TIMES, July 27, 2005, at C10.

88. *Id.*

89. CTR. FOR SCI. IN THE PUBLIC INTEREST, *supra* note 198, at 1.

90. *See generally id.* (The title of the report is a play on the NCAA's campaign to "Take a Kid to a Game.").

91. *NCAA Board OKs 12th Game; Decision Could Revive WVU-Herd Series*, CHARLESTON GAZETTE, Apr. 29, 2005, at P1B.

92. Jeff Miller, *NCAA Extends Brand's Deal; Board Also Approves Start of Academic Performance Guidelines*, DALLAS MORNING NEWS, Aug. 6, 2005, at 11C.

93. "Of course, many laws also produce side-effects and may do more harm than good. Policy choices should take these costs into account." Friedman, *supra* note 192, at 14.

94. *See* John Tierney, *Debunking the Drug War*, N.Y. TIMES, Aug. 9, 2005, at A19.

95. *Id.* (arguing that media exaggeration and law enforcement overreaction to amphetamine use makes the problem worse, not better).

96. Rutledge, *supra* note 158 (quoting Richard Keeling, physician and former director of health services at the University of Wisconsin-Madison).

97. *Id.*

98. *Id.*

99. *Id.*

100. Keith Barry, *Survey Offers Insight Into Freshman Substance Use*, TUFTS DAILY, Mar. 11, 2005. . . .

101. *Id.*

102. *Id.* (The administrators were commenting in light of an online questionnaire sent to freshmen. 600 students, or 47.1% of the Class of 2008, responded to the October, 2004 survey.)

103. MNOOKIN & WEISBERG, *supra* note 29, at 649.

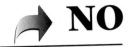
Underage Drinking: Why Do Adolescents Drink, What Are the Risks, and How Can Underage Drinking Be Prevented?

Alcohol is the drug of choice among youth. Many young people are experiencing the consequences of drinking too much, at too early an age. As a result, underage drinking is a leading public health problem in this country.

Each year, approximately 5,000 young people under the age of 21 die as a result of underage drinking; this includes about 1,900 deaths from motor vehicle crashes, 1,600 as a result of homicides, 300 from suicide, as well as hundreds from other injuries such as falls, burns, and drownings (1–5).

Yet drinking continues to be widespread among adolescents, as shown by nationwide surveys as well as studies in smaller populations. According to data from the 2005 Monitoring the Future (MTF) study, an annual survey of U.S. youth, three-fourths of 12th graders, more than two-thirds of 10th graders, and about two in every five 8th graders have consumed alcohol. And when youth drink they tend to drink intensively, often consuming four to five drinks at one time. MTF data show that 11 percent of 8th graders, 22 percent of 10th graders, and 29 percent of 12th graders had engaged in heavy episodic (or "binge[1]") drinking within the past two weeks (6) (see figure).

Research also shows that many adolescents start to drink at very young ages. In 2003, the average age of first use of alcohol was about 14, compared to about 17½ in 1965 (7,8). People who reported starting to drink before the age of 15 were four times more likely to also report meeting the criteria for alcohol dependence at some point in their lives (9). In fact, new research shows that the serious drinking problems (including what is called alcoholism) typically associated with middle age actually begin to appear much earlier, during young adulthood and even adolescence.

Other research shows that the younger children and adolescents are when they start to drink, the more likely they will be to engage in behaviors that harm themselves and others. For example, frequent binge drinkers (nearly 1 million high school students nationwide) are more likely to engage in risky behaviors, including using other drugs such as marijuana and cocaine, having sex with six or more partners, and earning grades that are mostly Ds and Fs in school (10).

From *Alcohol Alert*, number 67, January 2006, U.S. Department of Health and Human and Services.

Why Do Some Adolescents Drink?

As children move from adolescence to young adulthood, they encounter dramatic physical, emotional, and lifestyle changes. Developmental transitions, such as puberty and increasing independence, have been associated with alcohol use. So in a sense, just being an adolescent may be a key risk factor not only for starting to drink but also for drinking dangerously.

Risk-taking   Research shows the brain keeps developing well into the twenties, during which time it continues to establish important communication connections and further refines its function. Scientists believe that this lengthy developmental period may help explain some of the behavior which is characteristic of adolescence—such as their propensity to seek out new and potentially dangerous situations. For some teens, thrill-seeking might include experimenting with alcohol. Developmental changes also offer a possible physiological explanation for why teens act so impulsively, often not recognizing that their actions—such as drinking—have consequences.

Expectancies   How people view alcohol and its effects also influences their drinking behavior, including whether they begin to drink and how much. An adolescent who expects drinking to be a pleasurable experience is more likely to drink than one who does not. An important area of alcohol research is focusing on how expectancy influences drinking patterns from childhood through adolescence and into young adulthood (11–14). Beliefs about alcohol are established very early in life, even before the child begins elementary school (15). Before age 9, children generally view alcohol negatively and see drinking as bad, with adverse effects. By about age 13, however, their expectancies shift, becoming more positive (11,16). As would be expected, adolescents who drink the most also place the greatest emphasis on the positive and arousing effects of alcohol.

Sensitivity and tolerance to alcohol   Differences between the adult brain and the brain of the maturing adolescent also may help to explain why many young drinkers are able to consume much larger amounts of alcohol than adults (17) before experiencing the negative consequences of drinking, such as drowsiness, lack of coordination, and withdrawal/hangover effects (18,19). This unusual tolerance may help to explain the high rates of binge drinking among young adults. At the same time, adolescents appear to be particularly sensitive to the positive effects of drinking, such as feeling more at ease in social situations, and young people may drink more than adults because of these positive social experiences (18,19).

Personality characteristics and psychiatric comorbidity   Children   who begin to drink at a very early age (before age 12) often share similar personality characteristics that may make them more likely to start drinking. Young people who are disruptive, hyperactive, and aggressive—often referred to as having conduct problems or being antisocial—as well as those who are depressed, withdrawn, or anxious, may be at greatest risk for alcohol problems (20). Other behavior problems associated with alcohol use include rebelliousness (21), difficulty avoiding harm or harmful situations (22), and a host of other traits seen in young people who act out without regard for rules or the feelings of others (i.e., disinhibition) (23–25).

TREATMENT: AN UNMET NEED

A major unmet need exists in the treatment of alcohol use disorders: In 2002, 1.4 million youth met the criteria for alcohol abuse or dependence, but only 227,000 actually received any treatment for these problems (1).

Moreover, much of the treatment available today does not address the specific needs of adolescents (2). For example, most young people prefer easy access to treatment, with strategies tailored to their age group (3), and treatments that do not remove them from their home or academic settings (2). Youth perceive traditional services (e.g., alcoholism treatment programs, Alcoholics Anonymous) as less helpful than brief interventions tailored to their concerns (4). Consequently, alternative formats, attention to developmental transitions, and social marketing are needed to better address alcohol problems that emerge during adolescence.

Adolescent Treatment Interventions

Complex interventions have been developed and tested in adolescents referred for treatment of alcohol and other drug disorders. Many of these patients are likely to have more than one substance use disorder (e.g., alcohol and marijuana) and to have other psychiatric disorders as well (e.g., depression, anxiety, or conduct disorder). Brief interventions are, as a rule, delivered to adolescents in general medical settings (e.g., primary care clinics, emergency rooms) or in school-based settings. These settings offer an excellent opportunity for intervening with adolescents to address their drinking before they progress to serious alcohol use disorders and to prevent the development of alcohol-related problems (5).

References

1. **Substance Abuse and Mental Health Services Administration (SAMHSA).** *Results from the 2002 National Survey on Drug Use and Health: National Findings.* NHSDA Series H–22, DHHS Pub. No. SMA 03–3836. Rockville, MD: SAMHSA, Office of Applied Studies, 2003. . . .
2. **Brown, S.A.** Facilitating change for adolescent alcohol problems: A multiple options approach. In: Wagner, E.F., and Waldron, H.B., eds. *Innovations in Adolescent Substance Abuse Intervention.* Oxford, England: Elsevier Science, 2001. pp. 169–187
3. **Metrik, J.;** Frissell, K.C.; McCarthy, D.M.; et al. Strategies for reduction and cessation of alcohol use: What do adolescents prefer? *Alcoholism: Clinical and Experimental Research* 27:74–80, 2003. PMID: 12544009
4. **D'Amico, E.J.;** McCarthy, D.M.; Metrik, J.; and Brown, S.A. Alcohol-related services: Prevention, secondary intervention and treatment preferences of adolescents. *Journal of Child & Adolescent Substance Abuse* 14:61–80, 2004.
5. **Wagner, E.F.;** Brown, S.A.; Monti, P.; et al. Innovations in adolescent substance abuse intervention. *Alcoholism: Clinical and Experimental Research* 23:236–249, 1999. PMID: 10069552

Hereditary factors   Some of the behavioral and physiological factors that converge to increase or decrease a person's risk for alcohol problems, including tolerance to alcohol's effects, may be directly linked to genetics. For example, being a child of an alcoholic or having several alcoholic family members places a person at greater risk for alcohol problems. Children of alcoholics (COAs) are between 4 and 10 times more likely to become alcoholics themselves than are children who have no close relatives with alcoholism (26). COAs also are more likely to begin drinking at a young age (27) and to progress to drinking problems more quickly (9).

Research shows that COAs may have subtle brain differences which could be markers for developing later alcohol problems (28). For example, using high-tech brain-imaging techniques, scientists have found that COAs have a distinctive feature in one brainwave pattern (called a P300 response) that could be a marker for later alcoholism risk (29,30). Researchers also are investigating other brainwave differences in COAs that may be present long before they begin to drink, including brainwave activity recorded during sleep (31) as well as changes in brain structure (32) and function (33).

Some studies suggest that these brain differences may be particularly evident in people who also have certain behavioral traits, such as signs of conduct disorder, antisocial personality disorder, sensation-seeking, or poor impulse control (34–38). Studying how the brain's structure and function translates to behavior will help researchers to better understand how predrinking risk factors shape later alcohol use. For example, does a person who is depressed drink to alleviate his or her depression, or does drinking lead to changes in his brain that result in feelings of depression?

Other hereditary factors likely will become evident as scientists work to identify the actual genes involved in addiction. By analyzing the genetic makeup of people and families with alcohol dependence, researchers have found specific regions on chromosomes that correlate with a risk for alcoholism (39–41). Candidate genes for alcoholism risk also have been associated with those regions (42). The goal now is to further refine regions for which a specific gene has not yet been identified and then determine how those genes interact with other genes and gene products as well as with the environment to result in alcohol dependence. Further research also should shed light on the extent to which the same or different genes contribute to alcohol problems, both in adults and in adolescents.

Environmental aspects   Pinpointing a genetic contribution will not tell the whole story, however, as drinking behavior reflects a complex interplay between inherited and environmental factors, the implications of which are only beginning to be explored in adolescents (43). And what influences drinking at one age may not have the same impact at another. As Rose and colleagues (43) show, genetic factors appear to have more influence on adolescent drinking behavior in late adolescence than in mid-adolescence.

Environmental factors, such as the influence of parents and peers, also play a role in alcohol use (44). For example, parents who drink more and who view drinking favorably may have children who drink more, and an adolescent girl with an older or adult boyfriend is more likely to use alcohol and other drugs and to engage in delinquent behaviors (45).

Figure 1

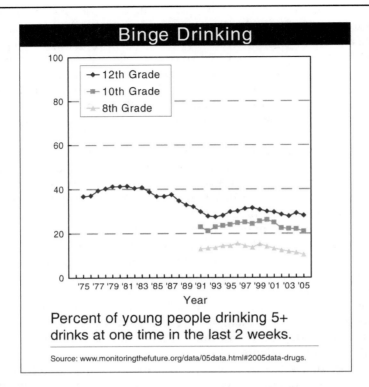

Binge Drinking

Percent of young people drinking 5+
drinks at one time in the last 2 weeks.

Source: www.monitoringthefuture.org/data/05data.html#2005data-drugs.

Researchers are examining other environmental influences as well, such as the impact of the media. Today alcohol is widely available and aggressively promoted through television, radio, billboards, and the Internet. Researchers are studying how young people react to these advertisements. In a study of 3rd, 6th, and 9th graders, those who found alcohol ads desirable were more likely to view drinking positively and to want to purchase products with alcohol logos (46). Research is mixed, however, on whether these positive views of alcohol actually lead to underage drinking.

What Are the Health Risks?

Whatever it is that leads adolescents to begin drinking, once they start they face a number of potential health risks. Although the severe health problems associated with harmful alcohol use are not as common in adolescents as they are in adults, studies show that young people who drink heavily may put themselves at risk for a range of potential health problems.

Brain effects   Scientists currently are examining just how alcohol affects the developing brain, but it's a difficult task. Subtle changes in the brain may be difficult to detect but still have a significant impact on long-term thinking and memory skills. Add to this the fact that adolescent brains are still maturing, and the study of alcohol's effects becomes even more complex. Research has shown that animals fed alcohol during this critical developmental stage continue to show long-lasting impairment from alcohol as they age (47). It's simply not known how alcohol will affect the long-term memory and learning skills of people who began drinking heavily as adolescents.

Liver effects   Elevated liver enzymes, indicating some degree of liver damage, have been found in some adolescents who drink alcohol (48). Young drinkers who are overweight or obese showed elevated liver enzymes even with only moderate levels of drinking (49).

Growth and endocrine effects   In both males and females, puberty is a period associated with marked hormonal changes, including increases in the sex hormones, estrogen and testosterone. These hormones, in turn, increase production of other hormones and growth factors (50), which are vital for normal organ development. Drinking alcohol during this period of rapid growth and development (i.e., prior to or during puberty) may upset the critical hormonal balance necessary for normal development of organs, muscles, and bones. Studies in animals also show that consuming alcohol during puberty adversely affects the maturation of the reproductive system (51).

Preventing Underage Drinking Within a Developmental Framework

Complex behaviors, such as the decision to begin drinking or to continue using alcohol, are the result of a dynamic interplay between genes and environment. For example, biological and physiological changes that occur during adolescence may promote risk-taking behavior, leading to early experimentation with alcohol. This behavior then shapes the child's environment, as he or she chooses friends and situations that support further drinking. Continued drinking may lead to physiological reactions, such as depression or anxiety disorders, triggering even greater alcohol use or dependence. In this way, youthful patterns of alcohol use can mark the start of a developmental pathway that may lead to abuse and dependence. Then again, not all young people who travel this pathway experience the same outcomes.

Perhaps the best way to understand and prevent underage alcohol use is to view drinking as it relates to development. This "whole system" approach to underage drinking takes into account a particular adolescent's unique risk and protective factors—from genetics and personality characteristics to social and environmental factors. Viewed in this way, development includes not only the adolescent's inherent risk and resilience but also the current conditions that help to shape his or her behavior (52).

Children mature at different rates. Developmental research takes this into account, recognizing that during adolescence there are periods of rapid growth and reorganization, alternating with periods of slower growth and integration of body systems. Periods of rapid transitions, when social or cultural factors most strongly influence the biology and behavior of the adolescent, may be the best time to target delivery of interventions (53). Interventions that focus on these critical development periods could alter the life course of the child (54), perhaps placing him or her on a path to avoid problems with alcohol.

To date, researchers have been unable to identify a single track that predicts the course of alcohol use for all or even most young people. Instead, findings provide strong evidence for wide developmental variation in drinking patterns within this special population (55,56).

Interventions for Preventing Underage Drinking

Intervention approaches typically fall into two distinct categories: (1) environmental-level interventions, which seek to reduce opportunities for underage drinking, increase penalties for violating minimum legal drinking age (MLDA) and other alcohol use laws, and reduce community tolerance for alcohol use by youth; and (2) individual-level interventions, which seek to change knowledge, expectancies, attitudes, intentions, motivation, and skills so that youth are better able to resist the pro-drinking influences and opportunities that surround them.

Environmental approaches include:

Raising the price of alcohol   A substantial body of research has shown that higher prices or taxes on alcoholic beverages are associated with lower levels of alcohol consumption and alcohol-related problems, especially in young people (57–60).

Increasing the minimum legal drinking age   Today all States have set the minimum legal drinking at age 21. Increasing the age at which people can legally purchase and drink alcohol has been the most successful intervention to date in reducing drinking and alcohol-related crashes among people under age 21 (61). NHTSA (1) estimates that a legal drinking age of 21 saves 700 to 1,000 lives annually. Since 1976, these laws have prevented more than 21,000 traffic deaths. Just how much the legal drinking age relates to drinking-related crashes is shown by a recent study in New Zealand. Six years ago that country lowered its minimum legal drinking age to 18. Since then, alcohol-related crashes have risen 12 percent among 18- to 19-year-olds and 14 percent among 15- to 17-year-olds (62). Clearly a higher minimum drinking age can help to reduce crashes and save lives, especially in very young drivers.

Enacting zero-tolerance laws   All States have zero-tolerance laws that make it illegal for people under age 21 to drive after *any* drinking. When the first eight States to adopt zero-tolerance laws were compared with nearby States without such laws, the zero-tolerance States showed a 21-percent greater decline in the proportion of single-vehicle night-time fatal crashes involving drivers under 21, the type of crash most likely to involve alcohol (63).

Stepping up enforcement of laws   Despite their demonstrated benefits, legal drinking age and zero-tolerance laws generally have not been vigorously enforced (64). Alcohol purchase laws aimed at sellers and buyers also can be effective (65), but resources must be made available for enforcing these laws.

Individual-focused interventions include:

School-based prevention programs The first school-based prevention programs were primarily informational and often used scare tactics; it was assumed that if youth understood the dangers of alcohol use, they would choose not to drink. These programs were ineffective. Today, better programs are available and often have a number of elements in common: They follow social influence models and include setting norms, addressing social pressures to drink, and teaching resistance skills. These programs also offer interactive and developmentally appropriate information, include peer-led components, and provide teacher training (66).

Family-based prevention programs Parent's ability to influence whether their children drink is well documented and is consistent across racial/ethnic groups (67,68). Setting clear rules against drinking, consistently enforcing those rules, and monitoring the child's behavior all help to reduce the likelihood of underage drinking. The Iowa Strengthening Families Program (ISFP), delivered when students were in grade 6, is a program that has shown long-lasting preventive effects on alcohol use (69,70).

Selected Programs Showing Promise

Environmental interventions are among the recommendations included in the recent National Research Council (NRC) and Institute of Medicine (IOM) report on underage drinking (71). These interventions are intended to reduce commercial and social availability of alcohol and/or reduce driving while intoxicated. They use a variety of strategies, including server training and compliance checks in places that sell alcohol; deterring adults from purchasing alcohol for minors or providing alcohol to minors; restricting drinking in public places and preventing underage drinking parties; enforcing penalties for the use of false IDs, driving while intoxicated, and violating zero-tolerance laws; and raising public awareness of policies and sanctions.

WHO DRINKS?

Rates of drinking and alcohol-related problems are highest among White and American Indian or Alaska Native youth, followed by Hispanic youth, African Americans, and Asians.

Prevalence rates of drinking for boys and girls are similar in the younger age groups; among older adolescents, however, more boys than girls engage in frequent and heavy drinking, and boys show higher rates of drinking problems.

The following community trials show how environmental strategies can be useful in reducing underage drinking and related problems.

The Massachusetts saving lives program   This intervention was designed to reduce alcohol-impaired driving and related traffic deaths. Strategies included the use of drunk driving checkpoints, speeding and drunk driving awareness days, speed-watch telephone hotlines, high school peer-led education, and college prevention programs. The 5-year program decreased fatal crashes, particularly alcohol-related fatal crashes involving drivers ages 15–25, and reduced the proportion of 16- to 19-year-olds who reported driving after drinking, in comparison with the rest of Massachusetts. It also made teens more aware of penalties for drunk driving and for speeding (72).

The community prevention trial program   This program was designed to reduce alcohol-involved injuries and death. One component sought to reduce alcohol sales to minors by enforcing underage sales laws; training sales clerks, owners, and managers to prevent sales of alcohol to minors; and using the media to raise community awareness of underage drinking. Sales to apparent minors (people of legal drinking age who appear younger than age 21) were significantly reduced in the intervention communities compared with control sites (73).

Communities mobilizing for change on alcohol   This intervention, designed to reduce the accessibility of alcoholic beverages to people under age 21, centered on policy changes among local institutions to make underage drinking less acceptable within the community. Alcohol sales to minors were reduced: 18- to 20-year-olds were less likely to try to purchase alcohol or provide it to younger teens, and the number of DUI arrests declined among 18- to 20-year-olds (74,75).

Multicomponent comprehensive interventions   Perhaps the strongest approach for preventing underage drinking involves the coordinated effort of all the elements that influence a child's life—including family, schools, and community. Ideally, intervention programs also should integrate treatment for youth who are alcohol dependent. Project Northland is an example of a comprehensive program that has been extensively evaluated.

Project Northland was tested in 22 school districts in northeastern Minnesota. The intervention included (1) school curricula, (2) peer leadership, (3) parental involvement programs, and (4) communitywide task force activities to address larger community norms and alcohol availability. It targeted adolescents in grades 6 through 12.

Intervention and comparison communities differed significantly in "tendency to use alcohol," a composite measure that combined items about intentions to use alcohol and actual use as well as in the likelihood of drinking "five or more in a row." Underage drinking was less prevalent in the intervention communities during phase 1; higher during the interim period (suggesting a "catch-up" effect while intervention activities were minimal); and again lower during phase 2, when intervention activities resumed (76).

Project Northland has been designated a model program by the Substance Abuse and Mental Health Services Administration (SAMHSA), and its materials have been adapted for a general audience. It now is being replicated in ethnically diverse urban neighborhoods.

Conclusion

Today, alcohol is widely available and aggressively promoted throughout society. And alcohol use continues to be regarded, by many people, as a normal part of growing up. Yet underage drinking is dangerous, not only for the drinker but also for society, as evident by the number of alcohol-involved motor vehicle crashes, homicides, suicides, and other injuries.

People who begin drinking early in life run the risk of developing serious alcohol problems, including alcoholism, later in life. They also are at greater risk for a variety of adverse consequences, including risky sexual activity and poor performance in school.

Identifying adolescents at greatest risk can help stop problems before they develop. And innovative, comprehensive approaches to prevention, such as Project Northland, are showing success in reducing experimentation with alcohol as well as the problems that accompany alcohol use by young people.

References

1. **National Highway Traffic Safety Administration (NHTSA).** *Traffic Safety Facts 2002: Alcohol.* DOT Pub. No. HS–809–606. Washington, DC: NHTSA, National Center for Statistics & Analysis, 2003. . . .

2. **Centers for Disease Control and Prevention (CDC),** National Center for Injury Prevention and Control (NCIPC). Web-Based Injury Statistics Query and Reporting System (WISQARS), 2004. . . .

3. **Smith, G.S.;** Branas, C.C.; and Miller, T.R. Fatal nontraffic injuries involving alcohol: A metaanalysis. *Annals of Emergency Medicine* 33:659–668, 1999. PMID: 10339681

4. **Levy, D.T.;** Miller, T.R.; and Cox, K.C. *Costs of Underage Drinking.* Washington, DC: U.S. Dept. of Justice, Office of Justice Programs, Office of Juvenile Justice and Delinquency Prevention, 1999. . . .

5. **Hingson, R.,** and Kenkel, D. Social, health, and economic consequences of underage drinking. In: National Research Council and Institute of Medicine. Bonnie, R.J., and O'Connell, M.E., eds. *Reducing Underage Drinking: A Collective Responsibility.* Washington, DC: National Academies Press, 2004. pp. 351–382. . . .

6. **Johnston, L.D.;** O'Malley, P.M.; Bachman, J.G.; and Schulenberg, J.E. *Monitoring the Future, National Survey Results on Drug Use, 1975–2004. Volume I: Secondary School Students.* NIH Pub. No. 05–5727. Bethesda, MD: National Institute on Drug Abuse, 2005. . . .

7. **Newes-Adeyi, G.;** Chiung, C.M.; Williams, G.D.; and Faden, V.B. *NIAAA Surveillance Report No. 74: Trends in Underage Drinking in the United States, 1991–2003.* Bethesda, MD: National Institute on Alcohol Abuse and Alcoholism, 2005. . . .

8. **Substance Abuse and Mental Health Services Administration (SAMHSA).** *Results from the 2002 National Survey on Drug Use and Health: National Findings.* NHSDA Series H–22, DHHS Pub. No. SMA 03–3836. Rockville, MD: SAMHSA, Office of Applied Studies, 2003. . . .

9. **Grant, B.F.,** and Dawson, D.A. Age at onset of drug use and its association with DSM–IV drug abuse and dependence: Results from the National Longitudinal Alcohol Epidemiologic Survey. *Journal of Substance Abuse* 10:163–173, 1998. PMID: 9854701

10. **Grunbaum, J.A.;** Kann, L.; Kinchen, S.; et al. Youth risk behavior surveillance—United States, 2003. *Morbidity and Mortality Weekly Report Surveillance Summary,*

May 21;53:1–96, 2004. Erratum in *MMWR*, 2004 June 25; 53:536. Erratum *MMWR Morbidity and Mortality Weekly Report* 2005 June 24; 54(24):608. PMID: 15152182

11. **Dunn, M.E.**, and Goldman, M.S. Empirical modeling of an alcohol expectancy memory network in elementary school children as a function of grade. *Experimental and Clinical Psychopharmacology* 4:209–217, 1996.

12. **Lang, A.R.**, and Strizke, W.G.K. Children and alcohol. In: Galanter, M., ed. *Recent Developments in Alcoholism, Vol. 11: Ten Years of Progress.* New York: Plenum Press, 1993. pp. 73–85. PMID: 8234939

13. **Smith, G.T.**; Goldman, M.S.; Greenbaum, P.E.; and Christiansen, B.A. Expectancy for social facilitation from drinking: The divergent paths of high-expectancy and low-expectancy adolescents. *Journal of Abnormal Psychology* 104:32–40, 1995. PMID: 7897051

14. **Zucker, R.A.**; Kincaid, S.B.; Fitzgerald, H.E.; and Bingham, C.R. Alcohol schema acquisition in preschoolers: Differences between children of alcoholics and children of nonalcoholics. *Alcoholism: Clinical and Experimental Research* 19:1011–1017, 1995. PMID: 7485810

15. **Noll, R.B.**; Zucker, R.A.; and Greenberg, G.S. Identification of alcohol by smell among preschoolers: Evidence for early socialization about drugs occurring in the home. *Child Development* 61:1520–1527, 1990. PMID: 2245743

16. **Dunn, M.E.**, and Goldman, M.S. Age and drinking-related differences in the memory organization of alcohol expectancies in 3rd, 6th, 9th, and 12th grade children. *Journal of Consulting and Clinical Psychology* 66:579–585, 1998. PMID: 9642899

17. **Johnston, L.D.**; O'Malley, P.M.; and Bachman, J.G. *Monitoring the Future, National Survey Results on Drug Use, 1975–2002. Volume I: Secondary School Students.* NIH Pub. No. 03–5375. Bethesda, MD: National Institute on Drug Abuse, 2003. . . .

18. **Spear, L.P.** The adolescent brain and age-related behavioral manifestations. *Neuroscience and Biobehavioral Reviews* 24:417–463, 2000.PMID: 10817843

19. **Spear, L.P.**, and Varlinskaya, E.I. Adolescence: Alcohol sensitivity, tolerance, and intake. In: Galanter, M., ed. *Recent Developments in Alcoholism, Vol. 17: Alcohol Problems in Adolescents and Young Adults: Epidemiology, Neurobiology, Prevention, Treatment.* New York: Springer, 2005. pp. 143–159. PMID: 15789864

20. **Zucker, R.A.**; Wong, M.M.; Puttler, L.I.; and Fitzgerald, H.E. Resilience and vulnerability among sons of alcoholics: Relationship to developmental outcomes between early childhood and adolescence. In: Luthar, S.S., ed. *Resilience and Vulnerability: Adaptation in the Context of Childhood Adversities.* New York: Cambridge University Press, 2003. pp. 76–103.

21. **Brook, J.S.**; Whiteman, M.; Finch, S.; and Cohen, P. Aggression, intrapsychic distress, and drug use: Antecedent and intervening processes. *Journal of the American Academy of Child & Adolescent Psychiatry* 34:1076–1084, 1995. PMID: 7665446

22. **Jones, S.P.**, and Heaven, P.C. Psychosocial correlates of adolescent drug-taking behaviour. *Journal of Adolescence* 21:127–134, 1998. PMID: 9585491

23. **Colder, C.R.**, and O'Connor, R. Attention bias and disinhibited behavior as predictors of alcohol use and enhancement reasons for drinking. *Psychology of Addictive Behaviors* 16:325–332, 2002. PMID: 12503905

24. **Moss, H.B.**, and Kirisci, L. Aggressivity in adolescent alcohol abusers: Relationship with conduct disorder. *Alcoholism: Clinical and Experimental Research* 19:642–646, 1995. PMID: 7573787

25. **Colder, C.R.**, and Chassin, L. Affectivity and impulsivity: Temperament risk for adolescent alcohol involvement. *Psychology of Addictive Behaviors* 11:83–97, 1997.

26. **Russell, M.** Prevalence of alcoholism among children of alcoholics. In: Windle, M., and Searles, J.S., eds. *Children of Alcoholics: Critical Perspectives.* New York: Guilford, 1990. pp. 9–38.

27. **Donovan, J.E.** Adolescent alcohol initiation: A review of psychosocial risk factors. *Journal of Adolescent Health* 35:529.e7–18, 2004.

28. **Tapert, S.F.**, and Schweinsburg, A.D. The human adolescent brain and alcohol use disorders. In: Galanter, M., ed. *Recent Developments in Alcoholism, Vol. 17: Alcohol Problems in Adolescents and Young Adults: Epidemiology, Neurobiology, Prevention, Treatment.* New York: Springer, 2005. pp. 177–197. PMID: 15789866

29. **Begleiter, H.**; Porjesz, B.; Bihari, B.; and Kissin, B. Event-related brain potentials in boys at risk for alcoholism. *Science* 255:1493–1496, 1984. PMID: 6474187

30. **Hill, S.Y.**, and Steinhauer, S.R. Assessment of prepubertal and postpubertal boys and girls at risk for developing alcoholism with P300 from a visual discrimination task. *Journal of Studies on Alcohol* 54:350–358, 1993. PMID: 8487544

31. **Dahl, R.E.**; Williamson, D.E.; Bertocci, M.A.; et al. Spectral analyses of sleep EEG in depressed offspring of fathers with or without a positive history of alcohol abuse or dependence: A pilot study. *Alcohol* 30:193–200, 2003. PMID: 13679113

32. **Hill, S.Y.**; De Bellis, M.D.; Keshavan, M.S.; et al. Right amygdala volume in adolescent and young adult offspring from families at high risk for developing alcoholism. *Biological Psychiatry* 49:894–905, 2001. PMID: 11377407

33. **Schweinsburg, A.D.**; Paulus, M.P.; Barlett, V.C.; et al. An fMRI study of response inhibition in youths with a family history of alcoholism. *Annals of the New York Academy of Sciences* 1021:391–394, 2004. PMID: 15251915

34. **Bauer, L.O.**, and Hesselbrock, V.M. P300 decrements in teenagers with conduct problems: Implications for substance abuse risk and brain development. *Biological Psychiatry* 46:263–272, 1999. PMID: 10418702

35. **Bauer, L.O.**, and Hesselbrock, V.M. Subtypes of family history and conduct disorder: Effects on P300 during the Stroop Test. *Neuropsychopharmacology* 21:51–62, 1999. PMID: 10379519

36. **Schuckit, M.A.** Biological, psychological and environmental predictors of the alcoholism risk: A longitudinal study. *Journal of Studies on Alcohol* 59:485–494, 1998. PMID: 9718100

37. **Schuckit, M.A.**, and Smith, T.L. Assessing the risk for alcoholism among sons of alcoholics. *Journal of Studies on Alcohol* 58:141–145, 1997. PMID: 9065891

38. **Tarter, R.E.**; Alterman, A.I.; and Edwards, K.L. Vulnerability to alcoholism in men: A behavior-genetic perspective. *Journal of Studies on Alcohol* 46:329–356, 1985. PMID: 4033133

39. **Reich, T.**; Edenberg, H.J.; Goate, A.; et al. Genome-wide search for genes affecting the risk for alcohol dependence. *American Journal of Medical Genetics* 81:207–215, 1998. PMID: 9603606

40. **Long, J.C.**; Knowler, W.C.; Hanson, R.L.; et al. Evidence for genetic linkage to alcohol dependence on chromosomes 4 and 11 from an autosome-wide scan in an American Indian population. *American Journal of Medical Genetics. Part B: Neuropsychiatric Genetics* 81:216–221, 1998. PMID: 9603607

41. **Foroud, T.**; Edenberg, H.J.; Goate, A.; et al. Alcoholism susceptibility loci: Confirmation studies in a replicate sample and further mapping. *Alcoholism: Clinical and Experimental Research* 24:933–945, 2000. PMID: 10923994

42. **Edenberg, H.J.**, and Kranzler, H.R. The contribution of genetics to addiction therapy approaches. *Pharmacology & Therapeutics 2005.* [Epub ahead of print] PMID: 16026844

43. **Rose, R.J.;** Dick, D.M.; Viken, R.J.; and Kaprio, J. Gene-environment interaction in patterns of adolescent drinking: Regional residency moderates longitudinal influences on alcohol use. *Alcoholism: Clinical and Experimental Research* 25:637–643, 2001. PMID: 11371711

44. **Halpern-Felsher, B.L.,** and Biehl, M. Developmental and environmental influences on underage drinking: A general overview. In: National Research Council and Institute of Medicine. Bonnie, R.J., and O'Connell, M.E., eds. *Reducing Underage Drinking: A Collective Responsibility.* Washington, DC: National Academies Press, 2004. pp. 402–416. . . .

45. **Castillo Mezzich, A.;** Giancola, P.R.; Lu, S.Y.K.S.; et al. Adolescent females with a substance use disorder: Affiliations with adult male sexual partners. *American Journal of Addictions* 8:190–200, 1999. PMID: 10506900

46. **Austin, E.W.,** and Knaus, C. Predicting the potential for risky behavior among those "too young" to drink as the result of appealing advertising. *Journal of Health Communications* 5:13–27, 2000. PMID: 10848029

47. **White, A.M.;** Jamieson-Drake, D.W.; and Swartzwelder, H.S. Prevalence and correlates of alcohol-induced blackouts among college students: Results of an e-mail survey. *Journal of American College Health* 51:122–131, 2002. PMID: 12638993

48. **Clark, D.B.;** Lynch, K.G.; Donovan, J.E.; and Block, G.D. Health problems in adolescents with alcohol use disorders: Self-report, liver injury, and physical examination findings and correlates. *Alcoholism: Clinical and Experimental Research* 25:1350–1359, 2001. PMID: 11584156

49. **Strauss, R.S.;** Barlow, S.E.; and Dietz, W.H. Prevalence of abnormal serum aminotransferase values in overweight and obese adolescents. *Journal of Pediatrics* 136:727–733, 2000. PMID: 10839867

50. **Mauras, N.;** Rogol, A.D.; Haymond, M.W.; and Veldhuis, J.D. Sex steroids, growth hormone, insulin-like growth factor-1: Neuroendocrine and metabolic regulation in puberty. *Hormone Research* 45:74–80, 1996. PMID: 8742123

51. **Dees, W.L.;** Srivastava, V.K.; and Hiney, J.K. Alcohol and female puberty: The role of intraovarian systems. *Alcohol Research & Health* 25(4):271–275, 2001. PMID: 11910704

52. **Sroufe, L.A.,** and Rutter, M. The domain of developmental psychopathology. *Child Development* 55:17–29, 1984. PMID: 6705619

53. **Greenough, W.T.;** Black, J.E.; and Wallace, C.S. Experience and brain development. *Child Development* 58:539–559, 1987. PMID: 3038480

54. **Masten, A.S.** Regulatory processes, risk, and resilience in adolescent development. *Annals of the New York Academy of Sciences* 1021:310–319, 2004. PMID: 15251901

55. **Steinman, K.J.,** and Schulenberg, J. A pattern-centered approach to evaluating substance use prevention programs. In: Damon, W.; Peck, S.C.; and Roeser, R.W.; eds. *New Directions for Child and Adolescent Development, Vol. 101: Person-Centered Approaches to Studying Development in Context.* San Francisco: Jossey-Bass, 2003. pp. 87–98

56. **Schulenberg J.;** O'Malley, P.M.; Bachman, J.G.; et al. Getting drunk and growing up: Trajectories of frequent binge drinking during the transition to young adulthood. *Journal of Studies on Alcohol* 57:289–304, 1996. PMID: 8709588

57. **Leung, S.F.,** and Phelps, C.E. My kingdom for a drink. . . . ? A review of estimates of the price sensitivity of demand for alcoholic beverages. In: Hilton, M.E., and Bloss, G., eds. *Economics and the Prevention of Alcohol-Related Problems.* NIAAA Research Monograph No. 25. Rockville, MD: National Institute on Alcohol Abuse and Alcoholism, 1993. pp. 1–31.

58. **Kenkel, D.S.**, and Manning, W.G. Perspectives on alcohol taxation. *Alcohol Health & Research World* 20(4):230–238, 1996.

59. **Chaloupka, F.J.**; Grossman, M.; and Saffer, H. The effects of price on the consequences of alcohol use and abuse. In: Galanter, M., ed. *Recent Developments in Alcoholism, Vol. 14: The Consequences of Alcoholism.* New York: Plenum Press, 1998. pp. 331–346. PMID: 9751952

60. **Cook, P.J.**, and Moore, M.J. The economics of alcohol abuse and alcohol-control policies. *Health Affairs* 21:120–133, 2002. PMID: 11900152

61. **Wagenaar, A.C.**, and Toomey, T.L. Effects of minimum drinking age laws: Review and analyses of the literature from 1960 to 2000. *Journal of Studies on Alcohol* (Suppl. 14):206–225, 2002. PMID: 12022726

62. **Kypri, K.**; Voas, R.B.; Langley, J.D.; et al. Minimum purchasing age for alcohol and traffic crash injuries among 15- to 19-year-olds in New Zealand. *American Journal of Public Health* 96:126–131, 2006.

63. **Hingson, R.**; Heeren, T.; and Winter, M. Lower legal blood alcohol limits for young drivers. *Public Health Reports* 109:738–744, 1994. PMID: 7800781

64. **Jones, R.K.**, and Lacey, J.H. *Alcohol and Highway Safety 2001: A Review of the State of Knowledge.* DOT Pub. No. HS-809-383. Washington, DC: National Highway Traffic Safety Administration, 2001. . . . .

65. **Preusser, D.F.**; Williams, A.F.; and Weinstein, H.B. Policing underage alcohol sales. *Journal of Safety Research* 25:127–133, 1994.

66. **National Institute on Alcohol Abuse and Alcoholism.** Interventions for alcohol use and alcohol use disorders in youth. *Alcohol Research & Health* 28(3):163–174, 2004/2005.

67. **Barnes, G.M.**; Reifman, A.S.; Farrell, M.P.; and Dintcheff, B.A. The effects of parenting on the development of adolescent alcohol misuse: A six-wave latent growth model. *Journal of Marriage and Family* 62:175–186, 2000.

68. **Steinberg, L.**; Fletcher, A.; and Darling, N. Parental monitoring and peer influences on adolescent substance use. *Pediatrics* 93(6 Pt 2):1060–1064, 1994. PMID: 8197008

69. **Spoth, R.L.**; Redmond, C.; and Shin, C. Randomized trial of brief family interventions for general populations: Adolescent substance use outcomes 4 years following baseline. *Journal of Consulting and Clinical Psychology* 69:627–642, 2001. PMID: 11550729

70. **Spoth, R.**; Redmond, C.; Shin, C.; and Azevedo, K. Brief family intervention effects on adolescent substance initiation: School-level growth curve analyses 6 years following baseline. *Journal of Consulting and Clinical Psychology* 72:535–542, 2004. PMID: 15279537

71. **National Research Council (NRC) and Institute of Medicine (IOM),** Committee on Developing a Strategy to Reduce and Prevent Underage Drinking. Bonnie, R.J., and O'Connell, M.E., eds. *Reducing Underage Drinking: A Collective Responsibility.* Washington, DC: National Academies Press, 2004. . . . .

72. **Hingson, R.W.**, and Howland, J. Comprehensive community interventions to promote health: Implications for college-age drinking problems. *Journal of Studies on Alcohol* (Suppl. 14):226–240, 2002. PMID: 12022727

73. **Holder, H.D.** Community prevention of alcohol problems. *Addictive Behaviors* 25:843–859, 2000. PMID: 11125775

74. **Wagenaar, A.C.**; Murray, D.M.; Gehan, J.P.; et al. Communities Mobilizing for Change on Alcohol: Outcomes from a randomized community trial. *Journal of Studies on Alcohol* 61:85–94, 2000. PMID: 10627101

75. **Wagenaar, A.C.;** Murray, D.M.; and Toomey, T.L. Communities Mobilizing for Change on Alcohol (CMCA): Effects of a randomized trial on arrests and traffic crashes. *Addiction* 95:209–217, 2000. PMID: 10723849

76. **Perry, C.L.;** Williams, C.L.; Komro, K.A.; et al. Project Northland: Long-term outcomes of community action to reduce adolescent alcohol use. *Health Education Research* 17:117–132, 2002. PMID: 11888042

POSTSCRIPT

Are Drinking Age Laws Effective?

In view of the fact that the majority of youths consume alcohol, is it a worthwhile endeavor to try to teach young people how to drink responsibly? Are young people capable of drinking responsibly? Can young people learn to moderate their behavior, especially as those behaviors apply to alcohol consumption. In some areas, young people have shown that they are capable of being responsible. Despite that many young people get into accidents when operating motor vehicles, most do not have accidents. Many parents trust their children with babysitters. Putting the care of our children into the hands of young people shows much trust. Many young people hold jobs and are very responsible in that regard. Young people are allowed to own firearms and most understand the importance of handling firearms responsibly.

In many ways young people are treated as adults. For example, one can join the military prior to age 21. Many young people are sent to war where they are placed in jeopardy. Eighteen-year-olds are allowed, and encouraged, to vote. One can marry and bear children long before age 21. If one can be legally allowed to go to war, get married, and produce children, one could ask the question whether it is hypocritical to prohibit those under age 21 from drinking alcohol.

Of course, there is a major difference between an 18-, 19-, or 20-year-old drinking alcohol than one who is age 14 or age 15. If older teens are given the message of responsible drinking, then younger teens may interpret that it is okay for them to drink if they do so responsibly. Presumably, maturity comes with age. For example, it has been clearly shown that the younger one is when drinking is initiated, the greater the likelihood that dependency may develop. Besides the obvious physical problems associated with heavy alcohol abuse, such as those of the liver and endocrine system, young people who drink also have behavioral problems like being disruptive, aggressive, and rebellious. Anxiety and depression are associated with youth drinking also. According to statistics from the federal government, there are 1.4 million youth who meet the criteria for alcohol abuse or dependency.

To prevent youth drinking, the U.S. Department of Health and Human Services report recommends that the price of alcohol should be increased and that there should be stricter enforcement of laws. In particular, it is suggested that there should be zero tolerance for underage drinking and for those individuals and establishments that sell alcohol. Among those under age 21, approximately 1,900 die from motor vehicle crashes, 1,600 due to homicide, and 300 more from suicide. These statistics substantiate the need for preventing underage drinking according to the U.S. Department of Health and Human Services. Judith McMullen points out the inconsistency in a policy that

95

forbids alcohol consumption prior to age 21. Young people between ages 18 and 21 have discretion when it comes to health care decisions, educational decisions, and smoking.

Articles that address some of the problems and issues of underage drinking include "Binge Drinking and Associated Health Risk Behaviors among High School Students," by Jacqueline Miller and others (*Pediatrics*, January 2007); "Societal Cost of Underage Drinking," by Ted Miller and associates (*Journal of Studies on Alcohol*, July 2006); and "High School Drinking and Its Consequences," by C.M. Arata and colleagues (*Adolescence*, 2003).

ISSUE 4

Are the Dangers of Ecstasy (MDMA) Overstated?

YES: Jacob Sullum, from "Sex, Drugs and Techno Music," *Reason* (January 2002)

NO: National Institute on Drug Abuse, from "MDMA (Ecstasy) Abuse," *National Institute on Drug Abuse Research Report* (March 2006)

ISSUE SUMMARY

YES: Jacob Sullum, a senior editor at *Reason* magazine, contends that the effects of drugs such as Ecstasy, particularly in regard to sexual behavior, are exaggerated. Sullum refers to the history of marijuana and how it was deemed a drug that would make people engage in behaviors that they would not typically engage in. Sullum feels that the public's reaction is unjustified.

NO: Club drugs such as Ecstasy allow partygoers to dance and remain active for long periods of time according to the National Institute on Drug Abuse (NIDA). However, Ecstasy may produce a number of adverse effects such as high blood pressure, panic attacks, loss of consciousness, seizures, and death. Moreover, Ecstasy can produce negative effects on the brain, resulting in confusion, depression, memory impairment, and attention difficulties.

Although national surveys of secondary students in the United States have shown a decrease in the use of Ecstasy (MDMA), 11 million persons have used the drug at least once and nearly one half million people used it in the past month. The number of people admitted to emergency rooms due to adverse reactions to Ecstasy and other club drugs are significant also. In the year 2005, almost 11,000 people visited emergency rooms due to Ecstasy. As for other club drugs or hallucinogens, there were 1,864 emergency room visits attributed to LSD, 1,861 emergency room visits due to GHB, 275 visits due to Ketamine (Special K), and 7,535 visits due to PCP.

According to some drug experts, Ecstasy use at rave parties and among gay and bisexual men is deeply embedded. One could argue that enforcing laws more tightly against club drugs like Ecstasy increases the likelihood that adverse effects will occur because there would be no oversight on the purity of the drugs. This raises the question of whether it would be better to educate individuals about the potential harm of Ecstasy or simply be more vigilant in preventing its use. One of the problems associated with buying illegal drugs is that they are not always what they are purported to be. One cannot be sure of the authenticity of the drug being purchased. Moreover, if one is sold a bogus drug, one has no legal recourse.

Because Ecstasy is used at rave parties, attempts to make these parties and similar activities illegal are occurring on the national level as well as on the local level. A bipartisan bill was introduced into the Senate "to prohibit an individual from knowingly opening, maintaining, managing, controlling, renting, leasing, making available for use, or profiting from any place for the purpose of manufacturing, distributing, or using any controlled substance, and for other purposes." This act is referred to as the "Reducing Americans' Vulnerability to Ecstasy Act of 2002" or the "RAVE Act." Penalties could include 20 years in prison or a fine of $250,000 or twice the gross receipts derived from each violation, whichever is more. One potential problem with the bill is that its language is broad enough to close down any business or establishment where any drug use or transaction occurs.

There is concern that Ecstasy use will lead to adverse physical reactions as well as reckless behavior. One consequence of Ecstasy use is dehydration due to a rise in body temperature (hyperthermia). According to the National Institute on Drug Abuse (NIDA), some of the other potential effects from Ecstasy include profuse sweating, teeth grinding, high blood pressure, anxiety, aggressiveness, muscle cramping, panic attacks, nausea, loss of consciousness, and seizures. Whether or not Ecstasy is addictive still remains a subject of debate. Similarly, whether or not Ecstasy causes brain damage continues to be debated.

The following selections debate whether the dangers of Ecstasy are overstated. The effects of Ecstasy and other club drugs represent a serious threat to the physical and emotional well-being of young people according to the National Institute on Drug Abuse. Jacob Sullum acknowledges that drugs like Ecstasy have the potential to cause harm. In addition, Sullum notes that many drugs sold as Ecstasy are something else entirely. However, he feels that warnings associated with drugs are blown out of proportion and that the dangers of Ecstasy are exaggerated.

YES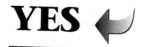

Jacob Sullum

Sex, Drugs, and Techno Music

[In 2001], the Chicago City Council decided "to crack down on wild rave parties that lure youngsters into environments loaded with dangerous club drugs, underage drinking and sometimes predatory sexual behavior," as the *Chicago Tribune* put it. The newspaper described raves as "one-night-only parties . . . often held in warehouses or secret locations where people pay to dance, do drugs, play loud music, and engage in random sex acts." Taking a dim view of such goings-on, the city council passed an ordinance threatening to jail building owners or managers who allowed raves to be held on their property. Mayor Richard Daley took the occasion to "lash out at the people who produce the huge rogue dance parties where Ecstasy and other designer drugs are widely used." In Daley's view, rave promoters were deliberately seducing the innocent. "They are after all of our children," he warned. "Parents should be outraged by this."

The reaction against raves reflects familiar anxieties about what the kids are up to, especially when it comes to sex. As the chemical symbol of raves, MDMA—a.k.a. Ecstasy—has come to represent sexual abandon and, partly through association with other "club drugs," sexual assault. These are not the only fears raised by MDMA. The drug, whose full name is methylene-dioxymethamphetamine, has also been accused of causing brain damage and of leading people astray with ersatz feelings of empathy and euphoria (concerns discussed later in this article). But the sexual angle is interesting because it has little to do with the drug's actual properties, a situation for which there is considerable precedent in the history of reputed aphrodisiacs.

A relative of both amphetamine and mescaline, MDMA is often described as a stimulant with psychedelic qualities. But its effects are primarily emotional, without the perceptual changes caused by LSD. Although MDMA was first synthesized by the German drug company Merck in 1912, it did not gain a following until the 1970s, when the psychonautical chemist Alexander Shulgin, a Dow researcher turned independent consultant, tried some at the suggestion of a graduate student he was helping a friend supervise. "It was not a psychedelic in the visual or interpretive sense," he later wrote, "but the lightness and warmth of the psychedelic was present and quite remarkable." MDMA created a "window," he decided. "It enabled me to see out, and to see my own insides, without distortions or reservations."

After observing some striking examples of people who claimed to have overcome serious personal problems (including a severe stutter and oppressive guilt) with the help of MDMA, Shulgin introduced the drug to a psychologist he knew who had already used psychedelics as an aid to therapy. "Adam," the pseudonym that Shulgin gave him (also a nickname for the drug), was on the verge of retiring, but was so impressed by MDMA's effects that he decided to continue working. He shared his techniques with other psychologists and psychiatrists, and under his influence thousands of people reportedly used the drug to enhance communication and self-insight. "It seemed to dissolve fear for a few hours," says a psychiatrist who tried MDMA in the early '80s. "I thought it would have been very useful for working with people with trauma disorders." Shulgin concedes that there was "a hint of snake-oil" in MDMA's reputed versatility, but he himself considered it "an incredible tool." He quotes one psychiatrist as saying, "MDMA is penicillin for the soul, and you don't give up penicillin, once you've seen what it can do."

Shulgin did not see MDMA exclusively as a psychotherapeutic tool. He also referred to it as "my low-calorie martini," a way of loosening up and relating more easily to others at social gatherings. This aspect of the drug came to the fore in the '80s, when MDMA became popular among nightclubbers in Texas, where it was marketed as a party drug under the name *Ecstasy*. The open recreational use of Ecstasy at clubs in Dallas and Austin brought down the wrath of the Drug Enforcement Administration [DEA], which decided to put MDMA in the same legal category as heroin. Researchers who emphasized the drug's psychotherapeutic potential opposed the ban. "We had no idea psychiatrists were using it," a DEA pharmacologist told *Newsweek* in 1985. Nor did they care: Despite an administrative law judge's recommendation that doctors be allowed to prescribe the drug, the ban on MDMA took effect the following year.

Thus MDMA followed the same pattern as LSD, moving from discreet psychotherapeutic use to the sort of conspicuous consumption that was bound to provoke a government reaction. Like LSD, it became illegal because too many people started to enjoy it. Although the DEA probably would have sought to ban any newly popular intoxicant, the name change certainly didn't help. In *Ecstasy: The MDMA Story*, Bruce Eisner quotes a distributor who claimed to have originated the name *Ecstasy*. He said he picked it "because it would sell better than calling it 'Empathy.' 'Empathy' would be more appropriate, but how many people know what it means?" In its traditional sense, *ecstasy* has a spiritual connotation, but in common usage it simply means intense pleasure—often the kind associated with sex. As David Smith, director of the Haight-Ashbury Free Clinic, observed, the name "suggested that it made sex better." Some marketers have been more explicit: A 1999 article in the *Journal of Toxicology* (headlined "SEX on the Streets of Cincinnati") reported an analysis of "unknown tablets imprinted with 'SEX'" that turned out to contain MDMA.

Hyperbolic comments by some users have reinforced Ecstasy's sexual connotations. "One enthusiast described the feeling as a six-hour orgasm!" exclaimed the author of a 2000 op-ed piece in Malaysia's *New Straits Times*, picking up a phrase quoted in *Time* a couple of months before. A column in *The Toronto Sun*, meanwhile, stated matter-of-factly that MDMA "can even make you feel like a six-hour orgasm." If simply taking MDMA makes you feel that way, readers might reasonably conclude, MDMA-enhanced sex must be indescribably good.

Another reason MDMA came to be associated with sex is its reputation as a "hug drug" that breaks down emotional barriers and brings out feelings of affection. The warmth and candor of people who've taken MDMA may be interpreted as flirtatiousness. More generally, MDMA is said to remove fear, which is one reason psychotherapists have found it so useful. The same effect could also be described as a loss of inhibitions, often a precursor to sexual liaisons. Finally, users report enhanced pleasure from physical sensations, especially the sense of touch. They often trade hugs, caresses, and back rubs.

Yet the consensus among users seems to be that MDMA's effects are more sensual than sexual. According to a therapist quoted by Jerome Beck and Marsha Rosenbaum in their book *Pursuit of Ecstasy*, "MDMA and sex do not go very well together. For most people, MDMA turns off the ability to function as a lover, to put it indelicately. It's called the love drug because it opens up the capacity to feel loving and affectionate and trusting." At the same time, however, it makes the "focusing of the body and the psychic energy necessary to achieve orgasm . . . very difficult. And most men find it impossible. . . . So it is a love drug but not a sex drug for most people."

Although this distinction is widely reported by users, press coverage has tended to perpetuate the connection between MDMA and sex. In 1985 *Newsweek* said the drug "is considered an aphrodisiac," while *Maclean's* played up one user's claim of "very good sexual possibilities." *Life* also cited "the drug's reputation for good sex," even while noting that it "blocks male ejaculation." More recently, a 2000 story about MDMA in *Time* began by describing "a classic Southeast Asian den of iniquity" where prostitutes used Ecstasy so they could be "friendly and outgoing." It warned that "because users feel empathetic, ecstasy can lower sexual inhibitions. Men generally cannot get erections when high on one, but they are often ferociously randy when its effects begin to fade." The story cited a correlation between MDMA use and "unprotected sex." A cautionary article in *Cosmopolitan* began with the account of "a 28-year-old lawyer from Los Angeles" who brought home a man with whom she felt "deeply connected" under the influence of MDMA. "We would have had sex, but he couldn't get an erection," she reported. "The next day, I was horrified that I had let a guy I couldn't even stand into my bed!"

Rape Drugs

MDMA has been linked not just to regrettable sexual encounters but to rapes in which drugs are used as weapons. The connection is usually made indirectly, by way of other drugs whose effects are quite different but which are also popular at raves and dance clubs. In particular, the depressants GHB and Rohypnol have acquired reputations as "date rape drugs," used to incapacitate victims to whom they are given surreptitiously. Needless to say, this is not the main use for these substances, which people generally take on purpose because they like their effects. It's not clear exactly how often rapists use GHB or Rohypnol, but such cases are surely much rarer than the hysterical reaction from the press and Congress (which passed a Date Rape Drug Prohibition Act [in 2001]) would lead one to believe. The public has nonetheless come to view these intoxicants primarily as instruments of assault, an impression that has affected the image of other "club drugs," especially MDMA.

Grouping MDMA with GHB and Rohypnol, a 2000 Knight Ridder story warned that the dangers of "club drugs" include "vulnerability to sexual assault." Similarly, the *Chicago Tribune* cited Ecstasy as the most popular "club drug" before referring to "women who suspect they were raped after they used or were slipped a club drug." In a *Columbus Dispatch* op-ed piece, pediatrician Peter D. Rogers further obscured the distinction between MDMA and the so-called rape drugs by saying that "Ecstasy . . . comes in three forms," including "GHB, also called liquid Ecstasy," and "Herbal Ecstasy, also known as ma huang or ephedra" (a legal stimulant), as well as "MDMA, or chemical Ecstasy." He asserted, without citing a source, that "so-called Ecstasy"—it's not clear which one he meant—"has been implicated nationally in the sexual assaults of approximately 5,000 teen-age and young adult women." Rogers described a 16-year-old patient who "took Ecstasy and was raped twice. She told me that she remembers the rapes but, high on the drug, was powerless to stop them. She couldn't even scream, let alone fight back." If Rogers, identified as a member of the American Academy of Pediatrics' Committee on Substance Abuse, had trouble keeping the "club drugs" straight, it's not surprising that the general public saw little difference between giving a date MDMA and slipping her a mickey.

As the alleged connections between MDMA and sex illustrate, the concept of an aphrodisiac is complex and ambiguous. A drug could be considered an aphrodisiac because it reduces resistance, because it increases interest, because it improves ability, or because it enhances enjoyment. A particular drug could be effective for one or two of these purposes but useless (or worse) for the others. Shakespeare observed that alcohol "provokes the desire, but it takes away the performance." Something similar seems to be true of MDMA, except that the desire is more emotional than sexual, a sense of closeness that may find expression in sex that is apt to be aborted because of difficulty in getting an erection or reaching orgasm. Also like alcohol, MDMA is blamed for causing people to act against their considered judgment. The concern is not just that people might have casual sex but that they might regret it afterward.

Surely this concern is not entirely misplaced. As the old saw has it, "Candy is dandy, but liquor is quicker." When drinking precedes sex, there may be a fine line between seducing someone and taking advantage, between lowering inhibitions and impairing judgment. But the possibility of crossing that line does not mean that alcohol is nothing but a trick employed by cads. Nor does the possibility of using alcohol to render someone incapable of resistance condemn it as a tool of rapists.

The closest thing we have to a genuine aphrodisiac—increasing interest, ability, and enjoyment—is Viagra, the avowed purpose of which is to enable people to have more and better sex. Instead of being deplored as an aid to hedonism, it is widely praised for increasing the net sum of human happiness. Instead of being sold on the sly in dark nightclubs, it's pitched on television by a former Senate majority leader. The difference seems to be that Viagra is viewed as a legitimate medicine, approved by the government and prescribed by doctors.

But as Joann Ellison Rodgers, author of *Drugs and Sexual Behavior*, observes, "there is great unease with the idea of encouraging sexual prowess. . . . At the very least, drugs in the service of sex do seem to subvert or at least trivialize important aspects of sexual experiences, such as love, romance, commitment, trust and health." If we've managed to accept Viagra and (to a lesser extent) alcohol as aphrodisiacs, it may be only because we've projected their darker possibilities onto other substances, of which the "club drugs" are just the latest examples.

Signal of Misunderstanding

The current worries about raves in some ways resemble the fears once symbolized by the opium den. The country's first anti-opium laws, passed by Western states in the late 19th century, were motivated largely by hostility toward the low-cost Chinese laborers who competed for work with native whites. Supporters of such legislation, together with a sensationalist press, popularized the image of the sinister Chinaman who lured white women into his opium den, turning them into concubines, prostitutes, or sex slaves. Although users generally find that opiates dampen their sex drive, "it was commonly reported that opium smoking aroused sexual desire," writes historian David Courtwright, "and that some shameless smokers persuaded 'innocent girls to smoke in order to excite their passions and effect their ruin.'" San Francisco authorities lamented that the police "have found white women and Chinamen side by side under the effects of this drug—a humiliating sight to anyone who has anything left of manhood." In 1910 Hamilton Wright, a U.S. diplomat who was a key player in the passage of federal anti-drug legislation, told Congress that "one of the most unfortunate phases of the habit of smoking opium in this country" was "the large number of women who [had] become involved and were living as common-law wives or cohabiting with Chinese in the Chinatowns of our various cities."

Fears of miscegenation also played a role in popular outrage about cocaine, which was said to make blacks uppity and prone to violence against whites, especially sexual assault. In 1910 Christopher Koch, a member of the Pennsylvania Pharmacy Board who pushed for a federal ban on cocaine, informed Congress that "the colored people seem to have a weakness for it. . . . They would just as leave rape a woman as anything else, and a great many of the southern rape cases have been traced to cocaine." Describing cocaine's effect on "hitherto inoffensive, law abiding negroes" in the *Medical Record*, Edward Huntington Williams warned that "sexual desires are increased and perverted."

Marijuana, another drug that was believed to cause violence, was also linked to sex crimes and, like opium, seduction. Under marijuana's influence, according to a widely cited 1932 report in *The Journal of Criminal Law and Criminology*, "sexual desires are stimulated and may lead to unnatural acts, such as indecent exposure and rape." The authors quoted an informant who "reported several instances of which he claimed to have positive knowledge, where boys had induced girls to use the weed for the purpose of seducing them." The federal Bureau of Narcotics, which collected anecdotes about marijuana's baneful effects to support a national ban on the drug, cited "colored students at the Univ. of Minn. partying with female students (white) smoking [marijuana] and getting their sympathy with stories of racial persecution. Result pregnancy." The bureau also described a case in which "two Negroes took a girl fourteen years old and kept her for two days in a hut under the influence of marijuana. Upon recovery she was found to be suffering from syphilis."

Drug-related horror stories nowadays are rarely so explicitly racist. A notable and surprising exception appears in the 2000 film *Traffic*, which is critical of the war on drugs but nevertheless represents the utter degradation of an upper-middle-class white teenager who gets hooked on crack by showing her having sex with a black man. Whether related to race or not, parental anxieties about sexual activity among teenagers have not gone away, and drugs are a convenient scapegoat when kids seem to be growing up too fast.

The link between drugs and sex was reinforced by the free-love ethos of the '60s counterculture that embraced marijuana and LSD. In the public mind, pot smoking, acid dropping, and promiscuous sex were all part of the same lifestyle; a chaste hippie chick was a contradiction in terms. When Timothy Leary extolled LSD's sex-enhancing qualities in a 1966 interview with *Playboy*, he fueled the fears of parents who worried that their daughters would be seduced into a decadent world of sex, drugs, and rock 'n' roll. The Charles Manson case added a sinister twist to this scenario, raising the possibility of losing one's daughter to an evil cult leader who uses LSD to brainwash his followers, in much the same way as Chinese men were once imagined to enthrall formerly respectable white girls with opium.

The alarm about the sexual repercussions of "club drugs," then, has to be understood in the context of warnings about other alleged aphrodisiacs, often identified with particular groups perceived as inferior, threatening, or both. The fear of uncontrolled sexual impulses, of the chaos that would result if we let our basic instincts run wild, is projected onto these groups and, by extension, their intoxicants. In the case of "club drugs," adolescents are both victims and perpetrators. Parents fear for their children, but they also fear them. When Mayor Daley warned that "they are after all of our children," he may have been imagining predators in the mold of Fu Manchu or Charles Manson. But the reality is that raves—which grew out of the British "acid house" movement, itself reminiscent of the psychedelic dance scene that emerged in San Francisco during the late '60s—are overwhelmingly a youth phenomenon.

The experience of moving all night to a throbbing beat amid flickering light has been likened to tribal dancing around a fire. But for most people over 30, the appeal of dancing for hours on end to the fast, repetitive rhythm of techno music is hard to fathom. "The sensationalist reaction that greets every mention of the word *Ecstasy* in this country is part of a wider, almost unconscious fear of young people," writes Jonathan Keane in the British *New Statesman*, and the observation applies equally to the United States. For "middle-aged and middle-class opinion leaders . . . E is a symbol of a youth culture they don't understand."

This is not to say that no one ever felt horny after taking MDMA. Individual reactions to drugs are highly variable, and one could probably find anecdotes suggesting aphrodisiac properties for almost any psychoactive substance. And it is no doubt true that some MDMA users, like the woman quoted in *Cosmo*, have paired up with sexual partners they found less attractive the morning after. But once MDMA is stripped of its symbolism, these issues are no different from those raised by alcohol. In fact, since MDMA users tend to be more lucid than drinkers, the chances that they will do something regrettable are probably lower.

I Love You Guys

Another alcohol-related hazard, one that seems to be more characteristic of MDMA than the risk of casual sex or rape, is the possibility of inappropriate emotional intimacy. The maudlin drunk who proclaims his affection for everyone and reveals secrets he might later wish he had kept is a widely recognized character, either comical or pathetic depending upon one's point of view. Given MDMA's reputation as a "love drug," it's natural to wonder whether it fosters the same sort of embarrassing behavior.

Tom Cowan, a systems analyst in his 30s, has used MDMA a few times, and he doesn't think it revealed any deep emotional truths. (All names of drug users in this story are pseudonyms.) "For me," he says, "it was almost too much of a fake. . . . It was too artificial for me. . . . I felt warm. I felt loved. All of those sensations came upon me. . . . I had all these feelings, but I knew that deep down I didn't feel that, so at the same time there was that inner struggle as far as just letting loose and just being. . . . That was difficult because of the fakeness about it for me." More typically, MDMA users perceive the warm feelings as real, both at the time and in retrospect. Some emphasize an enhanced connection to friends, while others report a feeling of benevolence toward people in general.

"I was very alert but very relaxed at the same time," says Alison Witt, a software engineer in her 20s. "I didn't love everybody. . . . It's a very social drug, and you do feel connected to other people, but I think it's more because it creates a sense of relaxation and pleasure with people you're familiar with." Walter Stevenson, a neuroscientist in his late 20s, gives a similar account: "I felt really happy to have my friends around me. I just enjoyed sitting there and spending time with them, not necessarily talking about anything, but not to the degree that I felt particularly attracted or warm to people I didn't know. I was very friendly and open to meeting people, but there wasn't anything inappropriate about the feeling."

Adam Newman, an Internet specialist in his 20s, believes his MDMA use has helped improve his social life. "It kind of catapulted me past a bunch of shyness and other mental and emotional blocks," he says. Even when he wasn't using MDMA, "I felt a lot better than I had in social interactions before." Bruce Rogers, a horticulturist in his 40s, says one thing he likes about MDMA is that "you can find something good in somebody that you dislike." He thinks "it would make the world a better place if everybody did it just once."

That's the kind of assertion, reminiscent of claims about LSD's earth-shaking potential, that tends to elicit skeptical smiles. But the important point is that many MDMA users believe the drug has lasting psychological benefits, even when it's taken in a recreational context—the sort of thing you don't often hear about alcohol.

Not surprisingly, people who use MDMA in clubs and at raves emphasize its sensual and stimulant properties, the way it enhances music and dancing. But they also talk about a sense of connectedness, especially at raves. Jasmine Menendez, a public relations director in her early 20s who has used MDMA both at raves and with small groups of friends, says it provides "a great body high. I lose all sense of inhibition and my full potential is released. . . . It allows me to get closer to people and to myself."

Too Much Fun

Euphoria is a commonly reported effect of MDMA, which raises the usual concerns about the lure of artificial pleasure. "It was an incredible feeling of being tremendously happy where I was and being content in a basic way," Stevenson recalls of the first time he felt MDMA's effects. He used it several more times after that, but it never became a regular habit.

Menendez, on the other hand, found MDMA "easy to become addicted to" because "you see the full potential in yourself and others; you feel like you won the lottery." She began chasing that feeling one weekend after another, often taking several pills in one night. "Doing e as much as I did affected my relationship with my mother," she says. "I would come home cracked out from a night of partying and sleep the whole day. She couldn't invite anyone over because I was always sleeping. She said that my party habits were out of control. We fought constantly. I would also go to work high from the party, if I had to work weekends. The comedown was horrible because I wanted to sleep and instead I had to be running around doing errands."

Menendez decided to cut back on her MDMA consumption, and recently she has been using it only on special occasions. "I think I've outgrown it finally," she says. "I used e to do some serious soul-searching and to come out of my shell, learning all I could about who I really am. I'm grateful that I had the experiences that I did and wouldn't change it for the world. But now, being 23, I'm ready to embrace mental clarity fully. Ecstasy is definitely a constructive tool and if used correctly can benefit the user. It changed my life for the better, and because of what I learned about myself, I'm ready to start a new life without it."

Sustained heavy use of MDMA is rare, partly because it's impractical. MDMA works mainly by stimulating the release of the neurotransmitter sero-tonin. Taking it depletes the brain's supply, which may not return to normal levels for a week or more. Some users report a hangover period of melancholy and woolly-headedness that can last a few days. As frequency of use increases,

MDMA's euphoric and empathetic effects diminish and its unpleasant side effects, including jitteriness and hangovers, intensify. Like LSD, it has a self-limiting quality, which is reflected in patterns of use. In a 2000 survey, 8.2 percent of high school seniors reported trying MDMA in the previous year. Less than half of them (3.6 percent) had used it in the previous month, and virtually none reported "daily" use (defined as use on 20 or more occasions in the previous 30 days). To parents, of course, any use of MDMA is alarming, and the share of seniors who said they'd ever tried the drug nearly doubled between 1996 and 2000, when it reached 11 percent.

Parental fears have been stoked by reports of sudden fatalities among MDMA users. Given the millions of doses consumed each year, such cases are remarkably rare: The Drug Abuse Warning Network counted nine MDMA-related deaths in 1998. The most common cause of death is dehydration and overheating. MDMA impairs body temperature regulation and accelerates fluid loss, which can be especially dangerous for people dancing vigorously in crowded, poorly ventilated spaces for hours at a time. The solution to this problem, well-known to experienced ravers, is pretty straightforward: avoid clubs and parties where conditions are stifling, take frequent rests, abstain from alcohol (which compounds dehydration), and drink plenty of water. MDMA also interacts dangerously with some prescription drugs (including monoamine oxidase inhibitors, a class of antidepressants), and it raises heart rate and blood pressure, of special concern for people with cardiovascular conditions.

Another hazard is a product of the black market created by prohibition: Tablets or capsules sold as Ecstasy may in fact contain other, possibly more dangerous drugs. In tests by private U.S. laboratories, more than one-third of "Ecstasy" pills turned out to be bogus. (The samples were not necessarily representative, and the results may be on the high side, since the drugs were submitted voluntarily for testing, perhaps by buyers who had reason to be suspicious.) Most of the MDMA substitutes, which included caffeine, ephedrine, and aspirin, were relatively harmless, but one of them, the cough suppressant dextromethorphan (DXM), has disturbing psychoactive effects in high doses, impedes the metabolism of MDMA, and blocks perspiration, raising the risk of overheating. Another drug that has been passed off as MDMA is paramethoxyamphetamine (PMA), which is potentially lethal in doses over 50 milligrams, especially when combined with other drugs. In 2000 the DEA reported 10 deaths tied to PMA. Wary Ecstasy users can buy test kits or have pills analyzed by organizations such as DanceSafe, which sets up booths at raves and nightclubs.

Nervous Breakdown

Generally speaking, a careful user can avoid the short-term dangers of MDMA. Of more concern is the possibility of long-term brain damage. In animal studies, high or repeated doses of MDMA cause degeneration of serotonin nerve receptors, and some of the changes appear to be permanent. The relevance of these studies to human use of MDMA is unclear because we don't know whether the same changes occur in people or, if they do, at what doses and with what practical consequences. Studies of human users, which often have serious methodological shortcomings, so far have been inconclusive.

Still, the possibility of lasting damage to memory should not be lightly dismissed. There's enough reason for concern that MDMA should no longer be treated as casually as "a low-calorie martini." If the fears of neurotoxicity prove to be well-founded and a safe dose cannot be estimated with any confidence, a prudent person would need a good reason—probably better than a fun night out—to take the risk. On the other hand, the animal research suggests that it may be possible to avoid neural damage by preventing hyperthermia or by taking certain drugs (for example, Prozac) in conjunction with MDMA. In that case, such precautions would be a requirement of responsible use.

However the debate about MDMA's long-term effects turns out, we should be wary of claims that it (or any drug) makes people "engage in random sex acts." Like the idea that certain intoxicants make people lazy, crazy, or violent, it vastly oversimplifies a complex interaction between the drug, the user, and the context. As MDMA's versatility demonstrates, the same drug can be different things to different people. Michael Buchanan, a retired professor in his early 70s, has used MDMA several times with one or two other people. "It's just wonderful," he says, "to bring closeness, intimacy—not erotic intimacy at all, but a kind of spiritual intimacy, a loving relationship, an openness to dialogue that nothing else can quite match." When I mention MDMA use at raves, he says, "I don't understand how the kids can use it that way."

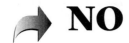
MDMA (Ecstasy) Abuse

What Is MDMA?

MDMA is an illegal drug that acts as both a stimulant and psychedelic, producing an energizing effect, as well as distortions in time and perception and enhanced enjoyment from tactile experiences. Typically, MDMA (an acronym for its chemical name 3,4-methylenedioxymethamphetamine) is taken orally, usually in a tablet or capsule, and its effects last approximately 3 to 6 hours. The average reported dose is one to two tablets, with each tablet typically containing between 60 and 120 milligrams of MDMA. It is not uncommon for users to take a second dose of the drug as the effects of the first dose begin to fade.

MDMA can affect the brain by altering the activity of chemical messengers, or neurotransmitters, which enable nerve cells in the brain to communicate with one another. Research in animals has shown that MDMA in moderate to high doses can be toxic to nerve cells that contain serotonin and can cause long-lasting damage to them. Furthermore, MDMA raises body temperature. On rare but largely unpredictable occasions, this has led to severe medical consequences, including death. Also, MDMA causes the release of another neurotransmitter, norepinephrine, which is likely the cause of the increase in heart rate and blood pressure that often accompanies MDMA use.

Although MDMA is known universally among users as ecstasy, researchers have determined that many ecstasy tablets contain not only MDMA but also a number of other drugs or drug combinations that can be harmful as well. Adulterants found in MDMA tablets purchased on the street include methamphetamine, caffeine, the over-the-counter cough suppressant dextromethorphan, the diet drug ephedrine, and cocaine. Also, as with many other drugs of abuse, MDMA is rarely used alone. It is not uncommon for users to mix MDMA with other substances, such as alcohol and marijuana.

A Brief History of MDMA

MDMA was developed in Germany in the early 1900s as a parent compound to be used to synthesize other pharmaceuticals. During the 1970s, in the United States, some psychiatrists began using MDMA as a psychotherapeutic tool, despite the fact that the drug had never undergone formal clinical trials nor

From *National Institute on Drug Abuse Research Report*, March 2006, U.S. Department of Health and Human and Services.

FROM THE DIRECTOR

*T*he so-called "club drug" MDMA continues to be used by millions of Americans across the country, despite evidence of its potential harmful effects. 3,4-methylenedioxymethamphetamine (MDMA, or ecstasy) has gained a deceptive reputation as a "safe" drug among its users. This illegal drug, which has both stimulant and psychedelic properties, is often taken for the feelings of well-being, stimulation, and the distortions in time and sensory perceptions that it produces. MDMA first became popular in the "rave" and all-night party scene, but its use has now spread to a wide range of settings and demographic subgroups. According to the 2004 National Survey on Drug Use and Health, more than 11 million people have tried MDMA at least once.

Myths abound about both the acute effects and long-term consequences of this drug, often called ecstasy or "X." Indeed, one reason for the rapid rise in the drug's popularity is that many young people believe that MDMA is a new safe drug. But MDMA is not new to the scientific community, as many laboratories began investigating this drug in the 1980s, and the picture emerging from their efforts is of a drug that is far from benign. For example, MDMA can cause a dangerous increase in body temperature that can lead to kidney failure. MDMA can also increase heart rate, blood pressure, and heart wall stress. Animal studies show that MDMA can damage specific neurons in the brain. In humans, the research is not conclusive at this time; however, a number of studies show that long-term, heavy MDMA users suffer cognitive deficits, including problems with memory.

NIDA-supported research is developing a clearer picture of the potential dangers of MDMA, and this Research Report summarizes the latest findings. We hope that this compilation of scientific information will inform readers and help the public recognize the risks of MDMA use.

Nora D. Volkow, M.D.
Director
National Institute on Drug Abuse

received approval from the U.S. Food and Drug Administration (FDA) for use in humans. In fact, it was only in late 2000 that the FDA approved the first small clinical trial for MDMA that will determine if the drug can be used safely with 2 sessions of ongoing psychotherapy under carefully monitored conditions to treat post-traumatic stress disorder. Nevertheless, the drug gained a small following among psychiatrists in the late 1970s and early 1980s, with some even calling it "penicillin for the soul" because it was perceived to enhance communication in patient sessions and reportedly allowed users to achieve insights about their problems. It was also during this time that MDMA first started becoming available on the street. In 1985, the U.S. Drug Enforcement Administration (DEA) banned the drug, placing it on its list of Schedule I drugs, corresponding to those substances with no proven therapeutic value.

What Is the Scope of MDMA Abuse in the U.S.?

It is difficult to determine the exact scope of this problem because MDMA is often used in combination with other substances, and does not appear in some traditional data sources, such as treatment admission rates.

More than 11 million persons aged 12 or older reported using ecstasy at least once in their lifetimes, according to the 2004 National Survey on Drug Use and Health. The number of current (use in past month) users in 2004 was estimated to be 450,000.

The Drug Abuse Warning Network, maintained by the Substance Abuse and Mental Health Services Administration, reported that mentions of MDMA in drug abuse-related cases in hospital emergency departments were 2,221 for the third and fourth quarters of 2003. The majority of patients who came to emergency departments mentioning MDMA as a factor in their admissions during that time were aged 18–20.

There is, however, some encouraging news from NIDA's Monitoring the Future (MTF) survey, an annual survey used to track drug abuse trends among adolescents in middle and high schools across the country. Between 2001 and 2005, annual ecstasy use decreased by 52 percent in 8th-graders, 58 percent in 10th-graders, and 67 percent in 12th-graders. Rates of lifetime MDMA use decreased significantly from 2004 to 2005 among 12th-graders.

In 2005, 8th-graders reported a significant decrease in perceived harmfulness in using MDMA occasionally. The MTF data also show that MDMA use extends across many demographic sub-groups. Among 12th-graders in 2005, for example, 3.9 percent of Whites, 3.0 percent of Hispanic students, and 1.4 percent of African-Americans reported using MDMA in the year prior to the survey.

Who Is Abusing MDMA?

MDMA first gained popularity among adolescents and young adults in the night-club scene or weekend-long dance parties known as raves. However, the profile of the typical MDMA user has been changing. Community-level data from NIDA's Community Epidemiology Work Group (CEWG), continued to report that use of MDMA has spread among populations outside the nightclub scene.

Reports also indicate that use is spreading beyond predominantly White youth to a broader range of ethnic groups. In Chicago, the drug continues to be predominantly used by White youth, but there are increasing reports of its use by African-American adults in their twenties and thirties. Also, indicators in New York suggest that both the distribution and use of club drugs are becoming more common in non-White communities.

Other NIDA research shows that MDMA has also become a popular drug among urban gay males. Reports have shown that some gay and bisexual men take MDMA and other club drugs in myriad venues. This is concerning given that the use of club drugs has been linked to high-risk sexual behaviors that may lead to HIV or other sexually transmitted diseases. Many gay males in big cities report using MDMA as part of a multiple-drug experience that includes marijuana, cocaine, methamphetamine, ketamine, and other legal and illegal substances.

What Are the Effects of MDMA?

MDMA has become a popular drug, in part because of the positive effects that a person may experience within an hour or so after taking a single dose. Those effects include feelings of mental stimulation, emotional warmth, empathy toward others, a general sense of well being, and decreased anxiety. In addition, users report enhanced sensory perception as a hallmark of the MDMA experience. Because of the drug's stimulant properties, when used in club or dance settings, MDMA can also enable users to dance for extended periods. However, there are some users who report undesirable effects immediately, including anxiety, agitation, and recklessness.

As noted, MDMA is not a benign drug. MDMA can produce a variety of adverse health effects, including nausea, chills, sweating, involuntary teeth clenching, muscle cramping, and blurred vision. MDMA overdose can also occur—the symptoms can include high blood pressure, faintness, panic attacks, and in severe cases, a loss of consciousness and seizures.

Because of its stimulant properties and the environments in which it is often taken, MDMA is associated with vigorous physical activity for extended periods. This can lead to one of the most significant, although rare, acute adverse effects—a marked rise in body temperature (hyperthermia). Treatment of hyperthermia requires prompt medical attention, as it can rapidly lead to muscle breakdown, which can in turn result in kidney failure. In addition, dehydration, hypertension, and heart failure may occur in susceptible individuals. MDMA can also reduce the pumping efficiency of the heart, of particular concern during periods of increased physical activity, further complicating these problems.

MDMA is rapidly absorbed into the human bloodstream, but once in the body, MDMA metabolites interfere with the body's ability to metabolize, or break down, the drug. As a result, additional doses of MDMA can produce unexpectedly high blood levels, which could worsen the cardiovascular and other toxic effects of this drug. MDMA also interferes with the metabolism of other drugs, including some of the adulterants that may be found in MDMA tablets.

In the hours after taking the drug, MDMA produces significant reductions in mental abilities. These changes, particularly those affecting memory, can last for up to a week, and possibly longer in regular users. The fact that MDMA markedly impairs information processing emphasizes the potential dangers of performing complex or skilled activities, such as driving a car, while under the influence of this drug.

Over the course of a week following moderate use of the drug, many MDMA users report feeling a range of emotions, including anxiety, restlessness, irritability, and sadness that in some individuals can be as severe as true clinical depression. Similarly, elevated anxiety, impulsiveness, and aggression, as well as sleep disturbances, lack of appetite, and reduced interest in and pleasure from sex have been observed in regular MDMA users. Some of these disturbances may not be directly attributable to MDMA, but may be related to some

EFFECTS OF MDMA

Reported Undesirable Effects

(up to 1 week post-MDMA, or longer):

- Anxiety
- Restlessness
- Irritability
- Sadness
- Impulsiveness
- Aggression
- Sleep disturbances
- Lack of appetite
- Thirst
- Reduced interest in and pleasure from sex
- Significant reductions in mental abilities

Potential Adverse Health Effects:

- Nausea
- Chills
- Sweating
- Involuntary jaw clenching and teeth grinding
- Muscle cramping
- Blurred vision
- Marked rise in body temperature (hyperthermia)
- Dehydration
- High blood pressure
- Heart failure
- Kidney failure
- Arrhythmia

Symptoms of MDMA Overdose:

- High blood pressure
- Faintness
- Panic attacks
- Loss of consciousness
- Seizures

of the other drugs often used in combination with MDMA, such as cocaine or marijuana, or to adulterants commonly found in MDMA tablets.

What Does MDMA Do to the Brain?

MDMA affects the brain by increasing the activity of at least three neurotransmitters (the chemical messengers of brain cells): serotonin, dopamine, and norepinephrine. Like other amphetamines, MDMA causes these neurotransmitters to be released from their storage sites in neurons, resulting in increased neurotransmitter activity. Compared to the very potent stimulant, methamphetamine, MDMA causes greater serotonin release and somewhat lesser dopamine release. Serotonin is a neurotransmitter that plays an important role in the regulation of mood, sleep, pain, appetite, and other behaviors. The excess release of serotonin by MDMA likely causes the mood elevating effects experienced by MDMA users. However, by releasing large amounts of serotonin, MDMA causes the brain to become significantly depleted of this important neurotransmitter, contributing to the negative behavioral aftereffects that users often experience for several days after taking MDMA.

Numerous studies in animals have demonstrated that MDMA can damage serotonin-containing neurons; some of these studies have shown these effects to be long lasting. This suggests that such damage may occur in humans as well; however, measuring serotonin damage in humans is more difficult. Studies have shown that some heavy MDMA users experience long-lasting confusion, depression, and selective impairment of working memory and attention processes. Such memory impairments have been associated with a decrease in serotonin metabolites or other markers of serotonin function. Imaging studies in MDMA users have shown changes in brain activity in regions involved in cognition, emotion, and motor function. However, improved imaging technologies and more research are needed to confirm these findings and to elucidate the exact nature of the effects of MDMA on the human brain.

It is also important to keep in mind that many users of ecstasy may unknowingly be taking other drugs that are sold as ecstasy, and/or they may intentionally use other drugs, such as marijuana, which could contribute to these behavioral effects. Additionally, most studies in people do not have behavioral measures from before the users began taking drugs, making it difficult to rule out pre-existing conditions. Factors such as gender, dosage, frequency and intensity of use, age at which use began, the use of other drugs, as well as genetic and environmental factors all may play a role in some of the cognitive deficits that result from MDMA use and should be taken into consideration when studying the effects of MDMA in humans.

Given that most MDMA users are young and in their reproductive years, it is possible that some female users may be pregnant when they take MDMA, either inadvertently or intentionally because of the misperception that it is a safe drug. The potential adverse effects of MDMA on the developing fetus are of great concern. Behavioral studies in animals have found significant adverse effects on tests of learning and memory from exposure to MDMA during a developmental period equivalent to the third trimester in humans. However, the effects of MDMA on animals earlier in development are unclear; therefore, more research is needed to determine what the effects of MDMA are on the developing human nervous system.

Is MDMA Addictive?

For some people, MDMA can be addictive. A survey of young adult and adolescent MDMA users found that 43 percent of those who reported ecstasy use met the accepted diagnostic criteria for dependence, as evidenced by continued use despite knowledge of physical or psychological harm, withdrawal effects, and tolerance (or diminished response), and 34 percent met the criteria for drug abuse. Almost 60 percent of people who use MDMA report withdrawal symptoms, including fatigue, loss of appetite, depressed feelings, and trouble concentrating.

MDMA affects many of the same neurotransmitter systems in the brain that are targeted by other addictive drugs. Experiments have shown that animals prefer MDMA, much like they do cocaine, over other pleasurable stimuli, another hallmark of most addictive drugs.

What Do We Know About Preventing MDMA Abuse?

Because social context and networks seem to be an important component of MDMA use, the use of peer-led advocacy and drug prevention programs may be a promising approach to reduce MDMA use among adolescents and young adults. High schools and colleges can serve as important venues for delivering messages about the effects of MDMA use. Providing accurate scientific information regarding the effects of MDMA is important if we hope to reduce the damaging effects of this drug. Education is one of the most important tools for use in preventing MDMA abuse.

Are There Effective Treatments for MDMA Abuse?

There are no specific treatments for MDMA abuse. The most effective treatments for drug abuse and addiction are cognitive behavioral interventions that are designed to help modify the patient's thinking, expectancies, and behaviors, and to increase skills in coping with life's stressors. Drug abuse recovery support groups may be effective in combination with behavioral interventions to support long-term, drug-free recovery. There are currently no pharmacological treatments for dependence on MDMA.

Access Information on the Internet

- What's new on the NIDA Web site
- Information on drugs of abuse
- Publications and communications (including NIDA NOTES)
- Calendar of events
- Links to NIDA organizational units
- Funding information (including program announcements and deadlines)
- International activities
- Links to related Web sites (access to Web sites of many other organizations in the field)

Where Can I Get More Scientific Information on MDMA?

To learn more about MDMA and other drugs of abuse, contact the National Clearinghouse for Alcohol and Drug Information (NCADI) at 800-729-6686. Information specialists are available to help you locate information and resources.

Fact sheets, including *InfoFacts*, on the health effects of MDMA, other drugs of abuse, and other drug abuse topics are available on the NIDA Web site . . . and can be ordered free of charge in English and Spanish from NCADI. . . .

References

Bolla, K.I.; McCann, U.D.; and Ricaurte, G.A. Memory impairment in abstinent MDMA ("Ecstasy") users. *Neurology* 51:1532–1537 (1998).

Broening, H.W.; Morford, L.L.; Inman-Wood, S.L.; Fukumura, M.; and Vorhees, C.V. 3,4-Methylenedioxymethamphetamine (Ecstasy)-induced learning and memory impairments depend on the age of exposure during early development. *The Journal of Neuroscience* 21:3228–3235 (2001).

Colado, M.I.; O'Shea, E.; Granados, R.; Misra, A.; Murray, T.K.; and Green, A.R.; A study of the neurotoxic effect of MDMA ('ecstasy') on 5-HT neurons in the brains of mothers and neonates following administration of the drug during pregnancy. *British Journal of Pharmacology* 121:827–833 (1997).

Community Epidemiology Work Group. *Epidemiologic Trends in Drug Abuse: Volume I.* Bethesda, MD. June 2005.

Cottler, L.B.; Womack, S.B.; Compton, W.M.; and Ben-Abdallah, A. Ecstasy abuse and dependence among adolescents and young adults: applicability and reliability of DSM-IV criteria. *Human Psychopharmacology* 16:599–606 (2001).

Curran, H.V.; and Travill, R.A. Mood and cognitive effects of ±3,4-methylene-dioxymethamphetamine (MDMA, 'ecstasy'): week-end 'high' followed by mid-week low. *Addiction* 92:821–831 (1997).

Dafters, R.I.; and Lynch, E. Persistent loss of thermo-regulation in the rate induced by 3,4-methylenedioxymethamphetamine (MDMA or "Ecstasy") but not by fenfluramine. *Psychopharmacology* 138:207–212 (1998).

Kish, S.J.; Furukawa, Y.; Ang, L.; Vorce, S.P.; and Kalasinsky, K.S. Striatal serotonin is depleted in brain of a human MDMA (Ecstasy) user. *Neurology* 55:294–296 (2000).

Koprich, J.B.; Chen, E.-Y.; Kanaan, N.M.; Campbell, N.G.; Kordower, J.H.; and Lipton, J.W. Prenatal 3,4-methylenedioxymethamphetamine (ecstasy) alters exploratory behavior, reduces monoamine metabolism, and increases forebrain tyrosine hydroxylase fiber density of juvenile rats. *Neurotoxicology and Teratology* 25: 509–517 (2003).

Lester, S.J.; Baggott, M.; Welm, S.; Schiller, N.B.; Jones, R.T.; Foster, E.; and Mendelson, J. Cardiovascular effects of 3,4-methylenedioxymethamphetamine: a double-blind, placebo-controlled trial. *Annals of Internal Medicine* 133:969–973 (2000).

Liechti, M.E.; and Vollenweider, F.X. Which neuroreceptors mediate the subjective effects of MDMA in humans? A summary of mechanistic studies. *Human Psychopharmacology* 16:589–598 (2001).

Lyles, J.; and Cadet, J.L. Methylenedioxymethamphetamine (MDMA, Ecstasy) neu-rotoxicity: cellular and molecular mechanisms. *Brain Research Reviews* 42:155–168 (2003).

McCann, U.D.; Eligulashvili, V.; and Ricaurte, G.A. (±)3,4-Methylenedioxymetham-phetamine ('Ecstasy')-induced serotonin neurotoxicity: clinical studies. *Neurop-sychobiology* 42:11–16 (2000).

Morgan, M.J. Ecstasy (MDMA): a review of its possible persistent psychological effects. *Psychopharmacology* 152:230–248 (2000).

Morgan, M.J. Memory deficits associated with recreational use of "ecstasy" (MDMA). *Psychopharmacology* 141:30–36 (1999).

National Institute on Drug Abuse. *Monitoring the Future: National Results on Adolescent Drug Use 2005.*

Obrocki, J.; Buchert, R.; Väterlein, O.; Thomasius, R.; Beyer, W.; and Schiemann, T. Ecstasy—long-term effects on the human central nervous system revealed by positron emission tomography. *British Journal of Psychiatry* 175:186–188 (1999).

Parrott, A.C.; and Lasky, J. Ecstasy (MDMA) effect upon mood and cognition: before, during and after a Saturday night dance. *Psychopharmacology* 139:261–268 (1998).

Reneman, L.; Booij, J.; Schmand, B.; van den Brink, W.; and Gunning, B. Memory disturbances in "Ecstasy" users are correlated with an altered brain serotonin neurotransmission. *Psychopharmacology* 148:322–324 (2000).

Schenk, S.; Gittings, D.; Johnstone, M.; and Daniela, E. Development, maintenance and temporal pattern of self-administration maintained by ecstasy (MDMA) in rats. *Psychopharmacology* 169:21–27 (2003).

Sherlock, K.; Wolff, K.; Hay, A.W.; and Conner, M. Analysis of illicit ecstasy tablets. *Journal of Accident and Emergency Medicine* 16:194–197 (1999).

Substance Abuse and Mental Health Services Administration, Office of Applied Studies. *Drug Abuse Warning Network, 2003: Interim National Estimates of Drug-Related Emergency Department Visits.* DAWN Series D-26, DHHS Publication No. (SMA) 04–3972. Rockville, MD (2004).

Thompson, M.R., Li, K.M., Clemens, K.J., Gurtman, C.G., Hunt, G.E., Cornish, J.L., and McGregor, I.S. Chronic fluoxetine treatment partly attenuates the long-term anxiety and depressive symptoms induced by MDMA ('Ecstasy') in rats. *Neuropsychopharmacology* 29(40):694–704, 2004.

Verkes, R.J.; Gijsman, H.J.; Pieters, M.S.M.; Schoemaker, R.C.; de Visser, S.; Kuijpers, M.; Pennings, E.J.M.; de Bruin, D.; Van de Wijngaart, G.; Van Gerven, J.M.A.; and Cohen, A.F. Cognitive performance and serotonergic function in users of ecstasy. *Psychopharmacology* 153:196–202 (2001).

Wareing, M.; Fisk, J.E.; and Murphy, P.N. Working memory deficits in current and previous users of MDMA ('ecstasy'). *British Journal of Psychology* 91:181–188 (2000).

POSTSCRIPT

Are the Dangers of Ecstasy (MDMA) Overstated?

There is little argument that mind-altering drugs can cause physical and emotional havoc for the user. People may become less inhibited and become involved in behaviors they would not typically do if they were not on drugs. It is not uncommon for Ecstasy users to open up emotionally. However, is one's use of Ecstasy and other so-called club drugs likely to increase these behaviors? Perhaps individuals who use these drugs are the types of people who would engage in reckless behavior regardless. In other words, is Ecstasy the reason people are more open or does Ecstasy provide the excuse to be more open?

The National Institute on Drug Abuse (NIDA) contends that these Ecstasy and other club drugs are deleterious. The fact that an increasing number of secondary students perceive Ecstasy as harmful illustrates its potential harm. In recent years, there has been a slight decrease in Ecstasy use by secondary students. Nonetheless, thousands of people visit emergency rooms as a result of an adverse reaction to Ecstasy. NIDA admits that additional research still needs to be conducted into the effects of Ecstasy, but that there is more than enough research to point to the dangers of Ecstasy.

Sullum argues that history shows that bringing attention to certain drugs results in their increased use. Young people would not know to alter their consciousness with certain drugs unless they were alerted to their effects. For example, how would one know that sniffing glue would affect one's consciousness unless that fact was established. However, if young people participate in an activity that is potentially harmful, one could argue that it is the government's responsibility to step in. At what point is too much information counterproductive? Balancing one's right to know about drugs with the publicity generated by informing the public about certain drugs is difficult.

The issue of whether or not we should be concerned about Ecstasy and other club drugs raises a number of interesting questions. For example, how much danger must a drug represent before it is considered too dangerous? Are exaggerating the effects of drugs like Ecstasy providing a disservice because other information about drugs that are especially harmful may be ignored? Should the government's focus be on prohibiting the use of Ecstasy at all costs or should the government try to educate people about its potential adverse effects?

At one time Ecstasy was used for therapeutic purposes. There has been a renewed interest in exploring the therapeutic benefits of Ecstasy. If Ecstasy has these types of benefits, can the drug be as bad as it is purported to be?

There are a number of articles that look at the benefits or dangers of Ecstasy and similar drugs. Two good articles are "Researchers Explore New Visions for Hallucinogens," by Susan Brown (*The Chronicle for Higher Education*, December 6, 2006) and "The Ups and Downs of Ecstasy," by Erika Check (*Nature*, May 13, 2004). Other informative articles on this issue include "Evidence for Significant Polydrug Use Among Ecstasy-Using College Students," by Eric Wish and colleagues (*Journal of American College Health*, 2006); "Research on Ecstasy Is Clouded by Errors," by Donald McNeil (*The New York Times*, December 2, 2003); and "Ecstasy Use Among Club Rave Attendees," by Amelia Arria and others (*Archives of Pediatrics and Adolescent Medicine*, March 2002). One group that sponsors research into the therapeutic benefits of Ecstasy and other drugs is the Multidisciplinary Association for Psychedelic Studies (MAPS). Its Web site is www.maps.org.

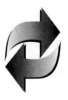

ISSUE 5

Should Pregnant Drug Users Be Prosecuted?

YES: Paul A. Logli, from "Drugs in the Womb: The Newest Battlefield in the War on Drugs," *Criminal Justice Ethics* (Winter/Spring 1990)

NO: Carolyn S. Carter, from "Perinatal Care for Women Who Are Addicted: Implications for Empowerment," *Health and Social Work* (August 2002)

ISSUE SUMMARY

YES: Paul A. Logli, an Illinois prosecuting attorney, argues that it is the government's duty to enforce every child's right to begin life with a healthy, drug-free mind and body. Logli maintains that pregnant women who use drugs should be prosecuted because they harm the life of their unborn children. He feels that it is the state's responsibility to ensure that every baby is born as healthy as possible.

NO: Carolyn Carter, a social work professor at Howard University, argues that the stigma of drug use during pregnancy has resulted in the avoidance of treatment. Carter asserts that the prosecution of pregnant drug users is unfair because poor women are more likely to be the targets of such prosecution. To enable pregnant women who use drugs to receive perinatal care, it is necessary to define their drug use as a health problem rather than as a legal problem.

T he effects that drugs have on a fetus can be mild and temporary or severe and permanent, depending on the extent of drug use by the mother, the type of substance used, and the stage of fetal development at the time the drug crosses the placental barrier and enters the bloodstream of the fetus. Both illegal and legal drugs, such as cocaine, crack, marijuana, alcohol, and nicotine, are increasingly found to be responsible for incidents of premature births, congenital abnormalities, fetal alcohol syndrome, mental retardation, and other serious birth defects. The exposure of the fetus to these substances and the long-term involuntary physical, intellectual, and emotional effects are disturbing. In addition, the medical, social, and economic costs to treat and care for babies who are exposed to or become addicted to drugs while in utero (in the uterus) warrant serious concern.

An important consideration regarding the prosecution of pregnant drug users is whether this is a legal problem or a medical problem. In recent years, attempts have been made to establish laws that would allow the incarceration of drug-using pregnant women on the basis of "fetal abuse." Some cases have been successfully prosecuted: Mothers have been denied custody of their infants until they enter appropriate treatment programs, and criminal charges have been brought against mothers whose children were born with drug-related complications. The underlying presumption is that the unborn fetus should be afforded protection against the harmful actions of another person, specifically the use of harmful drugs by the mother.

Those who profess that prosecuting pregnant women who use drugs is necessary insist that the health and welfare of the unborn child is the highest priority. They contend that the possibility that these women will avoid obtaining health care for themselves or their babies because they fear punishment does not absolve the state from the responsibility of protecting the babies. They also argue that criminalizing these acts is imperative to protect fetuses and newborns who cannot protect themselves. It is the duty of the legal system to deter pregnant women from engaging in future criminal drug use and to protect the best interests of infants.

Others maintain that drug use and dependency by pregnant women is a medical problem, not a criminal one. Many pregnant women seek treatment, but they often find that rehabilitation programs are limited or unavailable. Shortages of openings in chemical dependency programs may keep a prospective client waiting for months, during which time she will most likely continue to use the drugs to which she is addicted and prolong her fetus's drug exposure. Many low-income women do not receive drug treatment and adequate prenatal care due to financial constraints. Women who fear criminal prosecution because of their drug use may simply avoid prenatal care altogether.

Some suggest that medical intervention, drug prevention, and education—not prosecution—are needed for pregnant drug users. Prosecution, they contend, drives women who need medical attention away from the very help they and their babies need. Others respond that prosecuting pregnant women who use drugs will help identify those who need attention, at which point adequate medical and social welfare services can be provided to treat and protect the mother and child.

In the following selections, Paul A. Logli, arguing for the prosecution of pregnant drug users, contends that it is the state's responsibility to protect the unborn and the newborn because they are least able to protect themselves. He charges that it is the prosecutor's responsibility to deter future criminal drug use by mothers who he feels violate the rights of their potential newborns to have an opportunity for a healthy and normal life. Carolyn Carter contends that prosecuting pregnant drug users may be counterproductive to improving the quality of infant and maternal health. To help women who use drugs during pregnancy, it would be more helpful to identify the problem as a medical problem and not as a legal problem.

YES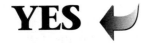

Paul A. Logli

Drugs in the Womb: The Newest Battlefield in the War on Drugs

Introduction

The reported incidence of drug-related births has risen dramatically over the last several years. The legal system and, in particular, local prosecutors have attempted to properly respond to the suffering, death, and economic costs which result from a pregnant woman's use of drugs. The ensuing debate has raised serious constitutional and practical issues which are far from resolution.

Prosecutors have achieved mixed results in using current criminal and juvenile statutes as a basis for legal action intended to prosecute mothers and protect children. As a result, state and federal legislators have begun the difficult task of drafting appropriate laws to deal with the problem, while at the same time acknowledging the concerns of medical authorities, child protection groups, and advocates for individual rights.

The Problem

The plight of "cocaine babies," children addicted at birth to narcotic substances or otherwise affected by maternal drug use during pregnancy, has prompted prosecutors in some jurisdictions to bring criminal charges against drug-abusing mothers. Not only have these prosecutions generated heated debates both inside and outside of the nation's courtrooms, but they have also expanded the war on drugs to a controversial new battlefield—the mother's womb.

A 1988 survey of hospitals conducted by Dr. Ira Chasnoff, Associate Professor of Northwestern University Medical School and President of the National Association for Perinatal Addiction Research and Education (NAPARE) indicated that as many as 375,000 infants may be affected by maternal cocaine use during pregnancy each year. Chasnoff's survey included 36 hospitals across the country and showed incidence rates ranging from 1 percent to 27 percent. It also indicated that the problem was not restricted to urban populations or particular racial or socio-economic groups. More recently a study at Hutzel Hospital in Detroit's inner city found that 42.7 percent of its newborn babies were exposed to drugs while in their mothers' wombs.

Paul A. Logli, "Drugs in the Womb: The Newest Battlefield in the War on Drugs," as appeared in Criminal Justice Ethics, Volume 9, Number 1, [Winter/Spring 1990] pp. 23–29. Reprinted by permission of The Institute for Criminal Justice Ethics, 555 West 57th Streedt, Suite 607, New York, NY 10019-1029.

The effects of maternal use of cocaine and other drugs during pregnancy on the mother and her newborn child have by now been well-documented and will not be repeated here. The effects are severe and can cause numerous threats to the short-term health of the child. In a few cases it can even result in death.

Medical authorities have just begun to evaluate the long-term effects of cocaine exposure on children as they grow older. Early findings show that many of these infants show serious difficulties in relating and reacting to adults and environments, as well as in organizing creative play, and they appear similar to mildly autistic or personality-disordered children.

The human costs related to the pain, suffering, and deaths resulting from maternal cocaine use during pregnancy are simply incalculable. In economic terms, the typical intensive-care costs for treating babies exposed to drugs range from $7,500 to $31,000. In some cases medical bills go as high as $150,000.

The costs grow enormously as more and more hospitals encounter the problem of "boarder babies"—those children literally abandoned at the hospital by an addicted mother, and left to be cared for by the nursing staff. Future costs to society for simply educating a generation of drug-affected children can only be the object of speculation. It is clear, however, that besides pain, suffering, and death the economic costs to society of drug use by pregnant women is presently enormous and is certainly growing larger.

The Prosecutor's Response

It is against this backdrop and fueled by the evergrowing emphasis on an aggressively waged war on drugs that prosecutors have begun a number of actions against women who have given birth to drug-affected children. A review of at least two cases will illustrate the potential success or failure of attempts to use existing statutes.

People v. Melanie Green.   On February 4, 1989, at a Rockford, Illinois hospital, two-day-old Bianca Green lost her brief struggle for life. At the time of Bianca's birth both she and her mother, twenty-four-year-old Melanie Green, tested positive for the presence of cocaine in their systems.

Pathologists in Rockford and Madison, Wisconsin, indicated that the death of the baby was the result of a prenatal injury related to cocaine used by the mother during the pregnancy. They asserted that maternal cocaine use had caused the placenta to prematurely rupture, which deprived the fetus of oxygen before and during delivery. As a result of oxygen deprivation, the child's brain began to swell and she eventually died.

After an investigation by the Rockford Police Department and the State of Illinois Department of Children and Family Services, prosecutors allowed a criminal complaint to be filed on May 9, 1989, charging Melanie Green with the offenses of Involuntary Manslaughter and Delivery of a Controlled Substance.

On May 25, 1989, testimony was presented to the Winnebago County Grand Jury by prosecutors seeking a formal indictment. The Grand Jury, however, declined to indict Green on either charge. Since Grand Jury proceedings in the State of Illinois are secret, as are the jurors' deliberations and votes, the reason for the decision of the Grand Jury in this case is determined more by conjecture than any direct knowledge. Prosecutors involved in the presentation observed that the jurors exhibited a certain amount of sympathy for the young woman who had been brought before the Grand Jury at the jurors' request. It is also likely that the jurors were uncomfortable with the use of statutes that were not intended to be used in these circumstances.

It would also be difficult to disregard the fact that, after the criminal complaints were announced on May 9th and prior to the Grand Jury deliberations of May 25th, a national debate had ensued revolving around the charges brought in Rockford, Illinois, and their implications for the ever-increasing problem of women who use drugs during pregnancy.

People v. Jennifer Clarise Johnson. On July 13, 1989, a Seminole County, Florida judge found Jennifer Johnson guilty of delivery of a controlled substance to a child. The judge found that delivery, for purposes of the statute, occurred through the umbilical cord after the birth of the child and before the cord was severed. Jeff Deen, the Assistant State's Attorney who prosecuted the case, has since pointed out that Johnson, age 23, had previously given birth to three other cocaine-affected babies, and in this case was arrested at a crack house. "We needed to make sure this woman does not give birth to another cocaine baby."

Johnson was sentenced to fifteen years of probation including strict supervision, drug treatment, random drug testing, educational and vocational training, and an intensive prenatal care program if she ever became pregnant again.

Support for the Prosecution of Maternal Drug Abuse

Both cases reported above relied on a single important fact as a basis for the prosecution of the drug-abusing mother: that the child was born alive and exhibited the consequences of prenatal injury.

In the Melanie Green case, Illinois prosecutors relied on the "born alive" rule set out earlier in *People v. Bolar.* In *Bolar* the defendant was convicted of the offense of reckless homicide. The case involved an accident between a car driven by the defendant, who was found to be drunk, and another automobile containing a pregnant woman. As a result, the woman delivered her baby by emergency caesarean section within hours of the collision. Although the newborn child exhibited only a few heart beats and lived for approximately two minutes, the court found that the child was born alive and was therefore a person for purposes of the criminal statutes of the State of Illinois.

The Florida prosecution relied on a live birth in an entirely different fashion. The prosecutor argued in that case that the delivery of the controlled substance occurred after the live birth via the umbilical cord and prior to the cutting of the cord. Thus, it was argued, that the delivery of the controlled substance occurred not to a fetus but to a person who enjoyed the protection of the criminal code of the State of Florida.

Further support for the State's role in protecting the health of newborns even against prenatal injury is found in the statutes which provide protection for the fetus. These statutes proscribe actions by a person, usually other than the mother, which either intentionally or recklessly harm or kill a fetus. In other words, even in the absence of a live birth, most states afford protection to the unborn fetus against the harmful actions of another person. Arguably, the same protection should be afforded the infant against intentional harmful actions by a drug-abusing mother.

The state also receives support for a position in favor of the protection of the health of a newborn from a number of non-criminal cases. A line of civil cases in several states would appear to stand for the principle that a child has a right to begin life with a sound mind and body, and a person who interferes with that right may be subject to civil liability. In two cases decided within months of each other, the Supreme Court of Michigan upheld two actions for recovery of damages that were caused by the infliction of prenatal injury. In *Womack v. Buckhorn* the court upheld an action on behalf of an eight-year-old surviving child for prenatal brain injuries apparently suffered during the fourth month of the pregnancy in an automobile accident. The court adopted with approval the reasoning of a New Jersey Supreme Court decision and "recognized that a child has a legal right to begin life with a sound mind and body." Similarly, in *O'Neill v. Morse* the court found that a cause of action was allowed for prenatal injuries that caused the death of an eight-month-old viable fetus.

Illinois courts have allowed civil recovery on behalf of an infant for a negligently administered blood transfusion given to the mother prior to conception which resulted in damage to the child at birth. However, the same Illinois court would not extend a similar cause of action for prebirth injuries as between a child and its own mother. The court, however, went on to say that a right to such a cause of action could be statutorily enacted by the Legislature.

Additional support for the state's role in protecting the health of newborns is found in the principles annunciated in recent decisions of the United States Supreme Court. The often cited case of *Roe v. Wade* set out that although a woman's right of privacy is broad enough to cover the abortion decision, the right is not absolute and is subject to limitations, "and that at some point the state's interest as to protection of health, medical standards and prenatal life, becomes dominant."

More recently, in the case of *Webster v. Reproductive Health Services,* the court expanded the state's interest in protecting potential human life by setting aside viability as a rigid line that had previously allowed state regulation only after viability had been shown but prohibited it before viability. The court goes on to say that the "fundamental right" to abortion as described in *Roe* is now accorded the lesser status of a "liberty interest." Such language surely supports a prosecutor's argument that the state's compelling interest in potential human life would allow the criminalization of acts which if committed by a pregnant woman can damage not just a viable fetus but eventually a born-alive infant. It follows that, once a pregnant woman has abandoned her right to abort and has decided to carry the fetus to term, society can well impose a duty on the mother to insure that the fetus is born as healthy as possible.

A further argument in support of the state's interest in prosecuting women who engage in conduct which is damaging to the health of a newborn child is especially compelling in regard to maternal drug use during pregnancy. Simply put, there is no fundamental right or even a liberty interest in the use of psycho-active drugs. A perceived right of privacy has never formed an absolute barrier against state prosecutions of those who use or possess narcotics. Certainly no exception can be made simply because the person using drugs happens to be pregnant.

Critics of the prosecutor's role argue that any statute that would punish mothers who create a substantial risk of harm to their fetus will run afoul of constitutional requirements, including prohibitions on vagueness, guarantees of liberty and privacy, and rights of due process and equal protection. . . .

In spite of such criticism, the state's role in protecting those citizens who are least able to protect themselves, namely the newborn, mandates an aggressive posture. Much of the criticism of prosecutorial efforts is based on speculation as to the consequences of prosecution and ignores the basic tenet of criminal law that prosecutions deter the prosecuted and others from committing additional crimes. To assume that it will only drive persons further underground is to somehow argue that certain prosecutions of crime will only force perpetrators to make even more aggressive efforts to escape apprehension, thus making arrest and prosecution unadvisable. Neither could this be accepted as an argument justifying even the weakening of criminal sanctions. . . .

The concern that pregnant addicts will avoid obtaining health care for themselves or their infants because of the fear of prosecution cannot justify the absence of state action to protect the newborn. If the state were to accept such reasoning, then existing child abuse laws would have to be reconsidered since they might deter parents from obtaining medical care for physically or sexually abused children. That argument has not been accepted as a valid reason for abolishing child abuse laws or for not prosecuting child abusers. . . .

The far better policy is for the state to acknowledge its responsibility not only to provide a deterrant to criminal and destructive behavior by pregnant addicts but also to provide adequate opportunities for those who might seek help to discontinue their addiction. Prosecution has a role in its ability to deter future criminal behavior and to protect the best interests of the child. The medical and social welfare establishment must assume an even greater responsibility to encourage legislators to provide adequate funding and facilities so that no pregnant woman who is addicted to drugs will be denied the opportunity to seek appropriate prenatal care and treatment for her addiction.

One State's Response

The Legislature of the State of Illinois at the urging of local prosecutors moved quickly to amend its juvenile court act in order to provide protection to those children born drug-affected. Previously, Illinois law provided that a court could assume jurisdiction over addicted minors or a minor who is generally declared neglected or abused.

Effective January 1, 1990, the juvenile court act was amended to expand the definition of a neglected or abused minor. . . .

> those who are neglected include . . . any newborn infant whose blood or urine contains any amount of a controlled substance. . . .

The purpose of the new statute is to make it easier for the court to assert jurisdiction over a newborn infant born drug-affected. The state is not required to show either the addiction of the child or harmful effects on the child in order to remove the child from a drug-abusing mother. Used in this context, prosecutors can work with the mother in a rather coercive atmosphere to encourage her to enter into drug rehabilitation and, upon the successful completion of the program, be reunited with her child.

Additional legislation before the Illinois Legislature is House Bill 2835 sponsored by Representatives John Hallock (R-Rockford) and Edolo "Zeke" Giorgi (D-Rockford). This bill represents the first attempt to specifically address the prosecution of drug-abusing pregnant women. . . .

The statute provides for a class 4 felony disposition upon conviction. A class 4 felony is a probationable felony which can also result in a term of imprisonment from one to three years.

Subsequent paragraphs set out certain defenses available to the accused.

> It shall not be a violation of this section if a woman knowingly or intentionally uses a narcotic or dangerous drug in the first twelve weeks of pregnancy and: 1. She has no knowledge that she is pregnant; or 2. Subsequently, within the first twelve weeks of pregnancy, undergoes medical treatment for substance abuse or treatment or rehabilitation in a program or facility approved by the Illinois Department of Alcoholism and Substance Abuse, and thereafter discontinues any further use of drugs or narcotics as previously set forth.

. . . A woman, under this statute, could not be prosecuted for self-reporting her addiction in the early stages of the pregnancy. Nor could she be prosecuted under this statute if, even during the subsequent stages of the pregnancy, she discontinued her drug use to the extent that no drugs were present in her system or the baby's system at the time of birth. The statute, as drafted, is clearly intended to allow prosecutors to invoke the criminal statutes in the most serious of cases.

Conclusion

Local prosecutors have a legitimate role in responding to the increasing problem of drug-abusing pregnant women and their drug-affected children. Eliminating the pain, suffering and death resulting from drug exposure in newborns must be a prosecutor's priority. However, the use of existing statutes to address the problem may meet with limited success since they are burdened with numerous constitutional problems dealing with original intent, notice, vagueness, and due process.

The juvenile courts may offer perhaps the best initial response in working to protect the interests of a surviving child. However, in order to address more serious cases, legislative efforts may be required to provide new statutes that will specifically address the problem and hopefully deter future criminal conduct which deprives children of their important right to a healthy and normal birth.

The long-term solution does not rest with the prosecutor alone. Society, including the medical and social welfare establishment, must be more responsive in providing readily accessible prenatal care and treatment alternatives for pregnant addicts. In the short term however, prosecutors must be prepared to play a vital role in protecting children and deterring women from engaging in conduct which will harm the newborn child. If prosecutors fail to respond, then they are simply closing the doors of the criminal justice system to those persons, the newborn, who are least able to open the doors for themselves.

Carolyn S. Carter

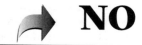 **NO**

Perinatal Care for Women Who Are Addicted: Implications for Empowerment

. . . Perinatal drug abuse is the use of alcohol and other drugs among women who are pregnant. The National Institute on Drug Abuse estimates that 5.5 percent of the women in the United States have used illicit drugs while pregnant, including cocaine, marijuana, heroin, and psychotherapeutic drugs that were not prescribed by a physician. More than 18 percent used alcohol during their pregnancy, and 20.4 percent smoked cigarettes.

Literature reports the increased use of drugs during pregnancy, using therapeutic communities and neighborhood context for addressing perinatal drug abuse; access barriers for low-income ethnic minority women who are addicted and pregnant; the importance of effective policy making; referrals to child protection services; and other responses to perinatal drug abuse.

Women who abuse drugs while pregnant face severe consequences, which include becoming stigmatized as immoral and deficient caregivers. A behavioral outcome of societal attitudes toward perinatal drug abuse is the degree to which the drug-taking behavior of pregnant women is criminalized. Criminalization refers to using legal approaches, such as incarceration, for medical problems of clients rather than referring them for treatment. Community response to the increasing number of women who give birth to infants addicted to crack cocaine, for example, has been to prosecute women for perinatal drug abuse. Similarly, the number of mentally ill inmates in jails and prisons is estimated as being twice that in state hospitals. Individuals in helping professions also display stigmatic attitudes toward perinatal drug abuse. Disparaging interactions with women in some perinatal care facilities, for example, include rude and judgmental comments to clients and violation of their confidentiality. Uncomfortable relationships with health care providers and fear of reprisal on the part of pregnant women who are addicted make women four times less likely to receive adequate care, thereby creating health risks for women who are addicted, their unborn fetuses, and their other children.

In this article I discuss contemporary responses to perinatal drug abuse, including ways in which the behavior of women who abuse drugs is criminalized

From *Health and Social Work*, vol. 27, issue 3, August 2002, pp. 166–174. Copyright © 2002 by National Association of Social Workers, Inc., Health & Social Work. Reprinted by permission. References omitted.

or subjected to legal interventions. Vignettes from an ethnographic study of 120 women who used heroin, crack cocaine, and methamphetamine while pregnant depict the attitudes and behaviors of health care providers, society at large, and women themselves toward maternal drug abuse. This article demonstrates how poor women and women of color encounter legal interventions—such as prosecution or reports to city or state child protective services (CPS)—more frequently for using drugs during pregnancy than their more affluent, white counterparts. Because criminalizing perinatal drug abuse presents substantial risks to the health of women and children, empowering strategies are suggested for redefining perinatal drug abuse less as a legal issue and more as a health concern. The strategies are consistent with elements of the national health plan of the U.S. Department of Health and Human Services (DHHS), such as creating access to health care and minimizing risks to maternal, infant, and child health.

Societal Attitudes Toward Perinatal Drug Abuse

Over the past 100 years, there has been an overall shift in obstetric medicine to a focus on fetal protection. In cases involving maternal drug abuse, the shift has sometimes resulted in adversarial attitudes with sentiment favoring the well-being of fetuses and against pregnant women. The following excerpts offer three perspectives toward perinatal drug abuse that have primary emphasis on unborn fetuses: The first comment reflects the attitudes of some drug dealers; the second statement is a common reaction of partners of pregnant women; and the third depicts the attitude of society at large.

> They [crack dealers] tell me that I shouldn't be doing this in the first place, but I'm gonna do it anyway. And they go, "You know it. I shouldn't even really sell you anything. I shouldn't sell you anything cause you're pregnant. I'm not gonna contribute to that."
>
> My baby came home with crack in her system, and he [baby's father who is himself a crack dealer] don't want to claim her now.
>
> I know one girl. She just smokes [crack] and doesn't give a damn. Her stomach is way out there, so she shouldn't be out there [using crack] anyway, cause people be like, "man, look, a pregnant woman!"

Negative attitudes like the ones in the vignettes above are pervasive and often based on assumed medical and developmental consequences of drugs on fetuses. The concerns are both supported and refuted by research. Studies of the effects of drug use on fetal development cite problems such as low birthweight, small head size, prematurity, and small size for gestational age. A study of 11,000 infants conducted by the Brown University School of Medicine, however, showed no increase in abnormalities at birth among children who had been exposed to cocaine in utero. Although the latter study has not followed the children into school age and is therefore inconclusive, other studies of adjustment among drug-exposed children also challenge the notion of devastating effects resulting from cocaine use during pregnancy. Coles concluded that the effects of the social environment are too often ignored in studies of perinatal drug abuse.

In addition to the pejorative attitudes toward women who abuse drugs during pregnancy based on ideas about adverse fetal development is the belief that drug use compromises the reproductive and caregiver roles of women. It is believed that women who abuse substances are unfit mothers undeserving of their children. Society sanctions women for failing to live up to preconceived gender-role expectations by using legal interventions, particularly against poor women of color who use drugs while they are pregnant.

Legal Interventions

Legal interventions for perinatal drug abuse may be increasing in the United States. Since 1985, 240 women in 35 states have been prosecuted for using alcohol or illegal drugs while pregnant. Eleven states have developed specific gestational-abuse statutes. The most comprehensive reporting system is in Minnesota and includes toxicological screening and "involuntary civil commitment" to drug rehabilitation of pregnant women who have used drugs. Before March 2001, eight states mandated that health care workers report neonates' positive drug toxicology as evidence of child abuse and neglect, thus paving the way for court proceedings and actions affecting the parental rights of mothers. On March 21, 2001, the U.S. Supreme Court ruled that it is unlawful to involuntarily test pregnant women who are suspected of drug abuse. In Ferguson v. City of Charleston, Charleston, South Carolina was a litigant in the Supreme Court case and, along with Florida, enforced the greatest number of legal interventions.

It is informative to place the legal interventions that occurred before the March 2001 judicial ruling within a sociocultural context. In doing so, it becomes clear that although illegal drug use is similar across class and racial lines, poor and ethnic minority women were more likely to be criminalized. The manner in which drug screening occurred is an example. Screenings commonly occurred during routine prenatal care, and the stated purpose was protecting fetuses. However, drug screenings were often limited to facilities that served low socioeconomic populations and populations of color, thus making screenings more detrimental for poor and pregnant women from ethnic minority groups.

Reports to CPS were disparate across cultural groups as well. A review of mandatory reporting of perinatal drug addiction in Florida showed that positive drug screening rates were almost equal among white and African American women and among women seen in clinics and private offices. Yet, reporting rates were much higher for African American women than for white women.

The procedures for prosecuting pregnant women for substance use were discretionary and reflected disparities across demographic groups. A 1987 review of court-ordered obstetrical interventions showed that 81 percent of the women were African American, Hispanic, or Asian and 24 percent did not speak English as a primary language. More recent study results indicate that pregnant African American women were nine times more likely to be prosecuted for substance use than pregnant white women.

Incarceration, like other legal approaches to perinatal drug abuse, also discriminated against poor women and women of color. Women with low incomes generally gave birth in public health settings. Delivering in these facilities increased their chances of incarceration compared with middle-and upper-income women who gave birth in private hospitals that rarely screened for illicit drugs. Public hospitals were more likely to have mandatory drug screenings and protocols that included reporting positive toxicology to CPS. Disclosing positive toxicology to CPS could result in incarceration. Disparities in the rate of incarceration extended to ethnic minority groups, with African American women facing the greatest burden of being imprisoned. Of the 41 pregnant women arrested for abusing drugs in South Carolina from 1989 to 1993, 40 were African American.

The American Medical Association (AMA) stated that drug addiction was an illness that required medical rather than legal intervention, and prosecution did not prevent harm to infants but it often resulted in harm. For example, fear of reprisal was a barrier to outreach and often deterred addicted pregnant women from receiving medical care. Avoiding medical care increased the risk of drug exposure before birth and ineffective parenting later. Also, women who abused drugs were more likely to physically abuse their children.

Legal interventions disregarded the treatment and advocacy roles of health care providers. For example, medical personnel often performed drug screenings without the informed consent of female patients, and the results were then used as evidence during criminal prosecutions. Addressing perinatal drug abuse through legal intervention was punitive. In large part, it operated on the assumption that although drug treatment programs for women were available in sufficient numbers, women had not made use of the services, and the research conclusively attested to the effectiveness of current drug programs for women with children. In fact, drug programs for women, and particularly pregnant women, were largely unavailable. Less than 1 percent of the federal antidrug budget was targeted for women, yet this minimal amount was expected to include women who were pregnant. Also, most drug interventions were designed with men in mind and overlooked the needs of women. Residential treatment programs, for example, rarely provided child care even though 80 percent of the women entering residential drug rehabilitation had children and half had their children living with them at the time they entered treatment. Consequently, mothers who were addicted to drugs, had other children for whom they provided primary care, and had no familial support, risked losing custody of their children by entering treatment.

Interventions based on legal ideology distorted client–worker relationships. Salient features of ethical client–helper relationships are establishing trust and respecting the confidentiality, dignity, and uniqueness of individuals. Women entering perinatal care could not be assured of these aspects of treatment. In the following scenarios involving two African American woman who were addicted to drugs, the clients' dignity and confidentiality were each violated while they received perinatal services:

> They [health care providers] look at you, they look at you foul and they tell me [sarcastic voice], "Oh, you're a crack user." And then they want to look at your record, and then this nurse look at it and this other nurse look at it, then this other nurse look at it, then . . . They talking all loud, everybody around.

> I know a lot of mothers say that they don't get prenatal care cause they feel like as soon as they walk through the door, they will be judged. "Oh you're a crack head. So why . . . did you get pregnant anyway?" So they don't get prenatal care . . . they are thinking how they gonna be looked at when they walk in the hospital door, like they are not good enough to be pregnant.

Experiences such as the ones above not only diminished the quality of services, but also restricted access by causing women to retreat before obtaining the care they sought.

The strained client–worker relationships precipitated by legal interventions also created parallel care systems that were not in the best interest of clients. Prototypes were nontraditional birthing methods. Parallel care also delayed registering the birth of children and reduced opportunities for health care providers to assist women in obtaining required immunizations and other follow-up care for their infants. In these ways, parallel systems for perinatal care placed both mothers who are addicted and infants at risk.

> I'm gonna have my baby at home and then I'm gonna register the birth at three or four months.

Health-Related Interventions

Health-related approaches to perinatal drug abuse are notably unlike legal interventions. As the Healthy People 2010 plan states, useful approaches to improving health build community partnerships and are systemic, multidisciplinary, absent of disparities across population groups, and attuned to the reciprocal relationship between individual health and community health. Reciprocal means community health is affected by the beliefs, attitudes, and behaviors of everyone in a given community and vice versa.

Components of Healthy People 2010—the national plan for improving public health in the United States—include two discrete goals, 467 objectives, and 28 focal areas. Among the focal areas of the plan are maternal, infant, and child health and substance abuse. Healthy People 2010 proposes to improve maternal, infant, and child health by decreasing maternal drug abuse. Because of the relevant focal areas and strategies of Healthy People 2010 and because the plan creates opportunities for individuals to make healthy lifestyle choices for themselves and their families, it has implications for developing empowerment strategies in perinatal care settings.

Implications for Empowerment

Of concern to social workers is that perinatal drug abuse, a health-related issue of families and children, is often criminalized. Basing perinatal approaches on empowerment strategies that target women who are addicted and health care providers promises to overcome legal interventions and address disparaging attitudes toward perinatal drug abuse.

Empowerment refers to increasing clients' personal, social, and political power so that they can change their situations and prevent reoccurrence of problems. Because empowerment theory emerged from efforts to develop more effective and responsive services for women and people of color, it is highly relevant to perinatal drug abuse.

The empowerment practice goals are helping client systems achieve a sense of personal power, become more aware of the connection between individual and community problems, develop helpful skills, and work toward social change. Studies cite the usefulness of empowerment practice in improving the contexts of human services organizations in ethnically diverse metropolitan areas and helping women of color in oppressed neighborhoods overcome unequal access to resources. Empowerment strategies include role playing as a technique for skills training, raising self-esteem, and helping women see the impact of the political environment on issues in their own lives. In empowerment practice, power is shared, clients are helped to "experience a sense of power" within helping relationships, and professionals are collaborators rather than superiors.

Perhaps the most empowering perinatal service about which social workers and their clients who are addicted can collaborate is helping women become alcohol and drug free. The specific strategies for motivating clients to seek drug rehabilitation, attain sobriety, and use relapse prevention measures are documented in the literature but are not a focus of this article. This article is concerned with empowering strategies for addressing the adverse attitudes and practices to which pregnant women who are addicted are often subjected. Examples include

- teaching pregnant women who are addicted to make formal complaints when they receive unprofessional services in perinatal care settings
- improving access by overcoming scheduling issues and advocating for adequate resources
- enhancing communication skills among women who are pregnant and addicted to drugs
- conducting culturally sensitive in-service training for health care providers
- addressing the unique issues of women of color
- promoting gender-sensitive programs
- overcoming systemic factors that create barriers to health care
- developing community partnerships with relevant groups
- recommending national policies that redefine perinatal drug abuse as a health issue.

Addressing Professional Attitudes and Practices

Social workers can help addicted women become empowered in perinatal care settings in which existing professional attitudes and practices are esteem lowering and potentially disempowering by conveying their own positive regard for the worth and dignity of individuals. This includes validating with clients that rude, judgmental, and other unethical practices are oppressive and unacceptable in health care settings. Collaborating with women about the best ways to file formal complaints against perinatal care personnel who fail to meet professional standards enhances women's personal power and is a model for social change.

Two of the most insurmountable barriers for low-income women seeking perinatal care are (1) the pejorative attitudes of providers and (2) the distrust of the health care system. Stressful interactions with health care providers can adversely affect the drug abuse recovery of women in perinatal care, further damage their self-esteem, and be intimidating as well.

The health of individuals and communities depends on access to quality health care. Case management approaches in which social workers appropriately assist in referring women who require perinatal care are potentially empowering because they facilitate access to services. Social workers can enhance their referrals by becoming knowledgeable about the practices and expectations for clients in perinatal care agencies and using the increased knowledge to improve clients' involvement in their own perinatal care regime. Examples are raising clients' general awareness of an agency's intake procedures and working collaboratively to overcome access barriers that are common in some perinatal care facilities. Access barriers include long waiting periods in facilities and scheduling problems—for example, consistently busy telephone lines and too few available appointments. Short-term strategies for overcoming barriers could involve scheduling appointments far in advance and adequately planning for such support services as extended child care, transportation, and meals when clients are scheduled for appointments. Long-term strategies should include advocating for increased resources.

By means of role playing or related techniques, addicted clients who require perinatal care can be taught more assertive, and thus personally empowering, means of communicating in health care settings. For instance, it is more useful for both clients and services professionals if a woman states, "Hello, I am [name] and I am here for my 3:00 appointment or the results of my lab work" than for her to say, "Hello, I am here for my appointment." Improved client communication may increase access and signal to providers that clients expect dignified, respectful services.

Health-related approaches to perinatal care have informed views on diversity. In-service training in which social workers help providers become more culturally sensitive to poor and ethnic minority clients is empowering because it can improve the overall environment of perinatal care settings. Our knowledge of human diversity and ethical commitment to ethnic-sensitive practice can enhance our role as trainers. Social workers understand, for instance, the usefulness of community intervention and how to use natural helping networks and extended families when working with poor families and families of color. Natural helpers, such as neighbors who can offer transportation or child care, are invaluable to perinatal drug abuse services. Lack of child care and transportation are access barriers that are personally disempowering to many women who require perinatal care.

It is also important to address the unique issues of women of color. For example, HIV infections are common among women who abuse intravenous drugs, but African American women are seven times more likely to die from

HIV/AIDS. Patient education on preventing HIV infections and other sexually transmitted diseases and planning for loss of parents and other effects of AIDS on families are important topics of discussion during perinatal care to African American women.

Counteracting Legal Interventions

Some experts believe the current political climate produces gender-biased, racist, and classist policies. An example is contemporary policy defining perinatal drug abuse as if it were strictly a legal issue and then targeting for prosecution poor women and women of color. Because of social workers' mandate to promote social justice, it is important that we advocate on behalf of vulnerable populations, for example, pregnant women who are addicted and their unborn children.

In recommending policies that foster adequate income, health insurance, and education, we can raise the socioeconomic status of mothers and, in turn, enhance the health status of drug-exposed babies. Being poor and less educated are linked to systemic issues like restricted access to health care, living in unsafe neighborhoods, inadequate housing, and limited opportunities to engage in health promotion. Many contemporary drug policies, however, blame women and divert attention from systemic forces, such as poverty, that promote substance abuse. A study of 1,000 substance abuse cases in four large cities showed that a sizable number of the parents lost their children to custodial care because of inadequate housing and poverty rather than explicit drug abuse. Healthy People 2010 embraces the empowering strategy of focusing on systemic factors that affect the health status of addicted women and their unborn fetuses.

Although it is important that social workers advocate for health-related perinatal care policies, it is even more empowering if the resulting programs are gender sensitive. Gender-sensitive perinatal programs take into account, among other factors, protecting women's physical health, access issues, and the rate of depression among women who are addicted. Depression, for example, is strongly correlated with high levels of personal stress, inadequate housing, lack of money for basic needs, and other factors associated with poverty. Because depressive symptoms are predictable among women who abuse drugs and can deter health-seeking behaviors, assessing depression in perinatal care settings is gender sensitive. Assessing depression is also a biopsychosocial strategy that favors health promotion. By treating depression, social workers can help clients in perinatal care settings overcome feelings of helplessness and become more available to engage in social change. Therefore, examining depression in perinatal care settings is personally, politically, and socially empowering to clients.

Social workers can intensify their perinatal advocacy efforts by developing community partnerships with CPS and perinatal care programs that fulfill the programs' missions while also protecting families and children. Perinatal toxicology screenings are allegedly designed to protect children, and CPS's primary mission is protecting children. However, between 1982 and 1989, when the number of substance abuse-related CPS cases doubled, child welfare agencies began separating children from their mothers solely on the basis of positive toxicology, without attempts to apply preventive measures or family rehabilitation. It is expedient that social workers help CPS and perinatal care providers refocus their dialogue on the needs of families within social and political contexts. Partnering agencies may then stop relying heavily on legal strategies and instead advocate for financial and other resources that can improve the health status of all family members—for example, by locating medical facilities in local communities and providing culturally specific health education. Because advocating community partnerships highlights the relatedness of individuals' problems and environmental conditions, it fulfills tenets of empowerment practice and Healthy People 2010.

Community partnerships that reach out to nontraditional partners can be among the most effective tools for improving health in communities. Social workers can further strengthen their campaigns to eliminate legal interventions for perinatal drug abuse by broadening their community partnerships with CPS and perinatal care programs to incorporate women, private companies, and community-based organizations such as criminal justice agencies, legal clinics, employment agencies, and churches. By providing research data, social workers can demonstrate to partners how legal means of "protecting" families and children are, in fact, injurious to them. Incarceration, for example, complicates birth outcomes in various ways. When women are released from prison, their own as well as their children's Medicaid eligibility is compromised for at least a month or more. If women and their children have chronic illnesses such as diabetes, HIV/AIDS, or hypertension, treatment adherence is essential, but health care is inaccessible without medical coverage. Women with low incomes, already at the highest risk of poor birth outcomes, are at greater risk of incarceration.

Once community partners are better informed, they can then educate politicians and other policymakers and thereafter solicit their help in adopting national policies that redefine perinatal drug abuse as a health-related issue. One example of such a policy is greater incentives for private corporations to develop partnerships with community-based drug rehabilitation organizations that accommodate mothers who are addicted as well as their children. Another is a policy that rewards medical schools for teaching students how to identify risk factors for substance use during pregnancy. In a survey of primary care physicians, only 17 percent could diagnose illicit drug use, a mere 30 percent were prepared to diagnose misuse of prescription drugs, and only 20 percent could confidently diagnose alcoholism. On the other hand, 82 percent of the physicians could identify patients with diabetes, and 83 percent could diagnose patients with hypertension. Increasing physicians' ability to identify risk factors for drug use during pregnancy is not only a preventive measure for improving maternal, infant, and child health, but a means of reinforcing among physicians and other health care providers the health-related definition of perinatal drug abuse.

Conclusion

Health care professionals and society at large exhibit negative attitudes toward women who abuse drugs. By means of empowerment strategies, social workers can potentially help clients who are addicted and pregnant to seek and complete perinatal treatment programs, improve the environment in which perinatal care services are provided, and advocate for policies that define perinatal drug abuse more as a health problem than a legal issue. Desired outcomes of these efforts are improved health care access and quality of life for families in which perinatal drug abuse is an issue.

POSTSCRIPT

Should Pregnant Drug Users Be Prosecuted?

Babies born with health problems as a result of their mothers' drug use is a tragedy that needs to be rectified. The issue is not whether this problem needs to be addressed but what course of action is best. The need for medical intervention and specialized treatment programs serving pregnant women with drug problems has been recognized. The groundwork has been set for funding and developing such programs. The Office of Substance Abuse Prevention is funding chemical dependency programs specifically for pregnant women in several states.

It has been argued that drug use by pregnant women is a problem that requires medical, not criminal, attention. One can contend the notion that pregnant drug users and their drug-exposed infants are victims of drug abuse. Critics contend that there is an element of discrimination in the practice of prosecuting women who use drugs during pregnancy because these women are primarily low-income, single, members of minorities, and recipients of public assistance. Possible factors leading to their drug use—poverty, unemployment, poor education, and lack of vocational training—are not addressed when the solution to drug use during pregnancy is incarceration. Moreover, many pregnant women are denied access to treatment programs.

Prosecution proponents contend that medical intervention is not adequate in preventing pregnant women from using drugs and that criminal prosecution is necessary. Logli argues that "eliminating the pain, suffering and death resulting from drug exposure in newborns must be a prosecutor's priority." He maintains that the criminal justice system should protect newborns and, if legal cause does exist for prosecution, then statutes should provide protection for the fetus. However, will prosecution result in more protection or less protection for the fetus? If a mother stops using drugs for fear of prosecution, then the fetus benefits. If the mother avoids prenatal care because of potential legal punishment, then the fetus suffers.

If women can be prosecuted for using illegal drugs such as cocaine and narcotics during pregnancy because they harm the fetus, then should women who smoke cigarettes and drink alcohol during pregnancy also be prosecuted? The evidence is clear that tobacco and alcohol place the fetus at great risk; however, most discussions of prosecuting pregnant drug users overlook women who use these drugs. Also, the adverse health effects from secondhand smoke are well documented. Should people be prosecuted if they smoke around pregnant women?

An excellent review of the effects of prenatal exposure to alcohol is "Alcohol and Pregnancy, Highlights from Three Decades of Research," by

Carrie L. Randall (*Journal of Studies on Alcohol*, vol. 62, 2001). Three articles that examine this issue thoroughly are "The Rights of Pregnant Women: The Supreme Court and Drug Testing," by Lawrence O. Gostin (*The Hastings Center Report*, September–October 2001); "Inside the Womb: Interpreting the Ferguson Case," by Samantha Weyrauch (*Duke Journal of Gender Law and Policy*, Summer 2002); and "Who Is the Guilty Party? Rights, Motherhood, and the Problem of Prenatal Drug Exposure," by Karen Zivi (*Law and Society Review*, vol. 34, no. 1, 2000).

ISSUE 6

Should Drug Addiction Be Considered a Disease?

YES: Lisa LeGrand, William Iacono, and Matt McGue, from "Predicting Addiction," *American Scientist* (March–April 2005)

NO: Jacob Sullum, from "H: The Surprising Truth About Heroin and Addiction," *Reason* (June 2003)

ISSUE SUMMARY

YES: Psychologists Lisa LeGrand, William Iacono, and Matt McGue maintain that certain personality characteristics, such as hyperactivity, acting-out behavior, and sensation-seeking may have their bases in genetics. LeGrand, Iacono, and McGue acknowledge the role of environment, but they feel that genes play a substantial role in drug-taking behavior.

NO: Jacob Sullum, a senior editor with *Reason* magazine, contends that drug addiction should not be considered a disease, a condition over which one has no control. Numerous individuals who have used drugs extensively have been able to stop drug use. Sullum maintains that drug use is a matter of behavior, not addiction. Classifying behavior as socially unacceptable does not prove that it is a disease.

Is drug addiction caused by an illness or disease, or is it caused by inappropriate behavioral patterns? This distinction is important because it has both legal and medical implications. Should people be held accountable for behaviors that stem from an illness over which they have no control? For example, if a person cannot help being an alcoholic and hurts or kills someone as a result of being drunk, should that person be treated or incarcerated? Likewise, if an individual's addiction is due to lack of self-control, rather than due to a disease, should taxpayer money go to pay for that person's treatment?

It can be argued that the disease concept of drug addiction legitimizes or excuses behaviors. If addiction is an illness, then blame for poor behavior can be shifted to the disease and away from the individual. Moreover, if drug addiction is incurable, can people ever be held responsible for their behavior?

Lisa LeGrand, William Iacono, and Matt McGue contend that addiction is caused by heredity, biochemistry, and environment influences. If drug addiction is the result of factors beyond the individual's control, then one should not be held responsible for one's behavior and that loss of control is not inevitable. Critics assert that many individuals have the ability of alcoholics to stop their abuse of drugs. For example, it has been shown that many cocaine and heroin users do not lose control while using these drugs. In their study of U.S. service personnel in Vietnam, epidemiologist Lee N. Robins and colleagues showed that most of the soldiers who used narcotics regularly during the war did not continue using them once they returned home. Many service personnel in Vietnam reportedly used drugs because they were in a situation they did not want to be in. Additionally, without the support of loved ones and society's constraints, they were freer to gravitate to behaviors that would not be tolerated by their families and friends.

Attitudes toward treating drug abuse are affected by whether it is perceived as an illness or as an act of free will. The disease concept implies that one needs help in overcoming addiction. By calling drug addiction a medical condition, the body is viewed as a machine that needs fixing; character and will become secondary. Also, by calling addiction a disease, the role of society in causing drug addiction is left unexplored. What roles do poverty, crime, unemployment, inadequate health care, and poor education have in drug addiction?

Jacob Sullum argues that the addictive qualities of drugs, especially heroin, are exaggerated. By claiming that certain drugs are highly addictive, it is easier to demonize those drugs and the people who use them. Sullum maintains that legal drugs such as alcohol and tobacco result in higher rates of addiction. Sullum also cites studies in which a number of heroin users are weekend users. This dispels the notion that heroin use always causes addiction.

According to the disease perspective, an important step for addicts to take in order to benefit from treatment is to admit that they are powerless against their addiction. They need to acknowledge that their drug addiction controls them and that drug addiction is a lifelong problem. The implication of this view is that addicts are never cured. Addicts must therefore abstain from drugs for their entire lives.

Is addiction caused by psychological or biological factors? Can drugs produce changes in the brain that result in drug addiction? How much control do drug addicts have over their use of drugs? In the following selections, LeGrand, Iacono, and McGue argue that addiction is a disease, whereas Sullum contends that the concept of drug addiction is a social construct, not based in science.

YES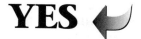

Lisa N. LeGrand, William G. Iacono, and Matt McGue

Predicting Addiction

In 1994, the 45-year-old daughter of Senator and former presidential nominee George McGovern froze to death outside a bar in Madison, Wisconsin. Terry McGovern's death followed a night of heavy drinking and a lifetime of battling alcohol addiction. The Senator's middle child had been talented and charismatic, but also rebellious. She started drinking at 13, became pregnant at 15 and experimented with marijuana and LSD in high school. She was sober during much of her 30s but eventually relapsed. By the time she died, Terry had been through many treatment programs and more than 60 detoxifications.

Her story is not unique. Even with strong family support, failure to overcome an addiction is common. Success rates vary by treatment type, severity of the condition and the criteria for success. But typically, fewer than a third of alcoholics are recovered a year or two after treatment. Thus, addiction may be thought of as a chronic, relapsing illness. Like other serious psychiatric conditions, it can cause a lifetime of recurrent episodes and treatments.

Given these somber prospects, the best strategy for fighting addiction may be to prevent it in the first place. But warning young people about the dangers of addiction carries little force when many adults drink openly without apparent consequences. Would specific warnings for individuals with a strong genetic vulnerability to alcoholism be more effective? Senator McGovern became convinced that his daughter possessed such a vulnerability, as other family members also struggled with dependency. Perhaps Terry would have taken a different approach to alcohol, or avoided it altogether, if she had known that something about her biology made drinking particularly dangerous for her.

How can we identify people—at a young enough age to intervene—who have a high, inherent risk of becoming addicted? Does unusual susceptibility arise from differences at the biochemical level? And what social or environmental factors might tip the scales for kids at greatest risk? That is, what kind of parenting, or peer group, or neighborhood conditions might encourage—or inhibit—the expression of "addiction" genes? These questions are the focus of our research.

Minnesota Twins

We have been able to answer some of these questions by examining the life histories of almost 1,400 pairs of twins. Our study of addictive behavior is

From *American Scientist*, vol. 93, March–April 2005, pp. 140–147. Copyright © 2005 by American Scientist. Reprinted by permission.

part of a larger project, the Minnesota Center for Twin Family Research (MCTFR), which has studied the health and development of twins from their pre-teen years through adolescence and into adulthood. Beginning at age 11 (or 17 for a second group), the participants and their parents cooperated with a barrage of questionnaires, interviews, brainwave analyses and blood tests every three years. The twin cohorts are now 23 and 29, respectively, so we have been able to observe them as children before exposure to addictive substances, as teenagers who were often experimenting and as young adults who had passed through the stage of greatest risk for addiction.

Studies of twins are particularly useful for analyzing the origins of a behavior like addiction. Our twin pairs have grown up in the same family environment but have different degrees of genetic similarity. Monozygotic or identical twins have identical genes, but dizygotic or fraternal twins share on average only half of their segregating genes. If the two types of twins are equally similar for a trait, we know that genes are unimportant for that trait. But when monozygotic twins are more similar than dizygotic twins, we conclude that genes have an effect.

This article reviews some of what we know about the development of addiction, including some recent findings from the MCTFR about early substance abuse. Several established markers can predict later addiction and, together with recent research, suggest a provocative conclusion: that addiction may be only one of many related behaviors that stem from the same genetic root. In other words, much of the heritable risk may be nonspecific. Instead, what is passed from parent to child is a tendency toward a group of behaviors, of which addiction is only one of several possible outcomes.

Markers of Risk

Personality

Psychologists can distinguish at-risk youth by their personality, family history, brainwave patterns and behavior. For example, certain personality traits do not distribute equally among addicts and nonaddicts: The addiction vulnerable tend to be more impulsive, unruly and easily bored. They're generally outgoing, sociable, expressive and rebellious, and they enjoy taking risks. They are more likely to question authority and challenge tradition.

Some addicts defy these categories, and having a certain personality type doesn't doom one to addiction. But such traits do place individuals at elevated risk. For reasons not completely understood, they accompany addiction much more frequently than the traits of being shy, cautious and conventional.

Although these characteristics do not directly cause addiction, neither are they simply the consequences of addiction. In fact, teachers' impressions of their 11-year-old students predicted alcohol problems 16 years later, according to a Swedish study led by C. Robert Cloninger (now at Washington University in St. Louis). Boys low in "harm avoidance" (ones who lacked fear and inhibition) and high in "novelty seeking" (in other words, impulsive, disorderly, easily bored and distracted) were almost 20 times more likely to have future alcohol problems than boys without these traits. Other studies of children in separate countries at different ages confirm that personality is predictive.

Family Background

Having a parent with a substance-abuse disorder is another established predictor of a child's future addiction. One recent and intriguing discovery from the MCTFR is that assessing this risk can be surprisingly straightforward, particularly for alcoholism. The father's answer to "What is the largest amount of alcohol you ever consumed in a 24-hour period?" is highly informative: The greater the amount, the greater his children's risk. More than 24 drinks in 24 hours places his children in an especially risky category.

How can one simple question be so predictive? Its answer is laden with information, including tolerance—the ability, typically developed over many drinking episodes, to consume larger quantities of alcohol before becoming intoxicated—and the loss of control that mark problematic drinking. It is also possible that a father who equivocates on other questions that can formally diagnose alcoholism—such as whether he has been unsuccessful at cutting down on his drinking or whether his drinking has affected family and work—may give a frank answer to this question. In our society, episodes of binge drinking, of being able to "hold your liquor," are sometimes a source of male pride.

Brainwaves

A third predictor comes directly from the brain itself. By using scalp electrodes to detect the electrical signals of groups of neurons, we can record characteristic patterns of brain activity generated by specific visual stimuli. In the complex squiggle of evoked brainwaves, the relative size of one peak, called P300, indicates addiction risk. Having a smaller P300 at age 17 predicts the development of an alcohol or drug problem by age 20. Prior differences in consumption don't explain this observation, as the reduced-amplitude P300 (P3-AR) is not a consequence of alcohol or drug ingestion. Rather, genes strongly influence this trait: P3-AR is often detectable in the children of fathers with substance-use disorders even before these problems emerge in the offspring. The physiological nature of P300 makes it an especially interesting marker, as it may originate from "addiction" genes more directly than any behavior.

Precocious Experimentation

Lastly, at-risk youth are distinguished by the young age at which they first try alcohol without parental permission. Although the vast majority of people try alcohol at some point during their life, it's relatively unusual to try alcohol *before* the age of 15. In the MCTFR sample of over 2,600 parents who had tried alcohol, only 12 percent of the mothers and 22 percent of the fathers did so before the age of 15. In this subset, 52 percent of the men and 25 percent of the women were alcoholics. For parents who first tried alcohol after age 19, the comparable rates were 13 percent and 2 percent, respectively. So, what distinguishes alcoholism risk is not *whether* a person tries alcohol during their teen years, but *when* they try it.

In light of these data, we cannot regard very early experimentation with alcohol as simply a normal rite of passage. Moreover, drinking at a young age often co-occurs with sex, the use of tobacco and illicit drugs, and rule-breaking behaviors. This precocious experimentation could indicate that the individual has inherited the type of freewheeling, impulsive personality that elevates the risk of addiction. But early experimentation may be a problem all by itself. It, and the behaviors that tend to co-occur with it, decrease the likelihood of sobriety-encouraging experiences and increase the chances of mixing with troubled peers and clashing with authority figures.

A General, Inherited Risk

Some of these hallmarks of risk are unsurprising. Most people know that addiction runs in families, and they may intuit that certain brain functions could differ in addiction-prone individuals. But how can people's gregarious-ness or their loathing of dull tasks or the age at which they first had sex show a vulnerability to addiction? The answer seems to be that although addiction risk is strongly heritable, the inheritance is fairly nonspecific. The inherited risk corresponds to a certain temperament or disposition that goes along with so-called *extertializing* tendencies. Addiction is only one of several ways this disposition may be expressed.

Externalizing behaviors include substance abuse, but also "acting out" and other indicators of behavioral under control or disinhibition. In childhood, externalizing traits include hyperactivity, "oppositionality" (negative and defiant behavior) and antisocial behavior, which breaks institutional and social rules. An antisocial child may lie, get in fights, steal, vandalize or skip school. In adult-hood, externalizing tendencies may lead to a personality marked by low constraint, drug or alcohol abuse, and antisocial behaviors, including irrespon-sibility, dishonesty, impulsivity, lawlessness and aggression. Antisociality, like most traits, falls on a continuum. A moderately antisocial person may never intentionally hurt someone, but he might make impulsive decisions, take physi-cal and financial risks or shirk responsibility.

It's worth reiterating that an externalizing disposition simply increases the risk of demonstrating problematic behavior. An individual with such ten-dencies could express them in ways that are not harmful to themselves and actually help society: Fire fighters, rescue workers, test pilots, surgeons and entrepreneurs are often gregarious, relatively uninhibited sensation-seekers—that is, moderate externalizers.

So a genetic inclination for externalizing can lead to addiction, hyperac-tivity, acting-out behavior, criminality, a sensation-seeking personality or *all* of these things. Although the contents of this list may seem haphazard, psy-chologists combine them into a single group because they all stem from the same *latent factor*. Latent factors are hypothesized constructs that help explain the observed correlations between various traits or behaviors.

For example, grades in school generally correlate with one another. People who do well in English tend to get good marks in art history, algebra and geol-ogy. Why? Because academic ability affects grades, regardless of the subject matter. In statistical lingo, academic ability is the "general, latent factor" and the course grades are the "observed indicators" of that factor. Academic ability is latent because it is not directly measured; rather, the statistician concludes that it exists and causes the grades to vary systematically between people.

Statistical analyses consistently show that externalizing is a general, latent factor—a common denominator—for a suite of behaviors that includes addiction. Furthermore, the various markers of risk support this conclusion: Childhood characteristics that indicate later problems with alcohol also point to the full spectrum of externalizing behaviors and traits. Thus, drinking alcohol before 15 doesn't just predict future alcohol and drug problems, but also future antisocial behavior. A parent with a history of excessive binge drinking is apt to have children not only with substance-use problems, but with behavioral problems as well. And a reduced-amplitude P300 not only appears in children with a familial risk for alcoholism, but in kids with a familial risk for hyperactivity, antisocial behavior or illicit drug disorders.

The associations between externalizing behaviors aren't surprising to clinicians. Comorbidity—the increased chance of having other disorders if you have one of them—is the norm, not the exception, for individuals and families. A father with a cocaine habit is more likely to find that his daughter is getting into trouble for stealing or breaking school rules. At first glance, the child's behavioral problems look like products of the stress, conflict and dysfunction that go with having an addict in the family. These are certainly aggravating factors. However, the familial and genetically informative MCTFR data have allowed us to piece together a more precise explanation.

Environment has a strong influence on a child's behavior—living with an addict is rife with challenges—but genes also play a substantial role. Estimates of the genetic effect on externalizing behaviors vary by indicator and age, but among older adolescents and adults, well over half of the differences between people's externalizing tendencies result from inheriting different genes.

Our analysis of the MCTFR data indicates that children inherit the general, latent factor of externalizing rather than specific behavioral factors. Thus, an antisocial mother does not pass on genes that code simply for antisocial behavior, but they do confer vulnerability to a range of adolescent disorders and behaviors. Instead of encounters with the law, her adolescent son may have problems with alcohol or drugs. The outcomes are different, but the same genes—expressed differently under different environmental conditions—predispose them both.

The Role of the Environment

Even traits with a strong genetic component may be influenced by environmental factors. Monozygotic twins exemplify this principle. Despite their matching DNA, their height, need for glasses, disease susceptibility or personality (just to name a few) may differ.

When one member of a monozygotic pair is alcoholic, the likelihood of alcoholism in the other is only about 50 percent. The high heritability of externalizing behaviors suggests that the second twin, if not alcoholic, may be antisocial or dependent on another substance. But sometimes the second twin is problem free. DNA is never destiny.

Behavioral geneticists have worked to quantify the role of the environment in addiction, but as a group we have done much less to specify it. Although we know that 50 percent of the variance in alcohol dependence comes from the environment, we are still in the early stages of determining what those environmental factors are. This ignorance may seem surprising, as scientists have spent decades identifying the environmental precursors to addiction and antisocial behavior. But only a small percentage of that research incorporated genetic controls.

Instead, many studies simply related environmental variation to children's eventual problems or accomplishments. A classic example of this failure to consider genetic influence is the repeated observation that children who grow up with lots of books in their home tend to do better in school. But concluding that books create an academic child assumes (falsely) that children are born randomly into families—that parent-child resemblance is purely social. Of course, parents actually contribute to their children's environment *and* their genes. Moreover, parents tend to provide environments that complement their children's genotypes: Smart parents often deliver both "smart" genes and an enriched environment. Athletic parents usually provide "athletic" genes and many opportunities to express them. And, unfortunately, parents with addiction problems tend to provide a genetic vulnerability coupled with a home in which alcohol or drugs are available and abusing them is normal.

To understand the true experiential origins of a behavior, one must first disentangle the influence of genes. By using genetically informative samples, we can subtract genetic influences and conclude with greater confidence that a particular environmental factor affects behavior. Using this approach, our data suggest that deviant peers and poor parent-child relationships exert true environmental influences that promote substance use and externalizing behaviors during early adolescence.

When considering the effect of environment on behavior, or any complex trait, it's helpful to imagine a continuum of liability. Inherited vulnerability determines where a person begins on the continuum (high versus low risk). From that point, psychosocial or environmental stressors such as peer pressure or excessive conflict with parents can push an individual along the continuum and over a disease threshold.

However, sometimes the environment actually modifies gene expression. In other words, the relative influence of genes on a behavior can vary by setting. We see this context-dependent gene expression in recent, unpublished work comparing study participants from rural areas (population less than 10,000) with those from more urban settings. Within cities of 10,000 or more, genes substantially influence which adolescents use illicit substances or show other aspects of the externalizing continuum—just as earlier research indicated. But in very rural areas, environmental (rather than genetic) factors overwhelmingly account for differences in externalizing behavior.

One way to interpret this finding is that urban environments, with their wider variety of social niches, allow for a more complete expression of genetically influenced traits. Whether a person's genes nudge her to substance use and rule-breaking, or abstinence and obedience, the city may offer more opportunities to follow those urges. At the same time, finite social prospects in the country may allow more rural parents to monitor and control their adolescents' activities and peer-group selection, thereby minimizing the impact of genes. This rural-urban difference is especially interesting because it represents a gene-by-environment interaction. The genes that are important determinants of behavior in one group of people are just not as important in another.

The Future of Addiction Research

This complex interplay of genes and environments makes progress slow. But investigators have the data and statistical tools to answer many important addiction-related questions. Moreover, the tempo of discovery will increase with advances in molecular genetics.

In the last fifteen years, geneticists have identified a handful of specific genes related to alcohol metabolism and synapse function that occur more often in alcoholics. But the task of accumulating the entire list of contributing genes is daunting. Many genes influence behavior, and the relative impor-tance of a single gene may differ across ethnic or racial populations. As a result, alcoholism-associated genes in one population may not exert a measur-able influence in a different group, even in well-controlled studies. There are also different pathways to addiction, and some people's alcoholism may be more environmental than genetic in origin. Consequently, not only is any one gene apt to have small effects on behavior, but that gene may be absent in a substantial number of addicts.

Nonetheless, some day scientists should be able to estimate risk by reading the sequence of a person's DNA. Setting aside the possibility of a futuristic dystopia, this advance will usher in a new type of psychology. Investigators will be able to observe those individuals with especially high (or low) genetic risks for externalizing as they respond, over a lifetime, to different types of environmental stressors.

This type of research is already beginning. Avshalom Caspi, now at the University of Wisconsin, and his colleagues divided a large group of males from New Zealand based on the expression level of a gene that encodes a neurotransmitter-metabolizing enzyme, monoamine oxidase A or MAOA. In combination with the life histories of these men, the investigators demonstrated that the consequences of an abusive home varied by genotype. The gene associ-ated with high levels of MAOA was protective—those men were less likely to show antisocial behaviors after childhood maltreatment than the low-MAOA group.

Further advances in molecular genetics will bring opportunities for more studies of this type. When investigators can accurately rank experimental participants by their genetic liability to externalizing, they will gain insight into the complexities of gene-environment interplay and answer several intriguing questions: What type of family environments are most at-risk chil-dren born into? When children with different genetic risks grow up in the same family, do they create unique environments by seeking distinct friends and experiences? Do they elicit different parenting styles from the same parents? Could a low-risk sibling keep a high-risk child from trouble if they share a close friendship? Is one type of psychosocial stressor more apt to lead to substance use while another leads to antisocial behavior?

Molecular genetics will eventually deepen our understanding of the biochemistry and biosocial genesis of addiction. In the interim, quantitative geneticists such as ourselves continue to characterize the development of behavior in ways that will assist molecular geneticists in their work. For example, if there is genetic overlap between alcoholism, drug dependence and antisocial behavior—as the MCTFR data suggest—then it may help to examine extreme externalizers, rather than simply alcoholics, when searching for the genes that produce alcoholism vulnerability.

Much Left to Learn

Although the MCTFR data have resolved some addiction-related questions, many others remain, and our team has just begun to scratch the surface of possible research. Our work with teenagers indicates that externalizing is a key factor in early-onset substance-use problems, but the path to later-life addiction may be distinct. Some evidence suggests that genes play a lesser role in later-onset addiction. Moreover, the markers of risk may vary. Being prone to worry, becoming upset easily and tending toward negative moods may, with age, become more important indicators. We don't yet know. However, the MCTFR continues to gather information about its participants as they approach their 30s, and we hope to keep following this group into their 40s and beyond.

Meanwhile, the evidence suggests that for early-onset addiction, most relevant genes are not specific to alcoholism or drug dependence. Instead, the same genes predispose an overlapping set of disorders within the externalizing spectrum. This conclusion has significant implications for prevention: Some impulsive risk-takers, frequent rule-breakers and oppositional children may be just as much at risk as early users.

At the same time, many kids with a genetic risk for externalizing don't seem to require any sort of special intervention; as it is, they turn out just fine. DNA may nudge someone in a certain direction, but it doesn't force them to go there.

Bibliography

Burt, S. A., M. McGue, R. F. Krueger and W. G. Iacono. 2005. How are parent-child conflict and childhood externalizing symptoms related over time? Results from a genetically informative cross-tagged study. *Development and Psychopathology* 17:1–21.

Caspi, A., J. McClay, T. E. Moffitt, J. Mill, J. Martin, I. W. Craig, A. Taylor and R. Poulton. 2002. Role of genotype in the cycle of violence in maltreated children. *Science* 297:851–854.

Cloninger, C. R., S. Sigvardsson and M. Bohman. 1988. Childhood personality predicts alcohol abuse in young adults. *Alcoholism: Clinical and Experimental Research* 12:494–505.

Hicks, B. M., R. F. Krueger, W. G. Iacono, M. McGue and C. J. Patrick. 2004. Family transmission and heritability of externalizing disorders: A twin-family study. *Archives of General Psychiatry* 61:922–928.

Iacono, W. G., S. M. Malone and M. McGue. 2003. Substance use disorders, externalizing psychopathology, and P300 event-related potential amplitude. *International Journal of Psychophysiology* 48:147–178.

Krueger, R. F., B. M. Hicks, C. J. Patrick, S. R. Carlson, W. G. Iacono and M. McGue. 2002. Etiologic connections among substance dependence, antisocial behavior, and personality: Modeling the externalizing spectrum. *Journal of Abnormal Psychology* 111:411–424.

Malone, S. M., W. G. Iacono and M. McGue. 2002. Drinks of the father: Father's maximum number of drinks consumed predicts externalizing disorders, substance use, and substance use disorders in preadolescent and adolescent offspring. *Alcoholism: Clinical and Experimental Research* 26:1823–1832.

McGovern, G. 1996. *Terry: My Daughter's Life-and-Death Struggle With Alcoholism.* New York: Random House.

McGue, M., W. G. Iacono, L. N. LeGrand, S. Malone and I. Elkins. 2001. The origins and consequences of age at first drink. I. Associations with substance-abuse disorders, disinhibitory behavior and psychopathology, and P3 amplitude. *Alcoholism: Clinical and Experimental Research* 25:1156–1165.

Porjesz, B., and H. Begleiter. 2003. Alcoholism and human electrophysiology. *Alcohol Research & Health* 27:153–160.

Turkheimer, E., H. H. Goldsmith and I.I. Gottesman. 1995. Some conceptual deficiencies in "developmental" behavioral genetics: Comment. *Human Development* 38:142–153.

Walden, B., M. McGue, W. G. Iacono, S. A. Burt and I. Elkins. 2004. Identifying shared environmental contributions to early substance use: The respective roles of peers and parents. *Journal of Abnormal Psychology* 113:440–450.

Jacob Sullum 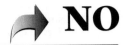 **NO**

H: The Surprising Truth About Heroin and Addiction

In 1992, *The New York Times* carried a front-page story about a successful businessman who happened to be a regular heroin user. It began: "He is an executive in a company in New York, lives in a condo on the Upper East Side of Manhattan, drives an expensive car, plays tennis in the Hamptons and vacations with his wife in Europe and the Caribbean. But unknown to office colleagues, friends, and most of his family, the man is also a longtime heroin user. He says he finds heroin relaxing and pleasurable and has seen no reason to stop using it until the woman he recently married insisted that he do so. "The drug is an enhancement of my life," he said. "I see it as similar to a guy coming home and having a drink of alcohol. Only alcohol has never done it for me."

The Times noted that "nearly everything about the 44-year-old executive . . . seems to fly in the face of widely held perceptions about heroin users." The reporter who wrote the story and his editors seemed uncomfortable with contradicting official anti-drug propaganda, which depicts heroin use as incompatible with a satisfying, productive life. The headline read, "Executive's Secret Struggle With Heroin's Powerful Grip," which sounds more like a cautionary tale than a success story. And *The Times* hastened to add that heroin users "are flirting with disaster." It conceded that "heroin does not damage the organs as, for instance, heavy alcohol use does." But it cited the risk of arrest, overdose, AIDS, and hepatitis—without noting that all of these risks are created or exacerbated by prohibition.

The general thrust of the piece was: Here is a privileged man who is tempting fate by messing around with a very dangerous drug. He may have escaped disaster so far, but unless he quits he will probably end up dead or in prison.

That is not the way the businessman saw his situation. He said he had decided to give up heroin only because his wife did not approve of the habit. "In my heart," he said, "I really don't feel there's anything wrong with using heroin. But there doesn't seem to be any way in the world I can persuade my wife to grant me this space in our relationship. I don't want to lose her, so I'm making this effort."

Judging from the "widely held perceptions about heroin users" mentioned by *The Times*, that effort was bound to fail. The conventional view of heroin,

From Reason, vol. 35, issue 12, June 2003, pp. 32–40. Copyright © 2003 by Reason Foundation. Reprinted by permission.

which powerfully shapes the popular understanding of addiction, is nicely summed up in the journalist Martin Booth's 1996 history of opium. "Addiction is the compulsive taking of drugs which have such a hold over the addict he or she cannot stop using them without suffering severe symptoms and even death," he writes. "Opiate dependence . . . is as fundamental to an addict's existence as food and water, a physio-chemical fact: an addict's body is chemically reliant upon its drug for opiates actually alter the body's chemistry so it cannot function properly without being periodically primed. A hunger for the drug forms when the quantity in the bloodstream falls below a certain level. . . . Fail to feed the body and it deteriorates and may die from drug starvation." Booth also declares that "everyone . . . is a potential addict"; that "addiction can start with the very first dose"; and that "with continued use addiction is a certainty."

Booth's description is wrong or grossly misleading in every particular. To understand why is to recognize the fallacies underlying a reductionist, drug-centered view of addiction in which chemicals force themselves on people—a view that skeptics such as the maverick psychiatrist Thomas Szasz and the psychologist Stanton Peele have long questioned. The idea that a drug can compel the person who consumes it to continue consuming it is one of the most important beliefs underlying the war on drugs, because this power makes possible all the other evils to which drug use supposedly leads.

When Martin Booth tells us that anyone can be addicted to heroin, that it may take just one dose, and that it will certainly happen to you if you're foolish enough to repeat the experiment, he is drawing on a long tradition of anti-drug propaganda. As the sociologist Harry G. Levine has shown, the original model for such warnings was not heroin or opium but alcohol. "The idea that drugs are inherently addicting," Levine wrote in 1978, "was first systematically worked out for alcohol and then extended to other substances. Long before opium was popularly accepted as addicting, alcohol was so regarded." The dry crusaders of the 19th and early 20th centuries taught that every tippler was a potential drunkard, that a glass of beer was the first step on the road to ruin, and that repeated use of distilled spirits made addiction virtually inevitable. Today, when a kitchen wrecked by a skinny model wielding a frying pan is supposed to symbolize the havoc caused by a snort of heroin, similar assumptions about opiates are even more widely held, and they likewise are based more on faith than facts.

Withdrawal Penalty

Beginning early in the 20th century, Stanton Peele notes, heroin "came to be seen in American society as the nonpareil drug of addiction—as leading inescapably from even the most casual contact to an intractable dependence, withdrawal from which was traumatic and unthinkable for the addict." According to this view, reflected in Booth's gloss and other popular portrayals, the potentially fatal agony of withdrawal is the gun that heroin holds to the addict's head. These accounts greatly exaggerate both the severity and the importance of withdrawal symptoms.

Heroin addicts who abruptly stop using the drug commonly report flu-like symptoms, which may include chills, sweating, runny nose and eyes, muscular aches, stomach cramps, nausea, diarrhea, or headaches. While certainly unpleasant, the experience is not life threatening. Indeed, addicts who have developed tolerance (needing higher doses to achieve the same effect) often voluntarily undergo withdrawal so they can begin using heroin again at a lower dose, thereby reducing the cost of their habit. Another sign that fear of withdrawal symptoms is not the essence of addiction is the fact that heroin users commonly drift in and out of their habits, going through periods of abstinence and returning to the drug long after any physical discomfort has faded away. Indeed, the observation that detoxification is not tantamount to overcoming an addiction, that addicts typically will try repeatedly before successfully kicking the habit, is a commonplace of drug treatment.

More evidence that withdrawal has been overemphasized as a motivation for using opiates comes from patients who take narcotic painkillers over extended periods of time. Like heroin addicts, they develop "physical dependence" and experience withdrawal symptoms when they stop taking the drugs. But studies conducted during the last two decades have consistently found that patients in pain who receive opioids (opiates or synthetics with similar effects) rarely become addicted.

Pain experts emphasize that physical dependence should not be confused with addiction, which requires a psychological component: a persistent desire to use the substance for its mood-altering effects. Critics have long complained that unreasonable fears about narcotic addiction discourage adequate pain treatment. In 1989, Charles Schuster, then director of the National Institute on Drug Abuse, confessed, "We have been so effective in warning the medical establishment and the public in general about the inappropriate use of opiates that we have endowed these drugs with a mysterious power to enslave that is overrated."

Although popular perceptions lag behind, the point made by pain specialists—that "physical dependence" is not the same as addiction—is now widely accepted by professionals who deal with drug problems. But under the heroin-based model that prevailed until the 1970s, tolerance and withdrawal symptoms were considered the hallmarks of addiction. By this standard, drugs such as nicotine and cocaine were not truly addictive; they were merely "habituating." That distinction proved untenable, given the difficulty that people often had in giving up substances that were not considered addictive.

Having hijacked the term addiction, which in its original sense referred to any strong habit, psychiatrists ultimately abandoned it in favor of substance dependence. "The essential feature of Substance Dependence," according to the American Psychiatric Association, "is a cluster of cognitive, behavioral, and physiological symptoms indicating that the individual continues use of the substance despite significant substance-related problems. . . . Neither tolerance nor withdrawal is necessary or sufficient for a diagnosis of Substance Dependence." Instead, the condition is defined as "a maladaptive pattern of substance use" involving at least three of seven features. In addition to tolerance and withdrawal, these include using more of the drug than intended; trying unsuccessfully to cut back; spending a lot of time getting the drug, using it, or recovering from its effects; giving up or reducing important social, occupational, or recreational activities because of drug use; and continuing use even while recognizing drug-related psychological or physical problems.

One can quibble with these criteria, especially since they are meant to be applied not by the drug user himself but by a government-licensed expert with whose judgment he may disagree. The possibility of such a conflict is all the more troubling because the evaluation may be involuntary (the result of an arrest, for example) and may have implications for the drug user's freedom. More fundamentally, classifying substance dependence as a "mental disorder" to be treated by medical doctors suggests that drug abuse is a disease, something that happens to people rather than something that people do. Yet it is clear from the description that we are talking about a pattern of behavior. Addiction is not simply a matter of introducing a chemical into someone's body, even if it is done often enough to create tolerance and withdrawal symptoms. Conversely, someone who takes a steady dose of a drug and who can stop using it without physical distress may still be addicted to it.

Simply Irresistible?

Even if addiction is not a physical compulsion, perhaps some drug experiences are so alluring that people find it impossible to resist them. Certainly that is heroin's reputation, encapsulated in the title of a 1972 book: *It's So Good, Don't Even Try It Once.*

The fact that heroin use is so rare—involving, according to the government's data, something like 0.2 percent of the U.S. population in 2001—suggests that its appeal is much more limited than we've been led to believe. If heroin really is "so good," why does it have such a tiny share of the illegal drug market? Marijuana is more than 45 times as popular. The National Household Survey on Drug Abuse indicates that about 3 million Americans have used heroin in their lifetimes; of them, 15 percent had used it in the last year, 4 percent in the last month. These numbers suggest that the vast majority of heroin users either never become addicted or, if they do, manage to give the drug up. A survey of high school seniors found that 1 percent had used heroin in the previous year, while 0.1 percent had used it on 20 or more days in the previous month. Assuming that daily use is a reasonable proxy for opiate addiction, one in 10 of the students who had taken heroin in the last year might have qualified as addicts. These are not the sort of numbers you'd expect for a drug that's irresistible.

True, these surveys exclude certain groups in which heroin use is more common and in which a larger percentage of users probably could be described as addicts. The household survey misses people living on the street, in prisons, and in residential drug treatment programs, while the high school survey leaves out truants and dropouts. But even for the entire population of heroin users, the estimated addiction rates do not come close to matching heroin's reputation. A 1976 study by the drug researchers Leon G. Hunt and Carl D. Chambers estimated there were 3 or 4 million heroin users in the United States, perhaps 10 percent of them addicts. "Of all active heroin users," Hunt and Chambers wrote, "a large majority are not addicts: they are not physically or socially dysfunctional; they are not daily users and they do not seem to require treatment." A 1994 study based on data from the National Comorbidity Survey estimated that 23 percent of heroin users never experience substance dependence.

The comparable rate for alcohol in that study was 15 percent, which seems to support the idea that heroin is more addictive: A larger percentage of the people who try it become heavy users, even though it's harder to get. At the same time, the fact that using heroin is illegal, expensive, risky, inconvenient, and almost universally condemned means that the people who nevertheless choose to do it repeatedly will tend to differ from people who choose to drink. They will be especially attracted to heroin's effects, the associated lifestyle, or both. In other words, heroin users are a self-selected group, less representative of the general population than alcohol users are, and they may be more inclined from the outset to form strong attachments to the drug.

The same study found that 32 percent of tobacco users had experienced substance dependence. Figures like that one are the basis for the claim that nicotine is "more addictive than heroin." After all, cigarette smokers typically go through a pack or so a day, so they're under the influence of nicotine every waking moment. Heroin users typically do not use their drug even once a day. Smokers offended by this comparison are quick to point out that they function fine, meeting their responsibilities at work and homey despite their habit. This, they assume, is impossible for heroin users. Examples like the businessman described by *The New York Times* indicate otherwise.

Still, it's true that nicotine's psychoactive effects are easier to reconcile with the requirements of everyday life than heroin's are. Indeed, nicotine can enhance concentration and improve performance on certain tasks. So one important reason why most cigarette smokers consume their drug throughout the day is that they can do so without running into trouble. And because they're used to smoking in so many different settings, they may find nicotine harder to give up than a drug they use only with certain people in secret. In one survey, 57 percent of drug users entering a Canadian treatment program said giving up their problem substance (not necessarily heroin) would be easier than giving up cigarettes. In another survey, 36 heroin users entering treatment were asked to compare their strongest cigarette urge to their strongest heroin urge. Most said the heroin urge was stronger, but two said the cigarette urge was, and 11 rated the two urges about the same.

In a sense, nicotine's compatibility with a wide range of tasks makes it more addictive than alcohol or heroin. But this is not the sort of thing people usually have in mind when they worry about addiction. Indeed, if it weren't for the health effects of smoking (and the complaints of bystanders exposed to the smoke), nicotine addiction probably would be seen as no big deal, just as caffeine addiction is. As alternative sources of nicotine that do not involve smoking (gum, patches, inhalers, beverages, lozenges, oral snuff) become popular not just as aids in quitting but as long-term replacements, it will be interesting to see whether they will be socially accepted. Once the health risks are dramatically reduced or eliminated, will daily consumption of nicotine still be viewed as shameful and declasse, as a disease to be treated or a problem to be overcome? Perhaps so, if addiction per se is the issue. But not if it's the medical, social, and psychological consequences of addiction that really matter.

The Needle and the Damage Done

To a large extent, regular heroin use also can be separated from the terrible consequences that have come to be associated with it. Because of prohibition, users face the risk of arrest and imprisonment, the handicap of a criminal record, and the violence associated with the black market. The artificially high price of heroin, perhaps 40 or 50 times what it would otherwise cost, may lead to heavy debts, housing problems, poor nutrition, and theft. The inflated cost also encourages users to inject the drug, a more efficient but riskier mode of administration. The legal treatment of injection equipment, including restrictions on distribution and penalties for possession, encourages needle sharing, which spreads diseases such as AIDS and hepatitis. The unreliable quality and unpredictable purity associated with the black market can lead to poisoning and accidental overdoses.

Without prohibition, then, a daily heroin habit would be far less burdensome and hazardous. Heroin itself is much less likely to kill a user than the reckless combination of heroin with other depressants, such as alcohol or barbiturates. The federal government's Drug Abuse Warning Network counted 4,820 mentions of heroin or morphine (which are indistinguishable in the blood) by medical examiners in 1999. Only 438 of these deaths (9 percent) were listed as directly caused by an overdose of the opiate. Three-quarters of the deaths were caused by heroin/morphine in combination with other drugs. Provided the user avoids such mixtures, has access to a supply of reliable purity, and follows sanitary injection procedures, the health risks of long-term opiate consumption are minimal.

The comparison between heroin and nicotine is also instructive when it comes to the role of drug treatment. Although many smokers have a hard time quitting, those who succeed generally do so on their own. Surprisingly, the same maybe true of heroin addicts. In the early 1960s, based on records kept by the Federal Bureau of Narcotics, sociologist Charles Winick concluded that narcotic addicts tend to "mature out" of the habit in their 30s. He suggested that "addiction may be a self limiting process for perhaps two-thirds of addicts." Subsequent researchers have questioned Winick's assumptions, and other studies have come up with lower estimates. But it's clear that "natural recovery" is much more common than the public has been led to believe.

In a 1974 study of Vietnam veterans, only 12 percent of those who were addicted to heroin in Vietnam took up the habit again during the three years after their return to the United States. (This was not because they couldn't find heroin; half of them used it at least once after their return, generally without becoming addicted again.) Those who had undergone treatment (half of the group) were just as likely to be re-addicted as those who had not. Since those with stronger addictions were more likely to receive treatment, this does not necessarily mean that treatment was useless, but it clearly was not a prerequisite for giving up heroin.

Despite its reputation, then, heroin is neither irresistible nor inescapable. Only a very small share of the population ever uses it, and a large majority of those who do never become addicted. Even within the minority who develop a daily habit, most manage to stop using heroin, often without professional intervention. Yet heroin is still perceived as the paradigmatic voodoo drug, ineluctably turning its users into zombies who must obey its commands.

Heroin in Moderation

The idea that drugs cause addiction was rejected in the case of alcohol because it was so clearly at odds with everyday experience, which showed that the typical drinker was not an alcoholic. But what the psychologist Bruce Alexander calls "the myth of drug-induced addiction" is still widely accepted in the case of heroin—and, by extension, the drugs compared to it—because moderate opiate users are hard to find. That does not mean they don't exist; indeed, judging from the government's survey results, they are a lot more common than addicts. It's just that people who use opiates in a controlled way are inconspicuous by definition, and keen to remain so.

In the early 1960s, however, researchers began to tentatively identify users of heroin and other opiates who were not addicts. "Surprisingly enough," a Northwestern University psychiatrist wrote in 1961, "in some cases at least, narcotic use may be confined to weekends or parties and the users may be able to continue in gainful employment for some time. Although this pattern often deteriorates and the rate of use increases, several cases have been observed in which relatively gainful and steady employment has been maintained for two to three years while the user was on what might be called a regulated or controlled habit."

A few years later, Harvard psychiatrist Norman Zinberg and David C. Lewis, then a medical resident, described five categories of narcotic users, including "people who use narcotics regularly but who develop little or no tolerance for them and do not suffer withdrawal symptoms." They explained that "such people are usually able to work regularly and productively. They value the relaxation and the 'kick' obtained from the drug, but their fear of needing more and more of the drug to get the same kick causes them to impose rigorous controls on themselves."

The example offered by Zinberg and Lewis was a 47-year-old physician with a successful practice who had been injecting morphine four times a day, except weekends, for 12 years. He experienced modest discomfort on Saturdays and Sundays, when he abstained, but he stuck to his schedule and did not raise his dose except on occasions when he was especially busy or tense. Zinberg and Lewis's account suggests that morphine's main function for him was stress relief: "Somewhat facetiously, when describing his intolerance of people making emotional demands on him, he said that he took 1 shot for his patients, 1 for his mistress, 1 for his family and 1 to sleep. He expressed no guilt about his drug taking, and made it clear that he had no intention of stopping."

Zinberg eventually interviewed 61 controlled opiate users. His criteria excluded both dabblers (the largest group of people who have used heroin) and daily users. One subject was a 41-year-old carpenter who had used heroin on weekends for a decade. Married 16 years, he lived with his wife and three children in a middle-class suburb. Another was a 27-year-old college student studying special education. He had used heroin two or three times a month for three years, then once a week for a year. The controlled users said they liked "the 'rush' (glow or warmth), the sense of distance from their problems, and the tranquilizing powers of the drug." Opiate use was generally seen as a social activity, and it was often combined with other forms of recreation. Summing up the lessons he learned from his research, Zinberg emphasized the importance of self-imposed rules dictating when, where, and with whom the drug would be used. More broadly, he concluded that "set and setting"—expectations and environment—play crucial roles in shaping a drug user's experience.

Other researchers have reported similar findings. After interviewing 12 occasional heroin users in the early 1970s, a Harvard researcher concluded that "it seems possible for young people from a number of different backgrounds, family patterns, and educational abilities to use heroin occasionally without becoming addicted." The subjects typically took heroin with one or more friends, and the most frequently reported benefit was relaxation. One subject, a 23-year-old graduate student, said it was "like taking a vacation from yourself . . . When things get to you, it's a way of getting away without getting away." These occasional users were unanimous in rejecting addiction as inconsistent with their self-images. A 1983 British study of 51 opiate users likewise found that distaste for the junkie lifestyle was an important deterrent to excessive use.

While these studies show that controlled opiate use is possible, the 1974 Vietnam veterans study gives us some idea of how common it is. "Only one-quarter of those who used heroin in the last two years used it daily at all," the researchers reported. Likewise, only a quarter said they had felt dependent, and only a quarter said heroin use had interfered with their lives. Regular heroin use (more than once a week for more than a month) was associated with a significant increase in "social adjustment problems," but occasional use was not.

Many of these occasional users had been addicted in Vietnam, so they knew what it was like. Paradoxically, a drug's attractiveness, whether experienced directly or observed secondhand, can reinforce the user's determination to remain in control. (Presumably, that is the theory behind all the propaganda warning how wonderful certain drug experiences are, except that the aim of those messages is to stop people from experimenting at all.) A neuroscientist in his late 20s who smoked heroin a couple of times told me it was "nothing dramatic, just the feeling that everything was OK for about six hours, and I wasn't really motivated to do anything." Having observed several friends who were addicted to heroin at one time or another, he understood that the experience could be seductive, but "that kind of seduction . . . kind of repulsed me. That was exactly the kind of thing that I was trying to avoid in my life."

Similarly, a horticulturist in his 40s who first snorted heroin in the mid-1980s said, "It was too nice." As he described it, "you're sort of not awake and you're not asleep, and you feel sort of like a baby in the cradle, with no worries, just floating in a comfortable cocoon. That's an interesting place to be if you don't have anything else to do. That's Sunday-afternoon-on-the-couch material." He did have other things to do, and after that first experience he used heroin only "once in a blue moon." But he managed to incorporate the regular use of another opiate, morphine pills, into a busy, productive life. For years he had been taking them once a week, as a way of unwinding and relieving the aches and pains from the hard manual labor required by his landscaping business. "We use it as a reward system," he said. "On a Friday, if we've been working really hard and we're sore and it's available, it's a reward. It's like, 'We've worked hard today. We've earned our money, we paid our bills, but we're sore, so let's do this. It's medicine.' "

Better Homes & Gardens

Evelyn Schwartz learned to use heroin in a similar way: as a complement to rest and relaxation rather than a means of suppressing unpleasant emotions. A social worker in her 50s, she injected heroin every day for years but was using it intermittently when I interviewed her a few years ago. Schwartz (a pseudonym) originally became addicted after leaving home at 14 because of conflict with her mother. "As I felt more and more alienated from my family, more and more alone, more and more depressed," she said, "I started to use [heroin] not in a recreational fashion but as a coping mechanism, to get rid of feelings, to feel OK. . . . I was very unhappy . . . and just hopeless about life, and I was just trying to survive day by day for many years."

But after Schwartz found work that she loved and started feeling good about her life, she was able to use heroin in a different way. "I try not to use as a coping mechanism," she said. "I try very hard not to use when I'm miserable, because that's what gets me into trouble. It's set and setting. It's not the drug, because I can use this drug in a very controlled way, and I can also go out of control." To stay in control, "I try to use when I'm feeling good," such as on vacation with friends, listening to music, or before a walk on a beautiful spring day. "If I need to clean the house, I do a little heroin, and I can clean the house, and it just makes me feel so good."

Many people are shocked by the idea of using heroin so casually, which helps explain the controversy surrounding a 2001 BBC documentary that explored why people use drugs. "Heroin is my drug of choice over alcohol or cocaine," said one user interviewed for the program. "I take it at weekends in small doses, and do the gardening." It may be unconventional, but using heroin to enliven housework or gardening is surely wiser than using it to alleviate grief, dissatisfaction, or loneliness. It's when drugs are used for emotional management that a destructive habit is apt to develop.

Even daily opiate use is not necessarily inconsistent with a productive life. One famous example is the pioneering surgeon William Halsted, who led a brilliant career while secretly addicted to morphine. On a more modest level, Schwartz said that even during her years as a self-described junkie she always held a job, always paid the rent, and was able to conceal her drug use from people who would have been alarmed by it. "I was always one of the best secretaries at work, and no one ever knew, because I learned how to titrate my doses," she said. She would generally take three or four doses a day: when she got up in the morning, at lunchtime, when she came home from work, and perhaps before going to sleep. The doses she took during the day were small enough so that she could get her work done. "Aside from the fact that I was a junkie," she said, "I was raised to be a really good girl and do what I'm supposed to do, and I did."

Schwartz, a warm, smart, hard-working woman, is quite different from the heroin users portrayed by government propaganda. Even when she was taking heroin every day, her worst crime was shoplifting a raincoat for a job interview. "I never robbed," she said. "I never did anything like that. I never hurt a human being. I could never do that. . . . I'm not going to hit anybody over the head. . . . I went sick a lot as a consequence. When other junkies would commit crimes, get money, and tighten up, I would be sick. Everyone used to say: 'You're terrible at being a junkie.' "

POSTSCRIPT

Should Drug Addiction Be Considered a Disease?

There is little debate that drug addiction is a major problem. Drug addiction wreaks havoc for society and ruins the lives of numerous individuals and people who care for them. Addressing the causes of drug addiction and what to do about people who become addicted is especially relevant. Views on whether or not drug addiction is a disease diverge. Because drug abuse can be viewed as a matter of free will or as a brain disorder, there are also different views on how society should deal with drug abusers. Should drug addicts be incarcerated or treated? Does it matter whether one is responsible for one's drug addiction?

One could argue that free will and the concept of a brain disorder both apply to drug addiction. What may start out as a matter of free will may turn into an illness. Likewise, drug use may start out as an occasional behavior that may become abusive. To illustrate this point, many people may use alcohol for recreational or social purposes, but their alcohol use may develop into a chronic, abusive pattern—one that the person cannot easily overcome. Initially, one can stop using alcohol without too much discomfort. As time passes, however, and alcohol consumption becomes more frequent and the amounts increase, stopping for many people becomes difficult. By its very definition, social drinkers can stop drinking at will. Alcoholics drink out of necessity.

Many people who use addictive drugs do not become dependent on them. Perhaps there are factors beyond free will and changes in the brain that account for these people to become dependent. Is it possible that social factors come into play? Can friends and colleagues and their attitudes about drugs influence whether a drug user becomes a drug abuser? In the final analysis, drug addiction may result from the interaction of numerous factors and not simply be a dichotomy between psychology and biology.

Stanton Peele, an outspoken critic of the disease concept, discusses this issue in "The Surprising Truth About Addiction" (*Psychology Today,* May/June 2004). In his book *Addiction Is a Choice*, Jeffrey Schaler argues against addiction as a disease. The opposite position is discussed in "Addiction Is a Brain Disease," by Alan Leshner (*Issues in Science and Technology*, Spring 2001). Other articles that explore whether addiction is a matter of biology are "Addiction Is a Disease," by John Halpern (*Psychiatric Times*, October 1, 2002) and "Addiction and Responsibility," by Richard J. Bonnie (*Social Research*, Fall 2001).

ISSUE 7

Should the Federal Government Play a Larger Role in Regulating Steroid Use?

YES: National Institute on Drug Abuse, from "Anabolic Steroid Abuse," *National Institute on Drug Abuse Research Report* (August 2006)

NO: Matthew J. Mitten, from "Drug Testing of Athletes—An Internal, Not External, Matter," *The New England Law Review* (Spring 2006)

ISSUE SUMMARY

YES: The National Institute on Drug Abuse (NIDA) warns that anabolic steroids produce numerous harmful side effects that can lead to stunted growth, breast development in males, excessive hair growth on women, acne, complications of the liver, and infections from nonsterile needles. Behaviorally, anabolic steroids have been associated with rage and aggression. According to NIDA, simply teaching about steroids does not deter their use.

NO: Matthew J. Mitten, a professor with the Marquette University Law School, feels that the federal government should not try to regulate the use of anabolic steroids. Rather, the various sports-governing bodies should be the regulators. Also, if athletes are aware of the risks of using anabolic steroids, then they could make the decision about whether to use these drugs. Allowing steroid use would essentially level the playing field for all athletes.

$\mathbf{A}$nabolic steroids are synthetic derivatives of the male hormone testosterone. Although they have legitimate medical uses, steroids are used increasingly by individuals to build up muscle quickly and to increase personal strength. Concerns over the potential negative effects of steroid use seem to be justified: an estimated 1 million Americans, including 4 percent of students in grades nine to twelve. Anabolic steroids users span all ethnic groups, nationalities, and socioeconomic groups. The emphasis on winning has led many athletes to take risks with steroids that are potentially destructive. Despite the widespread belief that anabolic steroids are used primarily by athletes, up to one-third of users are nonathletes who use these drugs to improve their physiques and self-images.

Society places much emphasis on winning, and to come out on top, many individuals are willing to make sacrifices—sacrifices that might compromise their health. Some people will do anything for the sake of winning. The sports headlines in many newspapers mention how various professional and Olympic athletes have used steroids. Drug testing is a major issue every time the Olympic competition is held. Besides the adverse physical consequences of steroids, there is the ethical question regarding fair play. Do steroids give competitors an unfair advantage? Should they be banned even if the side effects are not harmful? Do non-steroid users feel pressured to use these drugs to keep up with the competition? Would there be better regulation of steroibds if their use was permitted?

The short-term consequences of anabolic steroids are well documented. Possible short-term effects among men include testicular atrophy, sperm count reduction, impotency, baldness, difficulty urinating, and breast enlargement. Among women, some potential effects are deepening of the voice, breast reduction, menstrual irregularities, the growth of body hair, and clitoral enlargement. Both sexes may develop acne, swelling in the feet, reduced levels of high-density lipoproteins (the type of cholesterol that is good for the body), hypertension, and liver damage. Taking steroids as an adolescent will stunt one's growth. Also related to steroid use are psychological changes, including mood swings, paranoia and violent behavior.

Steroids' short-term effects have been researched thoroughly; however, their long-term effects have not been substantiated. The problem with identifying the long-term effects of anabolic steroids is the lack of systematic, long-term studies. Much of the information regarding steroids' long-term effects comes from personal reports, not well-conducted, well-controlled studies. However, personal stories and anecdotal evidence are often accepted as fact.

The American Medical Association opposes stricter regulation of anabolic steroids on two grounds. First, anabolic steroids have been used medically to improve growth and development, for certain types of anemia, breast cancer, endometriosis, and osteoporosis. If stricter regulations are imposed, people who may benefit medically from these drugs will have more difficulty acquiring them. Second, it is highly unlikely that illicit use of these drugs will cease if they are banned. By maintaining legal access to these drugs, more studies regarding their long-term consequences can be conducted.

In the following selections, the National Institute on Drug Abuse (NIDA) contends that people who use anabolic steroids are risking their mental and physical well-being. NIDA advocates more testing for anabolic steroids. Matthew Mitten argues that the government should not be in the business of testing for steroids. Mitten maintains that the various sports-governing bodies should be the groups responsible for steroid testing.

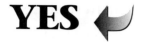
Anabolic Steroid Abuse

What Are Anabolic Steroids?

"Anabolic steroids" is the familiar name for synthetic substances related to the male sex hormones (e.g., testosterone). They promote the growth of skeletal muscle (anabolic effects) and the development of male sexual characteristics (androgenic effects) in both males and females. The term "anabolic steroids" will be used throughout this report because of its familiarity, although the proper term for these compounds is "anabolic-androgenic steroids."

Anabolic steroids were developed in the late 1930s primarily to treat hypogonadism, a condition in which the testes do not produce sufficient testosterone for normal growth, development, and sexual functioning. The primary medical uses of these compounds are to treat delayed puberty, some types of impotence, and wasting of the body caused by HIV infection or other diseases.

During the 1930s, scientists discovered that anabolic steroids could facilitate the growth of skeletal muscle in laboratory animals, which led to abuse of the compounds first by bodybuilders and weightlifters and then by athletes in other sports. Steroid abuse has become so widespread in athletics that it can affect the outcome of sports contests.

Illicit steroids are often sold at gyms, competitions, and through mail order operations after being smuggled into this country. Most illegal steroids in the United States are smuggled from countries that do not require a prescription for the purchase of steroids. Steroids are also illegally diverted from U.S. pharmacies or synthesized in clandestine laboratories.

What Are Steroidal Supplements?

In the United States, supplements such as tetrahydrogestrinone (THG) and androstenedione (street name "Andro") previously could be purchased legally without a prescription through many commercial sources, including health food stores. Steroidal supplements can be converted into testosterone or a similar compound in the body. Less is known about the side effects of steroidal supplements, but if large quantities of these compounds substantially increase testosterone levels in the body, then they also are likely to produce the same side effects as anabolic steroids themselves. The purchase of these supplements, with the notable exception of dehydroepiandrosterone (DHEA), became illegal after the passage in 2004 of amendments to the Controlled Substances Act.

From *National Institute on Drug Abuse Research Report*, August 2006. U.S. Department of Health and Human and Services.

What Is the Scope of Steroid Use in the United States?

The 2005 Monitoring the Future study, a NIDA-funded survey of drug use among adolescents in middle and high schools across the United States, reported that past year use of steroids decreased significantly among 8th- and 10th-graders since peak use in 2000. Among 12th-graders, there was a different trend—from 2000 to 2004, past year steroid use increased, but in 2005 there was a significant decrease, from 2.5 percent to 1.5 percent.

Steroid abuse affects individuals of various ages. However, it is difficult to estimate the true prevalence of steroid abuse in the United States because many data sources that measure drug abuse do not include steroids. Scientific evidence indicates that anabolic steroid abuse among athletes may range between one and six percent.

Why Do People Abuse Anabolic Steroids?

One of the main reasons people give for abusing steroids is to improve their athletic performance. Among athletes, steroid abuse has been estimated to be less that 6 percent according to surveys, but anecdotal information suggests more widespread abuse. Although testing procedures are now in place to deter steroid abuse among professional and Olympic athletes, new designer drugs constantly become available that can escape detection and put athletes willing to cheat one step ahead of testing efforts. This dynamic, however, may be about to shift if the saving of urine and blood samples for retesting at a future date becomes the standard. The high probability of eventual detection of the newer designer steroids, once the technology becomes available, plus the fear of retroactive sanctions, should give athletes pause.

Another reason people give for taking steroids is to increase their muscle size or to reduce their body fat. This group includes people suffering from the behavioral syndrome called muscle dysmorphia, which causes them to have a distorted image of their bodies. Men with muscle dysmorphia think that they look small and weak, even if they are large and muscular. Similarly, women with this condition think that they look fat and flabby, even though they are actually lean and muscular.

Some people who abuse steroids to boost muscle size have experienced physical or sexual abuse. In one series of interviews with male weightlifters, 25 percent who abused steroids reported memories of childhood physical or sexual abuse. Similarly, female weightlifters who had been raped were found to be twice as likely to report use of anabolic steroids or another purported muscle-building drug, compared with those who had not been raped. Moreover, almost all of those who had been raped reported that they markedly increased their bodybuilding activities after the attack. They believed that being bigger and stronger would discourage further attacks because men would find them either intimidating or unattractive.

Finally, some adolescents abuse steroids as part of a pattern of high-risk behaviors. These adolescents also take risks such as drinking and driving, carrying a gun, driving a motorcycle without a helmet, and abusing other illicit drugs. Conditions such as muscle dysmorphia, a history of physical or sexual abuse, or a history of engaging in high-risk behaviors have all been associated with an increased risk of initiating or continuing steroid abuse.

How Are Anabolic Steroids Abused?

Some anabolic steroids are taken orally, others are injected intramuscularly, and still others are provided in gels or creams that are applied to the skin. Doses taken by abusers can be 10 to 100 times higher than the doses used for medical conditions.

Cycling, Stacking, and Pyramiding

Steroids are often abused in patterns called "cycling," which involve taking multiple doses of steroids over a specific period of time, stopping for a period, and starting again. Users also frequently combine several different types of steroids in a process known as "stacking." Steroid abusers typically "stack" the drugs, meaning that they take two or more different anabolic steroids, mixing oral and/or injectable types, and sometimes even including compounds that are designed for veterinary use. Abusers think that the different steroids interact to produce an effect on muscle size that is greater than the effects of each drug individually, a theory that has not been tested scientifically.

Another mode of steroid abuse is referred to as "pyramiding." This is a process in which users slowly escalate steroid abuse (increasing the number of steroids or the dose and frequency of one or more steroids used at one time), reaching a peak amount at mid-cycle and gradually tapering the dose toward the end of the cycle. Often, steroid abusers pyramid their doses in cycles of 6 to 12 weeks. At the beginning of a cycle, the person starts with low doses of the drugs being stacked and then slowly increases the doses. In the second half of the cycle, the doses are slowly decreased to zero. This is sometimes followed by a second cycle in which the person continues to train but without drugs. Abusers believe that pyramiding allows the body time to adjust to the high doses, and the drug-free cycle allows the body's hormonal system time to recuperate. As with stacking, the perceived benefits of pyramiding and cycling have not been substantiated scientifically.

What Are the Health Consequences of Steroid Abuse?

Anabolic steroid abuse has been associated with a wide range of adverse side effects ranging from some that are physically unattractive, such as acne and breast development in men, to others that are life threatening, such as heart attacks and liver cancer. Most are reversible if the abuser stops taking the drugs, but some are permanent, such as voice deepening in females.

Most data on the long-term effects of anabolic steroids in humans come from case reports rather than formal epidemiological studies. From the case reports, the incidence of life-threatening effects appears to be low, but serious adverse effects may be underrecognized or underreported, especially since they may occur many years later. Data from animal studies seem to support this possibility. One study found that exposing male mice for one-fifth of their lifespan to steroid doses comparable to those taken by human athletes caused a high frequency of early deaths.

Hormonal System

Steroid abuse disrupts the normal production of hormones in the body, causing both reversible and irreversible changes. Changes that can be reversed include reduced sperm production and shrinking of the testicles (testicular atrophy). Irreversible changes include male-pattern baldness and breast development (gynecomastia) in men. In one study of male bodybuilders, more than half had testicular atrophy and/or gynecomastia.

In the female body, anabolic steroids cause masculinization. Breast size and body fat decrease, the skin becomes coarse, the clitoris enlarges, and the voice deepens. Women may experience excessive growth of body hair but lose scalp hair. With continued administration of steroids, some of these effects become irreversible.

Musculoskeletal System

Rising levels of testosterone and other sex hormones normally trigger the growth spurt that occurs during puberty and adolescence and provide the signals to stop growth as well. When a child or adolescent takes anabolic steroids, the resulting artificially high sex hormone levels can prematurely signal the bones to stop growing.

Cardiovascular System

Steroid abuse has been associated with cardiovascular diseases (CVD), including heart attacks and strokes, even in athletes younger than 30. Steroids contribute to the development of CVD, partly by changing the levels of lipoproteins that carry cholesterol in the blood. Steroids, particularly oral steroids, increase the level of low-density lipoprotein (LDL) and decrease the level of high-density lipoprotein (HDL). High LDL and low HDL levels increase the risk of atherosclerosis, a condition in which fatty substances are deposited inside arteries and disrupt blood flow. If blood is prevented from reaching the heart, the result can be a heart attack. If blood is prevented from reaching the brain, the result can be a stroke.

Steroids also increase the risk that blood clots will form in blood vessels, potentially disrupting blood flow and damaging the heart muscle so that it does not pump blood effectively.

Liver

Steroid abuse has been associated with liver tumors and a rare condition called peliosis hepatis, in which blood-filled cysts form in the liver. Both the tumors and the cysts can rupture, causing internal bleeding.

Skin

Steroid abuse can cause acne, cysts, and oily hair and skin.

Infections

Many abusers who inject anabolic steroids may use nonsterile injection techniques or share contaminated needles with other abusers. In addition, some steroid preparations are manufactured illegally under nonsterile conditions. These factors put abusers at risk for acquiring life-threatening viral infections, such as HIV and hepatitis B and C. Abusers also can develop endocarditis, a bacterial infection that causes a potentially fatal inflammation of the inner lining of the heart. Bacterial infections also can cause pain and abscess formation at injection sites.

What Effects Do Anabolic Steroids Have on Behavior?

Case reports and small studies indicate that anabolic steroids, when used in high doses, increase irritability and aggression. Some steroid abusers report that they have committed aggressive acts, such as physical fighting or armed robbery, theft, vandalism, or burglary. Abusers who have committed aggressive acts or property crimes generally report that they engage in these behaviors more often when they take steroids than when they are drug free. A recent study suggests that the mood and behavioral effects seen during anabolic-androgenic steroid abuse may result from secondary hormonal changes.

Scientists have attempted to test the association between anabolic steroids and aggression by administering high steroid doses or placebo for days or weeks to human volunteers and then asking the people to report on their behavioral symptoms. To date, four such studies have been conducted. In three, high steroid doses did produce greater feelings of irritability and aggression than did placebo, although the effects appear to be highly variable across individuals. In one study, the drugs did not have that effect. One possible explanation, according to the researchers, is that some but not all anabolic steroids increase irritability and aggression. Recent animal studies show an increase in aggression after steroid administration.

In a few controlled studies, aggression or adverse, overt behaviors resulting from the administration of anabolic steroid use have been reported by a minority of volunteers.

In summary, the extent to which steroid abuse contributes to violence and behavioral disorders is unknown. As with the health complications of steroid abuse, the prevalence of extreme cases of violence and behavioral disorders seems to be low, but it may be underreported or underrecognized.

Research also indicates that some users might turn to other drugs to alleviate some of the negative effects of anabolic steroids. For example, a study of 227 men admitted in 1999 to a private treatment center for addiction to heroin or other opioids found that 9.3 percent had abused anabolic steroids before trying any other illicit drug. Of these 9.3 percent, 86 percent first used opioids to counteract insomnia and irritability resulting from anabolic steroids.

POSSIBLE HEALTH CONSEQUENCES
OF ANABOLIC STEROID ABUSE

Hormonal System
- men
  - infertility
  - breast development
  - shrinking of the testicles
  - male-pattern baldness

- women
  - enlargement of the clitoris
  - excessive growth of body hair
  - male-pattern baldness

Musculoskeletal System
- short stature (if taken by adolescents)
- tendon rupture

Cardiovascular System
- increases in LDL; decreases in HDL
- high blood pressure
- heart attacks
- enlargement of the heart's left ventricle

Liver
- cancer
- peliosis hepatis
- tumors

Skin
- severe acne and cysts
- oily scalp
- jaundice
- fluid retention

Infection
- HIV/AIDS
- hepatitis

Psychiatric Effects
- rage, aggression
- mania
- delusions

Are Anabolic Steroids Addictive?

An undetermined percentage of steroid abusers may become addicted to the drugs, as evidenced by their continued abuse despite physical problems and negative effects on social relations. Also, steroid abusers typically spend large amounts of time and money obtaining the drugs, which is another indication that they may be addicted. Individuals who abuse steroids can experience withdrawal symptoms when they stop taking steroids, such as mood swings, fatigue, restlessness, loss of appetite, insomnia, reduced sex drive, and steroid cravings. The most dangerous of the withdrawal symptoms is depression, because it sometimes leads to suicide attempts. If left untreated, some depressive symptoms associated with anabolic steroid withdrawal have been known to persist for a year or more after the abuser stops taking the drugs.

What Can Be Done to Prevent Steroid Abuse?

Most prevention efforts in the United States today focus on athletes involved with the Olympics and professional sports; few school districts test for abuse of illicit drugs. It has been estimated that close to 9 percent of secondary schools conduct some sort of drug testing program, presumably focused on athletes, and that less than 4 percent of the Nation's high schools test their athletes for steroids. Studies are currently under way to determine whether such testing reduces drug abuse.

Research on steroid educational programs has shown that simply teaching students about steroids' adverse effects does not convince adolescents that they can be adversely affected. Nor does such instruction discourage young people from taking steroids in the future. Presenting both the risks and benefits of anabolic steroid use is more effective in convincing adolescents about steroids' negative effects, apparently because the students find a balanced approach more credible, according to the researchers.

NIDA-Funded Prevention Research Helps Reduce Steroid Abuse

A more sophisticated approach has shown promise for preventing steroid abuse among players on high school sports teams. The Adolescents Training and Learning to Avoid Steroids (ATLAS) program is showing high school football players that they do not need steroids to build powerful muscles and improve athletic performance. By educating student athletes about the harmful effects of anabolic steroids and providing nutrition and weight-training alternatives to steroid use, the ATLAS program has increased football players' healthy behaviors and reduced their intentions to abuse steroids. In the program, coaches and team leaders teach the harmful effects of anabolic steroids and other illicit drugs on immediate sports performance, and discuss how to refuse offers of drugs.

Studies show that 1 year after completion of the program, compared with a control group, ATLAS-trained students in 15 high schools had:

- Half the incidence of new abuse of anabolic steroids and less intention to abuse them in the future;
- Less abuse of alcohol, marijuana, amphetamines, and narcotics;
- Less abuse of "athletic enhancing" supplements;

- Less likelihood of engaging in hazardous substance abuse behaviors such as drinking and driving;
- Increased protection against steroid and other substance abuse. Namely, less interest in trying steroids, less desire to abuse them, better knowledge of alternatives to steroid abuse, improved body image, and increased knowledge of diet supplements.

The Athletes Targeting Healthy Exercise and Nutrition Alternatives (ATHENA) program was patterned after the ATLAS program, but designed for adolescent girls on sports teams. Early testing of girls enrolled in the ATHENA program showed significant decreases in risky behaviors. While preseason risk behaviors were similar among controls and ATHENA participants, the control athletes were three times more likely to begin using diet pills and almost twice as likely to begin abuse of other body-shaping substances, including amphetamines, anabolic steroids, and muscle-building supplements during the sports season. The use of diet pills increased among control subjects, while use fell to approximately half of the preseason levels among ATHENA participants. In addition, ATHENA team members were less likely to be sexually active, more likely to wear seatbelts, less likely to ride in a car with a driver who had been drinking, and they experienced fewer injuries during the sports season.

Both Congress and the Substance Abuse and Mental Health Services Administration have endorsed ATLAS and ATHENA as model prevention programs. These Oregon Health & Science University programs have been awarded the 2006 annual *Sports Illustrated* magazine's first-ever "Champion Award."

What Treatments Are Effective for Anabolic Steroid Abuse?

Few studies of treatments for anabolic steroid abuse have been conducted. Current knowledge is based largely on the experiences of a small number of physicians who have worked with patients undergoing steroid withdrawal. The physicians have found that supportive therapy is sufficient in some cases. Patients are educated about what they may experience during withdrawal and are evaluated for suicidal thoughts. If symptoms are severe or prolonged, medications or hospitalization may be needed.

Some medications that have been used for treating steroid withdrawal restore the hormonal system after its disruption by steroid abuse. Other medications target specific withdrawal symptoms—for example, antidepressants to treat depression and analgesics for headaches and muscle and joint pains.

Some patients require assistance beyond pharmacological treatment of withdrawal symptoms and are treated with behavioral therapies.

Where Can I Get Further Scientific Information About Steroid Abuse?

To learn more about anabolic steroids and other drugs of abuse, contact the National Clearinghouse for Alcohol and Drug Information (NCADI) at

800-729-6686. Information specialists are available to help you locate information and resources.

Fact sheets, including *InfoFacts*, on the health effects of anabolic steroids, other drugs of abuse, and other drug topics are available on the NIDA Web site . . . and can be ordered free of charge in English and Spanish from NCADI. . . .

References

Bahrke MS, Yesalis CE, Wright JE. Psychological and behavioral effects of endogenous testosterone and anabolic-androgenic steroids: an update. *Sports Med* 22(6):367–390, 1996.

Berning JM, Adams KJ, Stamford BA. Anabolic steroid usage in athletics: facts, fiction, and public relations. *J Strength Conditioning Res* 18(4):908–917, 2004.

Blue JG, Lombardo JA. Steroids and steroid-like compounds. *Clin Sports Med* 18(3):667–689, 1999.

Bronson FH, Matherne CM. Exposure to anabolic-androgenic steroids shortens life span of male mice. *Med Sci Sports Exerc* 29(5):615–619, 1997.

Brower KJ. Withdrawal from anabolic steroids. *Curr Ther Endocrinol Metab* 6:338–343, 1997.

Daly RC, et al. Neuroendocrine and behavioral effects of high-dose anabolic steroid administration in male normal volunteers. *Psychoneuroendocrinology* 28(3): 317–331, 2003.

Elliot D, Goldberg L. Intervention and prevention of steroid use in adolescents. *Am J Sports Med* 24(6):S46–S47, 1996.

Goldberg L, et al. Anabolic steroid education and adolescents: Do scare tactics work? *Pediatrics* 87(3):283–286, 1991.

Goldberg L, et al. Effects of a multidimensional anabolic steroid prevention intervention: The Adolescents Training and Learning to Avoid Steroids (ATLAS) Program. *JAMA* 276(19):1555–1562, 1996.

Goldberg L, et al. The ATLAS program: Preventing drug use and promoting health behaviors. *Arch Pediatr Adolesc Med* 154(4):332–338, 2000.

Gottfredson GD, et al. *The national study of delinquency prevention in schools.* Ellicott City, MD: Gottfredson Associates, Inc., 2000.

Green et al. NCAA study of substance use and abuse habits of college student-athletes. *Clin J Sport Med* 11(1):51–56, 2001.

Gruber AJ, Pope HG Jr. Compulsive weight lifting and anabolic drug abuse among women rape victims. *Compr Psychiatry* 40(4):273–277, 1999.

Gruber AJ, Pope HG Jr. Psychiatric and medical effects of anabolic-androgenic steroid use in women. *Psychother Psychosom* 69:19–26, 2000.

Hoberman JM, Yesalis CE. The history of synthetic testosterone. *Sci Am* 272(2): 76–81, 1995.

Leder BZ, et al. Oral androstenedione administration and serum testosterone concentrations in young men. *JAMA* 283(6):779–782, 2000.

The Medical Letter on Drugs and Therapeutics. Creatine and androstenedione—two "dietary supplements." 40(1039):105–106. New Rochelle, NY: The Medical Letter, Inc., 1998.

Middleman AB, et al. High-risk behaviors among high school students in Massachusetts who use anabolic steroids. *Pediatrics* 96(2):268–272, 1995.

Pope HG Jr, Kouri EM, Hudson MD. Effects of supraphysiologic doses of testosterone on mood and aggression in normal men: a randomized controlled trial. *Arch Gen Psychiatry* 57(2):133–140, 2000.

Porcerelli JH, Sandler BA. Anabolic-androgenic steroid abuse and psychopathology. *Psychiatr Clin North Am* 21(4):829–833, 1998.

Rich JD, Dickinson BP, Flanigan TP, Valone SE. Abscess related to anabolic-androgenic steroid injection. *Med Sci Sports Exerc* 31(2):207–209, 1999.

Stilger VG, Yesalis CE. Anabolic-androgenic steroid use among high school football players. *J Community Health* 24(2):131–145, 1999.

Su T-P, et al. Neuropsychiatric effects of anabolic steroids in male normal volunteers. *JAMA* 269(21):2760–2764, 1993.

Sullivan ML, Martinez CM, Gennis P, Gallagher, EJ. The cardiac toxicity of anabolic steroids. *Prog Cardiovasc Dis* 41(1):1–15, 1998.

Verroken M. Hormones and Sport. Ethical aspects and the prevalence of hormone abuse in sport. *J Endocrinol* 170(1):49–54, 2001.

Yesalis CE. *Anabolic steroids in sports and exercise,* 2nd edition. Champaign, IL: Human Kinetics. 2000.

Yesalis CE. Androstenedione. Sport dietary supplements update, 2000, *E-Sport-Med.com.*

Yesalis CE. Trends in anabolic-androgenic steroid use among adolescents. *Arch Pediatr Adolesc Med* 151(12):1197–1206.

Yesalis CE, Kennedy NJ, Kopstein AN, Bahrke MS. Anabolic-androgenic steroid use in the United States. *JAMA* 270(10):1217–1221, 1993.

Zorpette G. Andro angst. *Sci Am* 279(6):22–26, 1998.

Matthew J. Mitten

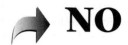 **NO**

Drug Testing of Athletes—An Internal, Not External, Matter

In today's society, the economic and intangible rewards for extraordinary athletic achievements and winning performances are substantial. Therefore, there is a significant incentive for athletes to maximize their onfield performance, which is the paramount objective of sports competition. Virtually all athletes use various artificial means to enhance their bodies' natural performance while playing their respective sports. Some athletes even use and publicly advertise artificial substances such as erectile dysfunction drugs to enhance their off-field performance.

Some substances and training techniques are not characterized as unfair competitive advantages, even if they are not universally available to all athletes because of their differing economic resources. It is generally permissible for athletes to ingest non-muscle building dietary supplements that facilitate athletic performance such as carbohydrates, electrolyte drinks, energy bars, vitamins, and minerals—and they are often encouraged to do so. Even the use of creatine as a muscle-building substance currently is not considered to be doping or an improper means of athletic performance enhancement.[1]

However, athletes' usage of federally controlled substances such as anabolic androgenic steroids, which include designer steroids such as THG (tetrahydrogestrinone) and steroid precursors is characterized as doping by sports governing bodies and punishable by sanctions if detected.[2] Anabolic androgenic steroids are synthetic variations of the male hormone testosterone that mimic its effects by having muscle-building (anabolic) and masculinizing (androgenic) characteristics with potentially harmful health consequences.[3] Steroids are a legitimate, therapeutic treatment for muscle-wasting conditions, but sports organizations prohibit their usage by athletes to enhance on-field performance. Also generally banned are steroid precursors such as androstenedione, which was admittedly used by former Major League Baseball ("MLB") player Mark McGwire.[4] These substances function like steroids after being ingested and metabolized by the body.[5] Sports organizations also ban and test for stimulants such as ephedrine and caffeine, which are contained in some over-the-counter products, because of their potential usage for unfair athletic performance enhancement.

Some athletes at all levels of sports competition are willing to use banned performance-enhancing drugs even though doing so violates the rules of the game, exposes them to sanctions, may adversely affect their health, and may violate federal and/or state law. Several former MLB and National Football League ("NFL") players such as Jose Canseco,[6] Ken Caminiti,[7] Bill Romanowski,[8] and Steve Courson[9] have admitted using anabolic steroids to enhance their on-field performances. Prominent Olympic athletes, for example, Ben Johnson and Jerome Young,[10] have tested positive for steroid usage and other Olympians are suspected or have been accused of using steroids. Approximately one percent of the 11,000 National Collegiate Athletic Association ("NCAA") student-athletes who are randomly tested each year test positive for usage of banned performance-enhancing substances.[11] According to a 2003 Center for Disease Control and Prevention survey of ninth through twelfth graders, steroid use by high school students has more than doubled from 1991 to 2003 to more than six percent.[12]

Anabolic steroids, when combined with vigorous physical training, do enhance athletic performance by making users bigger, stronger, and faster—while also reducing their recovery time after strenuous exercise. If steroids effectively enhance athletic performance, what is wrong with allowing athletes to take advantage of modern medicine and pharmacology? Athletes frequently are given painkillers and are fitted with artificial devices designed to enable continued participation in a sport despite an injury, which generally are considered to be acceptable practices. Although there is concern about potential health risks, libertarians point to the current lack of compelling medical evidence that steroid usage by adult athletes causes serious health risks beyond those already inherent in competitive sports. Some physicians and athletes, including World Cup champion skier Bode Miller, advocate allowing athletes to use steroids with medical supervision after full disclosure regarding their known health risks, rather than banning and imposing sanctions for their usage.[13]

Is there really an appropriate line that can be drawn between legitimate athletic performance enhancement through artificial means and unethical doping to achieve an unfair competitive advantage? And if so, who is the appropriate entity to draw this line? For example, athletes' usage of artificially created low-oxygen living environments in low altitude training areas currently is permitted; whereas, their use of erythropoietin ("EPO") to achieve similar effects on athletic performance are prohibited by sports governing bodies.

Perhaps it is easier to answer both questions by considering the second question first. Sports governing bodies have a legitimate interest in establishing uniform rules necessary to maintain the sport's integrity and image, to ensure competitive balance, and to protect athletes' health and safety. Although achieving maximum individual performance and winning is the objective of athletic competitions, the essence of sports is that all participants play by the same rules. Anti-doping rules are an integral part of the rules of the game, similar to rules regulating playing equipment, scoring competition results, and penalizing infractions. Even if a sport's rules of play are arbitrary (and they often are), the sport's governing body has the inherent authority to promulgate clearly defined rules to ensure fair play and enforce them in a uniform, non-discriminatory manner.

Even without medically conclusive evidence that steroid usage by athletes poses significant health risks, sports governing bodies have a rational basis for prohibiting their use to enhance athletic performance, especially since anabolic steroids are a federally controlled substance. Medical experts have identified several potential negative side effects of using anabolic steroids. Clinical experiments involving athletes' use of steroids solely to improve on-field performance would raise serious ethical issues. For example, East German athletes who were given steroids under medical supervision, which enabled them to win Olympic medals during the Cold War era, are now suffering serious adverse health effects.[14]

Courts and arbitration panels have upheld the legal authority of sports governing bodies (and educational institutions) to randomly drug test high school, college, and Olympic athletes.[15] These tribunals generally conclude that protecting the integrity of athletic competition and sports participants' health and safety outweighs athletes' legitimate privacy interests. In essence, sports governing bodies have broad discretion to determine their respective brands of athletic competition, which includes conditioning athlete eligibility on compliance with doping rules. An athlete who uses banned performance enhancing substances is deemed to be a "cheater," whose violation of the "rules of the game" may be punished by the sport's governing body. However, it is vitally important to ensure that competition results are not nullified without legitimate reason or that their athletic participation opportunities are not denied without appropriate justification. Thus, all athletes who fail a drug test or are otherwise accused of doping should have the right to a fair hearing before an impartial adjudicatory body or tribunal with adequate safeguards to ensure due process and equitable treatment.

Athletes who use prohibited substances directly expose themselves to potential adverse health consequences and indirectly expose others to similar risks. By nature, many athletes are risk takers who will adopt others' successful training methods—even dangerous ones—if doing so enhances their athletic performance. Thus, other athletes' actual or perceived usage of steroids creates a strong incentive to level the playing field, which may cause an athlete who would not otherwise ingest or inject steroids to do so.

Pharmacological performance-enhancing substances are banned because of their adverse effects on *both* athletes' health and competitive integrity. For example, the World Anti-Doping Agency ("WADA") Code only prohibits usage of a substance that satisfies at least two of the following criteria: 1) it enhances or has the potential to enhance sports performance; 2) it creates an actual or potential health risk; or 3) it violates the spirit of sport.[16] No single criterion is a sufficient reason for prohibiting usage. For example, the first criterion includes the use of creatine and artificial low-oxygen living environments, which are permitted because neither of the other criteria presently are deemed to be satisfied. Conversely, the use of anabolic steroids is prohibited because at least two, and arguably all three, of these criteria are satisfied.

The WADA Code governs Olympic sports competition.[17] It generally provides for strict liability and mandatory minimum suspensions for athletes' usage of banned substances.[18] Pursuant to a contract with the United States Olympic Committee, the United States Anti-Doping Agency ("USADA"), an independent entity, administers and oversees the drug-testing program for American Olympic sport athletes.[19] An athlete has the right to appeal USADA's finding of a doping violation to an independent arbitration tribunal and to seek a reduced sanction because of mitigating circumstances.[20]

The NCAA has a random drug testing protocol applicable to all student-athletes who participate in its member institutions' intercollegiate athletics program.[21] With approximately 375,000 student-athletes subject to testing, it is currently the world's largest athletics drug testing program.[22] Testing occurs during NCAA championships, Division 1-A football bowl games, and out-of-season. It provides for strict liability and a one-year suspension from participation in all NCAA sports (along with a loss of one year of athletics eligibility) for testing positive for a banned substance, with the right to an administrative appeal before members of the NCAA's Competitive Safeguards and Medical Aspects of Sports's Drug Education and Testing Subcommittee ("DETS").[23] Effective August 1, 2005, the NCAA's drug-testing protocol was modified to make it more consistent with the WADA Code by now allowing consideration of a reduced penalty based on the student-athlete's relative degree of fault for a doping violation.[24] The DETS may reduce the length of the suspension to one-half season of competition in the particular sport or determine that no suspension is appropriate based on extenuating circumstances.[25]

The NCAA's drug testing program is effectively reducing the usage of banned performance-enhancing substances (except amphetamines) by student-athletes. Survey results indicated that 4.9% of student-athletes used steroids in 1989; a 2005 survey reveals that this figure has dropped to 1.2%.[26] Factors causing this decline include the removal of steroid precursors from the open market; increased year-round drug testing; and more education programs for student-athletes. Approximately two-thirds of the student-athletes responding to the 2005 survey believe that the NCAA's drug testing program deters their peers from using steroids.[27] Other surveys indicate that its member institutions are generally satisfied with the NCAA process for adjudicating appeals of student-athlete positive drug tests.

Because of the large number of students participating in interscholastic athletics and the high cost of testing ($50 to $100 per test), no state high school athletics governing body presently requires testing for performance-enhancing drugs.[28] For the same reasons, very few school districts test for anabolic steroids. The California Interscholastic Federation, which regulates high school athletics, recently adopted a policy to curb steroid use.[29] It requires a student and his/her parents to agree in writing that the athlete will not use steroids without a physician's prescription and that coaches complete a certification program having a significant component regarding steroids and performance-enhancing dietary supplements.[30] It also prohibits school-related personnel and groups from selling, distributing, or advocating the use of muscle-building dietary supplements.[31]

Professional team sport athletes such as MLB, National Basketball Association ("NBA"), NFL, and National Hockey League ("NHL") players have chosen to unionize. Drug testing, which is a term or condition of employment, is a mandatory subject of collective bargaining. Unlike the governing bodies for non-unionized professional sports (or the USOC or the NCAA), the NBA, NFL, NHL, and MLB clubs and their respective commissioners cannot unilaterally impose a drug-testing program on their players.

As part of the Bay Area Laboratory Co-Operative ("BALCO") grand jury investigation into the illegal sale and distribution of designer steroid THC, several prominent MLB players were called to testify in December 2003 regarding whether they used anabolic steroids to enhance their athletic performance.[32] In the wake of this scandal, President Bush, in his 2004 State of the Union Address, urged professional sports leagues to voluntarily adopt more stringent drug policies that will effectively eliminate steroid usage and set a better example for America's youth.[33]

To protect public health and safety, the federal government recently has taken steps to restrict access to performance-enhancing drugs and prevent their usage by athletes (particularly youthful ones). Anabolic steroids have been federally regulated since 1990. However, many athletes used steroid precursors, which were sold as legal over-the-counter dietary supplements under the Dietary Supplement Health and Education Act of 1994.[34] Except for dehydroepiandrosterone ("DHEA"), steroid precursors are now regulated by the Anabolic Steroid Control Act of 2004,[35] which became effective on January 20, 2005. As reflected by the BALCO grand jury proceeding, the federal government also is actively prosecuting those who illegally provide performance-enhancing drugs to athletes.

In addition to these measures, there have been several 2005 Congressional committee hearings regarding professional athletes' usage of steroids and proposed federal laws to reduce their demand for these substances. These bills would establish a uniform random drug testing policy for professional athletes, with substantial fines imposed on sports organizations for failing to implement and comply with this policy.

The Clean Sports Act of 2005[36] is intended "to protect the integrity of professional sports and the health and safety of athletes generally," with the objectives of eliminating performance-enhancing substances from professional sports and reducing usage by children and teenagers.[37] This legislation would apply only to the NFL, NBA, NHL, and MLB as well as the United States Boxing Commission, which must develop drug testing policies and procedures as stringent as those of USADA.[38] However, the bill provides that all professional sports leagues should comply with these standards. Each athlete would be tested five times annually.[39] There is a mandatory two-year suspension for a first offense and a lifetime ban for a second offense, with the possibility of a reduced penalty for unknown or unsuspected usage of a banned substance.[40] The Director of the Office of National Drug Control Policy would be empowered to include other professional sports leagues or NCAA Division I and Division II colleges and athletes within the Act's coverage based on a determination that doing so would prevent the use of performance-enhancing substances by high school, college, or professional athletes.[41] Non-compliance with the Act's substantive provisions would constitute unfair or deceptive acts or practices in violation of the Federal Trade Commission Act with a potential civil penalty of $1,000,000 per violation.[42]

The Drug Free Sports Act[43] would cover Major League Soccer and the Arena Football League as well as the NFL, NBA, NHL, and MLB.[44] Players in these leagues would be randomly tested at least once per year with progressive penalties for positive tests (a minimum two-year suspension for the first offense and permanent suspension for the second offense) and a possible reduced suspension depending on the athlete's degree of fault for usage of prohibited substances.[45] The Secretary of Commerce would be directed to promulgate regulations requiring testing for steroids and other performance-enhancing substances and may fine a professional sports league $5,000,000 for failing to adopt testing policies and procedures consistent with the regulations.[46]

With some variations, similar bills titled the Professional Sports Integrity and Accountability Act[47] and the Professional Sports Integrity Act of 2005[48] have been introduced in the Senate and House, respectively. Other proposals also are being developed by members of Congress. For example, a bill introduced by Senators Jim Bunning and John McCain proposes a half-season suspension for a professional athlete's first positive drug test, which is a compromise intended to facilitate passage of a federal drug testing program applicable to the NFL, NBA, NHL, MLB, and minor league baseball.[49] It also has a provision urging professional sports leagues to erase player records achieved with the assistance of performance-enhancing drugs.

Congress has jurisdiction to establish a drug testing program for professional leagues based on its federal constitutional authority to regulate interstate commerce, and there are other potential bases for enacting such legislation. Nevertheless, professional athletes and their unions may assert that federally mandated drug testing violates their rights under the United States Constitution. Targeted drug testing of professional athletes but not other private employees is inconsistent treatment. However, the federal equal protection clause requires only a rational basis to justify treating professional athletes differently, which is satisfied by their prominence in American society and imitation by youths.

A more interesting issue is whether federal legislation mandating drug testing of adult professional athletes without an individualized suspicion of illegal drug usage constitutes an unreasonable "search" in violation of the Fourth Amendment. In recent years, the United States Supreme Court has upheld mandatory random drug testing of high school athletes for recreational drugs by public educational institutions to protect their health and safety.[50] Other courts have rejected college athletes' legal challenges to mandatory random drug testing for performance-enhancing and recreational drugs as a condition of participation in intercollegiate athletics.[51] The reasoning of this judicial precedent, which holds that random drug testing is an appropriate means of maintaining the integrity of amateur athletic competition and protecting athletes' health, likely also applies to professional sports.

Although Congress has valid regulatory authority, the proposed federal legislation would inappropriately interfere with the internal governance of professional sports, which historically has not been subject to direct government regulation, and the collective bargaining process. A federal sports doping law also would raise interesting questions regarding its application to, and effect on, players on Canadian teams in the NHL, NBA, and MLB. Athletic governing bodies are in the best position to establish appropriate drug testing programs to regulate the permissible bounds of competition and to protect athletes' health and safety. The primary harm that results from athletes' usage of banned performance-enhancing substances is to the sport's integrity. Thus, the sport's governing body should have the exclusive authority to establish doping violation sanctions that suspend or bar athletes from competition.

Market considerations, combined with political pressure, provide a strong incentive for professional sports leagues and their respective players unions to establish effective internal drug-testing programs. In January 2005, MLB clubs and the MLB Players Association established the first testing program for performance-enhancing drugs covering MLB players in response to pressure from Congress.[52] During the 2005 season, several players (approximately 1.5% of those subject to testing) tested positive for banned substances. Among them was Raphael Palmeiro, who testified under oath that he never used steroids during a March 2005 Congressional committee hearing.[53]

Current suspensions for a first drug testing violation are four games for NFL players, ten games for NBA players, and twenty games for NHL players. In response to the legislation proposed by Senators Bunning and McCain, MLB clubs and the players union recently agreed to a system of enhanced penalties for steroid use. First time offenders face a fifty game suspension for testing positive for the use of steroids, which is significantly more severe than the previous sanction of a ten-day suspension for MLB players. MLB's current fifty game suspension for a player's first positive test for steroids is proportionately similar to the corresponding NFL and NHL sanctions based on the length of their respective regular seasons.

As urged by proposed federal legislation, player records and competition results tarnished by the use of banned performance-enhancing substances should be nullified by athletic governing bodies. But this is a sanction that should be imposed only by the sport's governing body, not the federal government. For example, the World Boxing Association reinstated John Ruiz as its heavyweight champion because James Toney tested positive for performance-enhancing drugs after defeating Ruiz in an April 30, 2005 title fight.[54] Ruiz has also filed a $10 million lawsuit against Toney, alleging that Toney's use of steroids to enhance his strength and stamina caused Ruiz to lose the fight and suffer financial loss.

Rather than imposing an external drug-testing program on sports organizations, the federal government should focus on restricting access to performance-enhancing drugs that pose health risks and prosecuting those who distribute these substances illegally. In October 2005, BALCO founder Victor Conte, BALCO Vice President James Valente, and personal trainer Greg Anderson were sentenced to terms ranging from four months in federal prison to probation for distributing illegal, performance-enhancing substances to elite athletes.[55]

The federal government also has the authority to prosecute American athletes for violating controlled substances laws by knowingly using illegal performance-enhancing substances such as steroids. Criminal prosecution may be an appropriate means to punish professional athletes for the indirect harm caused to American youths who view them as role models and emulate their conduct. In Italy, athletes are subject to criminal prosecution for doping violations based on the illegal use of substances under Italian law.[56] Although the International Olympic Committee ("IOC") is opposed to using criminal law to punish sports doping, the Italian government declined the IOC's request to exempt athletes competing in the 2006 Winter Olympics in Turin from the country's anti-doping laws.[57]

As an alternative to criminal prosecution, Congress should consider authorizing the Internal Revenue Service to levy a special tax on the income of professional athletes who use federally controlled performance-enhancing substances illegally. This would create a strong economic disincentive for athletes to dope as a means of enhancing their performance and incomes. In my opinion, the revenues generated by this tax should be used to fund educational programs that warn youthful athletes about the health risks of using performance-enhancing substances and explain why their usage is banned by sports governing bodies.

Sports governing bodies and the federal government have important roles to play in eradicating the use of prohibited performance-enhancing substances by athletes. However, the differing regulatory roles of private sports governing bodies and the government should be complementary and consistent with their respective objectives, rather than overlapping and potentially conflicting. Drug testing and sanctioning of athletes should be an internal matter that is best handled by sports governing bodies, with the federal government having the exclusive authority to impose external criminal and/or economic penalties on athletes for doping offenses.

Notes

1. Creatine is not currently listed on any of the federal schedules of controlled substances. *See* 21 U.S.C. § 812 (2000); *see also* 21 C.F.R. § 1308.11-.15 (2005).

2. *See* WILL CARROLL, THE JUICE 178–79 (Ivan R. Dee ed. 2005) (distinguishing between violations of federal law and sports rules).

3. *See Anabolic Steroid Control Act of 2004: Hearing on H.R. 3866 Before Subcomm. on Crime, Terrorism, and Homeland Security of the H. Comm. on the Judiciary,* 108th Cong. 8 (2004) (statement of the Honorable Joseph Rannazzisi, Deputy Director of the Office of Diversion Control, Drug Enforcement Admin., U.S. Dep't of Justice); *see also* CARROLL, *supra* note 2, at 49–51, 54–56, 179.

4. CARROLL, *supra* note 2, at 11.

5. *Id.*

6. *Id.* at 44.

7. Jeff Zillgitt, *Because of Steroids, Baseball Needs a Change in Leadership*, USA TODAY.COM, Mar. 10, 2004. . . .

8. *I Used Steroids, Romo Tells '60 Minutes': LB of 4 NFL Champs Says He Received Substances from BALCO's Conte*, MSNBC.COM, Oct. 17, 2005. . . .

9. Ken Murray, *Steroid Heat Now Turns to NFL*, BALT. SUN, Mar. 30, 2005, at 1E, *available at* 2005 WLNR 4972231.

10. *All Relay Runners Except Young to Retain Sydney Golds*, USATODAY.COM, July 21, 2005. . . . *Report: Palmeiro Tested Positive for Stanozolol*, USATODAY.COM, Aug. 03, 2005. . . .

11. Matthew J. Mitten, *Is Drug Testing of Athletes Necessary?*, USA TODAY, Nov. 1 *2005*, (Magazine), at 60, *available at* 2005 WLNR 19188001.

12. *See* CTRS. FOR DISEASE CONTROL & PREVENTION, MORBIDITY AND MORTALITY WEEKLY REPORT: YOUTH RISK BEHAVIOR SURVEILLANCE—UNITED STATES, 2003, at 61 (2004). . . .

13. Erica Bulman, *Miller Will Compete in Olympics, Favors Legalizing Drugs in Sports*, ALPINE NEWS, Oct. 20, 2005. . . .

14. Mitten, *supra* note 11.

15. *See infra* notes 50–51 and accompanying text.

16. WORLD ANTI-DOPING AGENCY, WORLD ANTI-DOPING CODE 17 (2003). . . .

17. *See* Richard W. Pound, *A New Era Begins*, PLAY TRUE, Issue 1 2006 at 1. . . .

18. WORLD ANTI-DOPING AGENCY, *supra* note 16, at 8, 26.

19. U.S. Anti-Doping Agency, USADA History. . . . (last visited Apr. 10, 2006).

20. Mitten, *supra* note 11.

21. *Id.*

22. Press Release, NCAA, NCAA Launches College Basketball Web Site, (Nov. 19, 1999). . . .

23. NCAA, 2005-06 NCAA DIVISION I MANUAL: CONSTITUTION; OPERATING BYLAWS; ADMINISTRATIVE BYLAWS 338 (2005). . . .

24. Mitten, *supra* note 11.

25. *Id.*

26. Michelle Brutlag Hosick, *Latest Athlete Drug-Use Data Continue Downward Pattern*, NCAA NEWS ONLINE, Aug. 29, 2005. . . .

27. *Id.*

28. David Leon Moore, *As Steroid Use Doubles, A School Fights Back*, USA TODAY, May 5, 2005, at 1A, *available at* 2005 WLNR 7026098.

29. *See* CAL. INTERSCHOLASTIC FED'N, CONSTITUTION AND BYLAWS § 524 (2005). . . .

30. *Id.* § 22(B)(9)(d).

31. *Id.* § 22(B)(12).

32. *See, e.g.,* Jere Longman & William C. Rhoden, *Baseball; Inquiry on Steroid Use Gets Bonds Testimony*, N.Y. TIMES, Dec. 5, 2003, at D1.

33. *See* Address Before a Joint Session of the Congress on the State of the Union, 40 WEEKLY COMP. PRES. 94, 100 (Jan. 20, 2004).

34. *See* Dietary Supplement Health and Education Act of 1994, Pub. L. No. 103–417, 108 Stat. 4325, 4327 (codified as amended in scattered sections of 21 U.S.C.).

35. Pub. L. No. 108–358, 118 Stat. 1661 (codified as amended at 21 U.S.C. § 801).

36. S. Con. Res. 1114, 109th Cong. (2005).

37. *Id.* § 2(a)(8)-(b).

38. *Id.* § 4(b).

39. *Id.* § 4(b)(1).

40. *Id.* § 4(b)(7).

41. *Id.* § 5(c).

42. Clean Sports Act of 2005, S. Con. Res. 1114, 109th Cong. § 6(b)(2) (2005).

43. H.R. 1862, 109th Cong. (2005).

44. *Id.* § 2(2).

45. *Id.* § 3(1)-(4).

46. *Id.* §§ 3–5.

47. S. 1334, 109th Cong. (2005).

48. H.R. 2516, 109th Cong. (2005).

49. Howard Fendrich, *Tougher Drug Policy Worked out—Amphetamines Also on List of Banned Substances*, MEMPHIS COM. APPEAL, Nov. 16, 2005, at D8, *available at* 2005 WLNR 18571013.

50. *See, e.g.,* Bd. of Educ. of Indep. Sch. Dist. No. 92 v. Earls, 536 U.S. 822, 838 (2002); Vernonia Sch. Dist. 47J v. Acton, 515 U.S. 646, 664–65 (1995).

51. *See, e.g.,* Hill v. NCAA, 865 P.2d 633 (Cal. 1994); Brennan v. B'd. of Tr. for Univ. of Louisiana Sys., 691 So. 2d 324 (La. Ct. App. 1997).

52. Jack Curry, *Baseball Backs Stiffer Penalties for Steroid Use,* N.Y. TIMES, Nov. 16, 2005, at A1, *available at* 2005 WLNR 18489088.

53. Richard Sandomir, *Report: No Evidence of Perjury by Palmeiro,* N.Y. TIMES, Nov. 11, 2005, at D1, *available at* 2005 WLNR 18237200.

54. Associated Press, *Boxing; Toney Out: Ruiz Again the Champ,* N.Y. TIMES, May 18, 2005, at D6, *available at* 2005 WLNR 7826934.

55. David Kravets, *BALCO Founder Conte Sentenced to Eight Months,* CINCINNATI POST, Oct. 19, 2005, at B5, *available at* 2005 WLNR 16991875.

56. Greg Couch, *Olympic Stories Taking Shape: Americans Figure to Shine on Ice—Not in Hockey—and Slopes,* CHICAGO SUN-TIMES, Dec. 22, 2005, at 118, *available at* 2005 WLNR 20751838.

57. *Id.*

POSTSCRIPT

Should the Federal Government Play a Larger Role in Regulating Steroid Use?

There are several reasons why long-term research into the effects of anabolic steroids is lacking. First, it is unethical to give drugs to people that may prove harmful, even lethal. Also, the amount of steroids given to subjects in a laboratory setting may not replicate what illegal steroid users actually take. Users who take steroids illegally may take substantially more than that which subjects are given in a clinical trial. It is not uncommon for steroid users to "stack" their drugs, meaning they take several different steroids.

Second, to determine the true effects of drugs, double-blind studies need to be conducted. This means that neither the researcher nor the people receiving the drugs know whether the subjects are receiving the steroids or the placebos (inert substances). This approach is not practical with steroids because subjects can always tell if they received the steroids or the placebos. The effects of steroids could be determined by following up with people who are known steroid users. However, this method lacks proper controls. If physical or psychological problems appear in a subject, for example, it cannot be determined whether the problems are due to the steroids or to other drugs the person may have been taking. Also, the type of person who uses steroids may be the type of person who has emotional problems in the first place.

Even though the Drug Enforcement Administration estimates the black-market trade in anabolic steroids to be several hundred million dollars a year, one could argue that steroids are symptomatic of a much larger social problem. Society places much emphasis on appearance and performance. From the time we are children, we are bombarded with constant reminders that we must do better than the next person. If you want to make the varsity team, if you want that scholarship, if you want to be a professional athlete, then you need to do whatever it takes to get there. We are also constantly reminded of the importance of appearance—to either starve ourselves or pump ourselves up (or both) in order to satisfy the cultural ideal of beauty. If we cannot achieve these cultural standards through exercising, dieting, or drug use, then we can turn to surgery. Many males growing up are given the message that they should be "big and strong." One shortcut to achieving that look is through the use of steroids. Steroid use fits into the larger social problem of people not accepting themselves and their limitations.

Testing for steroid use is discussed Scott Laffe's article "Steroids: To Test or to Educate? Several School Districts Find a Will and a Way to Examine Their Athletes for Illegal Substance Use" (*School Administrator*, June 2006). The use of steroids in sports is dealt with in "Chemical Edge: The Risks of Performance-Enhancing Drug," by Marissa Saltzman (*Odyssey,* May 1, 2006); "Drugs and the Olympics" (*The Economist,* August 7, 2004); "Risks of Doping Often Overlooked for Rewards," by Mark Emmons (*San Jose Mercury News,* November 12, 2003); and "Can Drug Busters Beat New Steroids? It's Scientist Vs. Scientist as the Athens Olympics Approach," by Arlene Weintraub (*Business Week,* June 14, 2004). The dangers of steroids are discussed in "Anabolic Steroids and Dependence," by Helen Keane (*Contemporary Drug Problems,* Fall 2003). The effects of tetrahydrogestrinone (THG), another performance-enhancing drug is described in Deanna Franklin's article "FDA Warns About Dangers of THG: Banned Steroid" (*Pediatric News,* January 2004).

Internet References . . .

National Institute on Alcohol Abuse and Alcoholism (NIAAA)

This site provides research on the causes, consequences, treatment, and prevention of alcoholism and alcohol-related problems.

http://niaaa.nih.gov

American Medical Association (AMA)

Information regarding the development and promotion of standards in medical practice, research, and education are included through this website.

http://www.ama-assn.org

Columbia University College of Physicians and Surgeons Complete Home Medical Guide

This site provides information about health and medicine, including information dealing with psychotherapeutic drugs.

http://cpmcnet.columbia.edu/texts/guide/hmg06_005.html

American Psychological Association (APA)

Research concerning different psychological disorders and the various types of treatments, including drug treatments that are available, can be accessed through this site.

http://www.apa.org

CDC's Tobacco Information and Prevention Source

This location contains current information on smoking prevention programs. Much data regarding teen smoking can be found at this site.

http://www.cdc.gov/tobacco

Drugs and Social Policy

*E*xcept for the debate over whether laws prohibiting marijuana use should be relaxed, each debate in this section focuses on drugs that are already legal. Despite concerns over the effects of illegal drugs, the most frequently used drugs in society are legal drugs. Because of their prevalence and legal status, the social, psychological, and physical impact of drugs like tobacco, caffeine, alcohol, and prescription drugs are often minimized or negated. However, tobacco and alcohol cause far more death and disability than all illegal drugs combined.

The recent trend toward medical self-help raises questions of how much control one should have over one's health. The current tendency to identify nicotine as an addictive drug and to promote the moderate use of alcohol to reduce heart disease has generated much controversy. In the last several years the increase in consumers requesting prescription drugs for themselves and Ritalin for their children also has created much concern. Lastly, should marijuana be prescribed for people with certain illnesses for which some have suggested the drug could be beneficial?

- Are the Adverse Effects of Smoking Exaggerated?

- Should Laws Prohibiting Marijuana Use Be Relaxed?

- Are Psychotherapeutic Drugs Overprescribed for Treating Mental Illness?

- Do the Consequences of Caffeine Outweigh Its Benefits?

- Should School-age Children with Attention Deficit/Hyperactivity Disorder (ADHD) Be Treated with Ritalin and Other Stimulants?

- Do Consumers Benefit When Prescription Drugs Are Advertised?

ISSUE 8

Are the Adverse Effects of Smoking Exaggerated?

YES: Robert A. Levy and Rosalind B. Marimont, from "Lies, Damned Lies, and 400,000 Smoking-Related Deaths," *Regulation* (vol. 21, no. 4, 1998)

NO: Centers for Disease Control, from *The Health Consequences of Smoking: A Report of the Surgeon General* (2004)

ISSUE SUMMARY

YES: Robert A. Levy, a senior fellow at the Cato Institute, and Rosalind B. Marimont, a mathematician and scientist who retired from the National Institute of Standards and Technology, claim that the government distorts and exaggerates the dangers associated with cigarette smoking. Levy and Marimont state that factors such as poor nutrition and obesity are overlooked as causes of death among smokers. They note that cigarette smoking is harmful, but the misapplication of statistics should be regarded as "junk science."

NO: The 2004 Surgeon General's report on smoking states that the evidence pointing to the dangers of smoking is overwhelming. The report clearly links cigarette smoking to various forms of cancer, cardiovascular diseases, respiratory diseases, reproductive problems, and a host of other medical conditions.

Most people, including those who smoke, recognize that cigarette smoking is harmful. Because of tobacco's reputation as an addictive substance that jeopardizes people's health, many activists are requesting that more stringent restrictions be placed on it. As it stands now, cigarette packages are required to carry warnings describing the dangers of tobacco products. In many countries tobacco products cannot be advertised on television or billboards. Laws that prevent minors from purchasing tobacco products are being more vigorously enforced than they have ever been before. However, the World Health Organization feels that global leadership in curtailing the proliferation of cigarette smoking is lacking.

Defenders of the tobacco industry point to benefits associated with nicotine, the mild stimulant that is the chief active chemical in tobacco. In previous centuries, for example, tobacco was used to help people with a variety of ailments, including skin diseases; internal and external disorders; and diseases of the eyes, ears, mouth, and nose. Tobacco and its smoke were employed often by Native Americans for sacramental purposes. For users, nicotine provides a sense of euphoria, and smoking is a source of gratification that does not impair thinking or performance. One can drive a car, socialize, study for a test, and engage in a variety of activities while smoking. Nicotine can relieve anxiety and stress, and it can reduce weight by lessening one's appetite and by increasing metabolic activity. Many smokers assert that smoking cigarettes enables them to concentrate better and that abstaining from smoking impairs their concentration.

Critics paint a very different picture of tobacco products, citing some of the following statistics: Tobacco is responsible for about 30 percent of deaths among people between ages 35 and 69, making it the single most prominent cause of premature death in the developed world. The relationship between cigarette smoking and cardiovascular disease, including heart attack, stroke, sudden death, peripheral vascular disease, and aortic aneurysm, is well documented. Even as few as one to four cigarettes daily can increase the risk of fatal coronary heart disease. Cigarettes have also been shown to reduce blood flow and the level of high-density lipoprotein cholesterol, which is the beneficial type of cholesterol.

Cigarette smoking is strongly associated with cancer, accounting for over 85 percent of lung cancer cases and 30 percent of all deaths due to cancer. Cancer of the pharynx, larynx, mouth, esophagus, stomach, pancreas, uterus, cervix, kidney, and bladder has been related to smoking. Studies have shown that smokers have twice the rate of cancer than nonsmokers.

According to smokers' rights advocates, the majority of smokers are already aware of the potential harm of tobacco products; in fact, most smokers tend to overestimate the dangers of smoking. Adults should therefore be allowed to smoke if that is their wish. Many promote the idea that the Food and Drug Administration (FDA) and a number of politicians are attempting to deny smokers the right to engage in a behavior that they freely choose. On the other hand, tobacco critics maintain that due to the addictiveness of nicotine—the level of which some claim is manipulated by tobacco companies—smokers really do not have the ability to stop their behavior. That is, after a certain point, smoking cannot be considered freely chosen behavior.

In the following selections, Robert A. Levy and Rosalind B. Marimont argue that the scientific evidence demonstrating that tobacco use is harmful to smokers is disputable. Levy and Marimont state that smoking has been demonized unfairly. Cigarette smoking is not illegal and does not cause intoxication, violent behavior, or unemployment. "The Health Consequences of Smoking: A Report of the Surgeon General" identifies statistics that clearly demonstrate the high level of harm associated with cigarette smoking. Numerous bodily systems, ranging from the cardiovascular to the pulmonary to the digestive systems, are adversely affected by cigarette smoking.

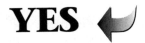

YES

**Robert A. Levy and
Rosalind B. Marimont**

Lies, Damned Lies, and 400,000
Smoking-Related Deaths

Truth was an early victim in the battle against tobacco. The big lie, repeated ad nauseam in anti-tobacco circles, is that smoking causes more than 400,000 premature deaths each year in the United States. That mantra is the principal justification for all manner of tobacco regulations and legislation, not to mention lawsuits by dozens of states for Medicaid recovery, class actions by seventy-five to eighty union health funds, similar litigation by thirty-five Blue Cross plans, twenty-four class suits by smokers who are not yet ill, sixty class actions by allegedly ill smokers, five hundred suits for damages from secondhand smoke, and health-related litigation by twelve cities and counties—an explosion of adjudication never before experienced in this country or elsewhere.

The war on smoking started with a kernel of truth—that cigarettes are a high risk factor for lung cancer—but has grown into a monster of deceit and greed, eroding the credibility of government and subverting the rule of law. Junk science has replaced honest science and propaganda parades as fact. Our legislators and judges, in need of dispassionate analysis, are instead smothered by an avalanche of statistics—tendentious, inadequately documented, and unchecked by even rudimentary notions of objectivity. Meanwhile, Americans are indoctrinated by health "professionals" bent on imposing their lifestyle choices on the rest of us and brainwashed by politicians eager to tap the deep pockets of a pariah industry.

The aim of this paper is to dissect the granddaddy of all tobacco lies—that smoking causes 400,000 deaths each year. To set the stage, let's look at two of the many exaggerations, misstatements, and outright fabrications that have dominated the tobacco debate from the outset.

Third-Rate Thinking About
Secondhand Smoke

"Passive Smoking Does Cause Lung Cancer, Do Not Let Them Fool You," states the headline of a March 1998 press release from the World Health Organization. The release begins by noting that WHO had been accused of suppressing its own study because it "failed to scientifically prove that there is an association between passive smoking . . . and a number of diseases, lung cancer in particular." Not true, insisted WHO. Smokers themselves are not the only ones who suffer health problems because of their habit; secondhand smoke can be fatal as well.

The press release went on to report that WHO researchers found "an estimated 16 percent increased risk of lung cancer among nonsmoking spouses of smokers. For workplace exposure the estimated increase in risk was 17 percent." Remarkably, the very next line warned: "Due to small sample size, neither increased risk was statistically significant." Contrast that conclusion with the hype in the headline: "Passive Smoking Does Cause Lung Cancer." Spoken often enough, the lie becomes its own evidence.

The full study would not see the light of day for seven more months, until October 1998, when it was finally published in the *Journal of the National Cancer Institute*. News reports omitted any mention of statistical insignificance. Instead, they again trumpeted relative risks of 1.16 and 1.17, corresponding to 16 and 17 percent increases, as if those ratios were meaningful. Somehow lost in WHO's media blitz was the National Cancer Institute's own guideline: "Relative risks of less than 2 [that is, a 100 percent increase] are considered small. . . . Such increases may be due to chance, statistical bias, or effects of confounding factors that are sometimes not evident." To put the WHO results in their proper perspective, note that the relative risk of lung cancer for persons who drink whole milk is 2.4. That is, the increased risk of contracting lung cancer from whole milk is 140 percent—more than eight times the 17 percent increase from secondhand smoke.

What should have mattered most to government officials, the health community and concerned parents is the following pronouncement from the WHO study: After examining 650 lung cancer patients and 1,500 healthy adults in seven European countries, WHO concluded that the "results indicate no association between childhood exposure to environmental tobacco smoke and lung cancer risk."

EPA's Junk Science

Another example of anti-tobacco misinformation is the landmark 1993 report in which the Environmental Protection Agency declared that environmental tobacco smoke (ETS) is a dangerous carcinogen that kills three thousand Americans yearly. Five years later, in July 1998, federal judge William L. Osteen lambasted the EPA for "cherry picking" the data, excluding studies that "demonstrated no association between ETS and cancer," and withholding "significant portions of its findings and reasoning in striving to confirm its *a priori* hypothesis." Both "the record and EPA's explanation," concluded the court, "make it clear that using standard methodology, EPA could not produce statistically significant results." A more damning assessment is difficult to imagine, but here are the court's conclusions at greater length, in its own words.

EPA publicly committed to a conclusion before research had begun; excluded industry [input thereby] violating the [Radon Research] Act's procedural requirements; adjusted established procedure and scientific norms to validate the Agency's public conclusion, and aggressively utilized the Act's authority to disseminate findings to establish a de facto regulatory scheme intended to restrict Plaintiff's products and to influence public opinion. In conducting the ETS Risk Assessment, EPA disregarded information and made findings on selective information; did not disseminate significant epidemiologic information; deviated from its Risk Assessment Guidelines; failed to disclose important findings and reasoning; and left significant questions without answers. EPA's conduct left substantial holes in the administrative record. While so doing, EPA produced limited evidence, then claimed the weight of the Agency's research evidence demonstrated ETS causes cancer.

—Flue-Cured Tobacco Coop. Stabilization Corp. v. United States Environmental Protection Agency, 4 F. Supp. 2d 435, 465–66 (M.D.N.C. 1998)

Hundreds of states, cities, and counties have banned indoor smoking—many in reaction to the EPA report. California even prohibits smoking in bars. According to Matthew L. Myers, general counsel of the Campaign for Tobacco-Free Kids, "the release of the original risk assessment gave an enormous boost to efforts to restrict smoking." Now that the study has been thoroughly debunked, one would think that many of the bans would be lifted. Don't hold your breath. When science is adulterated and debased for political ends, the culprits are unlikely to reverse course merely because they have been unmasked.

In reaction to the federal court's criticism EPA administrator Carol M. Browner said, "It's so widely accepted that secondhand smoke causes very real problems for kids and adults. Protecting people from the health hazards of secondhand smoke should be a national imperative." Like *Alice in Wonderland,* sentence first, evidence afterward. Browner reiterates: "We believe the health threats . . . from breathing secondhand smoke are very real." Never mind science; it is Browner's beliefs that control. The research can be suitably tailored.

For the EPA to alter results, disregard evidence, and adjust its procedures and standards to satisfy agency prejudices is unacceptable behavior, even to a first-year science student. Those criticisms are about honesty, carefulness, and rigor—the very essence of science.

Classifying Diseases as Smoking-Related

With that record of distortion, it should come as no surprise that anti-tobacco crusaders misrepresent the number of deaths due to smoking. Start by considering the diseases that are incorrectly classified as smoking-related. The Centers for Disease Control and Prevention (CDC) prepares and distributes information on smoking-attributable mortality, morbidity and economic costs (SAMMEC). In its *Morbidity and Mortality Weekly Report* for 27 August 1993, the CDC states that 418,690 Americans died in 1990 of various diseases that they contracted because, according to the government, they smoked.

Diseases are categorized as smoking-related if the risk of death for smokers exceeds that for nonsmokers. In the jargon of epidemiology, a relative risk that is greater than 1 indicates a connection between exposure (smoking) and effect (death). Recall, however, the National Cancer Institute's guideline: "Relative risks of less than two are considered small. . . . Such increases may be due to chance, statistical bias, or effects of confounding factors that are sometimes not evident." And the *Federal Reference Manual on Scientific Evidence* confirms that the threshold test for legal significance is a relative risk of two or higher. At any ratio below two, the results are insufficiently reliable to conclude that a particular agent (e.g., tobacco) caused a particular disease.

What would happen if the SAMMEC data were to exclude deaths from those diseases that had a relative risk of less than two for current or former smokers? Table 1 shows that 163,071 deaths reported by CDC were from diseases that should not have been included in the report. Add to that another 1,362 deaths from burn injuries—unless one believes that Philip Morris is responsible when a smoker falls asleep with a lit cigarette. That is a total of 164,433 misreported deaths out of 418,690. When the report is properly limited to diseases that have a significant relationship with smoking, the death total declines to 254,257. Thus, on this count alone, SAMMEC overstates the number of deaths by 65 percent.

Table 1

Disease Category	Relative Risk	Deaths From Smoking
Cancer of pancreas	1.1–1.8	2,931*
Cancer of cervix	1.9	647*
Cancer of bladder	1.9	2,348*
Cancer of kidney, other urinary	1.2–1.4	353
Hypertension	1.2–1.9	5,450
Ischemic heart disease (age 35–64)	1.4–1.8	15,535*
Ischemic heart disease (age 65+)	1.3–1.6	64,789
Other heart disease	1.2–1.9	35,314
Cerebrovascular disease (age 35–64)	1.4	2,681*
Cerebrovascular disease (age 65+)	1.0–1.9	14,610
Atherosclerosis	1.3	1,267*
Aortic aneurysm	1.3	448*
Other arterial disease	1.3	372*
Pneumonia and influenza	1.4–1.6	10,552*
Other respiratory diseases	1.4–1.6	1,063*
Pediatric diseases	1.5–1.8	1,711
Sub-total		160,071
Environmental tobacco smoke	1.2	3,000
Total		163,071

* Number of deaths for this category assumes population deaths distributed between current and former smokers in same proportion as in Cancer Prevention Survey CPS-II, provided by the American Cancer Society.

Calculating Excess Deaths

But there is more. Writing on "Risk Attribution and Tobacco-Related Deaths" in the 1993 *American Journal of Epidemiology,* T. D. Sterling, W. L. Rosenbaum, and J. J. Weinkam expose another overstatement—exceeding 65 percent—that flows from using the American Cancer Society's Cancer Prevention Survey (CPS) as a baseline against which excess deaths are computed. Here is how one government agency, the Office of Technology Assessment (OTA), calculates the number of deaths caused by smoking:

The OTA first determines the death rate for persons who were part of the CPS sample and never smoked. Next, that rate is applied to the total U.S. population in order to estimate the number of Americans who would have died if no one ever smoked. Finally, the hypothetical number of deaths for assumed never-smokers is subtracted from the actual number of U.S. deaths, and the difference is ascribed to smoking. That approach seems reasonable if one important condition is satisfied: The CPS sample must be roughly the same as the overall U.S. population with respect to those factors, other than smoking, that could be associated with the death rate. But as Sterling, Rosenbaum, and Weinkam point out, nothing could be further from the truth.

The American Cancer Society bases its CPS study on a million men and women volunteers, drawn from the ranks of the Society's members, friends, and acquaintances. The persons who participate are more affluent than average, overwhelmingly white, married, college graduates, who generally do not have hazardous jobs. Each of those characteristics tends to reduce the death rate of the CPS sample which, as a result, enjoys an average life expectancy that is substantially longer than the typical American enjoys.

Because OTA starts with an atypically low death rate for never-smokers in the CPS sample, then applies that rate to the whole population, its baseline for determining excess deaths is grossly underestimated. By comparing actual deaths with a baseline that is far too low, OTA creates the illusion that a large number of deaths are due to smoking.

That same illusion pervades the statistics released by the U.S. Surgeon General, who in his 1989 report estimated that 335,600 deaths were caused by smoking. When Sterling, Rosenbaum, and Weinkam recalculated the Surgeon General's numbers, replacing the distorted CPS sample with a more representative baseline from large surveys conducted by the National Center for Health Statistics, they found that the number of smoking-related deaths declined to 203,200. Thus, the Surgeon General's report overstated the number of deaths by more than 65 percent simply by choosing the wrong standard of comparison.

Sterling and his coauthors report that not only is the death rate considerably lower for the CPS sample than for the entire U.S. but, astonishingly, even smokers in the CPS sample have a lower death rate than the national average for both smokers and nonsmokers. As a result, if OTA were to have used the CPS death rate for smokers, applied that rate to the total population, then subtracted the actual number of deaths for all Americans, it would have found that smoking saves 277,621 lives each year. The authors caution, of course, that their calculation is sheer nonsense, not a medical miracle. Those "lives would be saved only if the U.S. population would die with the death rate of smokers in the affluent CPS sample."

Unhappily, the death rate for Americans is considerably higher than that for the CPS sample. Nearly as disturbing, researchers like Sterling, Rosenbaum, and Weinkam identified that statistical predicament many years ago; yet the government persists in publishing data on smoking-related deaths that are known to be greatly inflated.

Controlling for Confounding Variables

Even if actual deaths were compared against an appropriate baseline for non-smokers, the excess deaths could not properly be attributed to smoking alone. It cannot be assumed that the only difference between smokers and nonsmokers is that the former smoke. The two groups are dissimilar in many other respects, some of which affect their propensity to contract diseases that have been identified as smoking-related. For instance, smokers have higher rates of alcoholism, exercise less on average, eat fewer green vegetables, are more likely to be exposed to workplace carcinogens, and are poorer than nonsmokers. Each of those factors can be a "cause" of death from a so-called smoking-related disease; and each must be statistically controlled for if the impact of a single factor, like smoking, is to be reliably determined.

Sterling, Rosenbaum, and Weinkam found that adjusting their calculations for just two lifestyle differences—in income and alcohol consumption—between smokers and nonsmokers had the effect of reducing the Surgeon General's smoking-related death count still further, from 203,200 to 150,000. That means the combined effect of using a proper standard of comparison coupled with controls for income and alcohol was to lower the Surgeon General's estimate 55 percent—from 335,600 to 150,000. Thus, the original estimate was a disquieting 124 percent too high, even without adjustments for important variables like occupation, exercise, and nutritional habits.

What if smokers got plenty of exercise and had healthy diets while non-smokers were couch potatoes who consumed buckets of fast food? Naturally, there are some smokers and nonsmokers who satisfy those criteria. Dr. William E. Wecker, a consulting statistician who has testified for the tobacco industry, scanned the CPS database and found thousands of smokers with relatively low risk factors and thousands of never-smokers with high risk factors. Comparing the mortality rates of the two groups, Dr. Wecker discovered that the smokers were "healthier and die less often by a factor of three than the never-smokers." Obviously, other risk factors matter, and any study that ignores them is utterly worthless.

Yet, if a smoker who is obese; has a family history of high cholesterol, diabetes, and heart problems; and never exercises dies of a heart attack, the government attributes his death to smoking alone. That procedure, if applied to the other causal factors identified in the CPS study, would produce more than twice as many "attributed" deaths as there are actual deaths, according to Dr. Wecker.

For example, the same calculations that yield 400,000 smoking-related deaths suggest that 504,000 people die each year because they engage in little or no exercise. Employing an identical formula, bad nutritional habits can be shown to account for 649,000 excess deaths annually. That is nearly 1.6 million deaths from only three causes—without considering alcoholism, accidents, poverty, etc.—out of 2.3 million deaths in 1995 from all causes combined. And on it goes—computer-generated phantom deaths, not real deaths—constrained neither by accepted statistical methods, by common sense, nor by the number of people who die each year.

Adjusting for Age at Death

Next and last, we turn to a different sort of deceit—one pertaining not to the number of smoking-related deaths but rather to the misperception that those deaths are somehow associated with kids and young adults. For purposes of this discussion, we will work with the far-fetched statistics published by CDC—an annual average from 1990 through 1994 of 427,743 deaths attributable to tobacco. Is the problem as serious as it sounds?

At first blush, it would seem that more than 400,000 annual deaths is an extremely serious problem. But suppose that all of the people died at age ninety-nine. Surely then, the seriousness of the problem would be tempered by the fact that the decedents would have died soon from some other cause in any event. That is not far from the truth: while tobacco does not kill people at an average age of ninety-nine, it does kill people at an average age of roughly seventy-two—far closer to ninety-nine than to childhood or even young adulthood. Indeed, according to a 1991 RAND study, smoking "reduces the life expectancy of a twenty-year-old by about 4.3 years"—not a trivial concern to be sure, but not the horror that is sometimes portrayed.

Consider Table 2, which shows the number of deaths and age at death for various causes of death: The three nonsmoking categories total nearly 97,000 deaths—probably not much different than the correctly calculated number of smoking-related deaths—but the average age at death is only thirty-nine. As contrasted with a seventy-two-year life expectancy for smokers, each of those nonsmoking deaths snuffs out thirty-three years of life—our most productive years, from both an economic and child-rearing perspective.

Perhaps that is why the Carter Center's "Closing the Gap" project at Emory University examined "years of potential life lost" (YPLL) for selected diseases, to identify those causes of death that were of greatest severity and consequence. The results were reported by R.W. Amler and D.L. Eddins, "Cross-Sectional Analysis: Precursors of Premature Death in the United States," in the 1987 *American Journal of Preventive Medicine*. First, the authors determined for each disease the annual number of deaths by age group. Second, they multiplied for each age group the number of deaths times the average number of years remaining before customary retirement at age sixty-five. Then they computed YPLL by summing the products for each disease across age groups.

Table 2

Cause of Death	Number of Deaths per Year	Mean Age at Death
Smoking-attributed	427,743	72
Motor vehicle accidents	40,982	39
Suicide	30,484	45
Homicide	25,488	32

Source: Centers for Disease Control and Prevention

Table 3

Cause	Deaths	YPLL
Alcohol-related	99,247	1,795,458
Gaps in primary care*	132,593	1,771,133
Injuries (excluding alcohol-related)	64,169	1,755,720
Tobacco-related	338,022	1,497,161

* Inadequate access, screening and preventive interventions.

Thus, if smoking were deemed to have killed, say, fifty thousand people from age sixty through sixty-four, a total of 150,000 years of life were lost in that age group—i.e., fifty thousand lives times an average of three years remaining to age sixty-five. YPLL for smoking would be the accumulation of lost years for all age groups up to sixty-five.

Amler and Eddins identified nine major precursors of preventable deaths. Measured by YPLL, tobacco was about halfway down the list—ranked four out of nine in terms of years lost—not "the number one killer in America" as alarmists have exclaimed. Table 3 shows the four most destructive causes of death, based on 1980 YPLL statistics. Bear in mind that the starting point for the YPLL calculation is the number of deaths, which for tobacco is grossly magnified for all of the reasons discussed above.

According to Amler and Eddins, even if we were to look at medical treatment—measured by days of hospital care—nonalcohol-related injuries impose a 58 percent greater burden than tobacco, and nutrition-related diseases are more burdensome as well.

Another statistic that more accurately reflects the real health repercussions of smoking is the age distribution of the 427,743 deaths that CDC mistakenly traces to tobacco. No doubt most readers will be surprised to learn that—aside from burn victims and pediatric diseases—*tobacco does not kill a single person below the age of 35.*

Each year from 1990 through 1994, as shown in Table 4, only 1,910 tobacco-related deaths—less than half of 1 percent of the total—were persons below age thirty-five. Of those, 319 were burn victims and the rest were infants whose parents smoked. But the relationship between parental smoking and pediatric diseases carries a risk ratio of less than 2, and thus is statistically insignificant. Unless better evidence is produced, those deaths should not be associated with smoking.

Table 4

U.S. Smoking-Attributable Mortality by Cause and Age of Death
1990–1994 Annual Average

Age at Death	Pediatric Diseases	Burn Victims	All Other Diseases	Total
Under 1	1,591	19	0	1,610
1–34	0	300	0	300
35–49	0	221	21,773	21,994
50–69	0	286	148,936	149,222
70–74	0	96	62,154	62,250
75–84	0	133	120,537	120,670
85+	0	45	71,652	71,697
Totals	1,591	1,100	425,052	427,743

Source: Private communication from the Centers for Disease Control and Prevention

On the other hand, the National Center for Health Statistics reports that more than twenty-one thousand persons below age thirty-five died from motor vehicle accidents in 1992, more than eleven thousand died from suicide, and nearly seventeen thousand died from homicide. Over half of those deaths were connected with alcohol or drug abuse. That should put smoking-related deaths in a somewhat different light.

Most revealing of all, almost 255,000 of the smoking-related deaths—nearly 60 percent of the total—occurred at age seventy or above. More than 192,000 deaths—nearly 45 percent of the total—occurred at age seventy-five or higher. And roughly 72,000 deaths—almost 17 percent of the total—occurred at the age of 85 or above. Still, the public health community disingenuously refers to "premature" deaths from smoking, as if there is no upper age limit to the computation.

The vast overestimate of the dangers of smoking has had disastrous results for the health of young people. Risky behavior does not exist in a vacuum; people compare uncertainties and apportion their time, effort, and money according to the perceived severity of the risk. Each year, alcohol and drug abuse kills tens of thousands of people under the age of thirty-five. Yet according to a 1995 survey by the U.S. Department of Health and Human Services, high school seniors thought smoking a pack a day was more dangerous than daily consumption of four to five alcoholic beverages or using barbiturates. And the CDC reports that the number of pregnant women who drank frequently quadrupled between 1991 and 1995—notwithstanding that fetal alcohol syndrome is the largest cause of preventable mental retardation, occurring in one out of every one thousand births.

Can anyone doubt that the drumbeat of antismoking propaganda from the White House and the health establishment has deluded Americans into thinking that tobacco is the real danger to our children? In truth, alcohol and drug abuse poses an immensely greater risk and antismoking zealots bear a heavy burden for their duplicity.

Conclusion

The unvarnished fact is that children do not die of tobacco-related diseases, correctly determined. If they smoke heavily during their teens, they may die of lung cancer in their old age, fifty or sixty years later, assuming lung cancer is still a threat then.

Meanwhile, do not expect consistency or even common sense from public officials. Alcoholism contributes to crime, violence, spousal abuse, and child neglect. Children are dying by the thousands in accidents, suicides, and homicides. But states go to war against nicotine—which is not an intoxicant, has no causal connection with crime, and poses little danger to young adults or family members.

The campaign against cigarettes is not entirely dishonest. After all, a seasoning of truth makes the lie more digestible. Evidence does suggest that cigarettes substantially increase the risk of lung cancer, bronchitis, and emphysema. The relationship between smoking and other diseases is not nearly so clear, however; and the scare-mongering that has passed for science is appalling. Not only is tobacco far less pernicious than Americans are led to believe, but its destructive effect is amplified by all manner of statistical legerdemain—counting diseases that should not be counted, using the wrong sample as a standard of comparison, and failing to control for obvious confounding variables.

To be blunt, there is no credible evidence that 400,000 deaths per year—or any number remotely close to 400,000—are caused by tobacco. Nor has that estimate been adjusted for the positive effects of smoking—less obesity, colitis, depression, Alzheimer's disease, Parkinson's disease and, for some women, a lower incidence of breast cancer. The actual damage from smoking is neither known nor knowable with precision. Responsible statisticians agree that it is impossible to attribute causation to a single variable, like tobacco, when there are multiple causal factors that are correlated with one another. The damage from cigarettes is far less than it is made out to be.

Most important, the government should stop lying and stop pretending that smoking-related deaths are anything but a statistical artifact. The unifying bond of all science is that truth is its aim. When that goal yields to politics, tainting science in order to advance predetermined ends, we are all at risk. Sadly, that is exactly what has transpired as our public officials fabricate evidence to promote their crusade against big tobacco.

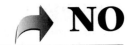

The Health Consequences of Smoking: A Report of the Surgeon General

Executive Summary

This report of the Surgeon General on the health effects of smoking returns to the topic of active smoking and disease, the focus of the first Surgeon General's report published in 1964. The first report established a model of comprehensive evidence evaluation for the 27 reports that have followed: for those on the adverse health effects of smoking, the evidence has been evaluated using guidelines for assessing causality of smoking with disease. Using this model, every report on health has found that smoking causes many diseases and other adverse effects. Repeatedly, the reports have concluded that smoking is the single greatest cause of avoidable morbidity and mortality in the United States.

Of the Surgeon General's reports published since 1964, only a few have comprehensively documented and updated the evidence on active smoking and disease. The 1979 report provided a broad array of information, and the 1990 report on smoking cessation also investigated major diseases caused by smoking. Other volumes published during the 1980s focused on specific groups of diseases caused by smoking, and the 2001 report was devoted to women and smoking. Because there has not been a recent systematic review of the full sweep of the evidence, the topic of active smoking and health was considered an appropriate focus for this latest report. Researchers have continued to identify new adverse effects of active smoking in their ongoing efforts to investigate the health effects of smoking. Lengthy follow-ups are now available for thousands of participants in long-term cohort (follow-up) studies.

This report also updates the methodology for evaluating evidence that the 1964 report initiated. Although that model has proved to be effective, this report establishes a uniformity of language concerning causality of associations so as to bring greater specificity to the findings of the report. Beginning with this report, conclusions concerning causality of association will be placed into one of four categories with regard to strength of the evidence: (1) sufficient to infer a causal relationship, (2) suggestive but not sufficient to infer a

From "The Health Consequences of Smoking: A Report of the Surgeon General," Centers for Disease Control, 2004. References omitted.

causal relationship, (3) inadequate to infer the presence or absence of a causal relationship, or (4) suggestive of no causal relationship.

This approach separates the classification of the evidence concerning causality from the implications of that determination. In particular, the magnitude of the effect in the population, the attributable risk, is considered under "implications" of the causal determination. For example, there might be sufficient evidence to classify smoking as a cause of two diseases but the number of attributable cases would depend on the frequency of the disease in the population and the effects of other causal factors.

This report covers active smoking only. Passive smoking was the focus of the 1986 Surgeon General's report and subsequent reports by other entities. The health effects of pipes and cigars, also not within the scope of this report, are covered in another report (NCI 1998).

In preparing this report, the literature review approach was necessarily selective. For conditions for which a causal conclusion had been previously reached, there was no attempt to cover all relevant literature, but rather to review the conclusions from previous Surgeon General's reports and focus on important new studies for that topic. The enormous scope of the evidence precludes such detailed reviews. For conditions for which a causal conclusion had not been previously reached, a comprehensive search strategy was developed. Search strategies included reviewing previous Surgeon General's reports on smoking, publications originating from the largest observational studies, and reference lists from important publications; consulting with content experts; and conducting focused literature searches on specific topics. For this report, studies through 2000 were reviewed.

In addition, conclusions from prior reports concerning smoking as a cause of a particular disease have been updated and are presented in this new format based on the evidence evaluated in this report (Table 1). Remarkably, this report identifies a substantial number of diseases found to be caused by smoking that were not previously causally associated with smoking: cancers of the stomach, uterine cervix, pancreas, and kidney; acute myeloid leukemia; pneumonia; abdominal aortic aneurysm; cataract; and periodontitis. The report also concludes that smoking generally diminishes the health of smokers.

Despite the many prior reports on the topic and the high level of public knowledge in the United States of the adverse effects of smoking in general, tobacco use remains the leading preventable cause of disease and death in the United States, causing approximately 440,000 deaths each year and costing approximately $157 billion in annual health-related economic losses. Nationally, smoking results in more than 5.6 million years of potential life lost each year. Although the rates of smoking continue to decline, an estimated 46.2 million adults in the United States still smoked cigarettes in 2001. In 2000, 70 percent of those who smoked wanted to quit. An increasingly disturbing picture of widespread organ damage in active smokers is emerging, likely reflecting the systemic distribution of tobacco smoke components and their high level of toxicity. Thus, active smokers are at higher risk for cataract, cancer of the cervix, pneumonia, and reduced health status generally.

Table 1

Diseases and Other Adverse Health Effects for which Smoking Is Identified as a Cause in the Current Surgeon General's Report

Disease	Highest Level Conclusion from Previous Surgeon General's Reports (year)	Conclusion from the 2004 Surgeon General's Report
Cancer		
Bladder cancer	"Smoking is a cause of bladder cancer; cessation reduces risk by about 50 percent after only a few years, in comparison with continued smoking." (1990, p. 10)	"The evidence is sufficient to infer a causal relationship between smoking and . . . bladder cancer."
Cervical cancer	"Smoking has been consistently associated with an increased risk for cervical cancer." (2001, p. 224)	"The evidence is sufficient to infer a causal relationship between smoking and cervical cancer."
Esophageal cancer	"Cigarette smoking is a major cause of esophageal cancer in the United States." (1982, p. 7)	"The evidence is sufficient to infer a causal relationship between smoking and cancers of the esophagus."
Kidney cancer	"Cigarette smoking is a contributory factor in the development of kidney cancer in the United States. The term 'contributory factor' by no means excludes the possibility of a causal role for smoking in cancers of this site." (1982, p. 7)	"The evidence is sufficient to infer a causal relationship between smoking and renal cell, [and] renal pelvis . . . cancers."
Laryngeal cancer	"Cigarette smoking is causally associated with cancer of the lung, larynx, oral cavity, and esophagus in women as well as in men. . . ." (1980, p. 126)	"The evidence is sufficient to infer a causal relationship between smoking and cancer of the larynx."
Leukemia	"Leukemia has recently been implicated as a smoking-related disease . . . but this observation has not been consistent." (1990, p. 176)	"The evidence is sufficient to infer a causal relationship between smoking and acute myeloid leukemia."
Lung cancer	"Additional epidemiological, pathological, and experimental data not only confirm the conclusion of the Surgeon General's 1964 Report regarding lung cancer in men but strengthen the causal relationship of smoking to lung cancer in women." (1967, p. 36)	"The evidence is sufficient to infer a causal relationship between smoking and lung cancer."
Oral cancer	"Cigarette smoking is a major cause of cancers of the oral cavity in the United States." (1982, p. 6)	"The evidence is sufficient to infer a causal relationship between smoking and cancers of the oral cavity and pharynx."
Pancreatic cancer	"Smoking cessation reduces the risk of pancreatic cancer, compared with continued smoking, although this reduction in risk may only be measurable after 10 years of abstinence." (1990, p. 10)	"The evidence is sufficient to infer a causal relationship between smoking and pancreatic cancer."
Stomach cancer	"Data on smoking and cancer of the stomach . . . are unclear." (2001, p. 231)	"The evidence is sufficient to infer a causal relationship between smoking and gastric cancers."

Table 1 (Continued)

Disease	Highest Level Conclusion from Previous Surgeon General's Reports (year)	Conclusion from the 2004 Surgeon General's Report
Cardiovascular diseases		
Abdominal aortic aneurysm	"Death from rupture of an atherosclerotic abdominal aneurysm is more common in cigarette smokers than in nonsmokers." (1983, p. 195)	"The evidence is sufficient to infer a causal relationship between smoking and abdominal aortic aneurysm."
Atherosclerosis	"Cigarette smoking is the most powerful risk factor predisposing to atherosclerotic peripheral vascular disease." (1983, p. 8)	"The evidence is sufficient to infer a causal relationship between smoking and subclinical atherosclerosis."
Cerebrovascular disease	"Cigarette smoking is a major cause of cerebrovascular disease (stroke), the third leading cause of death in the United States." (1989, p. 12)	"The evidence is sufficient to infer a causal relationship between smoking and stroke."
Coronary heart disease	"In summary, for the purposes of preventive medicine, it can be concluded that smoking is causally related to coronary heart disease for both men and women in the United States." (1979, p. 1–15)	"The evidence is sufficient to infer a causal relationship between smoking and coronary heart disease."
Respiratory diseases		
Chronic obstructive pulmonary disease	"Cigarette smoking is the most important of the causes of chronic bronchitis in the United States, and increases the risk of dying from chronic bronchitis." (1964, p. 302)	"The evidence is sufficient to infer a causal relationship between active smoking and chronic obstructive pulmonary disease morbidity and mortality."
Pneumonia	"Smoking cessation reduces rates of respiratory symptoms such as cough, sputum production, and wheezing, and respiratory infections such as bronchitis and pneumonia, compared with continued smoking." (1990, p. 11)	"The evidence is sufficient to infer a causal relationship between smoking and acute respiratory illnesses, including pneumonia, in persons without underlying smoking-related chronic obstructive lung disease."
Respiratory effects in utero	"In utero exposure to maternal smoking is associated with reduced lung function among infants. . . ." (2001, p. 14)	"The evidence is sufficient to infer a causal relationship between maternal smoking during pregnancy and a reduction of lung function in infants."
Respiratory effects in childhood and adolescence	"Cigarette smoking during childhood and adolescence produces significant health problems among young people, including cough and phlegm production, an increased number and severity of respiratory illnesses, decreased physical fitness, an unfavorable lipid profile, and potential retardation in the rate of lung growth and the level of maximum lung function." (1994, p. 41)	"The evidence is sufficient to infer a causal relationship between active smoking and impaired lung growth during childhood and adolescence." "The evidence is sufficient to infer a causal relationship between active smoking and the early onset of lung function decline during late adolescence and early adulthood. "

(continued)

Table 1 (Continued)

Disease	Highest Level Conclusion from Previous Surgeon General's Reports (year)	Conclusion from the 2004 Surgeon General's Report
		"The evidence is sufficient to infer a causal relationship between active smoking and respiratory symptoms in children and adolescents, including coughing, phlegm, wheezing, and dyspnea."
		"The evidence is sufficient to infer a causal relationship between active smoking and asthma-related symptoms (i.e., wheezing) in childhood and adolescence."
Respiratory effects in adulthood	"Cigarette smoking accelerates the age-related decline in lung function that occurs among never smokers. With sustained abstinence from smoking, the rate of decline in pulmonary function among former smokers returns to that of never smokers." (1990, p. 11)	"The evidence is sufficient to infer a causal relationship between active smoking in adulthood and a premature onset of and an accelerated age-related decline in lung function."
		"The evidence is sufficient to infer a causal relationship between sustained cessation from smoking and a return of the rate of decline in pulmonary function to that of persons who had never smoked."
Other respiratory effects	"Smoking cessation reduces rates of respiratory symptoms such as cough, sputum production, and wheezing, and respiratory infections such as bronchitis and pneumonia, compared with continued smoking." (1990, p. 11)	"The evidence is sufficient to infer a causal relationship between active smoking and all major respiratory symptoms among adults, including coughing, phlegm, wheezing, and dyspnea."
		"The evidence is sufficient to infer a causal relationship between active smoking and poor asthma control."
Reproductive effects		
Fetal death and stillbirths	"The risk for perinatal mortality—both stillbirth and neonatal deaths—and the risk for sudden infant death syndrome (SIDS) are increased among the offspring of women who smoke during pregnancy." (2001, p. 307)	"The evidence is sufficient to infer a causal relationship between sudden infant death syndrome and maternal smoking during and after pregnancy."
Fertility	"Women who smoke have increased risks for conception delay and for both primary and secondary infertility." (2001, p. 307)	"The evidence is sufficient to infer a causal relationship between smoking and reduced fertility in women."
Low birth weight	"Infants born to women who smoke during pregnancy have a lower average birth weight . . . than . . . infants born to women who do not smoke." (2001, p. 307)	"The evidence is sufficient to infer a causal relationship between maternal active smoking and fetal growth restriction and low birth weight."

Table 1 (Continued)

Disease	Highest Level Conclusion from Previous Surgeon General's Reports (year)	Conclusion from the 2004 Surgeon General's Report
Pregnancy complications	"Smoking during pregnancy is associated with increased risks for preterm premature rupture of membranes, abruptio placentae, and placenta previa, and with a modest increase in risk for preterm delivery." (2001, p. 307)	"The evidence is sufficient to infer a casual relationship between maternal active smoking and premature rupture of the membranes, placenta previa, and placental abruption." "The evidence is sufficient to infer a causal relationship between maternal active smoking and preterm delivery and shortened gestation."

Other effects

Disease	Highest Level Conclusion from Previous Surgeon General's Reports (year)	Conclusion from the 2004 Surgeon General's Report
Cataract	"Women who smoke have an increased risk for cataract." (2001, p. 331)	"The evidence is sufficient to infer a causal relationship between smoking and nuclear cataract."
Diminished health status/morbidity	"Relationships between smoking and cough or phlegm are strong and consistent; they have been amply documented and are judged to be causal . . . ." (1984, p. 47) "Consideration of evidence from many different studies has led to the conclusion that cigarette smoking is the overwhelmingly most important cause of cough, sputum, chronic bronchitis, and mucus hypersecretion." (1984, p. 48)	"The evidence is sufficient to infer a causal relationship between smoking and diminished health status that may be manifest as increased absenteeism from work and increased use of medical care services." "The evidence is sufficient to infer a causal relationship between smoking and increased risks for adverse surgical outcomes related to wound healing and respiratory complications."
Hip fractures	"Women who currently smoke have an increased risk for hip fracture compared with women who do not smoke." (2001, p. 321)	"The evidence is sufficient to infer a causal relationship between smoking and hip fractures."
Low bone density	"Postmenopausal women who currently smoke have lower bone density than do women who do not smoke." (2001, p. 321)	"In postmenopausal women, the evidence is sufficient to infer a causal relationship between smoking and low bone density."
Peptic ulcer disease	"The relationship between cigarette smoking and death rates from peptic ulcer, especially gastric ulcer, is confirmed. In addition, morbidity data suggest a similar relationship exists with the prevalence of reported disease from this cause." (1967, p. 40)	"The evidence is sufficient to infer a causal relationship between smoking and peptic ulcer disease in persons who are *Helicobacter pylori* positive."

Sources: U.S. Department of Health, Education, and Welfare 1964, 1967, 1979; U.S. Department of Health and Human Services 1980, 1982, 1983, 1984, 1989, 1990, 1994, 2001.

This new information should be an impetus for even more vigorous programs to reduce and prevent smoking. Smokers need to be aware that smoking carries far greater risks than the most widely known hazards. Health care providers should also use the new evidence to counsel their patients. For example, ophthalmologists may want to warn patients about the increased risk of cataract in smokers, and geriatricians should counsel their patients who smoke, even the oldest, to quit. This report shows that smokers who quit can lower their risk for smoking-caused diseases and improve their health status generally. Those who never start can avoid the predictable burden of disease and lost life expectancy that results from a lifetime of smoking. . . .

Major Conclusions

Forty years after the first Surgeon General's report in 1964, the list of diseases and other adverse effects caused by smoking continues to expand. Epidemiologic studies are providing a comprehensive assessment of the risks faced by smokers who continue to smoke across their life spans. Laboratory research now reveals how smoking causes disease at the molecular and cellular levels. Fortunately for former smokers, studies show that the substantial risks of smoking can be reduced by successfully quitting at any age. The evidence reviewed in this and prior reports of the Surgeon General leads to the following major conclusions:

1. Smoking harms nearly every organ of the body, causing many diseases and reducing the health of smokers in general.
2. Quitting smoking has immediate as well as long-term benefits, reducing risks for diseases caused by smoking and improving health in general.
3. Smoking cigarettes with lower machine-measured yields of tar and nicotine provides no clear benefit to health.
4. The list of diseases caused by smoking has been expanded to include abdominal aortic aneurysm, acute myeloid leukemia, cataract, cervical cancer, kidney cancer, pancreatic cancer, pneumonia, periodontitis, and stomach cancer.

POSTSCRIPT

Are the Adverse Effects of Smoking Exaggerated?

Much data indicate that smoking cigarettes is injurious to human health. For example, more than 400,000 people die from tobacco-related illnesses each year in the United States, costing the U.S. health care system billions of dollars annually. Not only does the smoker bear the cost of tobacco-related illness, so do millions of taxpayers.

Thousands more people develop debilitating conditions such as chronic bronchitis and emphysema. Levy and Marimont, however, question the accuracy of the data. How the data are presented and interpreted may affect how one feels about the issue of placing more restrictions on tobacco products. If cigarette smoking is demonized, as Levy and Marimont suggest, it is not difficult to influence people's positions on regulating tobacco. There is currently a great deal of antismoking sentiment in society because of how the statistics are presented. Levy and Marimont do not recommend that people use tobacco products; however, they state only that the consequences linked to it are exaggerated. If the health effects of cigarette smoking were not deemed as hazardous as they are, would people feel differently about smoking?

Despite the reported hazards of tobacco smoking, numerous proponents of smokers' rights assert that cigarette smoking is a matter of choice. However, many people could argue that smoking is not a matter of choice because smokers become addicted to nicotine. Others contend that the decision to start smoking is a matter of choice, but once tobacco dependency occurs, most smokers are in effect deprived of the choice to stop smoking. Yet, it has been shown that millions of smokers have been able to quit smoking. Contributing to the tobacco dilemma is the expansion of tobacco manufacturers into many developing countries and the proliferation of advertising despite its ban from television and radio. Print advertisements and billboards are popular tools for advertsing tobacco products.

Nevertheless, tobacco proponents maintain that people make all types of choices, and if the choices that people make are ultimately harmful, then that is their responsibility. A basic question is "do people have the right to engage in self-destructive behavior?" If people are looked down upon because they smoke cigarettes, then should people be looked down upon if they eat too much or exercise too little? Does one have the right to eat a half dozen double cheeseburgers, to be a couch potato, to drink until one passes out? At what point does one lose the right to engage in deleterious behaviors—assuming that the rights of others are not adversely affected?

A good overview of the incidence of smoking is described in *Trends in Tobacco Use* by the American Lung Association (January 2006). In addition, there are many articles that address the impact of tobacco on society. One article that focuses on reasons that teenagers smoke is "Too Many Kids Smoke," by Dianna Gordon (*State Legislatures,* March 2004). Kendall Morgan looks at the addictiveness of nicotine in "More Than a Kick" (*Science News,* March 22, 2003). Several times a year the SmokeFree Educational Services publishes *SmokeFree Air,* a newsletter describing actions that have been taken to limit smoking in public locations. Another article that looks at preventing cigarette use is "Effect of Increased Social Unacceptability on Reduction in Cigarette Consumption," by Benjamin Alamar and Stanton Glantz (*American Journal of Public Health,* August 2006).

ISSUE 9

Should Laws Prohibiting Marijuana Use Be Relaxed?

YES: Ethan A. Nadelmann, from "An End to Marijuana Prohibition," *National Review* (July 12, 2004)

NO: Office of National Drug Control Policy, from *Marijuana Myths and Facts: The Truth Behind 10 Popular Misconceptions* (2004)

ISSUE SUMMARY

YES: Ethan Nadelmann, founder and executive director of the Drug Policy Alliance, argues that law enforcement officials are overzealous in prosecuting individuals for marijuana possession. Eighty-seven percent of marijuana arrests are for possession of small amounts of the drug. The cost of marijuana enforcement to U.S. taxpayers ranges from $10–15 billion. In addition, punishments are unjust in that they vary greatly.

NO: The Office of National Drug Control Policy (ONDCP) contends that marijuana is not a harmless drug. Besides causing physical problems, marijuana affects academic performance and emotional adjustment. Moreover, dealers who grow and sell marijuana may become violent to protect their commodity.

Marijuana is the most commonly used illegal drug in the United States. Still the federal government maintains that it is a potentially dangerous substance. Also, its use represents a danger, not just to the user, but to others. The government claims that marijuana can be addictive and that more young people are in treatment for marijuana than for other illegal drugs.

The federal government argues that relaxing laws against marijuana use, even for medical purposes, is unwarranted. However, since the mid-1990s voters in California, Arizona, Oregon, Colorado, and other states have passed referenda to legalize marijuana for medical purposes. Despite the position of these voters, however, the federal government does not support the medical use of marijuana, and federal laws take precedence over state laws. A major concern of opponents of these referenda is that legalization of marijuana for medicinal purposes will lead to its use for recreational purposes.

Marijuana has been tested in the treatment of glaucoma, asthma, convulsions, epilepsy, and migraine headaches, and in the reduction of nausea, vomiting, and loss of appetite associated with chemotherapy treatments. Many medical professionals and patients believe that marijuana shows promise in the treatment of these disorders and others, including spasticity in amputees and multiple sclerosis.

Another consideration of relaxing marijuana laws, even for medical purposes, is what constitutes a legitimate medical use. For example, many people would agree that treating someone with marijuana who has glaucoma or is receiving chemotherapy would be a valid use of marijuana. Would smoking marijuana to get rid of a headache or because one has muscle soreness be reasonable medical uses for marijuana?

Advocates for relaxing marijuana laws feel that the drug is unfairly labeled as a dangerous drug. For example, many more people throughout the world die from tobacco smoking and alcohol than from marijuana. Yet using those products is not illegal. There are as many people in jail today for marijuana offenses as from cocaine, heroin, methamphetamine, Ecstasy, and all other illegal drugs combined, claims Nadelmann.

Another point raised by those people in favor of relaxing marijuana laws is that it would be easier to educate young people about marijuana's effects if it was legal. By simply keeping the drug illegal, the message is DON'T USE MARIJUANA, rather than how to reduce harms associated with it. Proponents such as Nadelmann and others do not advocate the unregulated use of marijuana. They favor a more reasoned, controlled approach.

Marijuana opponents argue that the evidence in support of marijuana as medically useful suffers from far too many deficiencies. The DEA, for example, believes that studies supporting the medical value of marijuana are scientifically limited, based on biased testimonies of ill individuals who have used marijuana, and grounded in the unscientific opinions of certain physicians, nurses, and other medical personnel. Furthermore, marijuana opponents feel that the safety of marijuana has not been established by reliable scientific data.

In the following selections, Ethan A. Nadelmann asserts that the federal government is overzealous in its enforcement of marijuana laws. Besides having approximately 700,000 people in jail for marijuana offenses, the government has set up needless political roadblocks to prevent the use of marijuana for medicinal purposes. The Office of National Drug Control Policy (ONDCP) argues that marijuana is far more dangerous than many young people realize. The ONDCP tries to dispel many of the myths associated with marijuana. The ONDCP maintains that marijuana should not be used for legal medical purposes because the current research on marijuana's medicinal benefits is inconclusive. Other drugs are available that preclude the need to use marijuana.

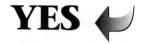

YES

Ethan A. Nadelmann

An End to Marijuana Prohibition

Never before have so many Americans supported decriminalizing and even legalizing marijuana. Seventy-two percent say that for simple marijuana possession, people should not be incarcerated but fined: the generally accepted definition of "decriminalization."[1] Even more Americans support making marijuana legal for medical purposes. Support for broader legalization ranges between 25 and 42 percent, depending on how one asks the question.[2] Two of every five Americans—according to a 2003 Zogby poll—say "the government should treat marijuana more or less the same way it treats alcohol: It should regulate it, control it, tax it, and only make it illegal for children."[3]

Close to 100 million Americans—including more than half of those between the ages of 18 and 50—have tried marijuana at least once.[4] Military and police recruiters often have no choice but to ignore past marijuana use by job seekers.[5] The public apparently feels the same way about presidential and other political candidates. Al Gore,[6] Bill Bradley,[7] and John Kerry[8] all say they smoked pot in days past. So did Bill Clinton, with his notorious caveat.[9] George W. Bush won't deny he did.[10] And ever more political, business, religious, intellectual, and other leaders plead guilty as well.[11]

The debate over ending marijuana prohibition simmers just below the surface of mainstream politics, crossing ideological and partisan boundaries. Marijuana is no longer the symbol of Sixties rebellion and Seventies permissiveness, and it's not just liberals and libertarians who say it should be legal, as William F. Buckley Jr. has demonstrated better than anyone. As director of the country's leading drug policy reform organization, I've had countless conversations with police and prosecutors, judges and politicians, and hundreds of others who quietly agree that the criminalization of marijuana is costly, foolish, and destructive. What's most needed now is principled conservative leadership. Buckley has led the way, and New Mexico's former governor, Gary Johnson, spoke out courageously while in office. How about others?

A Systemic Overreaction

Marijuana prohibition is unique among American criminal laws. No other law is both enforced so widely and harshly and yet deemed unnecessary by such a substantial portion of the populace.

Police make about 700,000 arrests per year for marijuana offenses.[12] That's almost the same number as are arrested each year for cocaine, heroin, methamphetamine, Ecstasy, and all other illicit drugs combined.[13] Roughly 600,000, or 87 percent, of marijuana arrests are for nothing more than possession of small amounts.[14] Millions of Americans have never been arrested or convicted of any criminal offense except this.[15] Enforcing marijuana laws costs an estimated $10–15 billion in direct costs alone.[16]

Punishments range widely across the country, from modest fines to a few days in jail to many years in prison. Prosecutors often contend that no one goes to prison for simple possession—but tens, perhaps hundreds, of thousands of people on probation and parole are locked up each year because their urine tested positive for marijuana or because they were picked up in possession of a joint. Alabama currently locks up people convicted three times of marijuana *possession* for 15 years to life.[17] There are probably—no firm estimates exist—100,000 Americans behind bars tonight for one marijuana offense or another.[18] And even for those who don't lose their freedom, simply being arrested can be traumatic and costly. A parent's marijuana use can be the basis for taking away her children and putting them in foster care.[19] Foreign-born residents of the U.S. can be deported for a marijuana offense no matter how long they have lived in this country, no matter if their children are U.S. citizens, and no matter how long they have been legally employed.[20] More than half the states revoke or suspend driver's licenses of people arrested for marijuana possession even though they were not driving at the time of arrest.[21] The federal Higher Education Act prohibits student loans to young people convicted of any drug offense;[22] all other criminal offenders remain eligible.[23]

This is clearly an overreaction on the part of government. No drug is perfectly safe, and every psychoactive drug can be used in ways that are problematic. The federal government has spent billions of dollars on advertisements and anti-drug programs that preach the dangers of marijuana—that it's a gateway drug, and addictive in its own right, and dramatically more potent than it used to be, and responsible for all sorts of physical and social diseases as well as international terrorism.[24,25] But the government has yet to repudiate the 1988 finding of the Drug Enforcement Administration's own administrative law judge, Francis Young, who concluded after extensive testimony that "marijuana in its natural form is one of the safest therapeutically active substances known to man."[26]

Is marijuana a gateway drug? Yes, insofar as most Americans try marijuana before they try other illicit drugs. But no, insofar as the vast majority of Americans who have tried marijuana have never gone on to try other illegal drugs, much less get in trouble with them, and most have never even gone on to become regular or problem marijuana users.[27] Trying to reduce heroin addiction by preventing marijuana use, it's been said, is like trying to reduce motorcycle fatalities by cracking down on bicycle riding.[28] If marijuana did not exist, there's little reason to believe that there would be less drug abuse in the U.S.; indeed, its role would most likely be filled by a more dangerous substance.

Is marijuana dramatically more potent today? There's certainly a greater variety of high-quality marijuana available today than 30 years ago. But anyone who smoked marijuana in the 1970s and 1980s can recall smoking pot that was just as strong as anything available today.[29] What's more, one needs to take only a few puffs of higher-potency pot to get the desired effect, so there's less wear and tear on the lungs.[30]

Is marijuana addictive? Yes, it can be, in that some people use it to excess, in ways that are problematic for themselves and those around them, and find it hard to stop. But marijuana may well be the least addictive and least damaging of all commonly used psychoactive drugs, including many that are now legal.[31] Most people who smoke marijuana never become dependent.[32] Withdrawal symptoms pale compared with those from other drugs. No one has ever died from a marijuana overdose, which cannot be said of most other drugs.[33] Marijuana is not associated with violent behavior and only minimally with reckless sexual behavior.[34] And even heavy marijuana smokers smoke only a fraction of what cigarette addicts smoke. Lung cancers involving only marijuana are rare.[35]

The government's most recent claim is that marijuana abuse accounts for more people entering treatment than any other illegal drug. That shouldn't be surprising, given that tens of millions of Americans smoke marijuana while only a few million use all other illicit drugs.[36] But the claim is spurious nonetheless. Few Americans who enter "treatment" for marijuana are addicted. Fewer than one in five people entering drug treatment for marijuana do so voluntarily.[37] More than half were referred by the criminal justice system.[38] They go because they got caught with a joint or failed a drug test at school or work (typically for having smoked marijuana days ago, not for being impaired), or because they were caught by a law-enforcement officer—and attending a marijuana "treatment" program is what's required to avoid expulsion, dismissal, or incarceration.[39] Many traditional drug treatment programs shamelessly participate in this charade to preserve a profitable and captive client stream.[40]

Even those who recoil at the "nanny state" telling adults what they can or cannot sell to one another often make an exception when it comes to marijuana—to "protect the kids." This is a bad joke, as any teenager will attest. The criminalization of marijuana for adults has not prevented young people from having better access to marijuana than anyone else. Even as marijuana's popularity has waxed and waned since the 1970s, one statistic has remained constant: More than 80 percent of high school students report it's easy to get.[41] Meanwhile, the government's exaggerations and outright dishonesty easily backfire. For every teen who refrains from trying marijuana because it's illegal (for adults), another is tempted by its status as "forbidden fruit."[42] Many respond to the lies about marijuana by disbelieving warnings about more dangerous drugs. So much for protecting the kids by criminalizing the adults.

The Medical Dimension

The debate over medical marijuana obviously colors the broader debate over marijuana prohibition. Marijuana's medical efficacy is no longer in serious dispute. Its use as a medicine dates back thousands of years.[43] Pharmaceutical products containing marijuana's central ingredient, THC, are legally sold in the U.S., and more are emerging.[44,45,46] Some people find the pill form satisfactory, and others consume it in teas or baked products. Most find smoking the easiest and most effective way to consume this unusual medicine,[47] but non-smoking consumption methods, notably vaporizers, are emerging.[48]

Federal law still prohibits medical marijuana.[49] But every state ballot initiative to legalize medical marijuana has been approved, often by wide margins—in California, Washington, Oregon, Alaska, Colorado, Nevada, Maine, and Washington, D.C.[50] State legislatures in Vermont,[51] Hawaii,[52] and Maryland[53] have followed suit, and many others are now considering their own medical marijuana bills—including New York,[54] Connecticut,[55] Rhode Island,[56] and Illinois.[57] Support is often bipartisan, with Republican governors like Gary Johnson and Maryland's Bob Ehrlich taking the lead.[58,59] In New York's 2002 gubernatorial campaign, the conservative candidate of the Independence party, Tom Golisano, surprised everyone by campaigning heavily on this issue.[60] The medical marijuana bill now before the New York legislature is backed not just by leading Republicans but even by some Conservative party leaders.[61]

The political battleground increasingly pits the White House—first under Clinton and now Bush—against everyone else. Majorities in virtually every state in the country would vote, if given the chance, to legalize medical marijuana.[62] Even Congress is beginning to turn; last summer about two-thirds of House Democrats and a dozen Republicans voted in favor of an amendment co-sponsored by Republican Dana Rohrabacher to prohibit federal funding of any Justice Department crackdowns on medical marijuana in the states that had legalized it.[63,64] (Many more Republicans privately expressed support, but were directed to vote against.) And federal courts have imposed limits on federal aggression: first in *Conant* v. *Walters*,[65] which now protects the First Amendment rights of doctors and patients to discuss medical marijuana, and more recently in *Raich* v. *Ashcroft*[66] and *Santa Cruz* v. *Ashcroft*,[67] which determined that the federal government's power to regulate interstate commerce does not provide a basis for prohibiting medical marijuana operations that are entirely local and non-commercial. (The Supreme Court let the *Conant* decision stand,[68] but has yet to consider the others.)

State and local governments are increasingly involved in trying to regulate medical marijuana, notwithstanding the federal prohibition. California, Oregon, Hawaii, Alaska, Colorado, and Nevada have created confidential medical marijuana patient registries, which protect bona fide patients and caregivers from arrest or prosecution.[69] Some municipal governments are now trying to figure out how to regulate production and distribution.[70] In California, where dozens of medical marijuana programs now operate openly, with tacit approval by local authorities, some program directors are asking to be licensed and regulated.[71,72] Many state and local authorities, including law enforcement, favor this but are intimidated by federal threats to arrest and prosecute them for violating federal law.[73]

The drug czar and DEA spokespersons recite the mantra that "there is no such thing as medical marijuana," but the claim is so specious on its face that it clearly undermines federal credibility.[74] The federal government currently provides marijuana—from its own production site in Mississippi—to a few patients who years ago were recognized by the courts as bona fide patients.[75]

No one wants to debate those who have used marijuana for medical purposes, be it Santa Cruz medical-marijuana hospice founder Valerie Corral or NATIONAL REVIEW's Richard Brookhiser.[76] Even many federal officials quietly regret the assault on medical marijuana. When the DEA raided Corral's hospice in September 2002, one agent was heard to say, "Maybe I'm going to think about getting another job sometime soon."

The Broader Movement

The bigger battle, of course, concerns whether marijuana prohibition will ultimately go the way of alcohol Prohibition, replaced by a variety of state and local tax and regulatory policies with modest federal involvement.[77] Dedicated prohibitionists see medical marijuana as the first step down a slippery slope to full legalization.[78] The voters who approved the medical-marijuana ballot initiatives (as well as the wealthy men who helped fund the campaigns[79]) were roughly divided between those who support broader legalization and those who don't, but united in seeing the criminalization and persecution of medical marijuana patients as the most distasteful aspect of the war on marijuana. (This was a point that Buckley made forcefully in his columns about the plight of Peter McWilliams, who likely died because federal authorities effectively forbade him to use marijuana as medicine.[80])

The medical marijuana effort has probably aided the broader anti-prohibitionist campaign in three ways. It helped transform the face of marijuana in the media, from the stereotypical rebel with long hair and tie-dyed shirt to an ordinary middle-aged American struggling with MS or cancer or AIDS.[81] By winning first Proposition 215, the 1996 medical-marijuana ballot initiative in California, and then a string of similar victories in other states, the nascent drug policy reform movement demonstrated that it could win in the big leagues of American politics.[82] And the emergence of successful models of medical marijuana control is likely to boost public confidence in the possibilities and virtue of regulating nonmedical use as well.

In this regard, the history of Dutch policy on cannabis (i.e., marijuana and hashish) is instructive. The "coffee shop" model in the Netherlands, where retail (but not wholesale) sale of cannabis is de facto legal, was not legislated into existence. It evolved in fits and starts following the decriminalization of cannabis by Parliament in 1976, as consumers, growers, and entrepreneurs negotiated and collaborated with local police, prosecutors, and other authorities to find an acceptable middle-ground policy.[83] "Coffee shops" now operate throughout the country, subject to local regulations.[84] Troublesome shops are shut down, and most are well integrated into local city cultures. Cannabis is no more popular than in the U.S. and other Western countries, notwithstanding the effective absence of criminal sanctions and controls.[85] Parallel developments are now underway in other countries.

Like the Dutch decriminalization law in 1976, California's Prop 215 in 1996 initiated a dialogue over how best to implement the new law.[86] The variety of outlets that have emerged—ranging from pharmacy-like stores to medical "coffee shops" to hospices, all of which provide marijuana only to people with a patient ID card or doctor's recommendation—play a key role as the most public symbol and manifestation of this dialogue. More such outlets will likely pop up around the country as other states legalize marijuana for medical purposes and then seek ways to regulate distribution and access. And the question will inevitably arise: If the emerging system is successful in controlling production and distribution of marijuana for those with a medical need, can it not also expand to provide for those without medical need?

Millions of Americans use marijuana not just "for fun" but because they find it useful for many of the same reasons that people drink alcohol or take pharmaceutical drugs. It's akin to the beer, glass of wine, or cocktail at the end of the workday, or the prescribed drug to alleviate depression or anxiety, or the sleeping pill, or the aid to sexual function and pleasure.[87] More and more Americans are apt to describe some or all of their marijuana use as "medical" as the definition of that term evolves and broadens. Their anecdotal experiences are increasingly backed by new scientific research into marijuana's essential ingredients, the cannabinoids.[88] Last year, a subsidiary of *The Lancet,* Britain's leading medical journal, speculated whether marijuana might soon emerge as the "aspirin of the 21st century," providing a wide array of medical benefits at low cost to diverse populations.[89]

Perhaps the expansion of the medical-control model provides the best answer—at least in the U.S.—to the question of how best to reduce the substantial costs and harms of marijuana prohibition without inviting significant increases in real drug abuse. It's analogous to the evolution of many pharmaceutical drugs from prescription to over-the-counter, but with stricter controls still in place. It's also an incrementalist approach to reform that can provide both the control and the reassurance that cautious politicians and voters desire.

In 1931, with public support for alcohol Prohibition rapidly waning, President Hoover released the report of the Wickersham Commission.[90] The report included a devastating critique of Prohibition's failures and costly consequences, but the commissioners, apparently fearful of getting out too far ahead of public opinion, opposed repeal.[91] Franklin P. Adams of the *New York World* neatly summed up their findings:

> Prohibition is an awful flop.
> We like it.
> It can't stop what it's meant to stop.
> We like it.
> It's left a trail of graft and slime
> It don't prohibit worth a dime
> It's filled our land with vice and crime,
> Nevertheless, we're for it.[92]

Two years later, federal alcohol Prohibition was history.

What support there is for marijuana prohibition would likely end quickly absent the billions of dollars spent annually by federal and other governments to prop it up. All those anti-marijuana ads pretend to be about reducing drug abuse, but in fact their basic purpose is sustaining popular support for the war on marijuana. What's needed now are conservative politicians willing to say enough is enough: Tens of billions of taxpayer dollars down the drain each year. People losing their jobs, their property, and their freedom for nothing more than possessing a joint or growing a few marijuana plants. And all for what? To send a message? To keep pretending that we're protecting our children? Alcohol Prohibition made a lot more sense than marijuana prohibition does today—and it, too, was a disaster.

Notes

1. Joel Stein, "The New Politics of Pot," *Time,* 4 November 2002. . . .

2. Ibid.; "Poll Finds Increasing Support For Legalizing Marijuana," *Alcoholism and Drug Abuse Weekly,* 15, No. 27 (2003): 8; Zogby International, "National Views on Drug Policy," (Utica, New York: Zogby, April 2003). The Poll was conducted during April 2003. Forty-one percent of respondents stated that marijuana should be treated in similar manner as alcohol.

3. Ibid.

4. Substance Abuse and Mental Health Services Administration, Department of Health and Human Services, *National Survey on Drug Use and Health, 2002* (Maryland: U.S. Department of Health and Humans Services, 2003): Table 1.31A.

5. Jesse Katz, "Past Drug Use, Future Cops," *Los Angeles Times*, 18 June 2000; "Alcohol and drug disqualification," . . . Military Advantage, 2004. . . .

6. Yvonne Abraham, "Campaign 2000/McCain: Crime and Drugs the Topic in South Carolina," *The Boston Globe,* 9 February 2000.

7. Greg Freeman, "Blagojevich's Pot Use Is Raising Eyebrows, But It Isn't Big News," *St. Louis Post-Dispatch*, 19 September 2002.

8. Bob Dart, "Democrat Hopefuls Pin Hearts on Sleeves; Political 'Oprahization' Means That Confession Is Good for the Poll," *The Austin American Statesman,* 8 December 2003.

9. John Stossel and Sam Donaldson, "Give Me a Break: Politicians Don't Always Do What They Say Or What They Do," *20/20 Friday,* ABC News, 25 August 2000.

10. Ibid.

11. See. . . .

12. Federal Bureau of Investigation, Division of Uniform Crime Reports, *Crime in the United States: 2002* (Washington, D.C.: U.S. Government Printing Office, 2003): 234. . . .

13. 840,000 arrests were made for all other drugs combined. Ibid.

14. Ibid.

15. There have been more than 11 million marijuana arrests made in the U.S. since 1970. See Federal Bureau of Investigation, *Uniform Crime Reports,* Washington, D.C.: Department of Justice, 1966–2002.

16. See. . . . See also Marijuana Policy Project, "Marijuana Prohibition Facts 2004," 2004 . . . (18 June 2004); Mitch Earleywine, *Understanding Marijuana: A New Look at the Scientific Evidence* (New York: Oxford University Press, 2002): 235.

17. The Alabama Sentencing Commission, *Recommendations for Reform of Alabama's Criminal Justice System 2003 Report* (Alabama: Alabama Sentencing Comission, March 2003): 22, 23.

18. Estimated by Marijuana Policy Project, based on Bureau of Justice Statistics, *Prisoners in 2001,* U.S. Department of Justice (Washington, D.C.: U.S. Government Printing Office, 2002); Bureau of Justice Statistics, U.S. Department of Justice, *Prison and Jail Inmates at Midyear 2001* (Washington, D.C.: U.S. Government Printing Office, 2002); Bureau of Justice Statistics, U.S. Department of Justice, *Profile of Jail Inmates, 1996* (Washington, D.C.: U.S. Government Printing Office, 1998); Bureau of Justice Statistics, U.S. Department of Justice, *Substance Abuse and Treatment, State and Federal Prisoners 1997* (Washington, D.C.: U.S. Government Printing Office, 1999). . . .

19. Judy Appel and Robin Levi, *Collateral Consequences: Denial of Basic Social Services Based on Drug Use* (California: Drug Policy Alliance, June 2003). . . .

20. Carl Hiassen, "New Rules Trap Immigrants with Old Secrets," *The Miami Herald,* 30 May 2004.

21. Paul Samuels and Debbie Mukamal, *After Prison: Roadblocks to Reentry: A Report on State Legal Barriers Facing People With Criminal Records* (New York: Legal Action Center, 2004). . . .

22. *Higher Education Act of 1998, U.S. Code,* Title 20, Sec. 1091.

23. According to data from the Department of Education analyzed by Students for Sensible Drug Policy, over 150,000 students have lost aid thus far due to the provision. See Greg Winter, "A Student Aid Ban for Past Drug Use is Creating a Furor," *The New York Times,* 13 March 2004; Alexandra Marks, "No Education Funds for Drug Offenders," *Christian Science Monitor,* 24 April 2001; John Kelly, "Students Seeking Aid Not Answering Drug Questions," *The Associated Press,* 21 March 2000.

24. See . . . .

25. Theresa Howard, "U.S. Crafts Anti-Drug Message," *USA Today,* 15 March 2004.

26. Drug Enforcement Administration, *In the Matter of Marijuana Rescheduling Petition* [Docket#86-22] (Washington, D.C.: U.S. Department of Justice, 6 September 1988): 57.

27. Based on data from *National Household Survey on Drug Abuse: Population Estimates 1994* (Rockville, MD: U.S. Department of Health and Human Services, 1995); *National Household Survey on Drug Abuse: Main Findings 1994* (Rockville, MD: U.S. Department of Health and Human Services, 1996). See also D.B. Kandel and M. Davies, "Progression to Regular Marijuana Involvement: Phenomenology and Risk Factors for Near-Daily Use," *Vulnerability to Drug Abuse,* Eds. M. Glantz and R. Pickens (Washington, D.C.: American Psychological Association, 1992): 211–253.

28. Lynn Zimmer and John P. Morgan, *Marijuana Myths, Marijuana Facts: A Review of the Scientific Evidence* (New York: Drug Policy Alliance, 1997): 37–38.

29. Ibid., 134–141.

30. Mitch Earleywine, *Understanding Marijuana: A New Look at the Scientific Evidence* (New York, Oxford University Press, 2002): 130.

31. Janet E. Joy, Stanley J. Watson Jr., and John A. Benson Jr., Eds., *Marijuana and Medicine: Assessing the Science Base* (Washington, D.C.: National Academy of Sciences Institute of Medicine, 1999): 89–91. . . .

32. See the findings of the Canadian Committee on Illegal Drugs . . . Pierre Claude Nolin, Chair, Senate Special Committee on Illegal Drugs, *Cannabis: Our Position for a Canadian Public Policy: Summary Report* (Ontario: Senate of Canada, 2002).

33. I Geenberg, "Psychiatric and Behavioral Observations of Casual and Heavy Marijuana Users," *Annals of the New York Academy of Sciences,* 282 (1976): 72–84; N. Solowij et al., "Biophysical Changes Associated with Cessation of Cannabis Use: A Single Case Study of Acute and Chronic Effects, Withdrawal and

Treatment," *Life Sciences* 56 (1995): 2127–2135; A.D. Bensusan, "Marihuana Withdrawal Symptoms," *British Journal of Medicine,* 3 (1971):112.

34. Numerous government commissions investigating the relationship between marijuana and violence have concluded that marijuana does not cause crime. See National Commission on Marihuana and Drug Abuse, *Marihuana: A Signal of Understanding* (Washington, D.C.: U.S. Government Printing Office, 1972): 77; Pierre Claude Nolin Chair, Senate Special Committee on Illegal Drugs, *Cannabis: Our Position for a Canadian Public Policy: Summary Report* (Ontario: Senate of Canada, 2002). See also Lynn Zimmer and John P. Morgan, *Marijuana Myths, Marijuana Facts: A Review of the Scientific Evidence* (New York: Drug Policy Alliance, 1997): 7, 88–91.

35. S. Sidney, C.P. Quesenberry, G.D. Friedman, and I.S. Tekawa, "Marijuana Use and Cancer Incidence," *Cancer Cause and Control* 8 (1997); 722–728; Lynn Zimmer and John P. Morgan, *Marijuana Myths, Marijuana Facts: A Review of the Scientific Evidence* (New York: Drug Policy Alliance, 1997): 7, 112–116; Mitch Earleywine, *Understanding Marijuana: A New Look at the Scientific Evidence* (New York, Oxford University Press, 2002): 155–158.

36. Substance Abuse and Mental Health Services Administration, Department of Health and Human Services, *National Survey on Drug Use and Health, 2002* (Maryland: U.S. Department of Health and Humans Services, 2003): 4, 5.

37. Substance Abuse and Mental Health Services Administration, *2003 Treatment Episode Data Set: 1992–2001,* National Admissions to Substance Abuse Treatment Services, DASIS Series: S-20 (Maryland: U.S. Department of Health and Human Services, 2003): 122.

38. Ibid.

39. Ibid.

40. Substance Abuse and Mental Health Services Administration, Department of Health and Human Services, "Coerced Treatment Among Youths: 1993 to 1998," *The DASIS Report,* 21 September 2001.

41. L.D. Johnston, P.M. O'Malley, and J.G. Bachman, *Monitoring the Future: National Results on Adolescent Drug Use: Overview of Key Findings, 2003* (Bethesda, Maryland: National Institute on Drug Abuse, 2004); Ann L. Pastore and Kathleen Maguire, Eds., U.S. Department of Justice, Bureau of Justice Statistics, *Sourcebook of Criminal Justice Statistics 2001* (Washington, D.C.: U.S. Government Printing Office, 2002): 173.

42. Svetlana Kolchik, "More Americans Used Illegal Drugs in 2001, U.S. Study Says," *USA Today,* 6 September 2002; Corky Newton, *Generation Risk: How to Protect Your Teenager from Smoking and Other Dangerous Behaviors* (New York: M. Evans and Company, 2001).

43. Ernest Abel, *Marijuana: The First Twelve Thousand Years* (New York: McGraw Hill, 1982); Martin Booth, *Cannabis: A History* (London: Doubleday, 2003); Janet E. Joy, Stanley J. Watson Jr., and John A. Benson Jr., Eds., *Marijuana and Medicine: Assessing the Science Base* (Washington, D.C.: National Academy of Sciences Institute of Medicine, 1999): 19. . . .

44. Janet E. Joy, Stanley J. Watson Jr., and John A. Benson Jr., Eds., *Marijuana and Medicine: Assessing the Science Base* (Washington, D.C.: National Academy of Sciences Institute of Medicine, 1999): 16. . . .

45. "Marijuana-Based Drug Developed to Treat MS," *Calgary Sun,* 12 May 2004.

46. Heather Stewart, "Late Again: GW's Cannabis-Based Painkiller," *The Guardian,* 1 May 2004.

47. See Janet E. Joy, Stanley J. Watson Jr., and John, A. Benson Jr., Eds., *Marijuana and Medicine: Assessing the Science Base* (Washington, D.C.: National Academy

of Sciences Institute of Medicine, 1999); 27–29; and Mitch Earleywine, *Understanding Marijuana: A New Look at the Scientific Evidence* (New York, Oxford University Press, 2002): 171.

48. Dale Gieringer, Joseph St. Laurent, and Scott Goodrich, "Cannabis Vaporizer Combines Efficient Delivery of THC with Effective Suppression of Pyrolytic Compounds," *Journal of Cannabis Therapeutics* 4(2004): 7–27. A British pharmaceutical company, GW Pharmaceuticals, has developed an oral spray to dispense cannabis to medical-marijuana patients. . . .

49. *Schedules of Controlled Substances, U.S. Code,* Title 21, Sec. 812.

50. Bill Piper et al., *State of the States: Drug Policy Reforms: 1996–2002* (New York: Drug Policy Alliance, 2003): 42. . . .

51. David Gram, "Vermont's Medical Marijuana Bill to Be Law," *Associated Press,* 20 May 2004.

52. Associated Press, "Hawaii Becomes First State to Approve Medical Marijuana Bill," *The New York Times,* 15 June 2000.

53. Craig Whitlock and Lori Montgomery, "Ehrlich Signs Marijuana Bill; Maryland Governor Weighs Independence, GOP Loyalty," *The Washington Post,* 23 May 2003; Angela Potter, "Maryland Governor Signs Medical Marijuana Bill Into Law," *Associated Press,* 22 May 2003.

54. Ellis Henican, "High Hopes for Pot," *Newsday,* 16 June 2004.

55. Ken Dixon, "State Urged to Legalize Medical Marijuana Use," *Connecticut Post,* 2 April 2004.

56. "Medical Marijuana in Rhode Island," *The Providence Journal,* 19 May 2004.

57. "Medical Marijuana Debate on Hold," *The State Journal-Register,* 3 March 2004.

58. Matthew Miller, "He Just Said No to the Drug War," *The New York Times Magazine,* 20 August 2000.

59. Richard Willing, "Attitudes Ease Toward Medical Marijuana," *USA Today,* 22 May 2003.

60. Seanne Adcox, "Golisano Proposes Medical Use of Marijuana," *New York Newsday,* 17 October 2002.

61. John H. Wilson, "Medical Marijuana Helps Serious Ill," *Albany Times Union,* 24 March 2004.

62. See Janet E. Joy, Stanley J. Watson Jr., and John A. Benson Jr., Eds., *Marijuana and Medicine: Assessing the Science Base* (Washington, D.C.: National Academy of Sciences Institutes of Medicine, 1999): 18; and Richard Schmitz and Chuck Thomas, *State-By-State Medical Marijuana Laws: How to Remove the Threat of Arrest* (Washington, D.C.: Marijuana Policy Project, 2001): Appendix D. . . .

63. Edward Epstein, "Bill to Protect Medicinal Pot Users Falls Short in House," *San Francisco Chronicle,* 24 July 2003.

64. In July 2004, a similar amendment was voted on and once again fell short of passage. . . .

65. See. . . .

66. The U.S. Supreme Court will hear *Raich v. Ashcroft* this fall . . . Eric Bailey, "State Set for Legal Showdown Over Pot," *Los Angeles Times,* 19 May 2004.

67. "Leave Medical Marijuana Group Alone, Judge Tells Government," *The New York Times,* 22 April 2004. . . .

68. Linda Greenhouse, "Supreme Court Roundup; Justices Say Doctors May Not Be Punished for Recommending Medical Marijuana," *The New York Times,* 15 October 2003.

69. National Organization for the Reform of Marijuana Laws, "Summary of active State Medical Marijuana Programs," July 2002. . . .

70. Laura Counts, "Oakland to Limit Marijuana Outlets," *Tri-Valley Herald,* 18 April 2004. Also see information on San Franciscos" Proposition. . . .

71. Amy Hilvers, "'Pot Club' Thrives in Oildale," *The Bakersfield Californian,* 26 May 2004.

72. Laura Counts, "Medical Marijuana Merchant Defies Oakland Order to Close," *The Oakland Tribune,* 2 June 2004.

73. Doug Bandow, "Where's the Compassion?," *National Review Online,* 19 December 2003. . . . See also Michael Gougis, "Medical Marijuana Tug of War: Lenient Sentences Underscore Conflicting State and Federal Pot Laws," *Daily News of Los Angeles,* 12 December 2003; Clarence Page, "Drug Warriors Trampling Rights of Medical Marijuana Proponents," *Salt Lake Tribune,* 12 February 2003.

74. Andrea Barthwell, "Haze of Myths Clouds Value of Medical 'Pot,'" *The Republican,* 27 July 2003; Alan W. Bock, "UNSPIN/Marijuana, Medicine, and Ed Rosenthal: The Issue: Medical Marijuana and Federal Law," *Orange County Register,* 9 February 2003; Ian Ith and Carol M. Ostrom, "Feds Pose Challenge to Use of Medical Marijuana," *The Seattle Times,* 16 September 2002; and Josh Richman, "Drug Czar Coolly Received in Bay Area; Federal Stance on Medical Marijuana Won't be Relaxed, Walters Says," *The Daily Review,* 18 November 2003.

75. David Brown, "NIH Panel Cautiously Favors Medical Study of Marijuana," *The Washington Post,* 21 February 1997; Ray Delgado, "Many Patients Call Government Marijuana Weak; Medicinal Cigarettes Loaded With Stems, Seeds, Researchers Say," *San Francisco Chronicle,* 16 May 2002; Lester Grinspoon and James B. Bakalar, *Marihuana: The Forbidden Medicine* (Connecticut: Yale University Press, 1997): 45–66.

76. Richard Brookhiser, "Drug Warriors Are Repeating Earlier Errors; Considering His Past Abuse, Bush Should Be Sympathetic to Reforms," *Chicago Sun-Times,* 25 May 2001; Richard Brookhiser, "In Dull Election, My Vote Is Going To Marijuana Man," *New York Observer,* 4 November 2002; Richard Brookhiser, "Madness of Pot Prohibition Claims Yet Another Victim," *New York Observer,* 24 July 2000; Richard Brookhiser, "The Sick Shouldn't Be Victims of the Drug War," *Buffalo News,* 20 July 2003; Richard Brookhiser, "Why I Support Medical Marijuana," Congressional Testimony, House Judiciary committee, Subcommittee on Crime, 6 March 1996. . . .

77. Raymond B. Fosdick, *Toward Liquor Control* (New York: Harper, 1993): David E. Kyvig, *Repealing national Prohibition,* 2nd Edition (Ohio: Kent State University Press, 2000).

78. John L. Mica, "Should the Federal Government Study the Effects of Medical Marijuana? Do Not Waste Taxpayers' Dollars," *Roll Call,* 21 June 1999.

79. George Soros, "The Drug War 'Cannot Be Won:' It's Time to Just Say No To Self-Destructive Prohibition," *The Washington Post,* 2 February 1997.

80. William F. Buckley Jr., "The Legal Jam," *National Review Online,* 15 May 2001; William F. Buckley, Jr., "Peter McWilliams, R.I.P.," *National Review,* 17 July 2000; William F. Buckley, Jr., "Reefer Madness," *National Review,* 14 July 2003.

81. Compare the photographs that accompany the following two articles: Tom Morganthau et al., "Should Drugs Be Legal?," *Newsweek,* 30 May 1988; Geoffrey Cowley et al., "Can Marijuana Be Medicine?," *Newsweek,* 3 February 1997.

82. Bill Piper et al., *State of the States: Drug Policy Reforms: 1996–2002* (New York: Drug Policy Alliance, 2003). . . .

83. Robert J. MacCoun and Peter Reuter, *Drug War Heresies: Learning from Other Vices, Times, and Places* (New York: Cambridge University Press, 2001): 238–264.

84. A.C.M. Jansen, "The Development of a 'Legal' Consumers' Market for Cannabis—the 'Coffee Shop' Phenomenon," *Between Prohibition and Legalization: The Dutch Experiment in Drug Policy,* E. Leuw and I. Haen Marshall, Eds., (New York: Kugler Publications, 1996).

85. Craig Reinarman, Peter D.A. Cohen, and Hendrien L. Kaal, "The Limited Relevance of Drug Policy: Cannabis in Amsterdam and in San Francisco," *American Journal of Public Health* 94 (2004): 836–842.

86. Michael Pollan, "Living With Medical Marijuana," *New York Times Magazine,* 20 July 1997.

87. See Pierre Claude Nolin, Chair, Senate Special Committee on Illegal Drugs, *Cannabis: Our Position for a Canadian Public Policy: Summary Report* (Ontario: Senate of Canada, 2002): Mitch Earleywine, *Understanding Marijuana: A New Look at the Scientific Evidence* (New York, Oxford University Press, 2002).

88. J. M. McPartland and E. B. Russo, "Cannabis and Cannabis Extracts: Greater Than the Sum of Their Parts?," *Journal of Cannabis Therapeutics* 1 (2001): 103–132; R. Mechoulam, L. A. Parker, and R. Gallily, "Cannabidiol: An Overview of Some Pharmacological Aspects," *Journal of Clinical Pharmacology,* 42 (2002): 11S–19S; R. G. Pertwee, "The Pharmacology and Therapeutic Potential of Cannabidiol," *Cannabinoids,* Ed. V. DiMarzo (The Netherlands: Kluwer Academic Publishers, 2004).

89. David Baker, Alan Thompson et al., "The Therapeutic Potential of Cannabis," *The Lancet Neurology,* 2 (2003): 294.

90. See . . . or the complete text of the Commission's report.

91. David E. Kyvig, *Repealing National Prohibition,* 2nd Edition (Ohio: Kent State University Press, 2000): 111–115.

92. As cited in David E. Kyvig, *Repealing National Prohibition,* 2nd Edition (Ohio: Kent State University Press, 2000): 114.

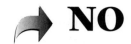

Marijuana & the Truth Behind 10 Popular Misperceptions

Introduction

Marijuana is the most widely used illicit drug in the United States. According to the National Survey on Drug Use and Health (formerly called the National Household Survey on Drug Abuse), 95 million Americans age 12 and older have tried "pot" at least once, and three out of every four illicit-drug users reported using marijuana within the previous 30 days.

Use of marijuana has adverse health, safety, social, academic, economic, and behavioral consequences. And yet, astonishingly, many people view the drug as "harmless." The widespread perception of marijuana as a benign natural herb seriously detracts from the most basic message our society needs to deliver: It is not OK for anyone—especially young people—to use this or any other illicit drug.

Marijuana became popular among the general youth population in the 1960s. Back then, many people who would become the parents and grandparents of teenage kids today smoked marijuana without significant adverse effects, so now they may see no harm in its use. But most of the marijuana available today is considerably more potent than the "weed" of the Woodstock era, and its users tend to be younger than those of past generations. Since the late 1960s, the average age of marijuana users has dropped from around 19 to just over 17. People are also lighting up at an earlier age. Fewer than half of those using marijuana for the first time in the late 1960s were under 18. By 2001, however, the proportion of under-18 initiates had increased to about two-thirds (67 percent).

Today's young people live in a world vastly different from that of their parents and grandparents. Kids these days, for instance, are bombarded constantly with pro-drug messages in print, on screen, and on CD. They also have easy access to the Internet, which abounds with sites promoting the wonders of marijuana, offering kits for beating drug tests, and, in some cases, advertising pot for sale. Meanwhile, the prevalence of higher potency marijuana, measured by levels of the chemical delta-9-tetrahydrocannabinol (THC), is increasing. Average THC levels rose from less than 1 percent in the mid-1970s to more than

From "Are Psychotherapeutic Drugs Effective for Treating Mental Illness", Office of National Drug Control Policy, 2004. References omitted.

6 percent in 2002. Sinsemilla potency increased in the past two decades from 6 percent to more than 13 percent, with some samples containing THC levels of up to 33 percent. . . .

Myth 1: Marijuana Is Harmless

Marijuana harms in many ways, and kids are the most vulnerable to its damaging effects. Use of the drug can lead to significant health, safety, social, and learning or behavioral problems, especially for young users. . . .

Short-term effects of marijuana use include memory loss, distorted perception, trouble with thinking and problem-solving, and anxiety. Students who use marijuana may find it hard to learn, thus jeopardizing their ability to achieve their full potential.

Cognitive Impairment

That marijuana can cause problems with concentration and thinking has been shown in research funded by the National Institute on Drug Abuse (NIDA), the federal agency that brings the power of science to bear on drug abuse and addiction. A NIDA-funded study at McLean Hospital in Belmont, Massachusetts, is part of the growing body of research documenting cognitive impairment among heavy marijuana users. The study found that college students who used marijuana regularly had impaired skills related to attention, memory, and learning 24 hours after they last used the drug.

Another study, conducted at the University of Iowa College of Medicine, found that people who used marijuana frequently (7 or more times weekly for an extended period) showed deficits in mathematical skills and verbal expression, as well as selective impairments in memory-retrieval processes. These findings clearly have significant implications for young people, since reductions in cognitive function can lead to poor performance in school. . . .

Mental Health Problems

Smoking marijuana leads to changes in the brain similar to those caused by cocaine, heroin, and alcohol. All of these drugs disrupt the flow of chemical neurotransmitters, and all have specific receptor sites in the brain that have been linked to feelings of pleasure and, over time, addiction. Cannabinoid receptors are affected by THC, the active ingredient in marijuana, and many of these sites are found in the parts of the brain that influence pleasure, memory, thought, concentration, sensory and time perception, and coordinated movement.

Particularly for young people, marijuana use can lead to increased anxiety, panic attacks, depression, and other mental health problems. One study linked social withdrawal, anxiety, depression, attention problems, and thoughts of suicide in adolescents with past-year marijuana use. Other research shows that kids age 12 to 17 who smoke marijuana weekly are three times more likely than non-users to have thoughts about committing suicide. A recently published longitudinal study showed that use of cannabis increased the risk of major depression fourfold, and researchers in Sweden found a link between marijuana use and an increased risk of developing schizophrenia.

According to the American Society of Addiction Medicine, addiction and psychiatric disorders often occur together. The latest National Survey on Drug Use and Health reported that adults who use illicit drugs were more than twice as likely to have serious mental illness as adults who did not use an illicit drug.

Researchers conducting a longitudinal study of psychiatric disorders and substance use (including alcohol, marijuana, and other illicit drugs) have suggested several possible links between the two: (1) people may use drugs to feel better and alleviate symptoms of a mental disorder; (2) the use of the drug and the disorder share certain biological, social, or other risk factors; or (3) use of the drug can lead to anxiety, depression, or other disorders. . . .

Long-Term Consequences

The consequences of marijuana use can last long after the drug's effects have worn off. Studies show that early use of marijuana is strongly associated with later use of other illicit drugs and with a greater risk of illicit drug dependence or abuse. In fact, an analysis of data from the National Household Survey on Drug Abuse showed that the age of initiation for marijuana use was the most important predictor of later need for drug treatment.

Regular marijuana use has been shown to be associated with other long-term problems, including poor academic performance, poor job performance and increased absences from work, cognitive deficits, and lung damage. Marijuana use is also associated with a number of risky sexual behaviors, including having multiple sex partners, initiating sex at an early age, and failing to use condoms consistently.

Myth 2: Marijuana Is Not Addictive

. . . According to the 2002 National Survey on Drug Use and Health, 4.3 million Americans were classified with dependence on or abuse of marijuana. That figure represents 1.8 percent of the total U.S. population and 60.3 percent of those classified as individuals who abuse or are dependent on illicit drugs.

The desire for marijuana exerts a powerful pull on those who use it, and this desire, coupled with withdrawal symptoms, can make it hard for long-term smokers to stop using the drug. Users trying to quit often report irritability, anxiety, and difficulty sleeping. On psychological tests they also display increased aggression, which peaks approximately one week after they last used the drug.

Many people use marijuana compulsively even though it interferes with family, school, work, and recreational activities. What makes this all the more disturbing is that marijuana use has been shown to be three times more likely to lead to dependence among adolescents than among adults. Research indicates that the earlier kids start using marijuana, the more likely they are to become dependent on this or other illicit drugs later in life. . . .

Myth 3: Marijuana Is Not as Harmful to Your Health as Tobacco

Although some people think of marijuana as a benign natural herb, the drug actually contains many of the same cancer-causing chemicals found in tobacco. Puff for puff, the amount of tar inhaled and the level of carbon monoxide absorbed by those who smoke marijuana, regardless of THC content, are three to five times greater than among tobacco smokers.

Consequently, people who use marijuana on a regular basis often have the same breathing problems as tobacco users, such as chronic coughing and wheezing, more frequent acute chest illnesses, and a tendency toward obstructed airways. And because respiratory problems can affect athletic performance, smoking marijuana may be particularly harmful to kids involved in sports.

Researchers at the University of California, Los Angeles, have determined that marijuana smoking can cause potentially serious damage to the respiratory system at a relatively early age. Moreover, in a review of research on the health effects of marijuana use, the researchers cited findings that show "the daily smoking of relatively small amounts of marijuana (3 to 4 joints) has at least a comparable, if not greater effect" on the respiratory system than the smoking of more than 20 tobacco cigarettes.

Recently, scientists in England produced further evidence linking marijuana use to respiratory problems in young people. A research team at the University of Birmingham found that regular use of marijuana, even for less than six years, causes a marked deterioration in lung function. . . .

Myth 4: Marijuana Makes You Mellow

. . . Research shows that kids who use marijuana weekly are nearly four times more likely than non-users to report they engage in violent behavior. One study found that young people who had used marijuana in the past year were more likely than non-users to report aggressive behavior. According to that study, incidences of physically attacking people, stealing, and destroying property increased in proportion to the number of days marijuana was smoked in the past year. Users were also twice as likely as non-users to report they disobey at school and destroy their own things.

In another study, researchers looking into the relationship between ten illicit drugs and eight criminal offenses found that a greater frequency of marijuana use was associated with a greater likelihood to commit weapons offenses; except for alcohol, none of the other drugs showed such a connection. . . .

Myth 5: Marijuana Is Used to Treat Cancer and Other Diseases

Under the Comprehensive Drug Abuse Prevention and Control Act of 1970, marijuana was established as a Schedule I controlled substance. In other words, it is a dangerous drug that has no recognized medical value.

Whether marijuana can provide relief for people with certain medical conditions, including cancer, is a subject of intense national debate. It is true that THC, the primary active chemical in marijuana, can be useful for treating some medical problems. Synthetic THC is the main ingredient in Marinol®, an FDA-approved medication used to control nausea in cancer chemotherapy patients and to stimulate appetite in people with AIDS. Marinol, a legal and safe version of medical marijuana, has been available by prescription since 1985.

However, marijuana as a smoked product has never proven to be medically beneficial and, in fact, is much more likely to harm one's health; marijuana smoke is a crude THC delivery system that also sends many harmful substances into the body. In 1999, the Institute of Medicine (IOM) published a review of the available scientific evidence in an effort to assess the potential health benefits of marijuana and its constituent cannabinoids. The review concluded that smoking marijuana is not recommended for any long-term medical use, and a subsequent IOM report declared, "marijuana is not a modern medicine." . . .

Myth 6: Marijuana Is Not as Popular as MDMA (Ecstasy) or Other Drugs among Teens Today

Recent survey data show that about 15 million people—6.2 percent of the U.S. population—are current marijuana users, and that nearly a third of them (4.8 million people) used the drug on 20 or more days in the past month. Among kids age 12 to 17, more than two million (8.2 percent) reported past-month marijuana use. By contrast, fewer than 250,000 young people (1 percent) reported past-month use of hallucinogens, and of that number, only half (124,000) had used MDMA.

The 2003 Monitoring the Future Study showed that marijuana is not only popular today, it has been the most widely used illicit drug among high school seniors for the entire 29 years of the study. Meanwhile, Ecstasy use among American teens appears to be declining after record increases. Between 2001 and 2003, past-month use of MDMA among students in the three grades surveyed dropped by more than half, from 1.8 percent to 0.7 percent (8th grade), 2.6 percent to 1.1 percent (10th grade), and 2.8 percent to 1.3 percent (12th grade). . . .

Myth 7: If I Buy Marijuana, I'm Not Hurting Anyone Else

Violence at Home

. . . The trade in domestically grown marijuana often turns violent when dealers have conflicts or when growers feel their crops are threatened. But drug criminals are not the only ones threatened by the violence of the marijuana trade.

Much of the marijuana produced in America is grown on public lands, including our national forests and parks—areas set aside to preserve wildlife habitats, provide playgrounds for our children, and serve as natural refuges for recreation. Traffickers grow their crops in these areas because the land is free and accessible, crop ownership is hard to document, and because growers are immune to asset forfeiture laws. Law enforcement officials report that many marijuana growers, seeking to protect their crops from busybodies and rival "pot pirates," surround their plots with crude booby traps, including fishhooks dangling at eye level, bear traps, punji sticks, and rat traps rigged with shotgun shells.

Most of the marijuana on America's public lands is grown in the vast national forests of California, where more than 540,000 plants were seized or eradicated on land managed by the U.S. Forest Service in 2003 alone. This figure does not include the 309,000 marijuana plants taken from Forest Service land in other states, nor does it take into account the hundreds of thousands of plants removed from land managed by other government agencies. For example, in 2003 more than 134,000 marijuana plants were seized or eradicated from areas in California administered by the U.S. Department of the Interior's Bureau of Land Management.

According to officers with the Forest Service and other agencies, many of California's illegal marijuana fields are controlled not by peace-loving flower children but by employees of Mexican drug-trafficking organizations carrying high-powered assault weapons. During the growing season, the officers say, the cartels smuggle hundreds of undocumented Mexican nationals into the U.S. to work the fields, bringing with them pesticides, equipment, and guns. Hunters, campers, and others have been threatened at gunpoint or fired upon after stumbling into these illegal gardens. . . .

Myth 8: My Kids Won't Be Exposed to Marijuana

. . . More than half (55 percent) of youths age 12 to 17 responding to the National Survey on Drug Use and Health in 2002 reported that marijuana would be easy to obtain. The survey indicated that most marijuana users got the drug from a friend, and that almost nine percent of youths who bought marijuana did so inside a school building. Moreover, nearly 17 percent of the young people surveyed said they had been approached by someone selling drugs in the past month. In the 2000 survey, more than a quarter of 12- to 17-year-olds (26.6 percent) reported that drug-selling occurs frequently in their neighborhoods.

Kids are also exposed to a relentless barrage of marijuana messages in the popular culture—in the music they listen to, the movies they watch, and the magazines they read. And then there's the Internet, a crowded landscape of pro-marijuana and drug legalization Web sites. More often than not, the culture glamorizes or trivializes marijuana use and fails to show the serious harm it can cause. . . .

Not Just an Inner-City Problem

Some people have the impression that kids in the inner city are those most likely to get involved with drugs. Research shows, however, that marijuana use among youth in cities, rural areas, and the suburbs is roughly the same, and that use rates are similar regardless of population density. For example, annual prevalence rates of marijuana use among 10th graders are 28 percent in non-urban areas, 29 percent in large metropolitan statistical areas, and 32 percent in other metropolitan areas.

Myth 9: There's Not Much Parents Can Do to Stop Their Kids from Experimenting with Marijuana

Many people are surprised to learn that parents are the most powerful influence on their children when it comes to drugs. By staying involved, knowing what their kids are doing, and setting limits with clear rules and consequences, parents can increase the chances their kids will stay drug free. Research shows that appropriate parental monitoring can reduce future drug use even among adolescents who may be prone to marijuana use, such as those who are rebellious, cannot control their emotions, and experience internal distress. . . .

Parental Involvement

Kids who learn about the risks of drugs from their parents or caregivers are less likely to use drugs than kids who do not. Parents can create situations that help them connect with their children and stay involved in their lives. Experts suggest that parents try to be home with their kids after school, if possible, because evidence indicates that the riskiest time for kids with regard to drug involvement is between the hours of 3 p.m. and 6 p.m. Parents who can't be home with their children should consider enrolling them in after-school programs, sports, or other activities, or arrange for a trusted adult to oversee them.

It's also important for families to participate in activities such as eating meals together; holding meetings in which each person gets a chance to talk; and establishing regular routines of doing something special (like taking a walk) that allow parents to talk to their kids. Opening channels of communication between parents and children, as well as between families and the greater community, gives young people greater confidence and helps them make healthy choices.

Myth 10: The Government Sends Otherwise Innocent People to Prison for Casual Marijuana Use

On the contrary, it is extremely rare for anyone, particularly first-time offenders, to get sent to prison just for possessing a small amount of marijuana. In most states, possession of an ounce or less of pot is a misdemeanor offense, and some states have gone so far as to downgrade simple possession of marijuana to a civil offense akin to a traffic violation.

. . . In 1997, according to the U.S. Department of Justice's Bureau of Justice Statistics (BJS), only 1.6 percent of the state inmate population had been convicted of a marijuana-only crime, including trafficking. An even smaller percentage of state inmates were imprisoned with marijuana *possession* as the only charge (0.7 percent). And only 0.3 percent of those imprisoned just for marijuana possession were first-time offenders.

More recent estimates from the BJS show that at midyear 2002, approximately 8,400 state prisoners were serving time for possessing marijuana in any amount. Fewer than half of that group, or about 3,600 inmates, were incarcerated on a first offense. In other words, of the more than 1.2 million people doing time in state prisons across America, only a small fraction were first-time offenders sentenced just for marijuana possession. And again, this figure includes possession of *any* amount.

On the federal level, prosecutors focus largely on traffickers, kingpins, and other major drug criminals, so federal marijuana cases often involve hundreds of pounds of the drug. Cases involving smaller amounts are typically handled on the state level. This is part of the reason why hardly anyone ends up in federal prison for simple possession of marijuana. The fact is, of all drug defendants sentenced in federal court for marijuana offenses in 2001, the vast majority were convicted of trafficking. Only 2.3 percent—186 people—were sentenced for simple possession, and of the 174 for whom sentencing information is known, just 63 actually served time behind bars. . . .

Conclusion

The clutter of messages about marijuana in the popular culture creates an atmosphere of confusion and sends kids mixed signals about the drug. But what should be clear is that no responsible person thinks young people should use marijuana. . . .

Parents can help keep their children away from marijuana by letting them know its dangers, and by monitoring their activities and staying involved in their lives. . . . Both of these Web sites are supported by the Office of National Drug Control Policy.

Schools and communities can also play an important role by providing activities that keep kids interested and involved in healthy, drug-free programs.

If you want to help dispel misperceptions and spread the truth about marijuana to help kids grow up drug-free, you can:

- Educate yourself about the dangers of marijuana and keep up with scientific research into its harmful effects. For a wealth of good information, visit the Web site for the National Institute on Drug Abuse at. . . .
- Help kids in trouble with marijuana get into drug treatment programs
- Be an advocate for better, more informed drugged-driving laws
- Support after-school programs and get involved in local anti-drug coalitions
- Stay informed about the marijuana laws in your state, and take a stand against changes in legislation that would increase the drug's availability in your community
- Support efforts to launch a student drug-testing program in your local schools

- See "What You Need to Know About Drug Testing in Schools," available by calling 800-666-3332. . . .
- To learn more about drug and alcohol abuse, visit the Substance Abuse & Mental Health Services Administration's National Clearinghouse for Alcohol and Drug Information at . . . or call its 24-hour hotline: 1-800-729-6686 or 1-800-788-2800

POSTSCRIPT

Should Laws Prohibiting Marijuana Use Be Relaxed?

The restrictive laws against marijuana, according to Nadelmann, has resulted in a burgeoning number of people in prison for marijuana offenses. Nadelmann does not contend that marijuana is a safe drug, but that legalizing it would enable officials to have better control over its use. In addition, he feels that the federal government prevents people from receiving medication that is both therapeutic and benign. The government's objection to marijuana, says Nadelmann, is based more on politics than scientific evidence.

From the federal government's perspective, promoting marijuana as a medicinal agent would be a mistake because it has not been proven medically useful or safe. Moreover, it feels that the availability of marijuana should not be predicated on personal accounts of its benefits or whether the public supports its use. Also, the federal government asserts that although studies show that marijuana may have medical value, much of that research has been based on bad scientific methodology and other deficiencies. The results of previous research, according to the federal government, do not lend strong credence to marijuana's medicinal value.

Some people have expressed concern about what will happen if marijuana is approved for medicinal use. Would it then become more acceptable for non-medical, recreational use? There is also a possibility that some people would misinterpret the government's message and think that marijuana cures cancer when, in fact, it would only be used to treat the side effects of the chemotherapy.

Despite its popularity, the federal government notes that parents should and can assert more influence on their children's desire to use marijuana. The government claims that marijuana is not the harmless drug that many proponents believe. Marijuana can have adverse effects, on mental health, on physical well-being, and on academic performance. In addition, thousands of young people enter substance abuse treatment for their addiction to marijuana. It is important, states the Office of National Drug Control Policy, to counteract how culture trivializes the dangers of marijuana use.

Many marijuana proponents contend that the effort to prevent the legalization of marijuana for medical use and nonmedical use is purely a political battle. Detractors maintain that the issue is purely scientific—that the data supporting marijuana's medical usefulness are inconclusive and scientifically unsubstantiated. And although the chief administrative law judge of the Drug Enforcement Administration (DEA) made a recommendation to change the status of marijuana from Schedule I to Schedule II, the DEA and other federal agencies are not compelled to do so, and they have resisted any change in the law.

A number of articles debate the merits of relaxing laws against marijuana use. David Wahlberg, in "Stronger Pot, Bigger Worries" (*The Sacramento Bee,* May 5, 2004), argues that one danger with marijuana today is that its potency has gotten increasingly stronger. In "Tokin' Politics: Making Marijuana Law reform An Election Issue" (*Heads,* May 2004), Paul Armentano writes that politicians have refused to relax marijuana laws because that decision would be politically unpopular. The ongoing dispute between the United States and Canada regarding marijuana laws is discussed by Donna Leinwand in "U.S., Canada Clash on Pot Laws" (*USA Today,* May 8, 2003). Articles that discuss whether or not marijuana should be legalized as a medication include "The Growing Debate on Medical Marijuana: Federal Power Vs. States Rights," by Alreen Hussein (*California Western Law Review,* vol. 37, no. 2, 2001) and "Cannabis Control: Costs Outweigh the Benefits," by Alex Wodak and others (*British Medical Journal,* January 12, 2002). Lester Grinspoon and James Bakalar's book *Marihuana, the Forbidden Medicine* (Yale University Press, 1997) provides a thorough history and overview of marijuana's medical benefits.

ISSUE 10

Are Psychotherapeutic Drugs Overprescribed for Treating Mental Illness?

YES: Leemon McHenry, from "Ethical Issues in Psychopharmacology," *Journal of Medical Ethics* (2006)

NO: Bruce M. Cohen, from "Mind and Medicine: Drug Treatments for Psychiatric Illness," *Social Research* (Fall 2001)

ISSUE SUMMARY

YES: Professor Leemon McHenry, a professor with the Philosophy Department at the California State University at Northridge, questions the effectiveness of psychiatric drugs, especially antidepressant drugs known as selective serotonin reuptake inhibitors (SSRIs). McHenry maintains that the increase in the prescribing of antidepressant drugs results from their promotion by the pharmaceutical industry. McHenry also argues that pharmaceutical companies should be more forthright in the efficacy of these drugs.

NO: Medical doctor Bruce M. Cohen maintains that psychiatric medicines are very beneficial in enabling individuals with a variety of illnesses to return to normal aspects of consciousness. Cohen points out that people with conditions such as anxiety, depression, and psychosis respond very well to medications. These types of drugs have been utilized successfully for hundreds of years.

One of the most common emotional problems in America is mental illness, especially depression. It is estimated that approximately 10 percent of Americans experience some type of depression during their lives. Although some of the newer antidepressant drugs such as Prozac, Paxil, and Zoloft have not been available that long, they account for billions of dollars in sales. Does this mean that more people are becoming mentally ill or are people more likely to be diagnosed with mental illness today?

Although antidepressant drugs were originally developed to treat depression—for which they are believed to be about 60 percent effective—these drugs are now prescribed for an array of other conditions. Some of these conditions include eating disorders like bulimia and obesity, obsessive-compulsive disorders, panic attacks, and anxiety. An important question about these drugs is currently under debate: Are they prescribed too casually? Some experts feel that physicians are giving psychotherapeutic drugs to patients who do not need chemical treatment to overcome their afflictions. Yale University professor Sherwin Nuland has argued that drugs like Prozac are relatively safe for its approved applications but that they are inappropriate for less severe problems.

As with most other drugs, psychotherapeutic drugs like antidepressants produce a number of adverse side effects. These effects include hypotension (low blood pressure), weight gain, and irregular heart rhythms. Other side effects that may be experienced are headaches, fatigue, profuse sweating, anxiety, reduced appetite, jitteriness, dizziness, stomach discomfort, nausea, sexual dysfunction, and insomnia. Because these drugs are relatively new, long-term side effects have yet to be determined.

Soon after Prozac was introduced, several lawsuits were filed against Eli Lilly and Company, the drug's manufacturer, due to Prozac's side effects. The drug was linked to violent and suicidal behavior. Some individuals charged with violent crimes have used the defense that Prozac made them act violently and that they should not be held accountable for their actions while on the drug. Prozac also has been implicated in a number of suicides, although it is unclear whether Prozac caused these individuals to commit suicide or whether they would have committed suicide anyway. Paxil and Zoloft, which were introduced after Prozac, reportedly have fewer side effects.

Psychiatrist Peter R. Breggin, who feels that antidepressant drugs are prescribed too frequently, has argued that they are used to replace traditional psychotherapy. Breggin claims that psychiatry has given in to the pharmaceutical companies. In contrast to psychiatry, antidepressant drugs are less expensive and more convenient. However, do these drugs get at the root of the problems that many people have? The United States Public Health Service recommends drug therapy for severe cases of depression but psychotherapy for mild or moderate cases of depression.

One may accept the use of drug therapy when one's medical condition is caused by a chemical imbalance. However, should drugs be employed to alter one's personality, to help one become more confident and less introverted? One could argue that if drugs help people with these personal qualities, then that is a healthy use of these drugs. Is using these drugs any different than people using cigarettes to relax or using alcohol to overcome one's shyness?

In the following selections, Leemon McHenry believes that psychotherapeutic drugs are overprescribed and that this is due to their heavy promotion by the pharmaceutical industry. Bruce M. Cohen argues that drugs such as antidepressants are invaluable drugs because they effectively treat anxiety, depression, and psychosis. The benefits of these drugs, claims Cohen, outweigh their potential side effects.

YES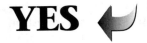

Leemon McHenry

Ethical Issues in Psychopharmacology

Now more than ever the moral and scientific integrity of psychopharmacology deserves close scrutiny. A behemoth pharmaceutical industry has created corporate psychiatry along with industry sponsored clinical research, direct to consumer marketing of antidepressants, ghost writing for medical journals and a major war for the market share. All the trappings are in place for marketing the disease rather than the cure. An illness intervention industry with no serious ethical commitment to health care threatens the most basic imperative of the medical art—"first, do no harm"—and demonstrates the weakness in the corporate model of medicine.

The Serotonin Hypothesis

The controversy over the serotonin hypothesis of depression lies at the very heart of the matter. Since, however, the pharmaceutical industry has an enormous financial interest in protecting the hypothesis, the problems with the theory are seldom discussed and less likely to reach publication. The epistemological virtue of science as the rigorous pursuit of truth has been corrupted by an industry that manipulates the process to its own advantage. Corporate psychiatrists become coconspirators by accepting a paradigm uncritically and by adopting the language game of chemical imbalance that entirely satisfies this purpose.

The serotonin hypothesis is a monoamine theory that advances the view that depression is caused by neurotransmitter system deficits. It was originally proposed in the late 1950s by George Ashcroft and Donald Eccleston at Edinburgh and gained further support from Alex Coppen at Surrey and Herman van Praag at Utrecht in the groundswell of early developments in biological psychiatry.[1-2] Low concentrations of serotonin, 5HT (5-hydroxytryptamine) or its main metabolite, 5-HIAA (5-hydroxyindole acetic acid), were found in autopsy studies of brains from suicide victims and in studies of cerebrospinal fluid from depressed patients.[3-6]

Although it might appear that the development of the new psychotropic drugs, the selective serotonin reuptake inhibitors (SSRIs), was the next logical step from the idea of serotonin deficiency, the actual history shows otherwise. The norepinephrine hypothesis of depression (another monoamine theory),

From *Journal of Medical Ethics*, vol. 32, 2006, pp. 405–410. Copyright © 2006 by BMJ Publishing Group. Reprinted by permission.

not the serotonin hypothesis, was the leading idea that guided research in psychopharmacology at the time, especially in the United States. The SSRIs were created when it became clear that drugs with an action on the serotonin system had a recognisably different effect from drugs active on the norepinephrine system. SSRIs function in the brain by blocking the breakdown or reuptake of serotonin from the synapse into the transmitting cell, thus leaving the serotonin active in the synapse for a longer period. "Selective" in "SSRI" suggests that the drug's action is clean or precise, but this is misleading as the drug has effects on a range of other neurotransmitter systems.

Although the serotonin theory might offer a compelling view within our physiochemical model of the brain, its main problem is over simlplicity in the overall neurochemical scenario. Even more to the point, however, it is probably false. The fact of the matter is that there never was a consistent body of evidence to support the theory. George Ashcroft, who was one of the pioneers in serotonin research, abandoned the idea of lowered serotonin levels by 1970. Ashcroft makes the crucial point: "What we believed was that 5-HIAA levels were probably a measure of functional activity of the systems and not a cause. It could just as well have been that people with depression had low activity in their system and that 5-HIAA was mirroring that and then when they got better it didn't necessarily go up."[9] With regard to Popperian and Kuhnian models of scientific advance, David Healy explains the survival of the monoamine theories despite a wealth of negative evidence. He describes them as erected on a quicksand of mistaken assumptions and apparently lacking in the mortar of supporting evidence.[10] Although there seems to be no question about the fact that SSRIs act on the serotonin system, what has not been established is an abnormality of serotonin metabolism in depression or that SSRIs correct a chemical Imbalance. Instead of going back to the proverbial drawing board with Ashcroft, however, the pharmaceutical company marketing departments revived the serotonin theory in the late 1980s and channelled all their financial might into promoting the SSRIs. It was a triumph of marketing over science. [11]

There are few neuroscientists today who would embrace the serotonin hypothesis. Whether this is true for prescribing physicians and psychiatrists is less clear. There are certainly those, perhaps the majority, who recognise that there are factors other than neurobiology involved in the aetiology, course and outcome of depressive disorders. My case against the serotonin hypothesis targets the manner in which this theory has been presented to the public by pharmaceutical Industry marketing.

The success of the SSRIs no more demonstrates the causal relationship between serotonin deficiency and depression than the relief provided by aspirin for the cause of a fever. The aspirin might treat the symptoms, but this does not provide any important information about the cause of the fever. Similarly, the fact that a patient's depression might be treated by an SSRI tells us nothing about the cause of the depression. Most of the supporting evidence for the serotonin hypothesis after the 1980s has been just exactly this. From the patients' response to the SSRIs, the inference is drawn that the cause of the disorder is a lack of serotonin. Drugs are used to probe and understand mental disorders yet this method functions entirely within the realm of symptomology. Nature refuses to reveal her true causes from the mere control of symptoms.

Depression is a complex mental disorder. Whether it is a disease with an organic origin is another matter. None the less, the current focus on neuro-chemical abnormality has produced a "depression puzzle," in which the pieces simply do not add up. First, reserpine, an antipsychotic, produces depressive symptoms by depleting the brain of complex amines. This should cause depression in all patients if the serotonin hypothesis were true, but it does not. Less than 20% of patients will become depressed. Second, Max Lurie and Harry Salzer used the antidepressant drug, isoniazid, in the 1950s with two out of three patients responding, but isoniazid has no action on the serotonin system (Healy,[8] p 52). So, the same kind of evidence (drug action) that is used in support of the serotonin hypothesis also counts against it. Third, there has been a gradual increase in depression around the world, culminating in what has been called the "era of depression" in the 1990s.[14] If, however, the serotonin hypothesis is true, this must be because there is a corresponding gradual increase in defective serotonergic systems around the world. There is no evidence for this implausible idea. Finally, twice as many women as men are likely to become depressed, whim must mean that women are born with a less effective serotonergic system. Again there is no evidence for this either.

Suppose that we dispose altogether of the serotonin hypothesis as an attempt to understand the aetiology of depression. What counts most in medicine are statistical correlations establishing varying degrees of reliability, and according to the advocates of SSRIs, their reliability (effectiveness and safety) is clearly established. The plain and simple fact of the matter (so it is said) is that millions of patients have been relieved of their debilitating depression, some of them in dramatic and unmistakable ways. How could this possibly be explained if the SSRIs are not effective treatments?

The clinical trials that form the basis of Food and Drug Administration (FDA) approval of SSRIs demonstrate repeatedly that these drugs show a clinically negligible advantage over inert placebo (sugar pills) in the treatment of depression. Here we must keep in mind that the data from clinical trials rank at the top of the hierarchy of evidence in the world of psychopharmacology. FDA approval, however, only requires that the drugs are better than nothing. According to the best data available, there is a less than 10% difference in the effect of FDA approved antidepressants versus placebo. [15-16] In some studies, placebo control groups duplicated 80% of the response to medication.[17-19] The studies that provide the desired results, embarrassingly minimal as they are, reach publication and appear in the databases of the pharmaceutical companies and the FDA. What the general public barely sees are many of the failures of clinical trials around the world and the clinical trials that are prematurely terminated due to adverse side effects. These failed studies never see the light of day because the pharmaceutical companies that fund the studies own the data that is produced from the contract research organisations and site management organisations. The control over the data also enables the companies to provide the spin on the data that favours their drugs.[20 21]

Marketing Depression

No one knows exactly how SSRIs work, if indeed they really do work at all. One plausible explanation is that they mask symptoms of depression in moderate cases that resolve themselves spontaneously. It is also well known that the more a drug is hyped in the mainstream media as a "miracle drug," the greater is the likelihood of a strong placebo effect. What is, however, fundamentally problematic from an ethical point of view is the over inflation of SSRI effectiveness and safety, questionable marketing strategies, and the megadose prescriptions that can alter brain chemistry and behaviour for the worse.

Pharmaceutical companies in their direct to consumer marketing continue to promote SSRIs in television advertisements with the catchy suggestion: "While the cause of depression is not known, you might be suffering from a chemical imbalance. Ask your physician about [SSRI trade name]." Website advertisements for certain SSRIs claim their non-habit-forming drugs "correct the chemical imbalance believed to cause the disorder" and include diagrams of how this "science" works. In this manner, the companies "grow the market" by increasing consumer awareness of depression and target larger populations for their drugs. Direct to consumer advertising increases the request rates of the drugs and brand choices as well the likelihood that these drugs will be prescribed by physicians and psychiatrists.

The idea of selling us depression, whether we are truly ill or not, has become an immensely lucrative strategy for selling SSRIs, a large part of which succeeds on the basis of the idea of chemical imbalance. The range of prescriptions for SSRIs has included severe, chronic depression (completely non-functional human beings); moderate cases of depression (precipitated by stress, loss of loved ones, rape, divorce, professional failure), and the completely ludicrous (the angst ridden, ill adjusted child, personality sculpting, and psychotherapeutic fashion). The marketing strategy plays on the public's desire for a quick fix for all the vicissitudes of life and the power of the suggestion contained in the easy to understand model of chemical imbalance. This phenomenon has been dubbed the "medicalisation of society"—a phrase coined to describe the belief that every problem requires medical treatment, which is particularly relevant in the case of antidepressants. A report by the UK House of Commons health committee attributes this to the activities of the pharmaceutical industry.[23] However, the strategy also works so well because of the public's ignorance of, and trust in, the institution of science—there will always be those who know these marvellous things beyond the reach of ordinary people and they offer these amazing solutions to problems that just yesterday we did not understand. SSRIs have been abused as lifestyle drugs or performance enhancement drugs in the manner of LSD, Viagra, or anabolic steroids. The pharmaceutical companies have benefited from this trend to the tune of ten billion dollars per year from sales of all SSRIs. The problem begins here. The industry is marketing the condition and then the lifelong commitment to their products.[24 25] Although patients might gain a short term solution from SSRI prescriptions, the long term harm is only just starting to come into focus for both individuals and the institution of medicine.

Marketing departments employ a strategy they call "evergreening" by beginning with one indication of a use for an SSRI and then moving on to explore other "green" pastures for potential markets. In order to convince people something is wrong with them that requires SSRI therapy, the marketing departments hire public relations firms to raise awareness of a newly approved indication, sometimes using celebrity spokespersons to pitch the idea. SSRIs were first marketed for depression, then for panic disorder, obsessive compulsive disorder, post traumatic stress disorder, seasonal affective disorder, generalised anxiety disorder, and social anxiety disorder. Other potential indications in the marketing strategy that show up in clinical trials include premature ejaculation and paedophilia (since we know SSRIs cause sexual dysfunction), premenstrual syndrome, writer's block, obesity, alcoholism, cocaine addiction, compulsive shopping, and smoking cessation.

Healy explains how the so called "depression epidemic" developed from psychiatric concerns over unrecognised and untreated depression in the 1960s and 1970s. National depression campaigns were mounted in the United States and the United Kingdom. These involved alerting physicians and third party payers in health care to the huge economic burdens of untreated depression and educational campaigns to shame physicians for failing to detect and treat depression (Healy,[8] p 43). The infusion of industry money into psychiatry means influence on the very definitions of psychological disorder that determine how a patient will be diagnosed and treated. In this manner, depression is understood to be a physiological disease that is treated by drugs like SSRIs and thereby gains the imprimatur of organisations like the American Psychiatric Association.

Pharmaceutical companies effectively control many professional conferences and medical journal publications, employ psychiatrists as "key opinion leaders" and pay them handsomely to sign on to publications ghost written by their own staff or medical communication agencies employed by the company. The practice of for profit, industry sponsored ghost writing has become a major concern since scientific journals are meant to be neutral arbiters of merit via the critical peer review process.[27-28] Marketing interests have, however, tainted some of the most distinguished journals in medicine, especially psychiatry. The marketing of depression has spread to the very highest levels now that the distinction between promotional materials and scientific objectivity has been blurred. Academics who are expected to be the legitimate authors of journal articles turn out to be little more than ornaments to a business rushing to gain blockbuster status for its drugs or instruments used in the competition between the various companies to dominate the market share.[29]

Is life really so much more stressful today than it was 20 or 30 years ago or has the marketing strategy of the pharmaceutical companies succeeded in convincing us that we are depressed and cannot cope without their drugs? Approximately 50 to 100 people per million were thought to be depressed before the creation of antidepressants; today our best estimates put the figure at 100,000 to 200,000 people per million (Healy,[8] p 20). A third possibility is that all these depressed people were previously walking the streets undiagnosed. If this was the idea of well intentioned psychiatrists forty years ago, it has been exploited with maximum financial results by pharmaceutical marketing departments.

Hidden Dangers

Within the controlled environment of clinical trials it is possible to limit variables to determine the efficacy of the study drug versus placebo and identify the likely cause of adverse reactions. With regard to the latter, this typically comes down to two possibilities: the underlying disorder or the study drug. Despite many cases in which the investigator identifies the study drug as the definite or probable cause of the adverse reaction, the pharmaceutical companies consistently blame the underlying disorder rather than the treatment. In the parlance of the industry, this is known as "defending the molecule." The more serious adverse reactions that show up in clinical trials and spontaneous reports include: akathisia; aggression; self mutilation; emotional blunting; worsening depression; withdrawal symptoms, and suicidality. The latter two were a major concern with the introduction of the SSRIs and have been the focus of considerable debate in the medical literature.

Given that the serotonin hypothesis of depression emerged partly from an examination of serotonin levels in suicide victims, there has been a theoretical resistance from the start to the very idea that SSRIs could be responsible for some cases of suicide. While it is clear that depressed patients are at a higher risk of suicide, what is particularly problematic for the claim that any suicidal thoughts or attempts while on an SSRI are always caused by the underlying disorder is the lack of any suicidal history in many of these patients. Moreover, some patients on SSRIs for indications other than depression or in healthy volunteer studies become suicidal. Numerous cases of this sort caused alarm among researchers in the early 1990s.[32-33] A common side effect of SSRIs is akathisia—a drug induced condition of extreme restlessness, insomnia, and agitation that is accompanied by compulsions to commit violence to oneself or to others.[34-36] Many patients will say that they "feel like a video on fast forward" or that they "just want to jump out of their skin" and see suicide as the only relief. The most disturbing cases on record concern functional individuals with moderate depression caused by some change of life who are prescribed an SSRI, become extremely agitated and restless, and then commit suicide within a matter of days or weeks—this being completely out of character with anything in their past. Patients of this sort are more than likely to be seen by primary care physicians who have not been trained to recognise the problem of akathisia. Their doctors will typically misdiagnose the symptoms as worsening depression and the suicides as a result of the underlying disorder—consistently with the approach of the marketing departments of the pharmaceutical companies.

The FDA and the drug companies have constantly argued that no causal relationship has been established between suicide and SSRIs despite the existence of many adverse drug experience reports. There are, however, indications that the sheer volume of these reports together with the ones from clinical trials are starting to command attention in psychiatry and general practice. Studies have been done by pharmaceutical companies that provide evidence for the causal relationship—namely, the method of determining causality: challenge, dechallenge, rechallenge, In this process a patient is given a drug and experiences a side effect (challenge), then the drug is discontinued and the side effect disappears (dechallenge), and finally the drug is reintroduced and the same side effect appears again (rechallenge). Suicidality is regularly coded as caused by the study drug by the investigators and the sponsor. What is even more revealing about the extent to which the pharmaceutical companies are willing to press the point is that discussions about side effects of drugs take on the character of something approaching a rigorous Humean scepticism with regard to the very meaning of the term "cause," but when the issue is efficacy the term suddenly has a perfectly clear meaning. SSRIs, we are told, do cause relief of depression. The serious side effects, such as suicidality, are merely unproved "associations."

In regulatory actions that were long overdue, the FDA issued a pair of warnings for SSRIs, both of which concern suicidality. On 22 March 2004, the FDA required antidepressant manufacturers to include in their label a warning statement that recommends close observation of adult and paediatric patients treated with these agents for worsening depression or the emergence of suicidality, "especially at the beginning of therapy or when the dose either increases or decreases." Then on 15 October 2004, the FDA, faced with public pressure from a recent action by UK regulators, followed up with the strongest warning possible—the "black box" warning—which describes the increased risk of suicidality in children and adolescents on SSRIs.[38][39]

Determining causality in SSRI/suicide cases is enormously complex. According to some studies we must distinguish between SSRI induced suicidality in children or adolescents, and adults: the former indicates a risk of suicide probably increased under SSRI therapy whereas the latter shows no increased risk.[40] The main evidence focuses attention on (1) the data comparing SSRI and tricyclics, which shows that users of SSRIs are not at any more risk of suicidality than those on tricyclics,[41] and (2) the failure of the SSRI/suicide cases to reach a statistical significance compared to placebo/suicide cases.[42][43][44] According to other studies the data from adult studies shows a twofold increase in the risk of fatal and non-fatal suicidal attempts in users of SSRIs compared to users of placebo, and this has been exactly what the data has shown since the introduction of the SSRIs.[45] Aursnes *et al* argue that Cipriani *et al* failed to convey the unanimous conclusion in the reviewed studies of an increased risk of suicidal attempts in adult patients on SSRIs.[46]

Many patients on SSRIs describe their experience as a "chemical prison." Once started on a regime, the attempt to reduce the dosage or discontinue the drug without experiencing severe adverse events can be very difficult. These include jolting electric zaps (paraesthesia); confusion; headaches; vomiting; dizziness; nausea; worsening depression; insomnia; irritability; emotional lability, including suicidality, and agitation that, when severe, can resemble a manic episode. A small percentage of patients claim they literally cannot get off the drugs even if they try and taper off the dosage. Pharmaceutical companies have vigorously maintained that SSRIs are not addictive and that what is believed to be withdrawal symptoms is really evidence that the drug is working. Since the adverse events that result from cessation of drug therapy are often confused with the re-emergence of the depressive illness, physicians typically advise their patients to continue their regime or increase the dosage. The most compelling evidence against the drugs, however, comes in the form of withdrawal symptoms in neonatals whose mothers were on SSRIs during pregnancy. In such cases, it is not possible to blame the adverse events on re-emergence of depression.[47-49]

The problem of withdrawal emerged first with paroxetine because of the great volume of reports on the adverse event reporting system. Paroxetine has a relatively short half life (21–24 hours) and shorter washout period compared to fluoxetine (4 to 16 days), so the withdrawal symptoms tend to be more severe upon abrupt discontinuation. In a feat of semantic opportunism, the maker of fluoxetine, Eli Lilly, launched a public relations campaign to replace "withdrawal symptoms" with "discontinuation symptoms." The alleged difference is that the latter does not imply addiction as with the case of alcohol or barbiturates. Over time, however, it has become more and more difficult to maintain this position despite the enormous amount of money that funded conferences and medical journal supplements on the topic.

The crux of the matter concerns the very meaning of "addiction." Psychiatrists who framed the definition in the third and fourth editions of *The Diagnostic and Statistical Manual of Mental Disorders* (DSM III and IV) had in mind diagnostic criteria identifying substance dependence—namely, maladaptive behaviour, euphoria, or compulsive drug seeking.[50] The classic cases of iatrogenic dependence in which the chemical system of the brain attempts to regain equilibrium no longer counts as addiction. This allowed the manufacturer of paroxetine, SmithKline Beecham (now GlaxoSmithKline), to claim in the patient's leaflet and in advertising that paroxetine is not addictive or habit forming. However, to patients suffering from withdrawal symptoms after discontinuing the drug, their physical dependence accorded with the common dictionary meaning of "addiction." In the *Oxford English Dictionary,* for example, "addiction" is defined as "the condition of taking drugs excessively and being unable to cease doing so without adverse effects".[51] In this latter sense, one can become "hooked" on SSRIs without exhibiting drug seeking behaviour or becoming completely non-functional.

For those who have followed the rise and fall of drugs in the marketplace, the SSRIs merely repeat a familiar pattern. The drug companies and regulators had claimed that benzodiazepines were not addictive for well over a decade, but eventually it was admitted that tranquilisers such as diazepam (Valium) were indeed addictive.[16] Glenmullen describes a "10–20–30" year pattern typical of side effects of popular psychiatric drugs—ten years for side effects to be identified, twenty years for enough data to accumulate to make the problem undeniable, and then thirty years for bureaucracies of regulatory agencies to make changes.[52] Of course, it still remains to be seen whether the SSRIs will follow this pattern to the same conclusion.

Conclusion

It is often claimed that corporations that are profit driven could not be expected to behave in any other manner than they do. The nature of business demands maximisation of the market share and shareholder value. Pharmaceutical companies, however, present themselves as responsible producers of health-care products. The very nature of the product involves trust in the science that produced it and an ethical commitment to the well-being of the patients who are their consumers. Despite appearances, nothing of this sort is true in the pharmaceutical industry.

As we have seen above, the serotonin hypothesis sold to consumers of pharmaceuticals is flawed. Making questionable claims for the efficacy and safety of SSRIs involves the pharmaceutical companies in further deception. Expanding the market for these drugs by creating dubious disease categories and then luring vulnerable individuals into SSRI therapy by direct to consumer advertising would represent, if perpetrated by a doctor, an abuse of the trust implicit in the relationship between patient and doctor.

I do not argue that SSRIs should be withdrawn from the market thus depriving clinicians and patients of this therapeutic option. Rather I argue that full disclosure of the data for efficacy and safety is a basic moral obligation of the pharmaceutical industry. Until such data is available to the public, prescribing clinicians and patients are relying on drug promotion rather than rigorous science. When Kant discusses the motivation of acting from duty as opposed to the motivation of self interest, he mentions the case of the merchant who keeps a fixed price for everyone so that a child who buys from him pays the same price as everyone else.[53] The only actions that have moral worth are those done from the motive of duty alone. And similarly, only when the pharmaceutical companies act from the motive of duty in fully disclosing all information they possess about the risks and benefits of their drugs do their actions have any moral worth.

The SSRI marketing story provides a lens through which we can view a much larger problem. The integrity of medicine is endangered by an industry that profits from illness and distorts the process of scientific inquiry by marketing strategy, public relations campaigns, and the sheer power of buying influence in high places. The House of Commons health committee in the UK has made the point: "It is not in the long term interest of industry for prescribers and the public to lose faith in it. We need an industry which is led by the values of scientists not those of its marketing force" (House of Commons health committee,[23] p 6). Medicine desperately needs to win back the territory lost to business. If and when it does, it is not likely to be a result of industry and government regulators facing up to the problems, but rather a matter of the sheer weight of legal actions filed by victims and public outcry about the moral concerns of the sort raised in this paper.

References

1. Healy D. *The antidepressant era*. Cambridge: Harvard University Press, 1997: 155–69.
2. Healy D. *The psychopharmacologists* [vols 1 and 3]. London: Altman, 2000.
3. Ashcroft GW, Sharman DF. 5-Hydroxyindoles in human cerebrospinal fluids. *Nature* 1960;186:1050–1.

4. Ashcroft GW, Crawford TBB, Stanton JB, *et al.* 5-Hydroxyindole compounds in the cerebrospinal fluid of patients with psychiatric or neurological diseases. *Lancet* 1966;**2**:1049–52.

5. Ashcroft GW, Eccleston D, Murry LG, *et al.* Modified amine hypothesis for the aetiology of affective illness. *Lancet* 1972;**2**:573–7.

6. Asberg M, Eriksson B, Martensson B, *et al.* Therapeutic effects of serotonin uptake inhibitors in depression. *J Clin Psychiatry* 1986;**47**(suppl 4):23–35S.

7. Kramer PD. *Listening to prozac.* New York: Penguin Books, 1993, especially ch 3.

8. Healy D. *Let them eat Prozac: the unhealthy relationship between the pharmaceutical industry and depression.* Toronto: James Lorimer, 2003.

9. Ashcroft G. The receptor enters psychiatry. In: Healy D, eds. *The psychopharmacologists* [vol 3]. London: Arnold, 2000:194.

10. Healy D. The structure of psychopharmacological revolutions. *Psychiatr Dev* 1987;**4**:349–76.

11. Antonuccio DO, Burns DD, Donton WG. Antidepressants: a triumph of marketing over science? *Prevention & Treatment.* . . .

12. Flores BH, Musselman DL, DeBattista C, *et al.* Biology of mood disorders. In: Schatzberg AF, Nameroff CB, eds. *Textbook of psychopharmacology* [3rd ed]. Washington DC: American Psychatric Publishing, 2004:718.

13. Nemeroff CB. The neurobiology of depression. *Scientific American* 1998; **278**:2–9.

14. Healy D. Psychopharmacology and the government of the self. . . .

15. Smith DC. Antidepressant efficacy. *Ethical Hum Sci Serv* 2000;**2**/3:215–16.

16. Medawar C. The antidepressant web: marketing depression and making medicines work. *Int J Risk Safety Med* 1997;**10**:86–91.

17. Kirsch I, Moore TJ, Scoboria A, *et al.* The emperor's new drugs: an analysis of antidepressant medication data submitted to the US Food and Drug Administration. *Prevention and Treatment.* . . .

18. Carroll BJ. Sertraline and the Cheshire cat in geriatric depression. *AM J Psychiatry* 2004;**161**:759.

19. Kirsch I, Moncrieff J. Efficacy of antidepressants in adults. *BMJ* 2005;**331**:155–7.

20. Bodenheimer T. Uneasy alliance: clinical investigators and the pharmaceutical industry. *N Engl J Med* 2000;**342**:1539–44 at 1541.

21. Whittington CJ, Kendall T, Fonagy P, *et al.* Selective serotonin reuptake inhibitors in childhood depression: systematic review of published versus unpublished data. *Lancet* 2004;**363**:1341–5.

22. Angell M. *The truth about the drug companies: how they deceive us and what to do about it.* New York: Random House, 2004:125.

23. House of Commons Health Committee. *The influence of the pharmaceutical industry vol 1.* London: The Stationery Office, 2005:100.

24. Wolfe SM. Profitably inventing new diseases. *Health Letter;* 2003;**19**:2–3.

25. Moynihan R, Cassels A. *Selling sickness: how the world's biggest pharmaceutical companies are turning us all into patients.* New York: Nation, 2005.

26. *SmithKlineBeecham's business plan guide December 1 1997—May 31, 1998.* . . .

27. Davidoff F, DeAngelis CD, Drazen JM, *et al.* Sponsorship, authorship, and accountability. *N Engl J Med* 2001;**345**:825–7.

28. Flanagin A, Carey LA, Fontanarosa PB, *et al.* Honorary authors and ghost authors in peer reviewed medical journals. *JAMA* 1998;**280**:222–4.

29. Healy D, Cattell D. Interface between authorship, industry and science in the domain of therapeutics. *Br J Psychiatry* 2003;**183**:22–7.

30. McHenry L. On the origin of great ideas: science in the age of big pharma. *Hastings Cent Rep* 2005;**35**:17–19.

31. Flynn P. *House of Commons official report:* col 1038. . . .

32. Teicher MH, Glod C, Cole JO. Suicidal preoccupation during fluoxetine treatment. *Am J Psychiatry* 1990;**147**:1380–1.

33. Masand P, Gupata S, Dewan M. Suicidal ideation related to fluoxetine treatment. *N Engl J Med* 1991;**324**:420.

34. LaPorta L. Sertraline-induced akathisia. *J Clin Psychopharmacology* 1993;**13**:219–20.

35. Healy D, Langmack C, Savage M. Suicide in the course of treatment of depression. *J Clin Psychopharmacology* 1999;**13**:94–9.

36. Breggin PR. *Toxic psychiatry: why therapy, empathy and love must replace the drugs, electroshock, and biochemical theories of the "new psychiatry."* New York: St Martin's Press, 1991:167.

37. Maris RRM. Suicide and neuropsychiatric adverse effects of SSRI medications: methodological issues. . . .

38. . . .

39. . . .

40. Cipriani A, Barbui C, Geddes JR. Suicide, depression, and antidepressants. *BMJ* 2005;**330**:373–4.

41. Martinez C, Riebrock S, Wise L, *et al.* Antidepressant treatment and the risk of fatal and non-fatal self harm in first episode depression: nested case control study. *BMJ* 2005;**330**:389–93.

42. Kahn A, Warner HA, Brown WA. Symptom reduction and suicide risk in patients treated with placebo in antidepressant clinical trials. *Arch Gen Psychiatry* 2000;**57**:311–17.

43. Khan A, Khan S, Kolts R, *et al.* Suicide rates in clinical trials of SSRIs, other antidepressants, and placebo: an analysis of FDA reports. *Am J Psychiatry* 2003;**160**:790–2.

44. Gunnell D, Saperia J, Ashby D. Selective serotonin reuptake inhibitors (SSRIs) and suicide in adults: meta-analysis of drug company data from placebo controlled, randomised controlled trials submitted to the MHRA's safety review. *BMJ* 2005;**330**:385–8.

45. Fergusson D, Doucette S, Glass KC, *et al.* Association between suicide attempts and selective serotonin reuptake inhibitors: systematic review of randomised controlled trials. *BMJ* 2005;**330**:396–9.

46. Aursnes I, Tvete IF, Goasemyr J, *et al.* Suicide attempts in clinical trials with paroxetine randomised against placebo. *BMC Medicine* 2005;**3**:14.

47. Nordeng H, Lindemann R, Perminov KV, *et al.* Neonatal withdrawal syndrome after in utero exposure to selective serotonin reuptake inhibitors. *Acta Poediatr* 2001;**90**:288–91.

48. Sanz EJ, De-las-Cuevas C, Kiuru A, *et al.* Selective serotonin reuptake inhibitors in pregnant women and neonatal withdrawal syndrome: a database analysis. *Lancet* 2005;**365**:482–7.

49. Medawar C, Hardon A. Medicines out of control? *Antidepressants and the conspiracy of goodwill.* Amsterdam: Aksant Academic Press, 2004:84.

50. American Psychiatric Association. *Diagnostic and statistical manual of mental disorders* [4th ed]. Washington, DC: APA, 2000:192–9.

51. Sykes JB. *The concise Oxford dictionary of current English*. Oxford: Clarendon Press, 1984:11.

52. Glenmullen J. *The antidepressant solution: a step by step guide to safely overcoming antidepressant withdrawal, dependence and "addiction."* New York: The Free Press, 2005:190–1.

53. Kant I. *The fundamental principles of the metaphysic of morals* [trans Abbott TK]. London: Longmans, Green and Co, 1946:15.

Bruce M. Cohen

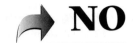 **NO**

Mind and Medicine: Drug Treatments for Psychiatric Illnesses

Psychiatric Disorders as Medical Illnesses

Psychiatric illnesses are conditions of the brain that lead to alternations in thinking, mood, and behavior. These illnesses are observed in cultures throughout the world and are probably at least as old as human beings. Recognizable features of psychiatric disorders are described in the texts of many early societies, including those of ancient Egypt, Israel, Greece, India, and China. Also ancient are attempts to treat people with disorders of cognition and emotion by what today would be called psychosocial therapies (including counseling, asylum, and exploration of thought) and psychopharmacologic therapies (that is, plant products or other drugs).

The most common symptoms experienced by those with psychiatric disorders fall into a few categories. Mood may be abnormally high or low. Irritability and anxiety are often felt. Thinking, and its expression in speech and other behaviors, may be illogical. Delusions, which are patently false beliefs not shared by others, can be present. Obsessions and compulsions may continuously haunt the sufferers. Prominent perceptual abnormalities may occur, the most common being hallucinations, which are false sensory percepts, usually the hearing of voices within one's own head. Finally, psychiatric disorders often are associated with changes of physiologic rhythms and the basic drives of life, with disrupted sleep, appetite, and energy.

Some symptoms of psychiatric disorders, notably depression or anxiety, seem to be extremes of normal states, just as hypertension is an extreme of blood pressure. Others, such as hallucinations, appear more distinct from normal experience, although most of us have occasionally thought we heard a voice when we were alone or saw a person when no one was there. These normal experiences are fleeting, while the symptoms of psychiatric disorders last from months to a lifetime.

Symptoms rarely occur alone. Rather, they tend to occur in recognizable clusters, called syndromes. Common syndromes in internal medicine include the pneumonias or congestive heart failure. The most common psychiatric syndromes include the depressive disorders, the anxiety disorders, and the

From Bruce M. Cohen, "Mind and Medicine: Drug Treatments for Psychiatric Illnesses," *Social Research*, vol. 68, no. 3 (Fall 2001). Copyright © 2001 by *Social Research*. Reprinted by permission.

psychotic disorders, such as bipolar disorders and schizophrenia. It is the latter that are most frequently associated with hallucinations and delusions.

Psychiatric disorders are medical illnesses. Like other medical disorders, they are due to the interaction of inherited and environmental factors that, together, lead to the development of illness. While the specific genes that predispose to psychiatric disorders have not yet been identified, the presence of these genes is thoroughly and convincingly documented from family, twin, and adoption studies. Similarly, subtle but repeatedly observed differences in the brain between those with and without psychiatric disorders are now documented by post mortem studies and observation of the brain during life using technologies such as magnetic resonance imaging (MRI), positron emission tomography (PET), and single photon emission computerized tomography (SPECT).

The explicit causes of most current cases of psychiatric disorder are not yet known, but numerous medical conditions that can cause psychiatric disorders are well documented. Over a century ago, many of the patients in psychiatric hospitals had infectious, nutritional, toxic, and hormonal conditions, such as syphilis, pellagra, lead poisoning, and hyper- and hypothyroidism which affected their thinking and mood. Today these medical disorders have responded well to preventive measures, based on diet and environmental advances, or to treatment with medications.

Psychiatric illnesses of unknown cause also tend to respond well to treatment, with success rates as high as those seen in other branches of medicine. Psychotherapeutic medication can restore to normal aspects of consciousness, including feeling, perception, and cognition. For this reason medication is at the core of treatment for most psychiatric disorders.

Drugs and the Brain

Taking drugs with the intent to change aspects of consciousness is very old and quite common. Alcohol, cocaine, opiates, and peyote have been used for thousands of years. These drugs appear to act on systems built into the brain to modulate behaviors associated with eating, sleeping, sexual activity, or other drives and rewards. Co-opting receptors and processes developed to respond to internal chemical messages, these external agents alter arousal, attention, emotional state, and thinking.

Foods can have effects on mood and cognition as well. Deficiencies of some nutrients, as noted, can lead to psychiatric illness, and the oldest recreational drugs are in essence food products or derivatives. Based on this history, numerous nutritional substances are currently being examined as possible treatments for psychiatric disorders.

Hormones, including thyroid, adrenal, and sex hormones, can have profound effects on brain function, drive, cognition, and feelings, and hormonal abnormalities, as was noted, can cause psychiatric symptoms. Hormone replacement—using hormones as drugs—can restore or, occasionally, disrupt mental function.

Further links between physiology, pharmacology, and psychology are evident from the effects of drugs given for purposes unrelated to brain function, but with unwanted actions there. For example, older antihistamines for allergies, which reached receptors throughout the body (including the brain), affected alertness, concentration, and memory. Newer agents were designed that were not absorbed into brain and, therefore, have few mental side effects.

These examples provide compelling evidence that drugs can change all the aspects of consciousness. This knowledge has been used for religious, recreational, and medicinal purposes for generations. With the revolution in organic chemistry, biochemistry, and molecular biology over the past hundred years, the development of new drugs targeted to specific illnesses, such as psychiatric disorders, has become more sophisticated and more successful.

Medication for Psychiatric Disorders

Medicinal treatments for psychiatric disorders are used throughout the world and have their origins in many ancient societies. The oldest documented of these medicinal preparations, made from the plant *Rauwolfia serpentina*, appears in Ayurmedic texts of India over 2,000 years ago. It was recommended for several medical illnesses including those whose description sounds much like the psychotic disorders: the schizophrenias and bipolar disorders. The active ingredient of this preparation was likely reserpine, which was isolated in the 1930s and used briefly but effectively to treat psychotic disorders in the 1950s. It was superseded by easier to use agents, the neuroleptic antipsychotic drugs (which will be described later), in the same decade.

Another "modern" treatment for psychiatric disorders, lithium, prescribed to patients with bipolar disorders, may also have been used in ancient times. Lithium is an element related to sodium and potassium. Like these elements, it most frequently occurs in nature as a salt, often appearing in spring waters. Between A.D. 100 and 300, during the Roman Empire, Arataeus, a physician from Cappadocia, and Soranus of Ephesus recommended waters from particular alkaline springs, which probably contained lithium, for the treatment of mania. While dose could not have been carefully controlled, their advice accords with the use of lithium today.

Eastern Hemisphere plant preparations containing opium have been used to alleviate pain for centuries, and in the late nineteenth and early twentieth centuries, opiate compounds isolated from these plants were used with limited efficacy for the treatment of psychotic disorders and severe depression. Similarly, coca leaves from the Western Hemisphere, chewed by generations for their energizing effects, yielded cocaine, used by Freud and others around 1900 for its stimulating and short-lived antidepressant effects.

None of these older medicinal preparations had strong and reliable enough therapeutic effects or tolerable toxicity for the routine treatment of patients with psychiatric disorders. Breakthroughs leading to the discovery of drugs currently in use, which have good safety and efficacy, occurred in the 1950s, with the introduction of the so-called tricyclic antidepressants, such as Tofranil (imipramine); neuroleptic antipsychotic drugs, such as Thorazine (chlorpromazine); and benzodiazepine anti-anxiety agents, such as Librium (chlordiazepoxide). These drugs revolutionized the care of people with psychiatric disorders, leading to the release of many patients from institutions and the return of others to productive lives.

These first modern medications were followed by many copies and by newer generations of psychotherapeutic drugs in the 1980s and 1990s. Examples include the serotonin specific re-uptake inhibitors, such as Prozac (fluoxetine), for depression; the atypical antipsychotic agents, such as Zyprex (olanzapine), for psychotic disorders; and the mood-stabilizing anticonvulsants, such as Depakote (valproate), for bipolar disorder.

The efficacy of these medications has been proved in numerous studies, including a large number of double-blind, placebo-controlled trials in which the drug being tested is compared to inactive substances, as well as compounds that have effects on the brain, such as sedation, that are not believed to address the key symptoms of psychiatric disorders. Neither the clinical investigator nor the patient knows which drug the patient is receiving. Few drugs in medicine have ever been as thoroughly tested and proven effective.

The proper use of these drugs leads to the successful treatment of most people with depressive disorders, anxiety disorders, schizophrenias and bipolar disorders, restoring them to their proper state of mind. As with all medications, there are side effects as well as therapeutic effects, but with careful use, beneficial effects far outweigh side effects for most people. The physical mechanisms underlying these drug effects and the return to normal consciousness are beginning to be understood, providing important information on the nature of psychiatric disorders and the relationship between brain and psyche.

Medications for Anxiety

In a lifetime, nearly one in six of us will experience a disorder in which anxiety is a prominent symptom. Current anti-anxiety medications, or anxiolytics, grew out of a recognition that alcohol, prized for the comfort and disinhibition it brought, could ease feelings of anxiety. Alcohol relieves distress or discomfort whether or not these feelings are pathological, as indicated by its common social use to relax couples on an evening out or large groups at a party.

Alcohol can provide some relief for those with disorders whose cardinal symptoms include anxiety. In these illnesses, feelings of anxiety may be nearly constant or may occur in attacks of panic. In either case the degree of anxiety is out of proportion to and may even bear no relationship to life events. Unfortunately, the relief is limited by the fast metabolism of alcohol and the tendency of the body to become tolerant to its effects. In fact, as the immediate action of alcohol fades, and as tolerance develops, those who drink for recreation or to medicate themselves for anxiety can find that a physiologic rebound opposite to the effects of alcohol occurs, and they become even more anxious.

From about 1900 on, recognizing the beneficial and toxic effects of alcohol, repeated attempts have been made to find chemical agents that share the calming or sedative effects of alcohol but lack its addictive qualities and the rebound that follows its use. These efforts have been only partially successful.

Early attempts to find safer and more effective compounds than alcohol for anxiety disorders and sedation led to discovery of the barbiturates. They were successful in producing anxiolytic effects, but toxic doses have tended to be close to therapeutic doses and tolerance and addiction are common. Barbiturates are still used for epilepsy and for sedation, but rarely in psychiatry for anxiety disorders.

In the 1950s, derivatives of mephenesin, chemically related to barbiturates, were developed and marketed under the names Miltown (meprobamate) and Equanil (tybamate). All these medications were superseded by compounds called benzodiazepine anxiolytics, which were developed in the late 1950s. The earliest of these, Librium (chlordiazepoxide) and Valium (diazepam), became exceedingly popular drugs, felt to have low risk of poisoning and to be associated only rarely with tolerance and addiction.

Today, a large number of long- and short-acting benzodiazepines are on the market as anxiolytics and sedatives. They are good and effective drugs that are neither as dangerous as alcohol or barbiturates nor as safe as early hopes and claims suggested. Tolerance is common and addiction not rare.

Like alcohol, benzodiazepines reduce anxiety whether or not an individual has an anxiety disorder. Used continuously, their anxiolytic effect tends to fade. While they often blunt the attacks or nagging presence of pathological anxiety, they rarely eliminate these symptoms entirely when used alone. Nevertheless, their powerful and consistent ability to reduce anxiety soon after they are ingested or injected suggests they may work by altering the very brain mechanisms that mediate anxiety.

Following years of fruitful study, the likely site through which the benzodiazepine anxiolytics have their clinical effects is known. Nerve cells (called neurons in the brain) process signals by both electrical and chemical means. Each cell receives chemical messages from other cells, sends electrical messages down its length, and secretes its own chemical compound or compounds, called neurotransmitters, on the cells it contacts. Neurotransmitters produce their effects by binding to specific proteins, called neurotransmitter receptors, which induce a cascade of chemical reactions in the cell to stimulate or reduce electrical activity each time a chemical signal is received.

Eighty to ninety percent of the neuron to neuron contacts in the brain involve one of two neurotransmitters: gama amino butyric acid (GABA) or glutamate. Glutamate is an excitatory neurotransmitter; its message makes a neuron more likely to fire an electrical signal. GABA is an inhibitory neurotransmitter; it quiets cells, making them less likely to fire a signal.

Benzodiazepines attach to some of the same receptors that bind the neurotransmitter GABA and change their characteristics, making them more sensitive to GABA. In this way, benzodiazepines amplify the GABA signal, shifting the overall balance between excitation and inhibition in the brain toward inhibition. At low doses, benzodiazepines may produce their calming anti-anxiety effect through this shift to inhibition. At high doses, inhibition becomes great enough to induce sleep, or at doses higher still, to cause coma.

GABA is used as a neurotransmitter throughout the brain, and benzodiazepines enhance its inhibitory effects globally in the brain. It is not known if such a widespread effect is needed for relief of anxiety in humans, or if a local effect in specific regions would suffice. Medical technology is not yet ready routinely to deliver drugs solely to where they are needed. This is a common problem in using drugs in patients. Brain cells can deliver chemicals precisely, but medications go throughout the body, both to where they are needed and where they are not.

Medication for Depression

Like anxiety disorders, depressive disorders are quite common, affecting over one in eight of the population, worldwide, in a lifetime. Symptoms of depression and anxiety often occur together, and for many people, so-called antidepressant drugs are a better long-term treatment of anxiety than are the anxiolytic drugs. In chemical structure and mechanism of action, however, the two classes of drugs are unrelated.

One might think that antidepressant drugs would be derived from stimulants, such as the amphetamines. Stimulants can raise mood in almost anyone and can be helpful in some cases of depression. Unfortunately, they are more often not helpful and even when they improve mood, only do so transiently. Like anxiolytics, their short-lived effects can lead to tolerance, craving, and addiction.

The earliest current antidepressants were discovered serendipitously in patients with tuberculosis who were treated with an antibiotic called iproniazide. Some of the patients not only had TB, but were severely depressed, until they received iproniazide. Tests in patients without TB, who suffered from depression, indicated that iproniazide was an effective therapeutic agent in relieving depression and restoring abnormalities of appetite, energy, and sleep that usually accompany this illness.

Pharmacologic studies determined that iproniazide was an inhibitor of an enzyme called monoamine oxidase, which metabolizes, and thereby inactivates, a group of chemical messengers that include norepinephrine (also called noradrenaline), serotonin, and dopamine. Like GABA, these compounds, which chemically are called monoamines, are used in the brain as neurotransmitters. Unlike GABA, the effects of which are rapid, appearing nearly instantaneously and ending as quickly, the effects of the monoamine neurotransmitters are slow by the standards of the brain, lasting seconds or longer once they are released. For this reason, it has been hypothesized that the monoamines set the "tone" of activity by region in the brain.

Inhibiting the breakdown of monoamines leads to a higher concentration of these neurotransmitters in the brain, which might be the means by which iproniazide relieved depression. Evidence supportive of this speculation arises from the mechanisms by which stimulants act to more transiently elevate mood. Specifically, stimulants cause the release of monoamine neurotransmitters in the brain; block the re-uptake of these neurotransmitters back into the cell that released them; or mimic the effects of the monoamine neurotransmitters at the receptor proteins that recognize their presence. Based on the success of iproniazide, more monoamine oxidase inhibitor drugs (all called by the acronym MAOI) like iproniazid were developed, tested, and proved to be effective antidepressants.

Soon after the introduction of MAOIs, a new and different class of antidepressants was independently discovered. These compounds were observed in a search for agents to treat psychotic disorders, such as schizophrenia. In the early 1950s, the first modern drugs for psychosis became available. They had a structure containing three rings of carbon and occasional nitrogen, sulfur, and oxygen atoms. Many such compounds were designed, synthesized, and tested, and a clever observer noted that one compound in particular, while it lacked effects to treat psychosis, seemed to brighten mood substantially in depressed patients. The compound, imipramine, proved to be a greatly successful antidepressant, still on the market over 40 years later. Other compounds structurally similar, with three rings and, therefore, called tricyclic antidepressants, or TCAs, were developed to treat depression. Like the MAOIs, they relieve all the symptoms of depression, not just the dysphoric mood of patients.

Also like MAOIs, TCAs appear to produce their effects through actions on monoamine neurotransmitters. Specifically, they inhibit the uptake of norepinephrine back into the cells that released it. This increases the amount of norepinephrine interacting with neurons and prolongs the time over which norepinephrine acts. They have a similar, but weaker, effect on the re-uptake of serotonin. They have little effect on dopamine, which is the reverse of stimulants, which have their greatest effects on dopamine release and re-uptake.

In the late 1980s, based on the success of the TCAs but searching for a new class of antidepressants, pharmaceutical companies designed drugs that preferentially blocked the re-uptake of serotonin, rather than norepinephrine. The first of these so-called serotonin-specific re-uptake inhibitors, or SSRIs, was Prozac (fluoxetine). It and other SSRIs developed later have been extraordinarily successful, in part because they have different side effects than the TCAs, being safer and seeming to be more comfortable for most people to take. This comfort has led to an increase in the prescription of antidepressants by primary care practitioners as well as psychiatrists, with many newly treated individuals feeling relief from depression and anxiety.

Antidepressants, whether MAOIs, TCAs, or SSRIs, do not seem to benefit those who do not have symptoms of a depressive disorder. The broad use and success of the SSRIs has suggested to some that they have mood-elevating effects in people whether or not the people treated are ill. This is unlikely, as most healthy people only suffer side effects from antidepressants. Rather, as depression is a common illness, like colds in children or high blood pressure in the elderly, and physicians more readily prescribe SSRIs than previous antidepressants, more people with depressive disorders, including milder disorders, are being treated and benefiting from treatment.

Looking to why the brain responds to antidepressants, the available evidence points strongly to drug effects mediated through the monoamine neurotransmitters norepinephrine and serotonin. Two classes of drugs, the MAOIs and the TCAs, discovered independently and serendipitously, have potent actions affecting these chemical signals. A third class of agents, the SSRIs, was developed on the theory that increased serotonin messages would relieve depression. Their success helps confirm the theory. Due to crosstalk, changes in either the serotonin or norepinephrine neurotransmitter system lead to changes in the other system. Furthermore, a role for both norepinephrine and serotonin is suggested by the fact that individual antidepressant drugs whose potency is specific to one or the other monoamine appear equally efficacious in the majority of people.

It is important to note that, while drug effects on serotonin and norepinephrine can relieve depression, this outcome is not direct and immediate. Unlike benzodiazepines for anxiety, or aspirin for headache, the therapeutic effects of antidepressants do not occur in minutes or hours. They require weeks of continued use. Somehow, the brain changes its state in response to the continued presence of drug and the consequent higher levels of monoamine neurotransmitters. Brain-imaging studies suggest that depression fades as regional brain activity changes in response to altered levels of monoamine neurotransmitters induced by antidepressant drugs.

Medications for Psychosis

Psychotic disorders are among the most disabling of illnesses, disturbing thinking, perception, mood, and their interconnections, and diminishing normal human interactions. Fortunately, modern antipsychotic medications are among the more efficacious treatments in medicine today, reversing all or most symptoms in the majority of people with psychotic disorders. The effect is so dramatic that some have called antipsychotic medications the penicillin of psychiatry.

The two most common psychotic illnesses, the schizophrenias and bipolar disorders, affect over one in one hundred people. They often strike the young and can prevent a normal life or reduce successful people to homelessness. Even milder forms or episodes of psychotic illnesses can disrupt relationships among spouses, relatives, and friends. Despite obvious symptoms, including delusions, hallucinations, disrupted speech and thinking, and disorganized behavior, those in the midst of psychosis often do not realize they are ill. This peculiar lack of insight, even in those who have had multiple episodes of illness and been well in between, is another aspect of the unusual state of mind and awareness accompanying these psychotic disorders.

Many patients understand their illnesses and understand the benefits and risks of treatment. In others, lack of insight leads to considerable discussion and debate between the patient and clinicians. When there is an immediate risk of harm to the patient or others due to the symptoms of illness, medication may be started even if the patient does not accept the need for treatment. This is not common. Occasionally, patients who know medications will ameliorate their symptoms choose not to be treated. This, too, is not common, as the symptoms of psychosis are extremely uncomfortable for most people.

Others observe the symptoms of illness, of course, and for many years physicians have tried to help those with psychotic disorders. Reserpine, given in *Rauwolfia serpentina* or as the isolated chemical, had beneficial effects, but at the risk of dangerously low blood pressure and strong sedation. Opiates were used to calm patients, but had minimal effects on the key symptoms of psychosis.

It was not until the early 1950s that the first specific, well-tolerated and effective medication for psychosis, Thorazine (chlorpromazine), was introduced. This medication, and others modeled after it, were so effective that the number of patients with psychotic disorders in hospitals began to drop substantially. With the development of even newer agents that had similar therapeutic effects but fewer side effects, decreases in hospitalization continue, despite a growing population.

The antipsychotic medications were discovered by design, partly from modifying known sedatives, but mostly by looking for agents related to anesthetics, which produced a profound calming effect but not loss of consciousness. The antipsychotic drugs, however, are not all sedatives and are not, as they were once called, major tranquilizers. Some are sedative and some not. Some reduce anxiety, and some can increase it. All work similarly in reducing the symptoms of psychosis, including disrupted thinking, mood, perception, and behavior. Only one, Clozaril (clozapine), may be on average modestly more efficacious than other antipsychotic drugs.

Those without psychotic disorders gain nothing but side effects from these drugs. The drugs have little effect on people with odd or idiosyncratic ideas and behaviors, unless they have the symptoms of schizophrenia or bipolar disorder.

Given that antipsychotic medications all tend to produce a similar therapeutic outcome and were designed to be pharmacologically similar to chlorpromazine, the original antipsychotic drug, it is not surprising that they share common mechanisms of action at a molecular level. Specifically, all antipsychotic drugs block signals at some but not all receptors for the chemical messengers dopamine, norepinephrine, and serotonin.

By blocking signals at these receptors, the antipsychotic drugs produce affects in several key areas of the brain. They change activity in the nucleus accumbens, which is involved, in part, in mediating a sense of reward; the amygdala, which is involved in determining a sense of threat, disquiet, or safety; the thalamus, which appears to be involved in coordinating aspects of thought, perception, and emotion; and the prefrontal cortex, which is the most developed of all areas of the human brain and is involved in attention, decision making, and keeping thoughts in consciousness.

Like the antidepressants, therapeutic effects of antipsychotic drugs can take weeks to develop. How the immediate effects of the antipsychotic drugs become longer term effects is not known. However, there is growing evidence that modulation of signals through the monoamine receptors affected by antipsychotic drugs leads to changes in the activity of GABAergic and glutaminergic cells, which mediate much of the function of the brain.

It is not surprising that even though the antipsychotic drugs have effects on only a few specific receptors in the brain, their use would change activity at many sites. Neurons that employ dopamine, norepinephrine, and serotonin as their chemical messengers are few, but they contact vast numbers of cells throughout the brain. In addition, because cells in the brain are interconnected in a dense network, a limited direct effect can translate into a broad distributed effect.

Most well-described functions of the brain, such as the processing of visual information or the control of movement, are handled by cells distributed across many different, but sometimes overlapping, areas of the brain. It is possible, and even likely, that emotions and thoughts are also a consequence of changes in the activity of specific groups of cells linked to one another but representing different aspects of feeling or cognition and existing in different locations within the brain. The wide distribution of neurons responding to antipsychotic drugs, and mediating their effects, illustrates this point.

Psychiatric Disorders, Psychotherapeutic Medication, and Consciousness

Medications are a key component of the treatment of most psychiatric disorders. They are not, of course, the sole treatment. Proper care requires attention to the psychological and social aspects of illness. These may represent environmental stressors that, unaddressed, can trigger illness in those predisposed. Also, psychological and social problems are frequently consequences of the disruption of mood, thought, and behavior caused by illness. Patients need support in reconstituting their lives and sense of self once their symptoms fade.

It is remarkable, however, just how powerful medications are in relieving the symptoms of psychiatric disorders. Along with genetic, structural, and functional evidence, the effects of drugs are compelling findings suggesting that psychiatric illnesses arise from abnormal activity of the brain; that is, they are medical disorders of the brain.

Arguments can be made for and against the recreational use of drugs. Society accepts some, such as alcohol, and not others, such as marijuana. By comparison, there is little basis for argument about the treatment of psychiatric disorders with medication. For most people, the benefits clearly outweigh the risks.

The effects of psychotherapeutic medications also speak to questions beyond that of the origin and nature of psychiatric disorders. They speak to the nature of consciousness.

Drugs can disturb all aspects of consciousness and drugs can restore aspects of consciousness. As drugs act on the structure, chemistry, and electrical activity of the brain, it is logical to conclude that all aspects of consciousness depend on physical states of the brain.

Evidence is growing as to the precise molecular sites at which drugs act, as well as on the specific changes that occur in cellular metabolism and the state of neural circuits during drug treatment. Pharmacologic studies point to particular regions of the brain or particular distributed groups of nerve cells as being involved in mediating mood, awareness, cognition, or the integration of experience. Studies of the consequences of lesions associated with epilepsy, tumors, strokes, and trauma also suggest that particular parts of the brain are necessary, if not sufficient, to determine aspects of consciousness. Results from pharmacology and pathology agree strongly on which areas are associated with which aspects of consciousness.

No simple connections are likely to exist between a molecule and a thought or a nerve cell and a mood. However, it is reasonable to expect that the state of networks of nerve cells in the brain may be closely related to conscious states of thinking or feeling. Drugs and medications can change the patterns of firing in neural circuits and the tone of neural activity in the brain. By doing so, they can alter those aspects of consciousness that make us most human. The study of drug effects will remain an important tool for designing and testing models of how mind may arise from brain. Equally or more important, the use of currently available drugs and the arrival of new drugs under development will continue to provide good treatments, and some day cures, for the devastating illnesses classified as psychiatric disorders.

POSTSCRIPT

Are Psychotherapeutic Drugs Overprescribed for Treating Mental Illness?

Many mental health practitioners maintain that psychotherapeutic drugs can be effective in treating the majority of people suffering from mental illness. However, there is a sharp disagreement about whether these drugs are prescribed too readily and whether they are taking the place of traditional talk therapy. Of course, this debate does not need focus on which type of treatment is best. Many people receive both drug therapy and psychotherapy. In addition, it has been shown that drug therapy and psychotherapy work best in conjunction with each other.

The debate regarding psychotherapeutic drugs has spurned other concerns. Should they be prescribed for common problems that people encounter on a daily basis, such as stress, feelings of anxiety, phobias, shyness, and obsessive-compulsive behavior? Many people experience these problems. A certain degree of anxiety, shyness, and compulsivity is not unusual. Should people rid themselves of these conditions even if they may incur adverse side effects?

The pursuit of happiness seems to be of paramount importance in our society. Yet, can one find happiness in a pill? Should one turn to pills to find happiness? Do these drugs represent a quick and easy fix and is it ethical to chemically alter an individual's mood and personality in order to be happy? Will psychopharmacology replace traditional psychotherapy? Is the rapid growth of antidepressant drugs a well-conceived promotion on the part of pharmaceutical companies? In a society that values solving problems quickly and easily, these drugs seem to effectively fulfill a need. However, do their advantages outweigh their disadvantages?

A popular slogan many years ago referred to "better living through chemistry." If a drug is available that will make people happier, more confident, and more socially adept, should that drug be available for people who would derive some degree of benefit from it? One concern is that some individuals may rely on drugs to remedy many of their problems rather than to work through those issues that caused the problems in the first place. It is much easier to drop a pill than to engage in self-exploration and self-reflection. One could make some analogy between psychotherapeutic drugs and other drugs. Many people now use alcohol, tobacco, over-the-counter medicines, and illegal drugs to cope with life's problems. Drugs, whether they are legal or illegal, are used increasingly for dealing with our daily problems.

One article that looked at the extensiveness of mood disorders is "Prevalence and Effects of Mood Disorders on Work Performance in a Nationally

Representative Sample of U.S. Workers," by Ronald Kessler and others (*American Journal of Psychiatry*, September 2006). Algis Valiunas comments on the role of drugs and the role of therapy in treating mental illness in "Sadness, Gladness—and Serotonin" (*Commentary*, January 2006). *Consumer Report* magazine (October 2004) assessed the advantages of drug therapy versus talk therapy and found that they work best when used in conjunction. Gordon Marino argues against psychotherapeutic drugs in "Altered States: Pills Alone Won't Cure the Blues" (*Commonweal*, May 21, 2004). The negative publicity regarding psychotherapeutic drugs may prevent young people from deriving their benefits according to Nancy Shute in "Teens, Drugs, and Sadness" (*U.S. News and World Report*, August 30, 2004). In his article "Is It Really Our Chemicals That Need Balancing?" (*Journal of American College Health*, July 2002), Christopher Bailey argues that society is falling into the trap of making minor problems into mental illnesses.

ISSUE 11

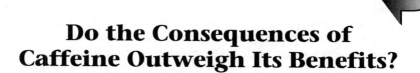

Do the Consequences of Caffeine Outweigh Its Benefits?

YES: James Thornton, from "Start Me Up," *Men's Health* (October 2004)

NO: Sally Satel, from "Is Caffeine Addictive?—A Review of the Literature," *American Journal of Drug and Alcohol Abuse* (November 2006)

ISSUE SUMMARY

YES: James Thornton from *Men's Health* describes caffeine as an addictive substance that results in withdrawal symptoms. The stimulating effects of caffeine are muted by tolerance that develops to the drug. One downside to caffeine is that it impedes one's ability to get to sleep. The lack of sleep may result in jitteriness and arrhythmias in adults. In large amounts caffeine can cause anxiety and panic attacks.

NO: According to medical doctor Sally Satel, caffeine may have addictive qualities but its dangers are overstated. Caffeine's addictive qualities are modest. Most caffeine users are able to moderate their consumption of caffeine. Headaches are one by-product of caffeine cessation. Very few people consume caffeine compulsively. Moreover, individuals who have difficulty moderating their caffeine use often have other psychiatric problems.

$\mathbf{C}$affeine is one of the most widely consumed legal drugs in the world. In the United States, more than 9 out of every 10 people drink some type of caffeinated beverage, mostly for its stimulating effects. Caffeine elevates mood, reduces fatigue, increases work capacity, and stimulates respiration. Caffeine often provides the lift people need to start the day. Although many people associate caffeine primarily with coffee, caffeine also is found in numerous soft drinks, over-the-counter medications, chocolate, and tea. Because caffeinated drinks are common in society and there are very few legal controls regarding the use of caffeine, its physical and psychological effects frequently are overlooked, ignored, or minimized.

In recent years coffee consumption has declined; however, the amount of caffeine being consumed has not declined appreciably because of the increase in caffeinated soft drink consumption. To reduce their levels of caffeine intake, many people have switched to decaffeinated drinks and coffee. Although this results in less caffeine intake, decaffeinated coffee still contains small amounts of caffeine.

Research studies evaluating the effects of caffeine consumption on personal health date back to the 1960s. In particular, the medical community has conducted numerous studies to determine whether or not there is a relationship between caffeine consumption and cardiovascular disease, because heart disease is the leading cause of death in many countries, including the United States. In spite of the many studies on this subject, a clear relationship between heart disease and caffeine is not yet apparent. Studies have yielded conflicting results. Rather than clarifying the debate regarding the consequences of caffeine, the research only adds to the confusion. As a result, studies suggesting that there is a connection between caffeine consumption and adverse physical and psychological effects have come under scrutiny by both the general public and health professions.

One serious limitation of previous research indicating that caffeine does have deleterious effects is that the research focused primarily on coffee use. There may be other ingredients in coffee besides caffeine that produce harmful effects. Moreover, an increasing percentage of the caffeine being consumed comes from other sources, such as soft drinks, tea, chocolate, antihistamines, and diet pills. Therefore, caffeine studies involving only coffee are not truly representative of the amount of caffeine that people ingest.

Another important criticism of caffeine research, especially studies linking caffeine use and heart disease, is gender bias. Until recently, research has focused primarily on the caffeine consumption of men. The bias in medical research is not limited to caffeine studies; men have traditionally been the primary group studied regarding many facets of health. This situation is changing. There is increasing research into the potential consequences of caffeine use on the fetus and nursing mother.

People who believe that drinking caffeine in moderation does not pose a significant health threat are critical of previous and current studies. This is particularly true of those studies that demonstrate a relationship between caffeine and heart disease. Critics contend that it is difficult to establish a definitive relationship between caffeine and heart disease due to a myriad of confounding variables. For example, cardiovascular disease has been linked to family history, a sedentary lifestyle, cigarette smoking, obesity, fat intake, and stress. Many individuals who consume large amounts of coffee also smoke cigarettes, drink alcohol, and are hard-driven. Several factors also affect caffeine's excretion from the body. Cigarette smoking increases caffeine metabolization, whereas the use of oral contraceptives and pregnancy slow down metabolization. Therefore, determining the extent to which caffeine use causes heart disease while adjusting for the influence of these other factors is difficult.

In the following selections, James Thornton of *Men's Health* cautions readers about the use of caffeine, even in moderate amounts. He claims that small amounts can cause panic and anxiety. In contrast, Sally Satel casts doubt on the negative effects associated with caffeine intake and that the effects of caffeine may not be as harmful as many people speculate.

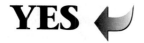

YES

James Thornton

Start Me Up

Caffeine. It's America's buzz word. And with spiked sodas and goosed gums, it's easier than ever to ingest. But is there a price for living a wired life? I'm an unnervous wreck. Stuporously groggy on this, the first full day of "Caffeine Cold Turkey," my head feels like it's been crushed in a vice. It's nearly impossible to think.

I slap myself three times, happy for the jolts of fleeting alertness each cheek sting provides. Alas, this exercise quickly proves too exhausting to continue. It's now 10:40 a.m., and I've been up since 8:45, nearly 2 full hours. Surely I've earned the right to take my first nap. But no: I shan't succumb to sleep's siren call so swiftly. I will struggle to stay awake till, at the very least, noonish. Given the headache, lethargy, and sundry other unpleasant symptoms involved so far in my withdrawal, you may be wondering about my reason for this exercise in abstention. Excellent question. Let's start with the basic truth that, God help me, I've become a slave to the bean. Our family's commercial-grade coffeemaker brews up to 10 cups at a time. When I first purchased this gizmo in the mid-'90s, I typically limited myself to 2 or 3 cups each morning. Over time, however, my usage incrementally escalated—3 cups gave way to 4, then 5, then 6, then . . . Honestly, I'm at a loss to explain how things got so out of whack. But for the past few years, my habit upon awakening has been to pack the basket with prodigious quantities of Colombian Supremo, hit the strongest brew button, then drink the resulting 10 cups of black coffee over the next hour. If the synapses of my brain can be compared to an obstinate mule team, then caffeine has become the lash that drives them. By lunch, I'm usually ready to follow up my morning dosage with one or two 12-ounce cans of Coke, nothing too serious. But by 5 o'clock, the workday done, I'm ready to resume heavy usage again—not to hone cognitive performance, but rather to boost physical endurance. As a masters swimmer averaging 17,000 yards a week, I've gotten in the habit of stopping off at a local convenience store en route to evening practice. Here I purchase and quickly down a 24-ounce cappuccino to goad my efforts in the pool. Unfortunately, I've become so habituated to my favorite drug that it no longer works terribly well for me. That's the main reason I decided to decaffeinate my body: I have a key swim meet coming

From *Men's Health*, vol. 19, issue 8, October 2004, pp. 172. Copyright © 2004 by Roland Press. Reprinted by permission.

up, and I've been concerned about my chances for some time. So concerned that I sought advice from Lawrence Armstrong, Ph.D., a professor of exercise at the University of Connecticut's human-performance lab and a longtime researcher into caffeine's sports-enhancing effects. "If you've developed a tolerance to caffeine" he told me, "you should try withdrawal until you become caffeine naive again, then come back to it for your meet, when it's likely you'll get a greater response per dose." That's the plan, anyway. Right now, I feel like a java junkie, even though, technically, I'm not one. Caffeine isn't a drug like amphetamines or cocaine, in that it doesn't act on the areas of the brain related to reward, motivation, and addiction. So I can't be "hooked" in the heroin sense of the word. On this, my first day of withdrawal, I absolutely crave caffeine, but I don't absolutely need it. It's now 11:18 a.m. What I do absolutely need is a nap. Though my personal usage is undeniably extreme, my affection for caffeine is hardly unique. According to Harriet de Wit, Ph.D., an associate professor of psychiatry at the University of Chicago, caffeine is by far the most widely used psychoactive drug in the world, easily surpassing both alcohol and nicotine. A study of java-drinking trends by the National Coffee Association (NCA) showed that, as of 2000, a record 79 percent of U.S. adults consumed coffee. As a nation, we down 350 million cups of coffee a day, with men swallowing significantly more than women. Of course, since many of us also imbibe tea, Big Gulps, and "energy" drinks such as Red Bull, these stats don't begin to measure the extent of America's buzz. Caffeine is ubiquitous. It's in everything from chocolate bars to over-the-counter analgesics, many cold remedies, and weight loss pills. There's even a new caffeinated gum on the market: Jolt Caffeine Energy Gum—available in Spearmint and Icymint. Two Chiclet-size pieces are capable of leaching, in about 5 minutes, 70 milligrams (mg)—or about a coffee cup's worth—of caffeine into the blood vessels under the tongue. (Coffee, by comparison, takes at least 45 minutes to produce peak caffeine levels in the bloodstream.)

Obviously, mankind has come a long way since Sufi priests made the first caffeinated drink out of coffee-bean husks, then used the liquid to fuel all-night religious ceremonies. Early Europeans witnessing these maniacal events dubbed the participants "whirling dervishes"—and the truth is, there's no shortage of us would-be dervishes around today.

So what exactly has made caffeine the Official Drug of the Human Race? The story of this plant-derived compound clearly begins with its action in the brain. Inside each human noggin, a slew of neurotransmitters and related compounds carry on cascading interactions that somehow result in everything from sleep to wakefulness, thoughts to emotions. Some of these molecules have a generally stimulating effect, while others work to dampen down nervous activity. Until about 20 years ago, scientists thought caffeine fell squarely into the brain-jazzing category. Then, in 1982, researchers discovered an evolutionary fluke: Caffeine's molecular structure is very similar to that of adenosine, an inhibitory brain substance found in many animals, including humans. "Animal studies have suggested that adenosine could be the 'somnolent,' or sleep-inducing, factor," explains Tom McLellan, Ph.D., a scientist at Defence R&D Canada in Toronto who studies caffeine for the Canadian military. "When people need sleep, their adenosine levels are high, which seems to trigger the brain into wanting to shut down." The longer you're awake, the more adenosine gradually accumulates in your brain. The growing surfeit, in turn, binds to specialized adenosine receptors, depressing nervous-system activity and making you groggy.

In ways that are not yet understood, getting enough sleep clears the chemical from your system, allowing you to begin the next day fully restored, your sleep debt paid in full. There is, however, an alternative to clearing adenosine: You can block it before it has a chance to make you sleepy. Caffeine does this by binding to adenosine receptors before the adenosine gets there. It's like jamming a toothpick into a keyhole so the key can't fit. To the holistic, health-food-store crowd, such molecular monkey-wrenching probably smacks of fooling Mother Nature in a way similar to pumping heifers full of bovine growth hormone. Surely we caffeine fiends can't keep doing this to ourselves day after day without having to pay some kind of penalty. Right?

The Health Impact

For decades, studies have attempted to find links between caffeine intake and a host of heavy-duty ailments, from heart disease to cancer. But no luck. The famed Framingham Heart Study, for example, concluded that caffeine consumption showed no influence on the rate of heart disease or stroke. Another investigation of 45,000 men published in *The New England Journal of Medicine* reached a similar conclusion. As for the cancer connection, a Norwegian study of 15,000 people found no significant correlation between coffee use and cancer, or any other disease, for that matter. The International Agency for the Research of Cancer reaffirmed this finding. "Caffeine, however, has been condemned by 'clean living' advocates because it has no nutritional value, is not needed for any physiologic function, and is commonly abused by the tired and stressed," concludes nutrition expert Nancy Clark, R.D., in a review paper published in *The Physician and Sportsmedicine.* "As a result, many coffee drinkers worry that their early-morning mugful will contribute to health problems. The truth is, coffee and other caffeinated beverages in moderation are not health demons." In fact, some health conditions may actually be helped by those judicious jolts of java. Harvard researchers recently connected caffeine intake to a reduced risk of type-2 diabetes, and just last year, scientists in Italy discovered that coffee may decrease a person's chances of developing oral or esophageal cancer.

The Emotional Effects

Even caffeine's greatest boosters have long acknowledged that in a certain subset of users, the drug can trigger unpleasant side effects, including anxiety and even panic attacks. Several years ago, University of Chicago researcher de Wit attended a lecture by German geneticist Jurgen Deckert, who reported his finding that a genetic variation in a type of adenosine receptor was strongly linked to panic disorder. "Since I knew that caffeine works on adenosine receptors," recalls de Wit, "I knew it would be easy to see whether this same gene variation is related to people's different responses to caffeine" In a study published in the journal *Neuropsychopharmacology,* de Wit and her colleagues gave 94 randomly selected volunteers 150 mg caffeine (the equivalent of 2 cups of coffee) or a placebo, then measured their responses in terms of mood, alertness, heart rate, and blood pressure. The researchers also genotyped each individual. On nearly all measures, from increased vigilance to relief from fatigue, caffeine proved to affect the test subjects identically. The only difference was that those with the specific genetic variation—about 30 percent of the total—reported anxiety, whereas the other 70 percent didn't. "What our data suggest," says de Wit, "is that if you have an unusual response to caffeine, there's probably a biological basis for why it's happening to you" Bottom line: If moderate doses of the bean give you the heebie-jeebies, it's best to cut it out entirely.

The Brain Benefits

Of all caffeine's purported effects, the one most touted by users themselves is its ability to provide a temporary mental edge. Unfortunately, for those who are hoping to ace a critical exam through a short-lived boost in IQ, the current evidence indicates that caffeine doesn't make you smarter. "What's been shown with caffeine is that it does have a dramatic effect on alertness," says McLellan, "but as you move to higher-order cognitive functioning, such as decision making, it doesn't really have an impact." Still, alertness is essential for most jobs, especially those in the military. In a new U.S. Air Force-funded study, researchers had 16 healthy men alternate 28 hours of consciousness with 14 hours of sleep for 1 month—an eccentric schedule designed to mimic shift work or jet lag. Every hour that the men were awake, they received tablets containing either a placebo substance or roughly 20 mg caffeine, the amount in 1/4 cup of coffee. The results proved unequivocal, with caffeine users consistently outperforming the placebo group on a host of computerized tests. The findings also showed something else—that it doesn't make sense to wake up and smell the coffee. "Caffeine had a very strong effect when delivered in small, incremental doses over time," says study author James Wyatt, Ph.D. "I hate to say it, but most of us have been using caffeine the wrong way." Wyatt bases his hypothesis on the fact that soporific adenosine levels are lowest when we first awake, precisely the time most of us reach for our Folgers. By the time adenosine starts to build, the morning caffeine spike is already waning. For those wedded to their caffeine fix, Wyatt recommends waiting till after lunch, when adenosine levels are starting to rise significantly. Thereafter, you'll get a more effective and consistent hit with small, regular doses, such as 1/4 cup per hour. It's important not to overdo it and end up compromising your ability to sleep at night. For most people, this probably means avoiding caffeine within 4 hours of bedtime. "Remember the big picture here," says Wyatt. "If everyone simply got 8.3 to 8.4 hours of quality sleep on a regular nightly basis, we wouldn't need caffeine in the first place."

The Endurance Angle

Studies have long shown that caffeine has ergogenic (i.e., sports-enhancing) effects in a multitude of activities, from swimming to tennis. The main effect seems to be improving endurance. In a 2002 study published in the *Journal of Applied Physiology*, McLellan and his colleagues found that the time it took for cyclists to exercise to exhaustion was significantly longer in those receiving caffeine than in those given a placebo. Moreover, this benefit was greatest in those who didn't use caffeine regularly. "More and more," says McLellan, "it's looking like caffeine works on motivation within the brain itself. It affects your perception of effort and makes you feel you're not working as hard as you might otherwise feel." It doesn't take whopping doses to get this effect. In McClellan's recent study of 9 men, the equivalent of 2 cups of coffee was sufficient to provide a longer exercise duration to exhaustion, with the consumption of more caffeine providing no additional benefit. If you're planning to try out the caffeine edge the next time you challenge a buddy, say, to five sets of tennis, keep in mind that coffee can sometimes trigger gastrointestinal distress, possibly because of acids and other components in the brew. In his studies for the Canadian military, McLellan found what he believes is an optimum delivery system: caffeinated gum. "I found it great, myself," he says. "It's really quick—the concentration peaks in 5 to 10 minutes. And it doesn't give me any stomach symptoms."

It's exactly 3 weeks since my last cup of coffee, and my system is presumably as caffeine-free now as the day I was born. The headaches and urge to hibernate that plagued me during the first 5 days of abstinence have faded, restoring a baseline normalcy—no less nor, alas, more energetic than I was during the long days of my high-octane dependency.

I stifle a yawn. In yesterday's mail, my secret weapon for my swim meet finally arrived: a dozen packs of Jolt Caffeine Energy Gum (available at convenience stores and . . .). In exactly 1/2 hour, I'll mount the starting blocks for the 500-yard freestyle at the Pennsylvania State Games. In preparation for this, I finally break my fast, popping a single piece of gum into my mouth. It takes a mere 10 minutes for the wad under my tongue to utterly obliterate any further urge to yawn.

Five minutes before the race, I chew a second piece, providing my system with the total caffeine equivalent of a single cup of coffee. The effect is nothing short of exhilarating. I explode off the blocks and find myself swimming with a remarkable degree of verve and indefatigability. When the splashing stops, I've placed first in the event—by 27 seconds—in the process swimming the second-fastest 500 of my life. Suspecting a possible fluke, I repeat the same two-hit caffeine-gum protocol for each race over the next 2 days. I easily win them all—the 100 backstroke, plus the 50, 100, and 200 freestyles—achieving close to lifetime bests in each race. True, this success hasn't come cheap. During the nights following both days of competition, I found it nearly impossible to sleep and, in fact, averaged no more than 3 fitful hours. And a day after getting home from the swim meet, I came down with the worst cold I've had in years. I'm sure the caffeine did not directly cause this. But could my immune system have been compromised by sleeplessness and by extraordinary effort made to seem effortless? In any event, this whole experience has given me a new appreciation—and respect—for a drink I'd come to think of as little more than hot brown water. Gone forever is my old gallon-a-day approach. From now on, I plan to keep my coffee drinking and gum chewing below moderate, saving occasional indulgences only for those times when this dervish truly needs to whirl.

Sally Satel

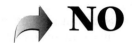 **NO**

Is Caffeine Addictive?—A Review of the Literature

Introduction

In July 2005, the Center for Science in the Public Interest, a Washington-based consumer advocacy group, called for the Food and Drug Administration (FDA) to mandate warning labels on caffeinated soda. The group's main concern was not only the association between soda and childhood obesity; it also judged caffeine to be a potentially dangerous substance. The Center suggested that "[C]affeinated drinks should bear a notice that reads 'This drink contains x grams of caffeine, which is a mildly addictive stimulant drug. Not appropriate for children'" (1).

Is caffeine addictive? Is it a harmful substance that compels the consumer to use at the risk of his well-being and despite a stated desire to refrain? Is it a "model drug of abuse" as the National Institute on Drug Abuse put it? (2). The answer is no. This paper summarizes evidence justifying this conclusion.

Impairment and Reinforcement

How does caffeine use fit into the DSM-IVR drug abuse schema? (3). A significant level of impairment is rarely a consequence of its consumption. Caffeine can be a factor in poor sleep, jitteriness, and arrhythmias in adults. Its effects on children, especially hyperactive ones, are not well known. However, in adults, too much caffeine produces sensations that are unpleasant (e.g., tremulousness, jitteriness) and may put a break on its consumption. Moreover, if caffeine were so intensely desirable, some individuals would likely self-administer caffeine supplements—available in 200 mg tablets—in doses exceeding the average caffeine intake of about 200 300 mg/day.

What about DSM IV-R dependence criteria? (4). Caffeine consumers do not display an inability to control consumption. Coffee drinking is weakly reinforcing, but this is not the same as saying that caffeine, as a substance, is reinforcing. Nehlig states that "the conditions under which caffeine functions as a reinforcer still are not clearly understood" (5).

From *American Journal of Drug and Alcohol Abuse*, vol. 32, issue 4, November 2006, pp. 493 502.

First, the possible reinforcing effects of coffee may not be the caffeine per se, but rather the pleasurable aroma and taste of coffee as well as the social environment that usually accompanies coffee consumption. Second, the desire to use repeatedly is most marked in heavy caffeine consumers (> 1000 mg/day) who also had histories of alcohol or drug abuse. For moderate caffeine users (130600 mg/day), caffeine reinforcement occurs in a smaller subset of consumers (6).

The author could find no reports of use that bear analogy to alcoholic-style drinking or chain smoking. Theoretically, an individual might be exquisitely sensitive to the effects of caffeine and be at risk for a more classical addiction, but if so, his sensitivity to caffeine would make the stimulating effects of the drug itself (e.g., jitteriness) too unpleasant to tolerate. Case reports of toxic levels involve deliberate or accidental overdoses of caffeine pills, not compulsive consumption of those pills or of coffee. In short, coffee drinking resembles more a dedicated habit than a compulsive addiction (7).

Animal studies permit analysis of the effects of caffeine on the brain. Nehlig has examined this question in depth and discovered that caffeine levels approximating human consumption do not activate brain reward circuits as do classic stimulants (8). Amphetamines, cocaine, and nicotine stimulate the release of dopamine in the shell of the nucleus accumbens, the key structure in the brain for reward, motivation, and addiction. However, caffeine has no effect on the shell of the nucleus accumbens. Moreover, the experimental rats received caffeine intravenously, a route well known to be more reinforcing than oral use.

An important question about the reinforcing properties of caffeine is whether ongoing use is a function of a drinker's enjoyment of caffeine-containing beverages—in which case, it is more like a loyal, pleasurable habit than a compulsion—or whether users consume it to avoid subtle withdrawal effects.

Caffeine Tolerance and Withdrawal

People use caffeine in a regular pattern—every morning or after dinner—but there is little evidence that such behavior is of a compulsive nature. Rather, caffeine drinkers are often dedicated to their coffee—they seek its warmth, flavor, aroma, and, sometimes, mildly stimulating benefits. They do not feel intense distress if it is unavailable; though, some will drink it in order to suppress withdrawal symptoms.

Tolerance. Daily caffeine drinkers quickly develop tolerance to the jitteriness, anxiety, and edginess occasionally reported by first time users of the substance. Rather than becoming tolerant to caffeine's desirable effects (wakefulness, alertness), most drinkers become tolerant to the negative ones. Notably, with standard drugs of abuse it generally takes additional drugs to achieve the desired effect of a high or a feeling of tranquility.

Withdrawal. Also called discontinuation syndroms, withdrawal occurs upon abruptly stopping the use of a drug (including some prescribed medications). This phenomenon occurs because the user's central nervous system has adapted to regular exposure to the substance.

Such physical dependence is a product of "neuroadaptation"—that is, central nervous system neurons adapt to compensate for the continuous presence of a substance in the brain tissue. In the case of opiate addiction, when the level drops below a certain point, the neurons "rebound" and the user experiences physical symptoms such as chills, shakes, stomach cramps, or vomiting. After a period of regular use, a person might "crave" opiates simply to stop the sickness, and not because he desires the high. By contrast, the essence of addiction (psychological dependence) is a craving for the drug and its compulsive use.

Caffeine withdrawal includes headache, lethargy, irritability, and mental fuzzy-headedness. Some or all can occur among many daily caffeine consumers who abruptly stop their intake (9). Sometimes doses as low as 100 mg/d can provoke these symptoms, though daily caffeine consumption among Americans is estimated at about 280 mg/d or the equivalent of 2–3 cups of coffee (10, 11). Symptoms begin twelve to twenty-four hours after sudden cessation of continuous use, reach a peak at twenty to forty-eight hours, and resolve after ingesting caffeine (12–14).

Thus, physical dependence denotes the need for a substance to achieve physiological homeostasis; the classic signs of this phenomenon are tolerance and withdrawal. It differs from addiction (also called psychological dependence or just "dependence" in DSM IV) in that the latter entails compulsive engagement in a behavior with negative consequences.

Studies on Withdrawal. Researchers use two standard techniques to assess the nature and frequency of withdrawal. One is to ask daily caffeine consumers whether they have ever stopped use abruptly and the effects of cessation. However, the problem with retrospective surveys is that recall is often unreliable and difficult to validate.

The second kind of study entails observation of regular consumers of caffeine who are switched, without their knowledge or the awareness of the rater, to a caffeine-free diet during a study period. Such double-blinded, prospective clinical studies assess experience in real-time by objective observers.

Survey Studies. There are ten published random surveys of caffeine withdrawal, with four of them involving hospitalized patients. Of the remaining six, two specifically recruited subjects who identified themselves as experiencing caffeine-withdrawal while two others simply recruited coffee drinkers (15, 16). In the first, Goldstein and Kaiser reported that 58 percent of the eighteen people in their survey who drank 5–10 cups of coffee per day felt "half awake" when they stopped and another 8 percent reported headaches after stopping (17). Hughes and colleagues found that 11 percent of those who had given up or reduced caffeine use in the past year experienced headache plus one other symptom which together produced "significant distress or impairment in social, occupational, or other important areas of functioning" (18).

The remaining two of the six surveys were both random samples of over 1000 participants who were not surveyed specifically for their caffeine use. Dews and colleagues reported on 11,112 subjects who responded to an ad unrelated to caffeine consumption. Sixty-one percent (6,815) claimed to be daily caffeine consumers and of these, 11 percent reported that they experienced symptoms such as headaches, irritability, and sleepiness when they stopped using caffeine abruptly (19). In the second survey, Kendler and Prescott reported on 1,642 women in a twin-registry study of genetic aspects of various conditions. Twenty-four percent claimed that in stopping or decreasing use, they developed a headache and at least one other symptom (20).

Experimental studies. In 2004, Juliano and Griffiths summarized forty-two double-blind trials (21). In these trials, subjects typically underwent placebo replacement for caffeine for various periods of time. The researchers then compare withdrawal symptoms in those who received a placebo versus those who continued to receive caffeine. The bulk of the studies showed that caffeine abstention resulted in the placebo group reporting higher rates of lethargy, fuzziness, and headache.

Three studies made a special effort to recruit subjects who were naive to the purpose of the study.

Hughes and colleagues recruited moderate to heavy coffee drinkers (about 5–7 cups/d) to participate in a study of the effects of different coffee strengths on mood, general performance, and preference for each beverage (22). The study was administered over a four-day period. Twenty-two subjects with no history of substance abuse or mental illness participated. Subjects consumed either 4 cups of decaf coffee only on Day 1 or caffeinated coffee only on Day 2 or vice versa. On Days 3 and 4, subjects were allowed to choose between decaf and caffeinated coffees. There were six 4-day sessions total. Overall, subjects preferred caffeinated coffee on the days they could chose. On experimental days when they were given decaf, 41 percent reported drowsiness, fatigue, and headache, though baseline levels of these symptoms were not reported.

Silverman and coworkers recruited sixty-two adults through ads promoting a study of the effect of foods—including caffeine on behavior and mood (23). The participants' average daily intake of caffeine was 235 mg/d. No participants with a history of psychiatric disorder were enrolled. The subjects participated in 2 two-day study periods that were one week apart. During each two-day period, they received either their usual caffeine dose in pill form or placebo pills. Fifty-two percent of those in the placebo condition reported moderate or severe headaches (2 percent baseline), while 8–11 percent complained about depression and anxiety.

Dews and his team used subjects who responded to an ad for various medical studies (24). Over half (6,815) of the 11,112 subjects were daily caffeine drinkers and of these, fifty-seven said they experienced difficulty in the past when they stopped use. Subjects for an experimental phase were selected from the fifty-seven; subjects with a psychiatric disorder within the last twelve months were excluded.

The fifty-seven subjects consumed an average of 200–300 mg caffeine/day with a maximum consumption of 550 mg. They were divided, randomly, into three experimental groups. The first (n = 18) was kept on a constant dose of caffeine throughout the observation period. In the second (n = 18), coffee was replaced with decaf, without their knowledge, after the first five days of the fourteen day study. Only six reported any symptoms within the first forty-eight hours of caffeine abstinence (one of them specifically reporting a "caffeine deprivation headache" on the first four days of withdrawal). Five others reported headache and lethargy on days 10 and 11.

Members of the third group (n = 20) were given progressively lower concentrations of caffeine (80 percent, 60, 40, 20, 0) on days 6–12. In that group, no consistent pattern of symptoms could be discerned. In many instances, the magnitude of the change registered was one-third of a point on a scale in which a single point indicated the change from "same as usual" to "slightly less than usual."

In Dews' study, three of seven subjects who claimed to experience "severe" withdrawal during the interview portion of the study, did not report any discomfort during the experimentally induced withdrawal segment of the trial. As the authors state: "It would appear that self-reports are an unreliable indicator of what is recognized by the same subject under double-blind conditions" (25). They conclude that caffeine withdrawal is not a clinically significant phenomenon and that many of the symptoms appear because subjects expect them to do so.

Methodological Problems

A number of methodological issues, in addition to the relatively small samples routinely used, complicate interpretation of clinical trials data. Foremost is whether the blind can be maintained, given the ability of drinkers to detect the presence of caffeine (26). Because blinding requires that neither the tester nor the participant know which drinks contain the active ingredient, the distinctive taste may make it impossible to preserve a blind. Additionally, there is evidence that research subjects will report in the desired direction of the person administering the study if it is known to them thus making it very difficult to obtain accurate data about caffeine effects and especially when reported withdrawal symptoms cannot be verified through a physical exam (27).

Second, it is important for studies to examine subjects who are representative of normal caffeine consumers. Particularly, a 1994 study by Strain and others, published in the prestigious Journal of the American Medical Association and one of the most widely cited studies on caffeine withdrawal, is problematic in this regard (28).

Not only was the study's sample size of eleven very small, the individuals were recruited through a newspaper ad specifically seeking subjects who deemed themselves "psychologically or physically dependent" upon caffeine. Therefore, the researchers chose an unrepresentative sample. Furthermore, the subjects' consent-to-participate form laid out the specific withdrawal symptoms, thus contaminating the blind and introducing expectation bias. In short, when the authors report that eight of the eleven subjects displayed "functional impairment" during the course of 2 two-day abstinence periods which were separated by one week, the finding is not obviously applicable to most caffeine consumers.

In addition, almost half of the subjects in the Strain study consumed their caffeine in the form of soft drinks. Given an average caffeine consumption of 300 mg/d, this means the subjects drank about ten cans of soda per day.

Additionally, the majority of the subjects had previous psychiatric problems, either alcohol or drug abuse and/or mood disorders. Such subjects may use caffeine to self-medicate depression-related lethargy and thus could experience an exaggerated withdrawal. They are more sensitive to the effects of caffeine, and may be prone to experience distress, to find strong emotional states hard to manage, and to act impulsively.

Lastly, the nature of a caffeine withdrawal syndrome is highly variable. For example, two studies examining the cardiovascular effects of abrupt caffeine cessation elicited reports of no symptoms (29, 30). In another study from Johns Hopkins, Suzette Evans and Roland Griffiths noted that twenty-four hours after cessation of high doses of caffeine (900 mg/d), subjects reported no withdrawal (31). Numerous other studies yield inconsistent observations and self-report (32–40).

Clinical Relevance: Should We Be Worried?

The American Psychiatric Association does not recognize caffeine dependence. Only caffeine withdrawal is mentioned in the Diagnostic and Statistical Manual; not as a formal diagnosis but rather as a diagnosis worthy of further study. However, the 5th edition of the manual is under construction—the final text is not expected until at least 2010—and some researchers such as Griffiths claim that dependence is a valid diagnosis and presumably seek its inclusion (41). Nonetheless, clinical indicators of dependence, such as difficulty curtailing or stopping the use of caffeine intake and consumption despite harm, have not been demonstrated let alone replicated (42).

The prevalence of caffeine withdrawal syndrome is unknown. Nonetheless, a clinician should keep in mind that the symptoms can appear in a patient who has abruptly stopped intake of food and fluids. The symptoms can be mistaken for depression or tension headache. Better yet, he can advise patients how to avoid symptoms by tapering caffeine before an elective procedure. If withdrawal has begun and is unpleasant, the clinician can administer caffeine tablets.

Conclusion

Caffeine is a mild stimulant that restores mental alertness or wakefulness during fatigue or drowsiness. Its use is widely acceptable because caffeine is rarely medically harmful (except perhaps in people who have particular physical conditions) and does not lead to social disruption of any kind. Abrupt discontinuation of a moderate amount (generally at least 3 cups of coffee per day; 7 cans of cola soft drink per day) can lead to bothersome symptoms, most notably headache, in some but not all people (43). These effects can be readily avoided by tapering the amount consumed. The only study in which withdrawal-related impairment appeared to be problematic was conducted using a small sample of patients chosen specifically because they believed they were dependent on caffeine and had high rates of remitted substance abuse and mood disorders.

In short, these subjects did not represent a random sample of caffeine drinkers and it is not possible to infer typical discontinuation symptoms from them.

Some have argued that continued caffeine use represents an attempt to suppress low grade withdrawal symptoms such as sleepiness and lethargy. In some moderate users, this is possible; however, in experimental contexts, the phenomenon is too inconsistent to constitute a reliably valid syndrome.

The common-sense use of the term addiction is that regular consumption is irresistible and that it creates problems. Caffeine use does not fit this profile. First, there is no harm to individuals or to society. Second, there is rarely a strong compulsion to use; more correctly the pattern of use can be described as a dedicated habit. Cessation of regular use may result in symptoms such as headache and lethargy. These are easily and reliably reversed by ingestion of caffeine. Avoidance of such symptoms, when they do occur, is easily accomplished by ingesting successively smaller doses of caffeine over about a week-long period.

Thus, caffeine use meets neither the common sense nor the scientific definitions of an addictive substance.

References

1. Center for Science in the Public Interest. CSPI Calls on FDA to Require Health Warnings on Sodas. . . .

2. Caffeine: A Model Drug of Abuse. National Institute on Drug Abuse, Research Monograph 1996; 162:73–75.

3. American Psychiatric Association. Diagnostic and Statistical Manual. 4th ed. 199.

4. American Psychiatric Association. Diagnostic and Statistical Manual. 4th ed. 197.

5. Nehlig A. Does caffeine lead to psychological dependence? Chemtech 1999; 29:30–35.

6. Nehlig A. Are we dependent upon coffee and caffeine? A review on human and animal data. Neuroscience and Biobehavioral Reviews 1999; 23: 563–576.

7. Daly JW. Caffeine has weak reinforcing properties, but with little or no evidence for upward dose adjustment possible because of the adverse effects of higher doses. Drug and Alcohol Dependence 1998; 51:199–206.

8. Juliano LM, Griffiths RR. A critical review of caffeine withdrawal: Empirical validation of symptoms and signs, incidence, severity, and associated features. Psychopharmacology 2004; 176:1–29.

9. Griffiths RR, Evans SM, Heishman SJ, Preston KL, Sannerud CA, Wolf B, Woodson PP. Low dose caffeine physical dependence in humans. Journal of Pharmacology and Experimental Therapeutics 1990; 255:1123–32.

10. Barone JJ, Roberts HR. Caffeine consumption. Food Chem Toxicol 1996; 34:119–129.

11. Dreisbach RH, Pfieffer C. Caffeine-withdrawal headache. The Journal of Laboratory and Clinical Medicine 1943; 28:1212–19.

12. Goldstein A, Kaiser S, Whitby O. Psychotropic effects of caffeine in man, IV: Quantitative and qualitative differences associated with habituation to coffee. Clinical Pharmacology and Therapeutics 1969; 10:489–97.

13. Strain EC, Mumford GK, Silverman K, Griffiths, RR. Caffeine dependence syndrome: Evidence from case histories and experimental evaluations. The Journal of the American Medical Association 1994; 272:1043–48.

14. Oberstar JV, Bernstein GA, Thuras PD. Caffeine use and dependence in adolescents: One year follow-up. Journal of Child & Adolescent Psychopharmacology 2002; 109:85–91.

15. Goldstein A, Kaizer S. Psychotropic effects of caffeine in man: A questionnaire survey of coffee drinking and its effects in a group of housewives. Clinical Pharmacology and Therapeutics 1969; 10:477–88.

16. Hughes JR, Oliveto AH, Liguori A, Carpenter J, Howard, T. Endorsement of DSM-IV dependence criteria among caffeine users. Drug and Alcohol Dependence 1998; 52:99–107.

17. Dews PB, Curtis G, Hanford K, O'Brien, CP. The frequency of caffeine withdrawal in a population-based survey and in a controlled, blinded pilot experiment. Psychopharmacology 1999; 39:1221–32.

18. Kendler KS, Prescott, CA. Caffeine intake, tolerance, and withdrawal in women: A population-based twin study. American Journal of Psychiatry 1999; 156:223–228.

19. Hughes J, Higgins S, Bickel WW, Hunt K, Fenwick JW, Gulliver SB, Mireault GC. Caffeine self-administration, withdrawal, and adverse effects among coffee drinkers. Archives of General Psychiatry 1991; 48:611–17.

20. Silverman K, Evans SM, Strain EC, Griffiths RR. Withdrawal syndrome after the double-blind cessation of caffeine consumption. New England Journal of Medicine 1992; 327:1109–1114.

21. Ibid., 1230.

22. Rosnthal R. Covert communication in the psychological experiment. Psychological Bulletin 1967; 67:356–67.

23. Robertson D, Wade D, Workman R, Woolsey R, Oates JA. Tolerance to the humoral and hemodynamic effects of caffeine in man. Journal of Clinical Investigation 1981; 67:1111–1117.

24. Ammon H, Bieck P, Mandalaz D, Verspohl E. Adaptation of blood pressure to continuous heavy coffee drinking in young volunteers. A double-blind crossover study. British Journal of Clinical Pharmacology 1983; 15:701–706.

25. Evans SM, Griffiths RR. Caffeine tolerance and choice in humans. Psychopharmacology 1992; 108:51–59.

26. Hughes JR, Oliveto AH, Higgins ST. Caffeine self-administration and subjective effects in adolescents. Experimental Clinical Psychopharmacology 1995; 3:364–70.

27. Liguori A, Hughes JR, Oliveto AH. Caffeine self-administration in humans: 1. Efficacy of cola vehicle. Experimental and Clinical Psychopharmacology 1997; 5:286–94.

28. Dews PB, O'Brien CP, Bergman J. Behavioral effects of caffeine: Dependence and related issues. 1998. (Unpublished version)

29. Hughes JR, Oliveto AH, Bickel WK, Higgins ST, Badger GJ. Caffeine self-administration and withdrawal: Incidence, individual differences and interrelationships. Drug and Alcohol Dependence 1993; 32:239–46.

30. Ibid., 614.

31. Juliano LM, Griffiths RR. Is caffeine a drug of dependence? Psychiatric Times 2001; 18(2).

32. Hughes JR, Oliveto AH, Helzer JE, Higgins ST, Bickel WK. Should caffeine abuse, dependence, or withdrawal be added to DSM-IV and ICD-10? American Journal of Psychiatry 1992; 149:33–40.

POSTSCRIPT

Do the Consequences of Caffeine Outweigh Its Benefits?

Although caffeine is commonly consumed by millions of people without much regard to its physical and psychological effects, many studies have questioned its safety. However, other studies have reported very few hazards. The basic question is whether or not people who drink several cups of coffee or other caffeinated beverages daily should be more concerned than they are. Are the claims of caffeine's benefits or hazards exaggerated?

Determining if certain foods or beverages promote disease or have health benefits can be trying because the research is unclear. Sometimes the research is contradictory. Many people become frustrated because quite a few of the things that we eat or drink are suspected of being unhealthy. For example, various reports indicate that the fat in beef can lead to various forms of cancer and heart disease, that we should consume less salt and sugar, that processed foods should be avoided, and that whole milk, butter, and margarine should be reduced or eliminated from our diets. If people paid attention to every report about the harmful effects of the foods and beverages they consumed, then they would not be able to eat much at all. What is the average consumer supposed to do?

A legitimate question is whether or not food studies are worth pursuing because so many of the products that are reportedly bad are enjoyed by millions of people. Some people claim they cannot start their day without caffeine. Caffeine is simply one more example of a commonly used product that has come under scrutiny. In addition, although the research is vast, it is inconclusive. One study, for instance, linked caffeine to pancreatic cancer, only to find later that the culprit was not caffeine but cigarette smoking. Research on caffeine's effects on cancers of the bladder, urinary tract, and kidney has also proven to be inconsistent and inconclusive. Because caffeinated products are consumed by millions of people, it is important to know if its dangers are significant or exaggerated. However, if professional researchers cannot agree about whether a product is safe or harmful, how can the average person know what to believe?

James Thornton from *Men's Health* claims that caffeine may cause dependence because it shares some of the same characteristics of cocaine, alcohol, and nicotine. They state that too much caffeine causes tolerance as well as withdrawal symptoms. Despite their concern, there are not support groups for people addicted to caffeine. Sally Satel counters that caffeine's adverse effects are overstated. Satel indicates that caffeine is a mild stimulant and not a dangerous drug that requires regulation. Furthermore, she indicates that caffeine may have possible benefits such as increased mental alertness and wakefulness.

The effects of caffeine during pregnancy are addressed in "Does Caffeine in Pregnancy Cause Birth Defects?" (*Child Health Alert*, June 2006). Jackie

Berning looks at the implications for athletes using caffeinated products in "Caffeine and Athletic Performance" (*Clinical Reference Systems*, May 24, 2006). Other articles that examine caffeine's psychological and physical effects are "Communicating the Message: Clarifying the Controversies About Caffeine," by Edith H. Hogan, Betsy A. Hornick, and Ann Bouchoux (*Nutrition Today*, January–February 2002); Brian Rowley's "The Buzz on Caffeine: The Latest Research on What's Brewing on This Popular Bodybuilding Pick-Me-Up, and How to Use It Wisely" (*Muscle and Fitness*, March 2002); Eric Metcalf's "Coffee to Go: Research Shows That Caffeine, in the Right Amount, Can Boost Performance Without Harming Your Health" (*Runner's World*, January 2002); and Jeff Novick's "Waking Up to the Effects of Caffeine: How Important Is That Morning Cup of Coffee?" (*Health Science*, Spring 2002).

ISSUE 12

Should School-Age Children with Attention Deficit/Hyperactivity Disorder (ADHD) Be Treated with Ritalin and Other Stimulants?

YES: Michael Fumento, from "Trick Question," *The New Republic* (February 3, 2003)

NO: Lawrence Diller, from "Ritalin and the Growing Influence of Big Pharma," *Psychotherapy Networker* (January/February 2005)

ISSUE SUMMARY

YES: Writer Michael Fumento disputes the idea that Ritalin is over-prescribed. He notes that there are many myths associated with Ritalin. It does not lead to abuse and addiction. Fumento argues that Ritalin is an excellent medication for ADHD. One reason it is not as accepted is because it has been demonized by various groups. It is possible that the drug is underutilized. Fumento contends that more students would benefit from Ritalin and other stimulants.

NO: Pediatrician and family therapist Lawrence Diller contends that Ritalin is overused because diagnosing ADHD is imprecise. Symptoms such as distractibility, inattention, and impulsivity are typical behaviors of many children. Moreover, it is unclear whether the use of Ritalin and other stimulants carries over to long-term academic success. Diller argues that the proliferation in the use of Ritalin stems from its promotion by the pharmaceutical industry.

The number one childhood psychiatric disorder in the United States is attention deficit/hyperactivity disorder, which affects approximately 6 million American school children. ADHD is characterized by inattentiveness, hyperactivity, and impulsivity. Many children are diagnosed as having only attention deficit disorder (ADD), which is ADHD without the hyperactivity. One commonly prescribed drug for ADHD is the stimulant Ritalin (generic name methylphenidate). American children consume 90 percent of all Ritalin produced worldwide. Only a very small percentage of European children are diagnosed with ADHD. Ritalin is therefore much less likely to be prescribed in Europe.

The use of stimulants to treat such behavioral disorders dates back to 1937. The practice of prescribing stimulants for behavioral problems increased dramatically beginning in 1970, when it was estimated that 150,000 American children were taking stimulant medications. It seems paradoxical for physicians to be prescribing a stimulant such as Ritalin for a behavioral disorder that already involves hyperactivity. However, Ritalin appears to be effective with many children, as well as with many adults, who suffer from this condition. Looking at this issue from a broader perspective, one needs to ask whether behavioral problems should be treated as a disease. Also, does Ritalin really address the problem? Or could it be covering up other maladies that otherwise should be treated?

Ritalin enhances the functioning of the brain's reticular activating system, which helps one to focus attention and to filter out extraneous stimuli. The drug has been shown to improve short-term learning. Ritalin also produces adverse effects such as insomnia, headaches, irritability, nausea, dizziness, weight loss, and growth retardation. Psychological dependence may develop, but physical dependence is unlikely. The effects of long-term Ritalin use are unknown.

Since 1990 the number of children receiving Ritalin has increased 500 percent. This large increase in the number of children diagnosed with ADHD may be attributed to a broader application of the criteria for diagnosing ADHD, heightened public awareness, and changes in American educational policy regarding schools' identifying children with the disorder. Some people feel that the increase in prescriptions for Ritalin reflects an increased effort to satisfy the needs of parents whose children exhibit behavioral problems. Ritalin has been referred to as "mother's little helper." Regardless of the reasons for the increase, many people question whether Ritalin is overprescribed and children are overmedicated or whether Ritalin is a miracle drug.

One problem with the increased prevalence of Ritalin prescriptions is that illegal use of the drug has also risen. There are accounts of some parents getting prescriptions for their children and then selling the drugs illegally. On a number of college campuses there are reports of students using Ritalin to get high or to stay awake in order to study. Historically, illegal use of Ritalin has been minimal, although officials of the Drug Enforcement Administration (DEA) are now concerned that its illegal use is proliferating. Problems with its use are unlikely to rival those of cocaine because Ritalin's effects are more moderate than those of cocaine or amphetamines.

The fact is that children now receive prescriptions for Ritalin rather readily. Frequently, parents will pressure their pediatricians into writing the prescriptions. One survey found that almost one-half of all pediatricians spent less than an hour assessing children before prescribing Ritalin. On the other hand, if there is a medication available that would remedy a problem, shouldn't it be prescribed? If a child's academic performance can improve through the use of Ritalin, should that child be denied the drug?

In the following selections, Michael Fumento maintains that ADHD is underdiagnosed in many instances. He asserts that Ritalin's bad reputation arises from many misconceptions regarding the drug. Lawrence Diller questions the effectiveness of Ritalin. He contends that it is overprescribed because of the way the drug is marketed.

YES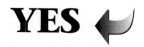

Michael Fumento

Trick Question

It's both right-wing and vast, but it's not a conspiracy. Actually, it's more of an anti-conspiracy. The subject is Attention Deficit Disorder (ADD) and Attention Deficit Hyperactivity Disorder (ADHD), closely related ailments (henceforth referred to in this article simply as ADHD). Rush Limbaugh declares it "may all be a hoax." Francis Fukuyama devotes much of one chapter in his latest book, *Our Posthuman Future*, to attacking Ritalin, the top-selling drug used to treat ADHD. Columnist Thomas Sowell writes, "The motto used to be: 'Boys will be boys.' Today, the motto seems to be: 'Boys will be medicated.'" And Phyllis Schlafly explains, "The old excuse of 'my dog ate my homework' has been replaced by 'I got an ADHD diagnosis.'" A March 2002 article in *The Weekly Standard* summed up the conservative line on ADHD with this rhetorical question: "Are we really prepared to redefine childhood as an ailment, and medicate it until it goes away?"

Many conservative writers, myself included, have criticized the growing tendency to pathologize every undesirable behavior—especially where children are concerned. But, when it comes to ADHD, this skepticism is misplaced. As even a cursory examination of the existing literature or, for that matter, simply talking to the parents and teachers of children with ADHD reveals, the condition is real, and it is treatable. And, if you don't believe me, you can ask conservatives who've come face to face with it themselves.

Myth: ADHD Isn't a Real Disorder

The most common argument against ADHD on the right is also the simplest: It doesn't exist. Conservative columnist Jonah Goldberg thus reduces ADHD to "ants in the pants." Sowell equates it with "being bored and restless." Fukuyama protests, "No one has been able to identify a cause of ADD/ADHD. It is a pathology recognized only by its symptoms." And a conservative columnist approvingly quotes Thomas Armstrong, Ritalin opponent and author, when he declares, "ADD is a disorder that cannot be authoritatively identified in the same way as polio, heart disease or other legitimate illnesses."

The Armstrong and Fukuyama observations are as correct as they are worthless. "Half of all medical disorders are diagnosed without benefit of a

From Michael Fumento, "Trick Question," *The New Republic*. vol. 228, no. 4 (February 3, 2003).

lab procedure," notes Dr. Russell Barkley, professor of psychology at the College of Health Professionals at the Medical University of South Carolina. "Where are the lab tests for headaches and multiple sclerosis and Alzheimer's?" he asks. "Such a standard would virtually eliminate all mental disorders."

Often the best diagnostic test for an ailment is how it responds to treatment. And, by that standard, it doesn't get much more real than ADHD. The beneficial effects of administering stimulants to treat the disorder were first reported in 1937. And today medication for the disorder is reported to be 75 to 90 percent successful. "In our trials it was close to ninety percent," says Dr. Judith Rapoport, director of the National Institute of Mental Health's Child Psychiatry Branch, who has published about 100 papers on ADHD. "This means there was a significant difference in the children's ability to function in the classroom or at home."

Additionally, epidemiological evidence indicates that ADHD has a powerful genetic component. University of Colorado researchers have found that a child whose identical twin has the disorder is between eleven and 18 times more likely to also have it than is a non-twin sibling. For these reasons, the American Psychiatric Association (APA), American Medical Association, American Academy of Pediatrics, American Academy of Child Adolescent Psychiatry, the surgeon general's office, and other major medical bodies all acknowledge ADHD as both real and treatable.

Myth: ADHD Is Part of a Feminist Conspiracy to Make Little Boys More Like Little Girls

Many conservatives observe that boys receive ADHD diagnoses in much higher numbers than girls and find in this evidence of a feminist conspiracy. (This, despite the fact that genetic diseases are often heavily weighted more toward one gender or the other.) Sowell refers to "a growing tendency to treat boyhood as a pathological condition that requires a new three R's—repression, re-education and Ritalin." Fukuyama claims Prozac is being used to give women "more of the alpha-male feeling," while Ritalin is making boys act more like girls. "Together, the two sexes are gently nudged toward that androgynous median personality . . . that is the current politically correct outcome in American society." George Will, while acknowledging that Ritalin can be helpful, nonetheless writes of the "androgyny agenda" of "drugging children because they are behaving like children, especially boy children." Anti-Ritalin conservatives frequently invoke Christina Hoff Sommers's best-selling 2000 book, *The War Against Boys*. You'd never know that the drug isn't mentioned in her book—or why.

"Originally I was going to have a chapter on it," Sommers tells me. "It seemed to fit the thesis." What stopped her was both her survey of the medical literature and her own empirical findings. Of one child she personally came to know she says, "He was utterly miserable, as was everybody around him. The drugs saved his life."

Myth: ADHD Is Part of the Public School System's Efforts to Warehouse Kids Rather Than to Discipline and Teach Them

"No doubt life is easier for teachers when everyone sits around quietly," writes Sowell. Use of ADHD drugs is "in the school's interest to deal with behavioral and discipline problems [because] it's so easy to use Ritalin to make kids compliant: to get them to sit down, shut up, and do what they're told," declares Schlafly. The word "zombies" to describe children under the effects of Ritalin is tossed around more than in a B-grade voodoo movie.

Kerri Houston, national field director for the American Conservative Union and the mother of two ADHD children on medication, agrees with much of the criticism of public schools. "But don't blame ADHD on crummy curricula and lazy teachers," she says. "If you've worked with these children, you know they have a serious neurological problem." In any case, Ritalin, when taken as prescribed, hardly stupefies children. To the extent the medicine works, it simply turns ADHD children into normal children. "ADHD is like having thirty televisions on at one time, and the medicine turns off twenty-nine so you can concentrate on the one," Houston describes. "This zombie stuff drives me nuts! My kids are both as lively and as fun as can be."

Myth: Parents Who Give Their Kids Anti-ADHD Drugs Are Merely Doping Up Problem Children

Limbaugh calls ADHD "the perfect way to explain the inattention, incompetence, and inability of adults to control their kids." Addressing parents directly, he lectures, "It helped you mask your own failings by doping up your children to calm them down."

Such charges blast the parents of ADHD kids into high orbit. That includes my Hudson Institute colleague (and fellow conservative) Mona Charen, the mother of an eleven-year-old with the disorder. "I have two non-ADHD children, so it's not a matter of parenting technique," says Charen. "People without such children have no idea what it's like. I can tell the difference between boyish high spirits and pathological hyperactivity. . . . These kids bounce off the walls. Their lives are chaos; their rooms are chaos. And nothing replaces the drugs."

Barkley and Rapoport say research backs her up. Randomized, controlled studies in both the United States and Sweden have tried combining medication with behavioral interventions and then dropped either one or the other. For those trying to go on without medicine, "the behavioral interventions maintained nothing," Barkley says. Rapoport concurs: "Unfortunately, behavior modification doesn't seem to help with ADHD." (Both doctors are quick to add that ADHD is often accompanied by other disorders that are treatable through behavior modification in tandem with medicine.)

Myth: Ritalin Is "Kiddie Cocaine"

One of the paradoxes of conservative attacks on Ritalin is that the drug is alternately accused of turning children into brain-dead zombies and of making them Mach-speed cocaine junkies. Indeed, Ritalin is widely disparaged as "kiddie cocaine." Writers who have sought to lump the two drugs together include Schlafly, talk-show host and columnist Armstrong Williams, and others whom I hesitate to name because of my long-standing personal relationships with them.

Mary Eberstadt wrote the "authoritative" Ritalin-cocaine piece for the April 1999 issue of *Policy Review*, then owned by the Heritage Foundation. The article, "Why Ritalin Rules," employs the word "cocaine" no fewer than twelve times. Eberstadt quotes from a 1995 Drug Enforcement Agency (DEA) background paper declaring methylphenidate, the active ingredient in Ritalin, "a central nervous system (CNS) stimulant [that] shares many of the pharmacological effects of amphetamine, methamphetamine, and cocaine." Further, it "produces behavioral, psychological, subjective, and reinforcing effects similar to those of d-amphetamine including increases in rating of euphoria, drug liking and activity, and decreases in sedation." Add to this the fact that the Controlled Substances Act lists it as a Schedule II drug, imposing on it the same tight prescription controls as morphine, and Ritalin starts to sound spooky indeed.

What Eberstadt fails to tell readers is that the DEA description concerns methylphenidate *abuse*. It's tautological to say abuse is harmful. According to the DEA, the drugs in question are comparable when "administered the same way at comparable doses." But ADHD stimulants, when taken as prescribed, are neither administered in the same way as cocaine nor at comparable doses. "What really counts," says Barkley, "is the speed with which the drugs enter and clear the brain. With cocaine, because it's snorted, this happens tremendously quickly, giving users the characteristic addictive high." (Ever seen anyone pop a cocaine tablet?) Further, he says, "There's no evidence anywhere in literature of [Ritalin's] addictiveness when taken as prescribed." As to the Schedule II listing, again this is because of the potential for it to fall into the hands of abusers, not because of its effects on persons for whom it is prescribed. Ritalin and the other anti-ADHD drugs, says Barkley, "are the safest drugs in all of psychiatry." (And they may be getting even safer: A new medicine just released called Strattera represents the first true non-stimulant ADHD treatment.)

Indeed, a study just released in the journal *Pediatrics* found that children who take Ritalin or other stimulants to control ADHD cut their risk of future substance abuse by 50 percent compared with untreated ADHD children. The lead author speculated that "by treating ADHD you're reducing the demoralization that accompanies this disorder, and you're improving the academic functioning and well-being of adolescents and young adults during the critical times when substance abuse starts."

Myth: Ritalin Is Overprescribed Across the Country

Some call it "the Ritalin craze." In *The Weekly Standard*, Melana Zyla Vickers informs us that "Ritalin use has exploded," while Eberstadt writes that "Ritalin use more than doubled in the first half of the decade alone, [and] the number of schoolchildren taking the drug may now, by some estimates, be approaching the *4 million mark."*

A report in the January 2003 issue of *Archives of Pediatrics and Adolescent Medicine* did find a large increase in the use of ADHD medicines from 1987 to 1996, an increase that doesn't appear to be slowing. Yet nobody thinks it's a problem that routine screening for high blood pressure has produced a big increase in the use of hypertension medicine. "Today, children suffering from ADHD are simply less likely to slip through the cracks," says Dr. Sally Satel, a psychiatrist, AEI fellow, and author of *PC, M.D.: How Political Correctness Is Corrupting Medicine.*

Satel agrees that some community studies, by the standards laid down in the APA's *Diagnostic and Statistical Manual of Mental Disorders (DSM)*, indicate that ADHD may often be over-diagnosed. On the other hand, she says, additional evidence shows that in some communities ADHD is *under*-diagnosed and *under*-treated. "I'm quite concerned with children who need the medication and aren't getting it," she says.

There *are* tremendous disparities in the percentage of children taking ADHD drugs when comparing small geographical areas. Psychologist Gretchen LeFever, for example, has compared the number of prescriptions in mostly white Virginia Beach, Virginia, with other, more heavily African American areas in the southeastern part of the state. Conservatives have latched onto her higher numbers—20 percent of white fifth-grade boys in Virginia Beach are being treated for ADHD—as evidence that something is horribly wrong. But others, such as Barkley, worry about the lower numbers. According to LeFever's study, black children are only half as likely to get medication as white children. "Black people don't get the care of white people; children of well-off parents get far better care than those of poorer parents," says Barkley.

Myth: States Should Pass Laws That Restrict Schools From Recommending Ritalin

Conservative writers have expressed delight that several states, led by Connecticut, have passed or are considering laws ostensibly protecting students from schools that allegedly pass out Ritalin like candy. Representative Lenny Winkler, lead sponsor of the Connecticut measure, told *Reuters Health*, "If the diagnosis is made, and it's an appropriate diagnosis that Ritalin be used, that's fine. But I have also heard of many families approached by the school system [who are told] that their child cannot attend school if they're not put on Ritalin."

Two attorneys I interviewed who specialize in child-disability issues, including one from the liberal Bazelon Center for Mental Health Law in Washington, D.C., acknowledge that school personnel have in some cases stepped over the line. But legislation can go too far in the other direction by declaring, as Connecticut's law does, that "any school personnel [shall be prohibited] from recommending the use of psychotropic drugs for any child." The law appears to offer an exemption by declaring, "The provisions of this section shall not prohibit *school medical staff* from recommending that a child be evaluated by an appropriate medical practitioner, or prohibit school personnel from consulting with such practitioner, with the consent of the parent or guardian of such child." [Emphasis added.] But of course many, if not most, schools have perhaps one nurse on regular "staff." That nurse will have limited contact with children in the classroom situations where ADHD is likely to be most evident. And, given the wording of the statute, a teacher who believed a student was suffering from ADHD would arguably be prohibited from referring that student to the nurse. Such ambiguity is sure to have a chilling effect on any form of intervention or recommendation by school personnel. Moreover, 20-year special-education veteran Sandra Rief said in an interview with the National Education Association that "recommending medical intervention for a student's behavior could lead to personal liability issues." Teachers, in other words, could be forced to choose between what they think is best for the health of their students and the possible risk of losing not only their jobs but their personal assets as well.

"Certainly it's not within the purview of a school to say kids can't attend if they don't take drugs," says Houston. "On the other hand, certainly teachers should be able to advise parents as to problems and potential solutions. . . . [T]hey may see things parents don't. My own son is an angel at home but was a demon at school."

If the real worry is "take the medicine or take a hike" ultimatums, legislation can be narrowly tailored to prevent them; broad-based gag orders, such as Connecticut's, are a solution that's worse than the problem.

The Conservative Case for ADHD Drugs

There are kernels of truth to every conservative suspicion about ADHD. Who among us has not had lapses of attention? And isn't hyperactivity a normal condition of childhood when compared with deskbound adults? Certainly there are lazy teachers, warehousing schools, androgyny-pushing feminists, and far too many parents unwilling or unable to expend the time and effort to raise their children properly, even by their own standards. Where conservatives go wrong is in making ADHD a scapegoat for frustration over what we perceive as a breakdown in the order of society and family. In a column in *The Boston Herald*, Boston University Chancellor John Silber rails that Ritalin is "a classic example of a cheap fix: low-cost, simple and purely superficial."

Exactly. Like most headaches, ADHD is a neurological problem that can usually be successfully treated with a chemical. Those who recommend or prescribe ADHD medicines do not, as *The Weekly Standard* put it, see them as "discipline in pill-form." They see them as pills.

In fact, it can be argued that the use of those pills, far from being liable for or symptomatic of the Decline of the West, reflects and reinforces conservative values. For one thing, they increase personal responsibility by removing an excuse that children (and their parents) can fall back on to explain misbehavior and poor performance. "Too many psychologists and psychiatrists focus on allowing patients to justify to themselves their troubling behavior," says Satel. "But something like Ritalin actually encourages greater autonomy because you're treating a compulsion to behave in a certain way. Also, by treating ADHD, you remove an opportunity to explain away bad behavior."

Moreover, unlike liberals, who tend to downplay differences between the sexes, conservatives are inclined to believe that there are substantial physiological differences—differences such as boys' greater tendency to suffer ADHD. "Conservatives celebrate the physiological differences between boys and girls and eschew the radical-feminist notion that gender differences are created by societal pressures," says Houston regarding the fuss over the boy-girl disparity among ADHD diagnoses. "ADHD is no exception."

But, however compatible conservatism may be with taking ADHD seriously, the truth is that most conservatives remain skeptics. "I'm sure I would have been one of those smug conservatives saying it's a made-up disease," admits Charen, "if I hadn't found out the hard way." Here's hoping other conservatives find an easier route to accepting the truth.

Lawrence Diller 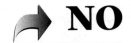 **NO**

Ritalin and the Growing Influence of Big Pharma

Nadine Lambert doesn't look the part of a radical firebrand, bent on undermining the pharmaceutical industry and sticking it to the power elite of the American child-psychiatry establishment. A pleasant, thoughtful, gray-haired academic, she's been a research psychologist in the department of education at the University of California at Berkeley since 1973, and now heads the department's School Psychology program. Lambert never planned on becoming the enfant terrible of the world of attention deficit/hyperactivity disorder (AD/HD) treatment. Her work in the field began quietly and methodically in the 1970s, when she became involved in a larger effort to develop special-education services for school-aged children. The original purpose of what became her life's work was a straightforward prevalence study to determine the relative number of handicapped and/or hyperactive children in San Francisco's East Bay area. From the mid-1970s to 1990, she regularly published scientific articles describing an ambitious research project that anticipated following these children to adulthood.

Then, in 1998, this dignified, middle-aged professor of educational psychology suddenly became the center of an academic firestorm. At the prestigious National Institutes of Health Consensus Conference on AD/HD, she announced the results of a study suggesting that use of Ritalin, one of the most routinely prescribed drugs for children in America, might contribute to later drug abuse. Her study of nearly 400 children with AD/HD showed that by the time children treated with Ritalin reached their mid-twenties, they had double the rates of cocaine abuse and cigarette smoking as young adults who hadn't taken it in childhood.

If Lambert had lobbed a grenade into her audience of child-psychiatry researchers, her report couldn't have been more explosive. For proponents of Ritalin and other psychiatric drugs for children—most of the attendees at the meeting—Lambert's findings had nightmarish implications. What if outraged parents now began to flood their offices, demanding to have their children taken off these medications and given alternative treatment? Perhaps even worse, if Lambert was right about Ritalin's dark potential, it meant that the

From *Psychotherapy Networker*, vol. 29, no. 1, January/February 2005, pp. 56+. Copyright © 2005 by Psychotherapy Networker. Reprinted by permission.

child-psychiatry establishment was wrong. Seriously wrong. Wrong all along. For the AD/HD researchers who'd long put their faith in Ritalin—even bet their careers on it—this was truly scary stuff.

Their fears were well-founded. The media picked up on the story and loudly questioned, as it had several times before, whether Ritalin was being overprescribed for children with AD/HD. But the tight-knit community of child-psychiatry researchers and academics wasn't about to roll over in defeat. Instead, within a year, child psychiatrist Joseph Biederman of Harvard Medical School, one of the country's most influential AD/HD researchers and a leading advocate for Ritalin use, announced the findings of a rebuttal study. His new research showed that kids prescribed Ritalin actually had an 85 percent lower rate of substance abuse four years later. The study further claimed that the medicated children were actually "protected" from engaging in later drug abuse.

Two subsequent studies by leading researchers Timothy Wilens, a long-time member of the Biederman team, and Russell Barkley, a professor of psychology at the University of South Carolina in Charleston and the world's leading theorist and arbiter of AD/HD, also took aim at the Lambert study. These studies differed in design from Lambert's and, as we'll see, also had numerous limitations. Nevertheless, the media obligingly switched course, now extensively touting the "protective benefits" of Ritalin. The pharmaceutical companies that manufacture Ritalin and similar stimulants reprinted the Biederman and Wilens papers and sent them to every pediatrician and child psychiatrist in the country.

Since this imbroglio, the National Institute of Drug Abuse (NIDA) has refused funding to Nadine Lambert, either to conduct further follow-up on her subjects or to analyze her current data more closely. Recently, a government official privately told her that her latest grant proposals have been harshly criticized during the peer-review process. Since the publication of her original study results, no major U.S. journal has been willing to publish either her new research or a fresh analysis of old research to rebut her critics. She's been dismissed in print by at least one prominent critic as an "outlier on the far end of a bell-shaped curve"—polite academese for a loose cannon, whose research is so fringy and unsubstantial that it can safely be ignored. But is it more appropriate to see her as the canary in the coal mine, sounding a warning about the unacknowledged dangers of one of the most widely prescribed drugs for children in America?

Do All Children Have AD/HD?

No one knows precisely how many children in the United States have AD/HD. As with all psychiatric conditions, there's no definitive test for AD/HD—no blood test or brain scan or even standardized psychological assessment that can unequivocally determine whether a particular child is or isn't affected. Much of the controversy roiling around AD/HD stems from the problem of diagnosis. In its milder forms, the disorder's symptoms of inattention, distractibility, impulsivity, and hyperactivity can look very much like the normal behavior of an active child.

Whatever the problems in diagnosis, Ritalin, along with newer sibling stimulants, have become the overwhelming treatment of choice for children who are "diagnosed" with AD/HD. Currently, nearly one in ten 11-year-old American boys takes some kind of stimulant medication—a classification that included Dexedrine or amphetamine and now includes drugs like Ritalin, Adderall, and Concerta. All told, the United States uses 80 percent of the world's stimulants. Critics of this trend point out that no other country addresses the behavior and school performance of children with such strong emphasis on psychiatric diagnosis and drug treatment.

But why *not* use these stimulants, when they seem to work wonders? This is the standard response of Ritalin's champions, who include legions of grateful parents and teachers across the country. Often, within minutes of taking the first dose, hyperactive Johnny metamorphoses into a different child—steady, focused, and compliant. Skills such as handwriting and following directions improve instantly. Indeed, thousands of studies, mostly of school-aged boys, prove the effectiveness of stimulants in helping children perform better at school and at home.

Ever since the first published report on the use of stimulants by kids in 1937, medical pundits have argued that drugs such as Ritalin operate differently in the brains of hyperactive kids as compared to normal kids—because the AD/HD brain is different. What else could explain how a stimulant could actually calm a child, rather than rev him up even more? It's easy to understand why the assertion that Ritalin calms only hyperactive kids carries so much weight in popular discourse.

But this claim is a myth. In fact, Ritalin and other stimulants improve *anybody's* ability to focus and pay attention to boring and difficult tasks. Studies from the National Institute of Mental Health in the 1970s proved that low-dose stimulants have the same effect on all children (and adults as well), whether or not they've been diagnosed with AD/HD. The hyperactive child who slows down on Ritalin appears calmer to parents and teachers, demonstrating that the Ritalin is working. Because the drug works so well, they conclude that the child must have AD/HD. But given Ritalin's universal effects on all children, by this logic it would follow that all children have AD/HD!

Understanding Ritalin's Effects

Ritalin may help everyone focus, but does it truly calm everyone? In fact, the "calming" effect of the drug on hyperactive kids is actually the result of their becoming more methodical in their performance, which, in turn, moderates their activity level. Indeed, normally active children also become less active when they're given the same low doses of stimulants as AD/HD kids get, though the activity slowdown in normal kids is less dramatic. Similarly, when AD/HD children take higher doses of stimulant medications, they react just like other children: both groups become overactive and agitated. Both normal kids and AD/HD kids complain that they feel "nervous" or "weird" on higher doses of stimulants.

Still, Ritalin undeniably helps hyperactive children. Surely, this pharmaceutical leg-up gives these youngsters a much better chance at achieving success as they grow into adolescence and adulthood. But, here's the rub. After nearly seven decades of prescribing Ritalin, Adderall, and similar stimulants for millions of children, we still don't know whether these drugs boost kids' chances for success later in life. Given the critical importance of this issue, why are we still so steeped in ignorance?

Part of the reason lies in the daunting challenge of systematically tracking children for a decade or more. In addition, since stimulants were introduced as a treatment for hyperactivity nearly seventy years ago, diagnostic categories for hyperactivity have changed dramatically. So it isn't clear that earlier studies of the impact of stimulants on hyperactivity examined the same population that today's researchers would be observing. Furthermore, studies done in the '60s and '70s were "naturalistic"—the children were separated into treated and control groups, based upon their families' choice of treatments—and not randomized, so they're vulnerable to being challenged by today's more stringent criteria.

Finally, while virtually all children taking stimulants in the '70s and '80s stopped taking them at around age 13, when hyperactivity tends to fade on its own, current standards of care mandate that many adolescents continue to take these meds through high school, and even into college. Indeed, the only new long-term-prospective randomized study in the United States lasted just 14 months, because doctors felt ethically bound not to deny AD/HD children access to stimulants required by the American standard of care. So the disappointing outcomes of earlier studies are easily dismissed by medication proponents, who maintain that outmoded definitions of AD/HD, changing standards of care, and lack of randomization render the older studies useless.

Still, a handful of AD/HD treatment studies were published in the late 1980s and early 1990s, tracking children prospectively from school age into young adulthood. These studies also showed disappointing results for Ritalin: children treated with stimulants did no better (in fact, they did slightly worse) than AD/HD kids who hadn't taken Ritalin. In this older research, all three groups of AD/HD kids studied—those getting only medication, those getting only family counseling and special education, and those getting a combined treatment of drug and nondrug interventions—did far worse than normal kids, as gauged by rates of high-school graduation, delinquency, and drug use. The most rigorous study, done by psychiatrist James Satterfield and his wife Breena Satterfield, a social worker, concluded that the medication-only children did the poorest and the combined-treatment group did the best at 10- and 15-year follow-ups.

This isn't to say that stimulants do no good whatsoever. Based on my 27 years of practice, I personally suspect that stimulants can help a kid get through the most difficult years when he's in mandatory schooling. But I believe that long-term outcomes are far more affected by learning problems and emotional problems that have roots in family and community factors.

Researchers and practitioners alike have long been concerned that Ritalin use in childhood could lead to later drug abuse. Lambert didn't invent this issue to annoy the psychiatric cognoscenti or frighten the general public.

Ritalin is a very powerful agent, classified by the U.S. Drug Enforcement Administration as a Schedule II drug, the strictest category of potentially abusable drugs that doctors are legally allowed to prescribe. Ritalin is a stimulant that's similar in molecular structure to "speed" (amphetamine), "crank" (methamphetamine) and crack cocaine—all drugs with devastating addictive potential. Laboratory animals, when given the choice of pressing a lever that sends a pellet of food into the cage or one that delivers a methylphenidate (Ritalin and Concerta) or amphetamine (Adderall and Dexedrine), quickly learn to choose the drug lever, ultimately starving to death and exhibiting bizarre behavior along the way.

Studies in normal adult volunteers taking one oral dose of Ritalin show very early signs of addiction when given a second dose of the drug several weeks later. Measures of eye-blink and heart rates—subtle markers of addiction—rise in adult humans who take the second dose of medication. As disturbing as these studies are, they haven't generated similar research on kids who take stimulants. No one had quite so clearly and bluntly linked this basic science of stimulant addiction to the real world of hyperactive kids and teens until Lambert announced her findings at the 1998 NIH Consensus Conference on AD/HD.

Why, then, has Lambert's study been so roundly dismissed? Her critics contend that her work is simply not up to snuff scientifically, pointing to her study's lack of randomization and the questionable validity of her control groups. Even though her naturalistic approach was state of the art for that time, there's no question that Lambert's study subjects weren't randomized into drug and nondrug treatment groups. Thus, despite her prodigious efforts to document the similarities between the two groups, it's quite possible that the sicker and more severely affected kids received Ritalin, while children with milder AD/HD didn't. If so, it's logical to conclude that the kids who received the drug might have gone on to have drug-abuse and other problems later in life simply because they were more troubled to begin with. This well-known study effect, called the "severity bias," could have tilted the scales toward negative outcomes for the drug-treated group. This failure to randomize has also plagued other older studies showing poorer outcomes for young people who took Ritalin as kids.

Lambert's findings have also been criticized for failing to take into account another childhood problem—conduct disorder. This disorder involves a pattern of delinquent behavior such as stealing, cheating, vandalism, physical violence, truancy, trouble with the law, and cruelty to animals. In his published critique, Russell Barkley suggests that the kids who took Ritalin in Lambert's study and showed higher levels of substance abuse later on actually suffered from conduct disorder in addition to hyperactivity. In other words, the medicated kids abused drugs later on not because the Ritalin had sensitized them to other drugs, but because their conduct disorder (which made it more likely that Ritalin would be prescribed for them in the first place) made them more susceptible to substance abuse. Lambert retorts that Barkley's reasoning is circular in that kids who abuse drugs invariably also have conduct disorder, regardless of what originally contributed to their drug use.

While Lambert's study is certainly imperfect, what's been ignored in most discussions of her work is that the studies cited as rebuttals to her conclusions are susceptible to the same kinds of criticisms. Both Biederman's study and Wilens's metanalysis were retrospective investigations that were also marred by nonrandomization and inadequate controls. Moreover, Biederman's conclusions were based on subjects still in their teens who were still taking medication, while Lambert tracked her subjects' drug use into their mid-twenties. Even Barkley's study wasn't randomized.

In fact, a dirty little secret of psychology research is that most studies are plagued with methodological difficulties, because it's still notoriously difficult to institute unimpeachable controls. "The field is a quagmire," observes long-time AD/HD research psychologist Stephen Hinshaw, also of the University of California at Berkeley. "No study can be absolutely free of the possibility of bias or some other unknown variable in the assignment of controls."

So if the studies that are intended to put the definitive kibosh on Lambert's work are similarly flawed, why can't she get the support she needs to conduct further research on the issues raised? After all, her research was considered vital enough to be funded for 20 years by the NIDA and the California Tobacco-Related Disease Research Program. In addition, one would think that her conclusions are dramatic and disquieting enough to prompt other researchers to reexamine them, utilizing more careful controls and randomization procedures. Why is this unlikely to happen, at least in the United States?

The answer, I believe, has much to do with the politics of American psychiatry and the influence of the multibillion-dollar psychopharmacology industry on scientific debates within the field. Joseph Biederman and his colleagues at the Pediatric Psychopharmacology Clinic of the Massachusetts General Hospital, along with Russell Barkley and other psychiatric specialists in AD/HD, are at the center of a seismic shift in the direction of American psychiatry. During the last 20 years, the field has largely reversed course in its thinking about children's behavioral problems, from assigning causation to the child's family and environment to assigning causation to the child's presumably malfunctioning brain. Certainly, once AD/HD children begin taking stimulants, the immediate and often global improvement in their behavior reinforces this brain-based line of reasoning, though it be logically flawed. Aspirin improves a headache, but no one says that a headache is caused by an "aspirin-deficiency."

This erroneous belief in biological causality is hugely profitable for the pharmaceutical industry, which now earns more than a billion dollars a year from sales of Ritalin, Adderall, and other AD/HD drugs. The runaway popularity of stimulants depends, in turn, upon the benediction they receive from leading academic experts, who receive major research funding from more than a half dozen of the world's largest pharmaceutical companies. These days, virtually all leading psychiatry researchers are biologically oriented scientists, who accept funding from pharmaceutical companies. Indeed, drug companies now supply 60 percent of all funding for biomedical research, and that percentage is undoubtedly much higher in the field of psychiatry.

Still, many doctors, both in and out of academic medicine, are troubled by the depth of the clinical research/drug industry connection. In 2001, Marcia Angell, then editor of the *New England Journal of Medicine,* wrote a stinging editorial entitled "Is Academic Medicine for Sale?" Charging that academic medical institutions are "growing increasingly beholden to industry," she pointed to the potentially corrupting ties binding medical research institutions to drug companies. "There is now considerable evidence that researchers with ties to drug companies are indeed more likely to report results that are favorable to the products of those companies than researchers without such ties," she wrote. "When the boundaries between industry and academic medicine become as blurred as they now are, the business goals of industry influence the mission of the medical schools in multiple ways."

From Therapy to Psychopharmacology

The truth is that we don't yet know whether Ritalin use makes kids more likely to abuse drugs later on, whether it protects them from later substance abuse, or whether it does neither. What we have are two sets of data, both significantly flawed. One set is accorded great weight and significance by the scientific powers-that-be, while the other is energetically trashed. The data in line with the most powerful economic interests and most influential academic voices are extolled as good science—even "truth"—while the other data are consigned to the dust heap of scientific irrelevance and the author placed under the research equivalent of house arrest.

We may never learn for certain whether Ritalin contributes to, or protects against, later drug abuse—at least not in any study from the United States. Ritalin, Adderall, and similar drugs have become such accepted treatments for AD/HD that it's now considered unethical to withhold them in any randomized, double-blind trial. "Treatment with stimulants has become the standard of care in this country," says University of California at Berkeley psychologist Hinshaw. "Running a study that withheld stimulants for a long time—the 10 or 15 years needed to check for later drug abuse—would be medically unethical in the United States."

But in Western Europe, where doctors don't assign an AD/HD diagnosis to as wide a swath of behaviors as do American physicians and are less apt to use stimulants to treat the disorder, there may still be opportunities to study the question. "The Germans are doing such a study right now," says Hinshaw, "but it'll take years, or we may never know."

Meanwhile, Lambert, who's now spent nearly 30 years of her life following and analyzing her group of AD/HD kids, tries to stay focused and productive. She continues to seek funding sources, but from philanthropic organizations rather than institutional medicine. She also continues to teach at Berkeley and to write rebuttals to the criticisms of her work, hoping to find a larger forum. "I'm just trying to get answers—it's what keeps me going," she says. But without funds to pursue her long-term AD/HD project, she doubts that she can continue the work. "I'm now aiming for a foreign journal like the *Canadian Journal of Psychiatry,*" she says. "I doubt that I can get a fair review in this country."

Even though I think Lambert's study has real merit and should be extended, I personally believe that neither the biologically sensitizing nor the protective potential of Ritalin is as important an influence on future drug abuse as environmental factors. Having prescribed Ritalin for 25 years—and having seen its short-term benefits a thousand times—my own observation suggests that a child's family and neighborhood are more important than the use of any medication in predicting whether a child will later abuse drugs. If I believed that Ritalin had a strong sensitizing impact on drug abuse, I'd never have prescribed it to most of the children I've treated with the drug.

Ironically though, the focus on Ritalin as hero or villain suggests just how far the debate has shifted over the years from the influence of the external environment on kids' lives to the internal environment of their individual brain chemistry. As a field, our attention has become increasingly diverted from the roles of family conflict, community breakdown, and poverty as the overriding factors leading to substance abuse in young people. As passions for and against drug interventions grow, they tend to drown out discussion of nonpharmaceutical interventions for children—family therapy, behavioral interventions, school-based and community-based programs—that have a proven record of effectiveness in decreasing drug abuse. These days, it isn't just the power and money of Big Pharma setting the agenda: it's also our own professional culture, which seems more and more enthralled by the biochemical fix.

POSTSCRIPT

Should School-Age Children with Attention Deficit/Hyperactivity Disorder (ADHD) Be Treated with Ritalin and Other Stimulants?

To satisfy their own emotional needs, many parents push their physicians into diagnosing their children with ADHD. Some of these parents believe that their children will benefit if they are labeled ADHD. The pressure for children to do well academically in order to get into the right college and graduate school is intense. Some parents feel that if their children are diagnosed with ADHD, then they may be provided special circumstances or allowances such as additional time when taking college entrance examinations. Some parents also realize that if their children are identified as having ADHD, then their children will be eligible for extra services in school. In some instances, the only way to receive such extra help is to be labeled with a disorder. Also, some teachers favor the use of Ritalin and other stimulants to control students' behavior. During the last few years, there has been increasing emphasis on controlling school budgets. The result is larger class sizes and higher student-to-teacher ratios. Thus, it should not be surprising that many teachers welcome the calming effect of Ritalin and other stimulants on students whose hyperactivity is disruptive to the class.

Whether or not drug therapy should be applied to behavioral problems raises another concern. What is the message that children are receiving about the role of drugs in society? Perhaps children will generalize the benefits of using legal drugs like Ritalin to remedy life's problems to using alcohol or illegal drugs to deal with other problems that they may be experiencing. Children may find that it is easier to drink alcohol or ingest a pill rather than to put the time and effort into resolving personal problems. For many adults, drugs seem to represent a shortcut to correcting life's difficulties. Through its reliance on drugs, is American society creating a wrong impression for its children, an illusion of believing that there is a pill for every ill?

When to prescribe Ritalin and other stimulants for children also places physicians in a quandary. They may see the benefit of helping students function more effectively in school. However, are physicians who readily prescribe Ritalin unintentionally promoting an antihumanistic, competitive environment in which performance matters regardless of cost? On the other hand, is it the place of physicians to dictate to parents what is best for their children? Should physicians acquiesce to the desires of parents who want to place their children on these drugs? In the final analysis, will the increase in prescriptions for Ritalin and other stimulants result in benefits for the child, for the parents, and for society?

Two articles that question the validity of Attention Deficit/Hyperactivity Disorder are Rachel Ragg's "School Uniformity" (*Ecologist,* November 2006) and Jonathon Leo's "Broken Brains or Flawed Studies? A Critical Review of ADHD Neuroimaging Research" (*The Journal of Mind and Behavior,* Winter 2003). The effects of Ritalin are examined in "ADHD: A Research Study," by Judy Broadway in *Education Today* (2006). How Ritalin functions is reviewed in "Methylphenidate: Mechanism of Action and Clinical Update" by Lawrence Scahill, Deirdre Carroll, and Kathleen Burke (*Journal of Child and Adolescent Psychiatric Nursing,* April–June 2004). Jeff Evans reports on the role of stimulants in school performance in "ADHD Medications Affect School Attendance and Substance Abuse: Retrospective Studies" (*Family Practice News,* April 1, 2004).

ISSUE 13

Do Consumers Benefit When Prescription Drugs Are Advertised?

YES: Merrill Matthews Jr., from "Advertising Drugs Is Good for Patients," *Consumers Research Magazine* (August 2001)

NO: Robert Langreth and Matthew Herper, from "Pill Pushers: How the Drug Industry Abandoned Science for Salesmanship," *Forbes* (May 8, 2006)

ISSUE SUMMARY

YES: Merrill Matthews, a health policy advisor with the American Legislative Exchange Council, argues that the advertising of prescription drugs directly to consumers will result in better-informed consumers. Additionally, communication between doctors and patients may improve because patients will be more knowledgeable about drugs.

NO: Writers Robert Langreth and Matthew Herper contend that the pharmaceutical industry spends much more money promoting drugs that are similar to existing drugs rather than researching how to develop new and better drugs. The top ten pharmaceutical companies spend twice as much money on marketing and administration as on research. Too often, claim Langreth and Herper, the excessive marketing of drugs creates demand even when the demand is not present.

One of the most lucrative businesses in the world today is the prescription drug business. Billions of dollars are spent every year for prescription drugs in the United States alone. But, the *only* way for consumers to obtain a prescribed drug is through a physician. In the early 1980s drug companies in the United States began to advertise directly to the consumer. It is logical for drug companies to advertise to physicians because they are responsible for writing prescriptions. However, is it logical for pharmaceutical manufacturers to advertise their drugs directly to consumers? Are consumers capable of making informed, rational decisions regarding their pharmaceutical needs? Do consumers derive any benefits when prescription drugs are advertised?

An increasing number of individuals are assuming more responsibility for their own health care. In the United States, over one-third of all prescriptions are written at the request of patients. Also, many patients do not take their doctors' prescriptions to pharmacies to be filled. Both of these scenarios raise the question of whether consumers are adequately educated to make decisions pertaining to their pharmaceutical needs or to assess risks associated with prescription drugs. Evidence suggests that many are not. Prescription drugs, for example, cause more worksite accidents than illegal drugs do.

Some commentators, however, argue that there are several advantages to directly advertising drugs to consumers. One advantage is that direct advertisements make consumers better informed about the benefits and risks of certain drugs. For example, it is not unusual for a person to experience side effects from a drug without knowing that the drug was responsible for the side effects. Advertisements can provide this information. Another advantage for consumers is that they may learn about medications that they might not have known existed. Furthermore, advertising lowers the cost of prescription drugs because consumers are able to ask their physicians to prescribe less expensive drugs than the physician might be inclined to recommend. Finally, prescription drug advertising allows consumers to become more involved in choosing the medications that they need or want.

Critics argue that there are a number of risks associated with the direct advertising of prescription drugs. One concern is with the content of drug advertisements. Consumers may not pay enough attention to information detailing a drug's adverse effects. Also, sometimes a drug's benefits are exaggerated. Another problem is that there are many instances in which drugs that have been approved by the Food and Drug Administration (FDA) for one purpose have been promoted for other purposes. Is the average consumer capable of understanding the purposes of the drugs that are being advertised?

Opponents of direct-to-consumer drug advertisements express concern with the way in which the information in the advertisements is presented. Promotions for drugs that appear as objective reports are often actually slick publicity material. In such promotions, medical experts are shown providing testimony regarding a particular drug. Many consumers may not be aware that these physicians have financial ties to the pharmaceutical companies. Celebrities—in whom the public often places its trust despite their lack of medical expertise—are used to promote drugs also. Finally, the cost of the drugs advertised, a major concern to most consumers, is seldom mentioned in the advertisements.

In the following selections, Merrill Matthews argues that the marketing of prescription drugs helps consumers because they lower the cost of drugs and they effectively inform consumers about the benefits of new drugs. Robert Langreth and Matthew Herper do not believe that consumers gain from prescription drug advertising. Pharmaceutical companies are more interested in promoting drugs than developing drugs that are medically beneficial.

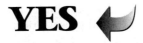

YES

Merrill Matthews, Jr.

Advertising Drugs Is
Good for Patients

Many health policy experts believe that direct-to-consumer (DTC) advertising by pharmaceutical companies misinforms gullible consumers, encourages drug overconsumption, increases health care costs, strains doctor-patient relationships and undermines the quality of patient care. For example:

- The American College of Physicians and the American Society of Internal Medicine, in a joint policy statement, wrote: "We are concerned that advertising will result in increased consumption of these highly advertised drugs; though their use may be neither appropriate nor necessary." The organizations also wrote: "Many times, physicians will give in to the demand and when they don't, often patients will 'doctor shop' until they find a physician who will prescribe the medication."
- Sen. Tim Johnson (D-S.D.) also questioned the growth of DTC. "Is the information value worth the yearly increases in drug costs that advertising inevitably causes? Are patients getting the best individual choices of medicines or just the best advertised ones? Are generic drugs, often an excellent cost-effective alternative, getting equal consideration?"
- Finally, members of the Committee on Bioethical Issues of the Medical Society of the State of New York wrote: "Direct drug advertising provides no real benefit to patients, is potentially harmful, and is costly. We therefore urge the U.S. Food and Drug Administration to review and strengthen its policies concerning this practice."

Are these criticisms accurate? In some cases, yes. For example, DTC advertising does encourage more drug consumption—which can lower some health care costs when drug therapy precludes the need for other, more expensive therapies.

However, the above-mentioned concerns largely are misdirected. They focus on the evolving pharmaceutical marketplace when in fact the whole health care system is in transition. And direct-to-consumer pharmaceutical ads are a response to the transitional process, not the cause of it.

The U.S. health care system has reached a cross-roads, and the direction the country takes will determine the type, availability and quality of care for years to come. Pharmaceutical advertising pre-supposes that health care consumers can make choices for themselves—and that's the type of health care system people want. Those who have no choice in health care have no need of advertising.

A health care system in transition   America is in the forefront of the information economy. One of the hallmarks of this new economy is access to much more information by many more people. Patients have much greater access to health care information, especially through the Internet and through advertising. Indeed, the most important change occurring in the health care system is this access to information. According to health care consultant Lyn Siegel:

- About 25% of on-line information is related to health;
- More than 50% of adults who go on the Web use it for health care information; and
- More than 26% of people who go to disease-oriented Web sites ask their doctors for a specific brand of medication. Thus information is driving the transition to a patient-directed health care system.

A generation ago physicians were the possessors of all medical information. Patients went to physicians and accepted evaluations and diagnoses almost without question. Patients who want second opinions and physicians who gracefully accede to their wishes are relatively new phenomena.

In a physician-directed health care system:

- Physicians have all the extant medical knowledge and skills;
- Physicians perform all patient examinations;
- Patients accept their physicians' diagnoses and insurers pay for the care;
- Hospitals admit patients based on physicians' orders and pharmacists fill the prescriptions; and,
- Drug and medical device companies market to the physicians who control all access to patients.

In this model, no one reaches patients without a physician's consent. The physician-directed system worked well for several decades. The vast majority of working Americans had good health insurance benefits that protected them, their families and their assets from catastrophic losses due to a major accident or illness. Third-party payers were generous in their reimbursement policies while doctors and hospitals could do only so much. Whatever doctors recommended, insurers covered.

Once the amazing medical advances of the 1970s and 1980s began to appear, health care costs began to soar. Insured workers and seniors on Medicare were insulated from the cost of care, and so had little incentive to control health care spending. Employers and the government, who paid most health care bills, desperately sought cost-control mechanisms. That's when managed care came in. Its proponents claimed that managed care could lower the cost of comprehensive health care coverage, in part by controlling utilization. While the arguments continue over how well managed care controlled costs and whether it sacrificed quality to achieve savings, the growth in health care spending did slow during the 1990s. Recently, though, the rate of growth has escalated and engendered fears of more double-digit increases in health care spending.

Meanwhile, the expansion of managed care helped to undermine the physician-directed health care system. Insurers and employers gained the power to question and even override doctors' decisions, which put doctors in an uncomfortable and unsatisfactory position.

Patients also reacted negatively. Many believed their doctors were willing or able to give them only the level of care their insurers would cover. This distrust undermined the doctor-patient relationship and spurred patients to seek health care information directly, rather than from their doctor or insurer. Thus health care consumers began to exploit the information economy.

Increasingly, patients are entering the health care system armed with information—and sometimes misinformation. They may not know how to practice medicine, but many know something about their medical condition and the options available to them. And they raise questions if the doctor follows a different path from the one they expect.

As Dr. Thomas R. Reardon, past president of the American Medical Association, has insightfully noted: "Patients themselves are also creating a strong impetus for change. Disillusioned by restrictions on coverage and care, they are increasingly demanding choice of physician, hospital, and even type of health plan. More than ever, patients see physicians as the essential point of trust in a changing system, and demand choice and stability in their vital relationships with their doctors. . . . At the same time, patients themselves are becoming better educated, not only about insurance options but also about medical treatments. Today, thanks to the Internet, trends in product advertising, and the massive proliferation of medical information, patients are better equipped to take part in their care than ever before. Rather than simplifying the physician's job, however, this increased patient knowledge base is creating new challenges."

We are transitioning toward a patient-directed health care system—if the federal and state governments don't intervene—in which all of the components cater to the patient, rather than the physician. It is impossible to overstate the magnitude of the change. We aren't there yet, but the system is moving—or being pulled—in that direction.

In the new system, insurers and employers, doctors and other health care providers, researchers and pharmaceutical companies will view the patient rather than the provider as the primary consumer. And in the new system:

- Insurers will have to create products that consumers rather than their employers want;
- Doctors will have to please their patients rather than insurers, reinvigorating the weakened doctor-patient relationship; and
- Pharmaceutical and medical device companies increasingly will market directly to the consumers who use their products.

Because health care consumers are becoming better informed, they will, on balance, make better decisions. And they will want even more information. But how do companies and providers reach individuals with the information the latter want and need? One way is through advertising.

Every Sunday newspaper is filled with advertising flyers for department stores, office products, computers, cars, food and clothing. Yet people don't complain they can't afford food because all the grocery stores advertise. And does anyone really think they would be able to get a computer for less money if none of the computer manufacturers and retail outlets advertised?

In virtually every sector of the economy, those with products or services to sell must get information to those who will buy. Advertising is the vehicle for getting information to the intended customers. It tells prospective customers about product availability, quality and cost—the information those prospects need in order to make comparisons. While some people may consider it annoying if they are not looking for a particular product, those in the market for the advertised item often will pay close attention to ads and other marketing techniques such as direct mail and communication from sales representatives.

The general assumption is that advertising raises the costs of products. This assumption recently has entered the debate over the impact of drug companies' advertisements aimed at consumers. But advertising can—and should— lower costs. For example, according to economist John Calfee of the American Enterprise Institute:

> A pioneering study compared the prices of eye-glasses in states that either permitted or restricted advertising for eyeglass services. Prices were about 25% higher where advertising was restricted or banned (and prices were highest for the least educated consumers). A later study by the Federal Trade Commission (FTC) staff showed that product quality in the states without advertising was not higher despite the higher prices. Studies also found higher prices in the absence of advertising for such diverse products as gasoline, prescription drugs and legal services.

How is it that advertising can actually lower prices? Most products have certain fixed costs, plus some variable costs. While variable costs are imputed to each item produced, fixed costs are divided by the number of products sold. The goal of advertising is to expand consumer awareness and increase sales. The more items sold, the greater the economies of scale and the lower the fixed costs per consumer.

Holman Jenkins of the Wall Street Journal explains the rationale: "The media also complain about advertising as if this were an extra cost borne by drug users. Drug companies spend on advertising because it's profitable—it pays for itself by generating additional sales, allowing development costs to be spread over a larger number of users. The average price to each user is lower."

In the absence of competition, advertising might raise prices. But in the absence of competition, vendors would likely raise prices whether they advertised or not. Competition keeps manufacturers from charging as much as they would like, except in cases where there is an unusually high demand for a particular product (as when everyone decides they want a Cabbage Patch doll, a Tickle Me Elmo or a Furby for Christmas). Thus, even when advertising doesn't increase sales, vendors cannot add the cost on top of the product if there are other competitively priced alternatives on the market.

DTC ads and the health care system   Putting information in the hands of consumers who didn't have that information before is a revolutionary business—and revolutions engender change. Critics know this and raise concerns that DTC advertising will increase health care spending, strain doctor-patient relationships and confuse consumers and patients. Worst of all, they believe going directly to the consumer is only a drug company technique to increase prices and therefore profits. Are any of these concerns valid?

Will DTC advertising increase health care spending?   Probably, but that is not necessarily bad. Increased health care spending is bad only when it is wasteful and inefficient. For example, if doctors were to prescribe medicines for patients who had no medical need, that would be wasteful—and unethical. However, very few doctors would prescribe medicines their patients do not need. In fact, a new *Prevention* magazine survey found that about half of those who talk to a doctor as a result of a DTC ad receive no drug therapy.

A greater concern is that patients, having seen an expensive brand-name drug advertised, will want it rather than a generic equivalent. When patients or their doctors choose brand names over generics, their choices may increase total health care spending. But, again, that may not be bad. The brand name may be higher in quality or slightly different in composition. And it may have fewer side effects. Thus it may offer additional benefits, in which case the additional cost may be justified.

If an expansion of DTC advertising means that we are treating more people who otherwise might have just suffered in pain or endured a debilitating condition, then increased medical spending is positive. Some have argued that increased drug spending may lower total health care costs if less expensive drug therapy replaces more expensive surgery or other procedures. This may be true for individual patients, but it cannot be aggregated to apply to the whole health care system. Total spending will continue to rise because the American health care system will continue to do more and more for patients.

Will DTC advertising strain the doctor-patient relationship?   Historically, doctors informed and patients performed. That is, doctors diagnosed and issued instructions that patients followed—or at least were supposed to. With more information at the patients' fingertips, that relationship is changing. Patients are asking questions, and doctors are beginning to see the questions as opportunities to enhance patients' understanding and sense of responsibility about their own health. (The author himself has asked a physician about an advertised prescription drug, and neither he nor the doctor saw anything unusual or unethical about the exchange.)

Doctors may have to take more time to discuss with their patients why Drug A, which the patient saw advertised on TV, would not in the doctor's opinion be as good a choice as Drug B. Cost, efficacy and suitability all may play a role in that discussion. Some irascible patients may refuse to accept the doctor's advice. But this occurs even without DTC advertising. Indeed, current DTC advertising is very subtle. No announcer tells the audience to demand Drug A from a doctor because it has been clinically proven to be better than

Drug B. DTC ads tend to convey too little information rather than too much. This may change, but the medical community already is learning to deal with people who come to the doctor not just as patients but as consumers.

Will DTC ads confuse patients?   Economist John Calfee contends that three decades of research on advertising has led to two basic understandings:

> First, advertising has an unsuspected power to improve consumer welfare. As a market-perfecting mechanism, advertising arises spontaneously to attack serious defects in the marketplace. Advertising is an efficient and sometimes irreplaceable mechanism for bringing consumers information that would otherwise languish on the sidelines. Advertising's promise of more and better information also generates ripple effects in the market. These include enhanced incentives to create new information and develop better products. Theoretical and empirical research has demonstrated what generations of astute observers had known intuitively, that markets with advertising are far superior to markets without advertising.
>
> The second finding is that competitive advertising is fundamentally a self-correcting process. Some people may find this surprising. Well-informed observers once thought that unregulated advertising would bring massive distortion of consumer information and decisions. Careful research, however, has shown these fears to be groundless. Self-correcting competitive forces in advertising generate markets in which information is richer and more fundamentally balanced than can be achieved through detailed controls over advertising and information.

Is DTC just a way to increase drug prices?   Drug companies advertise for the same reason every other company and industry advertises: to increase sales with a view to increasing profits. The consumer benefit is that, as competition grows, prices usually fall. By contrast, in the absence of marketing, prices would not go down, but up. Just consider under which scenario a manufacturer is more likely to charge high prices for low quality: where there is no advertising and consumers have no way to comparison-shop without taking their own time to go from store to store to compare price and quality, or where advertising takes that information directly to the consumer? It is not advertising that increases the price of products, it's the lack of it. High prices thrive in an atmosphere of ignorance. If critics want to see the price of prescription drugs fall, they should encourage even more advertising and competition.

The missing ingredient: value   As long as patients are insulated from the cost of medical care and doctors stand between patients and their prescriptions, the health care marketplace cannot work exactly like a normal market in which consumers demand from vendors quality, service and reasonable prices—that is, value.

But the U.S. health care system can take on some of the dynamics of a market, and in fact is already doing so. There is some competition; there is some DTC advertising; and prices at least for some health care products and services are relatively low.

As we continue to move into a patient-directed system, market forces may become more apparent. For example, if most people chose to combine a Medical Savings Account (MSA) for small expenses with a catastrophic health insurance policy for large expenses, patients would pay for their prescription drugs out of the MSA and thus be more cost-conscious.

In addition, the realization is growing in Washington that the current tax subsidy for health insurance causes problems. As a result, Congress may pass a tax credit that will help the uninsured purchase a policy. This in turn may lead to a fundamental shift in the type of health insurance policy people purchase—and facilitate the move to a patient-directed system.

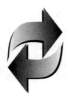

**Robert Langreth
and Matthew Herper**

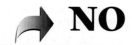

Pill Pushers: How the Drug Industry Abandoned Science for Salesmanship

Novartis employs some of the best medical researchers in the world, and they have created such lifesavers as Gleevec, which treats a deadly form of leukemia. But what is the fourth-biggest seller in the Novartis medicine cabinet? No lifesaver. It's Lamisil, a pill for—horrors!—toenail fungus. The main effect of the fungus is that it turns the toenail yellow; it can hurt, but no one has died of this inconvenience. But a few people may have died taking Lamisil. Federal regulators have linked the drug to 16 cases of liver failure, including 11 deaths. Novartis says most of the patients had preexisting illnesses or were also on other drugs.

Yet 10 million Americans have taken Lamisil, which costs $850 for a three-month treatment. They have been lured by a grotesque cartoon creature called Digger the Dermatophyte, a squat, yellow fellow with a dumb-guy New York accent. In TV ads he lifts a toenail as if it were the hood of a car, then creeps beneath it to declare, "I'm not leavin'!"

TNS Media Intelligence calculates that Novartis has spent $236 million on Lamisil ads in three years (Novartis says it has spent only $100 million). The first run, which featured Digger being crushed by a giant Lamisil tablet, so overstated the drug's benefit that regulators objected and the company had to pull the spots; the drug fully cures the problem in only 38% of patients. But the ad blitz undeniably was effective: Lamisil sales jumped 19% to $1.2 billion worldwide in 2004 and held steady last year.

Lamisil's rise points up what is wrong with the drug industry today: the triumph of salesmanship over science. The industry spends a fortune to create and sell a raft of me-too remedies aimed at quelling sometimes trivial maladies, even as research pipelines run dry, patents on old drugs expire and critical areas of medicine go underserved. Sometimes the marketing improves health;

From *Forbes Magazine*, May 8, 2006, pp. 94, 96–98, 100, 102. Reprinted by permission of Forbes Magazine, © 2006 Forbes Media Inc.

Americans would probably be better off if more of them were hounded into taking pills to lower cholesterol and blood pressure. Sometimes the result is the reverse, as when side effects from an overhyped and overprescribed medicine are fatal.

"The dominance of marketing over research has done real damage to company pipelines," says Jurgen Drews, former research chief for Roche. A decade ago he predicted a research slump; it has arrived. A total of 87 major drugs with $31 billion in combined annual sales have lost patent protection since 2002, but new drugs aren't arriving fast enough to replace them. Only 20 were cleared by the Food & Drug Administration last year, down from 53 a decade ago.

Drugmakers, says Maryland psychiatrist Jack E. Rosenblatt, editor of *Currents in Affective Illness*, "don't seem to realize that this is not toothpaste or shampoo, that they are dealing with something that can really hurt people."

The industry's malaise is certainly visible on Wall Street. The ten largest drugmakers have lost $130 billion in combined market value in two years, a 12% decline at a time when the S&P 500 Index is up 12%. They have endured scandal after scandal over drug safety and dubious sales practices. A total of 17 drugs have been recalled in the past decade. Wyeth's withdrawal of diet drug Redux in 1997 led to $22 billion in damages and counting (FORBES, *Apr. 10*).

Vioxx could yet eclipse that. Merck's new-generation painkiller—touted to consumers at a cost of $550 million over five years—was recalled in September 2004 when a study showed that patients on it for 18 months had double the risk of heart attacks. In the ensuing legal onslaught 10,000 suits have been filed, seeking billions in damages and accusing the company of misleading doctors and the feds. Last month Merck lost a $13.5 million verdict to one heart attack survivor, its second defeat in five cases tried. There are more potential lawsuits lurking where these came from.

The drug industry, of course, rejects the criticisms. Novartis says its Lamisil spending "absolutely" "in no way" has taken away resources from research into more serious diseases and that it spends far more on its cancer drugs. "Absolutely, marketing doesn't trump science—this is a science-driven industry," says Scott Lassman, a lawyer for Pharma, the industry trade group. He says makers have taken steps to curb any excesses and give ads a "more sober tone." Pfizer research chief Martin Mackay says, "We are thought of as monsters, but I don't know of a single case where we have been driven to take risks on a compound because of a marketing push. I would not let it happen."

Says Bristol-Myers Squibb Chief Executive Peter Dolan: "The biggest disconnect for me is between how the industry is portrayed and how people in it actually feel about what they do."

Yet Big Pharma's focus on marketing is undeniable, and it spends hugely on it. The top ten drug firms invest $42 billion a year on research, 14% of sales—yet they plow more than twice that much into marketing and administration. In a decade drug firms have almost tripled the ranks of salespeople calling on physicians, to 100,000, according to Verispan. That's one seller for every 9 docs; in 1996 it was one for 18. Often they encourage unauthorized off-label uses or sponsor "continuing medical education" sessions to stoke more prescriptions and broaden a drug's patient base.

❧❦❧

Even the research lab is more marketing-driven than ever. More than $9 billion a year in research spending goes to clinical trials of drugs that are already approved or may soon be—often to snare new ad slogans. That is up 90% in four years, says Goldman Sachs. Some of these ad-driven trials are skewed to pit the sponsor's full-strength product against a weaker dose of a rival pill. Yet drugmakers have failed to begin two-thirds of the 1,200 post-marketing trials required by the FDA.

The slogan-geared trials provide fodder for an explosion in consumer advertising of drugs, which had been highly restricted for decades before rules were eased in the 1990s. Ad spending in the U.S. has soared eightfold in nine years to $4.8 billion, says Nielsen Monitor-Plus, TV spots ply supposed low-risk, quick fixes to millions of people: Try Zoloft to get happy; gobble a state-of-the-art pain pill when aspirin would work fine. Drugs designed for narrow sets of patients end up in the hands of a far broader audience.

"It creates demand where there's not even disease there," complains internist Robert Centor of the University of Alabama. Drug giants "do it in a devious way," he says. "I wish they didn't spend all that money on marketing."

Merck's marketing of the painkiller Vioxx was, in retrospect, all too successful, contributing to the multibillion-dollar liability now looming over the company. Vioxx, part of a new class of drugs known as COX-2 inhibitors, had been intended for only the small slice of patients who can't stomach aspirin. But it ended up in the hands of 20 million people, driven by ad spending of $550 million in five years, says ad tracker TNS. Some spots had 1970s Olympic figure skater Dorothy Hamill twirling on the ice.

Vioxx's chief rival, Celebrex from Pfizer, also reached a far broader market because of splashy ads. About 60% of patients on the drugs had low ulcer risk and might have fared just as well on older generics, say researchers at the University of Chicago and Stanford. Pfizer says most gastrointestinal complications occur in patients who are not at high risk.

"People would come in asking for—demanding [a COX-2 inhibitor]—and sometimes threaten to find a new doctor if I didn't prescribe it," says physician John Abramson, a clinical instructor at Harvard Medical School who has consulted for plaintiff lawyers. "Vioxx wasn't a bad drug for everyone, it was a bad drug for certain patients," says Chris D. Robbins of Arxcel, which consults to pharmacy benefit managers. "Unfortunately, people saw the ads and started demanding the drugs from their doctors."

TV ads for prescription drugs were rare until Aug. 12, 1997, when the FDA lifted restrictions to let spots run without lengthy disclaimers of nasty side effects. Three days later Schering-Plough began a prime-time campaign for its antihistamine Claritin, featuring smiling folks frolicking in hay fields to the tune of Irving Berlin's "Blue Skies." Schering upped the ante in 1998 with one of the first celebrity pitches, by TV personality Joan Lunden. Claritin sales climbed 50% in 1997 and 30% more in 1998, hitting $2.3 billion. Schering's stock-market value approached $90 billion by mid-1999. Claritin lost patent protection in 2002. No problem: Schering was ready with Clarinex, a look-alike successor that still brings in $646 million in annual sales, even though its predecessor is sold over-the-counter at one-tenth of the price. The shift didn't help enough: Schering had a mediocre pipeline, and today its market cap is down by two-thirds to $27 billion.

⋯◈⋯

Other companies followed with ads for antidepressants, heartburn drugs, painkillers and impotence pills. Pfizer found its erectile dysfunction pitchman in Senator Bob Dole, then age 75. Wall Street cheered the changes. "We had the whole financial community focused on blockbusters and maximizing the revenues and aggressive marketing," says Daniel Vasella, chief executive of Novartis, which TNS Media Intelligence says has spent $235 million in three years advertising Zelnorm. (Novartis disputes the amount.) The drug, which treats irritable bowel syndrome, costs $200 a month.

In the rush to find big sellers, many companies fell into a herd mentality and focused on the same few common ailments, says Genentech Chief Arthur Levinson. "Everyone was doing the same thing, so the chances of success got smaller and smaller." Big Pharma "said we were nuts" to test a cancer drug that targeted only 25% of breast cancer patients, Levinson recalls. Now the drug, Herceptin, is near $1 billion in annual sales. "If you are developing novel drugs, you don't need sales forces of tens of thousands."

Some drug firms stopped researching in critical areas even as they focused on pop pills. Eli Lilly & Co. had dominated the antibiotic field for decades, and new remedies are badly needed to kill drug-resistant superbugs. Yet in the 1990s the company sold off three promising antibiotics and antifungals, two of which went on to win approval. Lilly exited antibiotic research entirely in 2002, believing the chances of success were higher with antivirals. The next year Lilly and partner Icos spent $243 million launching their me-too pill for erectile dysfunction, Cialis. Barry Eisenstein, who headed Lilly's antibiotic program from 1992 to 1996, says drugs for chronic conditions, like Prozac, are seen as "a much better and easier business proposition." Lilly says that any contention that it didn't pursue antibiotics to chase mass-market blockbusters is simply not valid.

⋯◈⋯

The "easiest profits" come from me-too drugs, says John Santa, medical director at Oregon Health & Science University. Genuine discovery is a risky business, "more like drilling for oil." Instead of prospecting for real cures, some companies repackage old drugs with the minimal tweaks needed to get a new patent. Then they stage exhaustive trials aimed at unearthing some slender advantage that can be cited in advertising.

One throwback, the Lunesta sleeping pill from Sepracor that came out early last year, is based on a remedy first approved in Europe two decades ago. It is very similar to Ambien, which is made by Sanofi-Aventis and racks up U.S. sales of $1.6 billion annually (on an ad budget of $130 million). Lunesta garnered $330 million in sales in its first nine months on the market thanks to TV spots featuring a diaphanous cartoon butterfly flitting in and out of moonlit bedrooms. Tagline: "Leave the rest to Lunesta." Sepracor spent $215 million last year advertising Lunesta, says TNS.

To differentiate Lunesta from Ambien, Sepracor tested its drug versus a placebo in 1,600 patients for six months, something Ambien's maker hadn't bothered to do. The trials let Sepracor claim in print ads that Lunesta "is the first and only hypnotic approved for long-term use."

Prescriptions for sleeping pills are up 48% in five years to 43 million prescriptions annually, driven by the huge ad spending for Ambien and Lunesta. Sales are up 140% in the same period to $2.76 billion. Yet the newer drugs "are no better than older ones costing about one-tenth as much," says John Abramson of Harvard. "Has insomnia become an epidemic in the past five years? Or are the makers skillfully leading Americans [to] an expensive drug?" he asks. Sepracor points to an Institute of Medicine report highlighting insomnia as a serious problem.

⁘

Astrazeneca, faced with patent expiration on its blockbuster for acid reflux, Prilosec—touted as "the purple pill"—tweaked it a bit to create "the new purple pill," Nexium. AstraZeneca studied high doses of Nexium in five trials totaling 12,000 patients. All this to show the drug helped the esophagus heal in an extra one in 20 patients, compared with Prilosec or competitor Prevacid.

The payoff: Nexium now is touted as "the healing purple pill," hawked in ubiquitous TV spots. In one, a sterling-haired man in black cites the "exciting news" from one of the studies and concludes, "Better is better." Nexium is the third-best-selling drug in the world, according to IMS Health, with $5.7 billion in sales and an ad budget of $226 million last year. Never mind that some of the trials were stacked: In three of the big trials AstraZeneca pitted high doses of Nexium versus half the dose of Prilosec; it never bothered to test whether twice the Prilosec dose would be equally effective. AstraZeneca says there are "clear differences" between the two purple pills and notes that one equal-dose study showed a statistical advantage for Nexium in esophageal healing.

In another instance AstraZeneca staged trials that fizzled but used them for a new ad claim anyway. Before it won approval in August 2003, AstraZeneca studied its Lipitor look-alike, Crestor, for cholesterol reduction, in 24,000 patients, hoping to prove superiority. But the only dose of Crestor that clearly beat Lipitor turned out to cause kidney problems and never won FDA approval. Nonetheless, after Crestor's debut AstraZeneca used ads featuring a voiceover by the stentorian actor Patrick Stewart of *Star Trek: The Next Generation*, in Seussian rhyme: "When Crestor performed in a head-to-head test, its lowering effect was clearly the best."

That claim brought a rebuke from the FDA in March 2005. The company halted the ads, but it now is testing Crestor in 30,000 more patients. AstraZeneca notes that Crestor is the only statin shown to clear plaque out of the arteries.

The drug industry has begun to restrain its own advertising. Last June Bristol-Myers Squibb took a first step, announcing that it would wait a year after drugs hit the market to begin running ads, leaving time for doctors to learn about a medicine and for side effects to crop up. Companies are now submitting ads to the FDA before they run and are more clearly stating big risks.

But myriad drugmakers have plenty of ways to game the system. In the market for new schizophrenia treatments Lilly and Johnson & Johnson and others have run 21 head-to-head trials—and 90% of the time the conclusions favor the sponsor's drug, according to research in the *American Journal of Psychiatry*. Nine studies compared Lilly's Zyprexa to Johnson & Johnson's Risperdal. All five Lilly-paid trials favored Zyprexa; three of four J&J studies favored Risperdal. Lilly stands by its high scientific standards and says the results highlight the need for more independent studies. Another analysis, in *Archives of Internal Medicine*, tallied 56 studies of painkillers; not once was the sponsor's drug deemed inferior.

"The comparative studies are a joke. They are comical. A lot of the scientific literature these days is worthless," says psychiatrist Jack E. Rosenblatt. "The whole process has been corrupted," says British bone researcher Aubrey Blumsohn. "It is getting worse as the financial stakes are rising."

⊷⟨✿⟩⊶

Blumsohn contends Procter & Gamble for years refused to supply raw data for a 2003 study he led comparing its drug Actonel to Merck's competing drug, Fosamax, even after he became suspicious that Procter's analysis was skewed in favor of Actonel. "It was a process of intimidation," says Blumsohn, who was suspended from his job at the University of Sheffield after he complained to the British press. (He recently left after agreeing to an undisclosed settlement.) Procter & Gamble says it "always" provided Blumsohn with "unfiltered access to all of the data that was relevant." "This issue is about a relationship fraught with misunderstanding, and we regret that," a spokesman says. Procter is now providing Dr. Blumsohn with additional data.

Despite the profusion of dubious trials, drugmakers often don't conduct crucial studies to ensure new drugs are truly safe as they move out to a mass market. This year Trasylol, a Bayer drug used to prevent bleeding during heart surgery, has emerged as yet another problem medication. In December Bayer promised annual sales of the drug, then at $280 million, would surge to $600 million.

But a study of 4,000 surgery patients found that the drug, at $1,400 per dose, posed more than twice as much risk of kidney failure as cheaper generic alternatives, as well as more heart attacks and strokes. Replacing Trasylol with generics would prevent 10,000 cases of kidney failure each year, says clinical researcher Dennis Mangano, who led the study at the nonprofit Ischemia Research & Education Foundation in San Bruno, Calif.

Bayer says its own studies of 6,500 patients haven't found any link between the drug and kidney failure, heart attack or stroke, and that it is working with the FDA to evaluate the Mangano report and another study linking the drug to serious adverse events. "Bayer's highest priority and concern is patient safety," says a spokeswoman.

⋅⊰⊙⊱⋅

Mangano, who also did the first study to raise concerns about the cardiovascular risk of Pfizer's Bextra (pulled from the market in April 2005), spent $35 million of his foundation's endowment to painstakingly gather the Trasylol data over four years. Few independent researchers have the money to perform such definitive safety studies. His foundation used to do clinical trials for the industry, but drug companies don't call much anymore, he says. "There is no incentive for companies to find problems with safety once a drug is approved. It is just downside risk," he says. The result is worrisome: "We find out a drug is unsafe when the bodies accumulate."

THE LURE OF OFF-LABEL

The most dubious drug sales practice is off-label marketing—pushing drugs for unproven (and unapproved) uses. Johnson & Johnson's Scios division is under federal investigation for the marketing and promotion of its heart drug Natrecor.

The intravenous drug is approved for one-time use to relieve the symptoms of patients with severe, acute heart failure. But some doctors say Scios pushed Natrecor for weekly "tune-ups," a use that is totally unproven and potentially dangerous—and that Scios even advocated setting up special outpatient clinics as new profit centers.

Two Scios sales reps made such a pitch to the Albert Einstein College of Medicine teaching hospital in the Bronx N.Y. in 2001 says David Brown, head of clinical cardiology at the time. Their 30-minute presentation detailed how the hospital could profit by opening a clinic that gave regular doses of Natrecor. "I was approached by them with the idea that it is a profit center based on the [Medicare] reimbursement," Brown says. Medicare paid doctors up to $600 for each visit plus the cost of the drug.

Brown declined, as did a colleague. But such clinics were becoming widespread. When Brown took a new job at SUNY stony Brook in 2004, he found that a Natrecor infusion clinic had opened up. The clinic closed shortly after he clamped down on the practice.

Soon after J&J acquired Scios for $2.4 billion in 2003, it seemed to brag about the dubious use in a report to investors: "Natrecor is increasingly administered in less invasive clinical settings like outpatient clinics." A J&J news release boasted that weekly outpatient use of Natrecor "led to positive clinical outcomes" in a 210 patient study. In fact, the study failed to prove an effect.

Eventually J&J set up a toll-free line to help doctors with reimbursement and sent out a 46-page Natrecor billing guide. But Medicare officials decided in March 2005 to halt payments for repeated Natrecor use, aiming to discourage the practice.

Scios also sponsored a special "supplement" to the Journal *Reviews in Cardiovascular Medicine* in fall 2004. MedReviews, the New York firm that published the journal promises on its Web site to put together "a supplement that achieves your marketing objectives." One eight-page article in the supplement emphasizes in its abstract and conclusion that Natrecor may be "safe and effective" for outpatient use. MedReviews says the supplement was "educational," and not promotional in nature. Johnson & Johnson says it abided by FDA guidelines and that the articles were developed by independent experts.

Tulane University cardiologist Thierry Le Jemtel, who wrote a different article in the same supplement, says MedReviews offered to ghostwrite his article for him, but he demurred. MedReviews says it doesn't typically use ghostwriters. J&J wouldn't answer whether ghostwriters were invoked

—M.H. and R.L.

POSTSCRIPT

Do Consumers Benefit When Prescription Drugs Are Advertised?

Opponents of prescription drug advertising contend that drug companies' promotions are frequently inaccurate or deceptive. Furthermore, they maintain that drug companies are more interested in increasing their profits, not in truly providing additional medical benefit to the average consumer. Drug companies do not deny that they seek to make profits from their drugs, but they argue that they are offering an important public service by educating the public about new drugs through their advertisements. Also, after investing millions of dollars into developing and testing new drugs, should not pharmaceutical companies profit from the sale of these drugs?

An important issue is whether or not the average consumer is capable of discerning information distributed by pharmaceutical companies. Are people without a background in medicine, medical terminology, or research methods sufficiently knowledgeable to understand literature disseminated by drug companies? With the help of the Internet and other media, prescription drug advertising proponents maintain that the average consumer is capable of understanding information about various drugs. On the other hand, will most people take the time to follow up on drugs that are advertised? And, if people do not take the time to read about drugs they see advertised in the media, is that the fault of the drug companies?

Some critics argue that restricting drug advertisements is a moot point because consumers cannot obtain prescriptions without the approval of their physicians. Yet, in numerous instances physicians acquiesce to the wishes of their patients and write prescriptions upon the request of the patient. If in this way patients receive prescriptions that are not appropriate for their needs, who is responsible: the patient, the physician, or the drug manufacturer and advertiser? Is the role of the physician to dictate to the patient what drugs are appropriate or is it the role of the physician to explain to the patient the various options and then let the patient decide what to do?

When drug manufacturers introduce a new drug, they get a patent on the drug to protect their investment. Drug companies, therefore, receive financial rewards for introducing new drugs. Of course, drug companies also take financial risks when developing new drugs. One could argue that drug companies should be awarded for the financial risks they take. However, some critics maintain that many of these new drugs are merely "me-too" drugs that are similar to existing drugs and that they do not provide any additional benefit. Are consumers being fooled into requesting more expensive drugs that are no better than drugs already on the market?

A retrospective look into prescription drug advertising is dealt with in "Are Direct to Consumer Advertisements of Prescription Drugs Educational?: Comparing 1992 to 2002," by Timothy Curry, Jeff Jarosch, and Shelley Pacholok in the *Journal of Drug Education* (2005). Michelle Meadows discusses ways to reduce the cost of prescription drugs in "Saving Money on Prescription Drugs," in *FDA Consumer* (September–October 2005). Two excellent articles that explore the benefits of prescription drug advertising are "Americans Find Prescription Drug Advertising Helpful, Survey Says" (*Biotech Business Week*, March 1, 2004) and "Media and Message Effects on DTC Prescription Drug Print Advertising Awareness," by Martin S. Roth in *Journal of Advertising Research* (June 2003).

Internet References . . .

National Clearinghouse for Alcohol and Drug Information (NCADI)

Information regarding a variety of drugs as well as research published by the federal government is available through this site. Up-to-date developments in drug use are available through NCADI.

http://www.health.org

The Weiner Nusim Foundation

This private foundation located in Connecticut publishes information regarding drug education. The information is free.

http://www.weinernusim.com

DrugHelp

This site, a service of the American Council for Drug Education (an affiliate of Phoenix House Foundation), provides information, counsel and referral to treatment centers.

http://www.drughelp.org

Partnership for a Drug-Free America

Extensive information on the effects of drugs and the extent of drug use by young people are discussed at this website.

http://www.drugfreeamerica.org

National Council on Alcoholism and Drug Dependence

This site contains objective information and referral for individuals, families and others seeking intervention and treatment.

http://www.ncadd.org

Drug Prevention and Treatment

In spite of their legal consequences and the government's interdiction efforts, drugs are widely available and used. Two common ways of dealing with drug abuse is to incarcerate drug users and to intercept drugs before they enter the country. However, many drug experts believe that more energy should be put into preventing and treating drug abuse. An important step toward prevention and treatment is to find out what contributes to drug abuse and how to nullify these factors.

By educating young people about the potential hazards of drugs and by developing an awareness of social influences that contribute to drug use, many drug-related problems may be averted. The debates in this section focus on different prevention and treatment issues such as the effect that tobacco advertisements have on smoking behavior, whether schools should drug test students, and the effectiveness of drug abuse treatment.

- Does Secondhand Smoke Endanger the Health of Nonsmokers?

- Is Alcoholism Hereditary?

- Should Marijuana Be Approved for Medical Use?

- Should Schools Drug Test Students?

- Does Drug Abuse Treatment Work?

- Is Abstinence an Effective Strategy for Drug Education?

ISSUE 14

Does Secondhand Smoke Endanger the Health of Nonsmokers?

YES: U.S. Department of Health and Human Services, from *The Health Consequences of Involuntary Exposure to Tobacco Smoke: A Report of the Surgeon General* (2006)

NO: J. B. Copas and J. Q. Shi, from "Reanalysis of Epidemiological Evidence on Lung Cancer and Passive Smoking," *British Medical Journal* (February 12, 2000)

ISSUE SUMMARY

YES: According to the Surgeon General's report on secondhand smoke, in 2005 more than 3,000 adult nonsmokers died from lung cancer, 46,000 from coronary heart disease, and about 430 newborns from sudden infant death syndrome. In addition, children exposed to secondhand smoke have an increased risk of acute respiratory infections, ear problems, and severe asthma. Simply separating smokers from nonsmokers or having separately ventilated areas for smoking is ineffective.

NO: Statisticians J. B. Copas and J. Q. Shi argue that research demonstrating that secondhand smoke is harmful is biased. They contend that many journals are more likely to publish articles if secondhand smoke is shown to be deleterious and that the findings of many studies exaggerate the adverse effects of secondhand smoke.

The movement to restrict secondhand smoke is growing. Smoking is banned on all commercial airplane flights within the continental United States. Canada, Australia, and many other countries have enacted similar bans. Smoking is prohibited or restricted in all federal public areas and workplaces. The right to smoke in public places is quickly being eliminated. Is this fair, considering tobacco's addictive hold over smokers? Former surgeon general C. Everett Koop and many researchers point out that smoking is an addiction that is as difficult to overcome as an addiction to cocaine or heroin.

Should smokers be penalized—prevented from smoking or isolated from nonsmokers—for having a nicotine addiction?

Articles describing passive smoking or secondhand smoking can be confusing because several terms frequently are used to describe it. *Passive smoking* has been referred to as involuntary smoking, and the smoke itself has been identified as both *secondhand smoke* and *environmental tobacco smoke*, or *ETS*. Secondhand smoke can be further broken down into *mainstream smoke* and *sidestream smoke*. Mainstream smoke is the smoke that the smoker exhales. Sidestream smoke is the smoke that comes off the end of the tobacco product as it burns. Sidestream smoke has higher concentrations of carbon monoxide and other gases than mainstream smoke. Scientists also believe that sidestream smoke contains more carcinogens than mainstream smoke.

The issue of passive smoking is extremely divisive. On one side of the debate are the nonsmokers, who strongly believe that their rights to clean air are compromised by smokers. Their objections are based on more than aesthetics; it is not simply a matter of smoke being unsightly, noxious, or inconvenient. Nonsmokers are becoming more concerned about the toxic effects of secondhand smoke. Groups of nonsmokers and numerous health professionals have initiated a massive campaign to educate the public on the array of health-related problems that have been associated with inhaling secondhand smoke.

On the other side are smokers, who believe that they should have the right to smoke whenever and wherever they wish. This group is backed by the tobacco industry, which has allocated vast sums of money and resources to conduct research studies on the effects of secondhand smoke. Based on the results of these studies, smoking rights groups claim that the health concerns related to secondhand smoke are based on emotion, not scientific evidence. They argue that there are too many variables involved to determine the exact impact of secondhand smoke. For example, to what extent does a polluted environment or a poorly ventilated house contribute to the health problems attributed to secondhand smoke? Isolating the effects of secondhand smoke is difficult, and any studies concluding that secondhand smoke is harmful are questionable.

Many smokers who acknowledge that smoking may have adverse effects on health argue that their freedoms should not be limited. They feel that they should have the right to engage in behaviors that affect only themselves, even if those behaviors are unhealthy. Some smokers reason that if smoking behavior is regulated, perhaps other personal behaviors also will become regulated. They fight against the regulation of smoking because they believe that behavior regulation is a potentially harmful trend.

In the following sections, the Surgeon General's Report stresses that the dangers associated with secondhand smoke are clear. Secondhand smoke, says the report, causes medical conditions ranging from sudden infant death syndrome to asthma to lung cancer. J. B. Copas and J. Q. Shi maintain that much of the information about the health hazards of secondhand smoke has been distorted and accepted as fact without adequate critical questioning.

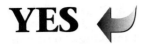
The Health Consequences
of Involuntary Exposure to
Tobacco Smoke: A Report
of the Surgeon General

Foreword

This twenty-ninth report of the Surgeon General documents the serious and deadly health effects of involuntary exposure to tobacco smoke. Secondhand smoke is a major cause of disease, including lung cancer and coronary heart disease, in healthy nonsmokers.

In 2005, it was estimated that exposure to secondhand smoke kills more than 3,000 adult nonsmokers from lung cancer, approximately 46,000 from coronary heart disease, and an estimated 430 newborns from sudden infant death syndrome. In addition, secondhand smoke causes other respiratory problems in nonsmokers such as coughing, phlegm, and reduced lung function. According to the CDC's National Health Interview Survey in 2000, more than 80 percent of the respondents aged 18 years or older believe that secondhand smoke is harmful and nonsmokers should be protected in their workplaces.

Components of chemical compounds in secondhand smoke, including nicotine, carbon monoxide, and tobacco-specifc carcinogens, can be detected in body fluids of exposed nonsmokers. These exposures can be controlled. In 2005, CDC released the *Third National Report on Human Exposure to Environmental Chemicals*, which found that the median cotinine level (a metabolite of nicotine) in nonsmokers had decreased across the life stages: by 68 percent in children, 69 percent in adolescents, and 75 percent in adults, when samples collected between 1999 and 2002 were compared with samples collected a decade earlier. These dramatic declines are further evidence that smoking restrictions in public places and workplaces are helping to ensure a healthier life for all people in the United States.

However, too many people continue to be exposed, especially children. The recent data indicate that median cotinine levels in children are more than twice those of adults, and non-Hispanic blacks have levels that are more than twice as high as those of Mexican Americans and non-Hispanic whites. These disparities need to be better understood and addressed.

From The Surgeon General, 2006.

Research reviewed in this report indicates that smoke-free policies are the most economic and effective approach for providing protection from exposure to secondhand smoke. But do they provide the greatest health impact. Separating smokers and nonsmokers in the same airspace is not effective, nor is air cleaning or a greater exchange of indoor with outdoor air. Additionally, having separately ventilated areas for smoking may not offer a satisfactory solution to reducing workplace exposures. Policies prohibiting smoking in the workplace have multiple benefits. Besides reducing exposure of nonsmokers to secondhand smoke, these policies reduce tobacco use by smokers and change public attitudes about tobacco use from acceptable to unacceptable.

Research indicates that the progressive restriction of smoking in the United States to protect nonsmokers has had the additional health impact of reducing active smoking. In November 2005, CDC's Tobacco-Free Campus policy took full effect in all facilities owned by CDC in the Atlanta area. As the Director of the nation's leading health promotion and disease prevention agency, I am proud to support this effort. With this commitment, CDC continues to protect the health and safety of all of its employees and serves as a role model for workplaces everywhere.

Julie Louise Gerberding, M.D., M.P.H.
Director
Centers for Disease Control and Prevention
and
Administrator
Agency for Toxic Substances and Disease Registry

Preface
(from the Surgeon General, U.S. Department of Health and Human Services)
Twenty years ago when Dr. C. Everett Koop released the Surgeon General's report, *The Health Consequences of Involuntary Smoking,* it was the first Surgeon General's report to conclude that involuntary exposure of nonsmokers to tobacco smoke causes disease. The topic of involuntary exposure of nonsmokers to secondhand smoke was first considered in Surgeon General Jesse Steinfeld's 1972 report, and by 1986, the causal linkage between inhaling secondhand smoke and the risk for lung cancer was clear. By then, there was also abundant evidence of adverse effects of smoking by parents on their children.

Today, massive and conclusive scientific evidence documents adverse effects of involuntary smoking on children and adults, including cancer and cardiovascular diseases in adults, and adverse respiratory effects in both children and adults. This 2006 report of the Surgeon General updates the 1986 report, *The Health Consequences of Involuntary Smoking,* and provides a detailed review of the epidemiologic evidence on the health effects of involuntary exposure to tobacco smoke. This new report also uses the revised standard language of causality that was applied in the 2004 Surgeon General's report, *The Health Consequences of Smoking.*

Secondhand smoke is similar to the mainstream smoke inhaled by the smoker in that it is a complex mixture containing many chemicals (including formaldehyde, cyanide, carbon monoxide, ammonia, and nicotine), many of which are known carcinogens. Exposure to secondhand smoke causes excess deaths in the U.S. population from lung cancer and cardiac related illnesses. Fortunately, exposures of adults are declining as smoking becomes increasingly restricted in workplaces and public places. Unfortunately, children continue to be exposed in their homes by the smoking of their parents and other adults. This exposure leads to unnecessary cases of bronchitis, pneumonia and worsened asthma. Among children younger than 18 years of age, an estimated 22 percent are exposed to secondhand smoke in their homes, with estimates ranging from 11.7 percent in Utah to 34.2 percent in Kentucky.

As this report documents, exposure to secondhand smoke remains an alarming public health hazard. Approximately 60 percent of nonsmokers in the United States have biologic evidence of exposure to secondhand smoke. Yet compared with data reviewed in the 1986 report, I am encouraged by the progress that has been made in reducing involuntary exposure in many workplaces, restaurants, and other public places. These changes are most likely the major contributing factors to the more than 75 percent reduction in serum cotinine levels that researchers have observed from 1988 to 1991. However, more than 126 million nonsmokers are still exposed. We now have substantial evidence on the efficacy of different approaches to control exposure to secondhand smoke. Restrictions on smoking can control exposures effectively, but technical approaches involving air cleaning or a greater exchange of indoor with outdoor air cannot. Consequently, nonsmokers need protection through the restriction of smoking in public places and workplaces and by a voluntary adherence to policies at home, particularly to eliminate exposures of children. Since the release of the 1986 Surgeon General's report, the public's attitude and social norms toward secondhand smoke exposure have changed significantly—a direct result of the growing body of scientific evidence on the health effects of exposure to secondhand smoke that is summarized in this report.

Finally, clinicians should routinely ask about secondhand smoke exposure, particularly in susceptible groups or when a child has had an illness caused by secondhand smoke, such as pneumonia. Because of the high levels of exposure among young children, their exposure should be considered a significant pediatric issue. Additionally, exposure to secondhand smoke poses significant risks for people with lung and heart disease. The large body of evidence documenting that secondhand smoke exposures produce substantial and immediate effects on the cardiovascular system indicates that even brief exposures could pose significant acute risks to older adults or to others at high risk for cardiovascular disease. Those caring for relatives with heart disease should be advised not to smoke in the presence of the sick relative.

An environment free of involuntary exposure to secondhand smoke should remain an important national priority in order to reach the *Healthy People 2010* objectives.

Richard Carmona, M.D., M.P.H., F.A.C.S.
Surgeon General

Executive Summary

The topic of passive or involuntary smoking was first addressed in the 1972 U.S. Surgeon General's report (*The Health Consequences of Smoking*, U.S. Department of Health, Education, and Welfare [USDHEW] 1972), only eight years after the first Surgeon General's report on the health consequences of active smoking (USDHEW 1964). Surgeon General Dr. Jesse Steinfeld had raised concerns about this topic, leading to its inclusion in that report. According to the 1972 report, nonsmokers inhale the mixture of sidestream smoke given off by a smoldering cigarette and mainstream smoke exhaled by a smoker, a mixture now referred to as "secondhand smoke" or "environmental tobacco smoke." Cited experimental studies showed that smoking in enclosed spaces could lead to high levels of cigarette smoke components in the air. For carbon monoxide (CO) specifically, levels in enclosed spaces could exceed levels then permitted in outdoor air. The studies supported a conclusion that "an atmosphere contaminated with tobacco smoke can contribute to the discomfort of many individuals" (USDHEW 1972, p. 7). The possibility that CO emitted from cigarettes could harm persons with chronic heart or lung disease was also mentioned.

Secondhand tobacco smoke was then addressed in greater depth in Chapter 4 (Involuntary Smoking) of the 1975 Surgeon General's report, *The Health Consequences of Smoking* (USDHEW 1975). The chapter noted that involuntary smoking takes place when nonsmokers inhale both sidestream and exhaled mainstream smoke and that this "smoking" is "involuntary" when "the exposure occurs as an unavoidable consequence of breathing in a smoke-filled environment" (p. 87). The report covered exposures and potential health consequences of involuntary smoking, and the researchers concluded that smoking on buses and airplanes was annoying to nonsmokers and that involuntary smoking had potentially adverse consequences for persons with heart and lung diseases. Two studies on nicotine concentrations in nonsmokers raised concerns about nicotine as a contributing factor to atherosclerotic cardiovascular disease in nonsmokers.

The 1979 Surgeon General's report, *Smoking and Health: A Report of the Surgeon General* (USDHEW 1979), also contained a chapter entitled "Involuntary Smoking." The chapter stressed that "attention to involuntary smoking is of recent vintage, and only limited information regarding the health effects of such exposure upon the nonsmoker is available" (p. 11–35). The chapter concluded with recommendations for research including epidemiologic and clinical studies. The 1982 Surgeon General's report specifically addressed smoking and cancer (U.S. Department of Health and Human Services [USDHHS] 1982). By 1982, there were three published epidemiologic studies on involuntary smoking and lung cancer, and the 1982 Surgeon General's report included a brief chapter on this topic. That chapter commented on the methodologic difficulties inherent in such studies, including exposure assessment, the lengthy interval during which exposures are likely to be relevant, and accounting for exposures to other carcinogens. Nonetheless, the report concluded that "Although the currently available evidence is not sufficient to conclude that passive or involuntary smoking causes lung cancer in nonsmokers, the evidence does raise concern about a possible serious public health problem" (p. 251).

Involuntary smoking was also reviewed in the 1984 report, which focused on chronic obstructive pulmonary disease and smoking (USDHHS 1984). Chapter 7 (Passive Smoking) of that report included a comprehensive review of the mounting information on smoking by parents and the effects on respiratory health of their children, data on irritation of the eye, and the more limited evidence on pulmonary effects of involuntary smoking on adults. The chapter began with a compilation of measurements of tobacco smoke components in various indoor environments. The extent of the data had increased substantially since 1972. By 1984, the data included measurements of more specific indicators such as acrolein and nicotine, and less specific indicators such as particulate matter (PM), nitrogen oxides, and CO. The report reviewed new evidence on exposures of nonsmokers using biomarkers, with substantial information on levels of cotinine, a major nicotine metabolite. The report anticipated future conclusions with regard to respiratory effects of parental smoking on child respiratory health.

Involuntary smoking was the topic for the entire 1986 Surgeon General's report, *The Health Consequences of Involuntary Smoking* (USDHHS 1986). In its 359 pages, the report covered the full breadth of the topic, addressing toxicology and dosimetry of tobacco smoke; the relevant evidence on active smoking; patterns of exposure of nonsmokers to tobacco smoke; the epidemiologic evidence on involuntary smoking and disease risks for infants, children, and adults; and policies to control involuntary exposure to tobacco smoke. That report concluded that involuntary smoking caused lung cancer in lifetime nonsmoking adults and was associated with adverse effects on respiratory health in children. The report also stated that simply separating smokers and nonsmokers within the same airspace reduced but did not eliminate exposure to secondhand smoke. All of these findings are relevant to public health and public policy (Table 1). The lung cancer conclusion was based on extensive information already available on the carcinogenicity of active smoking, the qualitative similarities between secondhand and mainstream smoke, the uptake of tobacco smoke components by nonsmokers, and the epidemiologic data on involuntary smoking. The three major conclusions of the report (Table 1), led Dr. C. Everett Koop, Surgeon General at the time, to comment in his preface that "the right of smokers to smoke ends where their behavior affects the health and well-being of others;

Table 1

Major Conclusions of the 1986 Surgeon General's Report, *The Health Consequences of Involuntary Smoking*

---

1. Involuntary smoking is a cause of disease, including lung cancer, in healthy nonsmokers.

2. The children of parents who smoke compared with the children of nonsmoking parents have an increased frequency of respiratory infections, increased respiratory symptoms, and slightly smaller rates of increase in lung function as the lung matures.

3. The simple separation of smokers and nonsmokers within the same air space may reduce, but does not eliminate, the exposure of nonsmokers to environmental tobacco smoke.

Source: U.S. Department of Health and Human Services 1986, p. 7.

furthermore, it is the smokers' responsibility to ensure that they do not expose nonsmokers to the potential [*sic*] harmful effects of tobacco smoke" (USDHHS 1986, p. xii).

Two other reports published in 1986 also reached the conclusion that involuntary smoking increased the risk for lung cancer. The International Agency for Research on Cancer (IARC) of the World Health Organization concluded that "passive smoking gives rise to some risk of cancer" (IARC 1986, p. 314). In its monograph on tobacco smoking, the agency supported this conclusion on the basis of the characteristics of sidestream and mainstream smoke, the absorption of tobacco smoke materials during an involuntary exposure, and the nature of dose-response relationships for carcinogenesis. In the same year, the National Research Council (NRC) also concluded that involuntary smoking increases the incidence of lung cancer in nonsmokers (NRC 1986). In reaching this conclusion, the NRC report cited the biologic plausibility of the association between exposure to secondhand smoke and lung cancer and the supporting epidemiologic evidence. On the basis of a pooled analysis of the epidemiologic data adjusted for bias, the report concluded that the best estimate for the excess risk of lung cancer in nonsmokers married to smokers was 25 percent, compared with nonsmokers married to nonsmokers. With regard to the effects of involuntary smoking on children, the NRC report commented on the literature linking secondhand smoke exposures from parental smoking to increased risks for respiratory symptoms and infections and to a slightly diminished rate of lung growth.

Since 1986, the conclusions with regard to both the carcinogenicity of secondhand smoke and the adverse effects of parental smoking on the health of children have been echoed and expanded (Table 2). In 1992, the U.S. Environmental Protection Agency (EPA) published its risk assessment of secondhand smoke as a carcinogen (USEPA 1992). The agency's evaluation drew on toxicologic information on secondhand smoke and the extensive literature on active smoking. A comprehensive meta-analysis of the 31 epidemiologic studies of secondhand smoke and lung cancer published up to that time was central to the decision to classify secondhand smoke as a group A carcinogen—namely, a known human carcinogen. Estimates of approximately 3,000 U.S. lung cancer deaths per year in non-smokers were attributed to secondhand smoke. The report also covered other respiratory health effects in children and adults and concluded that involuntary smoking is causally associated with several adverse respiratory effects in children. There was also a quantitative risk assessment for the impact of involuntary smoking on childhood asthma and lower respiratory tract infections in young children.

In the decade since the 1992 EPA report, scientific panels continued to evaluate the mounting evidence linking involuntary smoking to adverse health effects (Table 2). The most recent was the 2005 report of the California EPA (Cal/EPA 2005). Over time, research has repeatedly affirmed the conclusions of the 1986 Surgeon General's reports and studies have further identified causal associations of involuntary smoking with diseases and other health disorders. The epidemiologic evidence on involuntary smoking has markedly expanded since 1986, as have the data on exposure to tobacco smoke in the

Table 2

Selected Major Reports, Other Than Those of the U.S. Surgeon General, Addressing Adverse Effects from Exposure to Tobacco Smoke

Agency	Publication	Place and date of publication
National Research Council	*Environmental Tobacco Smoke: Measuring Exposures and Assessing Health Effects*	Washington, D.C United States 1986
International Agency for Research on Cancer (IARC)	*Monographs on the Evaluation of the Carcinogenic Risk of Chemicals to Humans: Tobacco Smoking (IARC Monograph 38)*	Lyon, France 1986
U.S. Environmental Protection Agency (EPA)	*Respiratory Health Effects of Passive Smoking: Lung Cancer and Other Disorders*	Washington, D.C. United States 1992
National Health and Medical Research Council	*The Health Effects of Passive Smoking*	Canberra, Australia 1997
California EPA (Cal/EPA), Office of Environmental Health Hazard Assessment	*Health Effects of Exposure to Environmental Tobacco Smoke*	Sacramento, California United States 1997
Scientific Committee on Tobacco and Health	*Report of the Scientific Committee on Tobacco and Health*	London, United Kingdom 1998
World Health Organization	*International Consultation on Environmental Tobacco Smoke (ETS) and Child Health. Consultation Report*	Geneva, Switzerland 1999
IARC	*Tobacco Smoke and Involuntary Smoking (IARC Monograph 83)*	Lyon, France 2004
Cal/EPA, Office of Environmental Health Hazard Assessment	*Proposed Identification of Environmental Tobacco Smoke as a Toxic Air Contaminant*	Sacramento, California United States 2005

many environments where people spend time. An understanding of the mechanisms by which involuntary smoking causes disease has also deepened.

As part of the environmental health hazard assessment, Cal/EPA identified specific health effects causally associated with exposure to secondhand smoke. The agency estimated the annual excess deaths in the United States that are attributable to secondhand smoke exposure for specific disorders: sudden infant death syndrome (SIDS), cardiac-related illnesses (ischemic heart disease), and lung cancer (Cal/EPA 2005). For the excess incidence of other health outcomes, either new estimates were provided or estimates from the 1997 health hazard assessment were used without any revisions (Cal/EPA 1997). Overall, Cal/EPA estimated that about 50,000 excess deaths result annually from exposure to secondhand smoke (Cal/EPA 2005). Estimated annual excess deaths for the total U.S. population are about 3,400 (a range of 3,423 to 8,866) from lung cancer, 46,000 (a range of 22,700 to 69,600) from cardiac-related illnesses, and

430 from SIDS. The agency also estimated that between 24,300 and 71,900 low birth weight or preterm deliveries, about 202,300 episodes of childhood asthma (new cases and exacerbations), between 150,000 and 300,000 cases of lower respiratory illness in children, and about 789,700 cases of middle ear infections in children occur each year in the United States as a result of exposure to secondhand smoke.

This new 2006 Surgeon General's report returns to the topic of involuntary smoking. The health effects of involuntary smoking have not received comprehensive coverage in this series of reports since 1986. Reports since then have touched on selected aspects of the topic: the 1994 report on tobacco use among young people (USDHHS 1994), the 1998 report on tobacco use among U.S. racial and ethnic minorities (USDHHS 1998), and the 2001 report on women and smoking (USDHHS 2001). As involuntary smoking remains widespread in the United States and elsewhere, the preparation of this report was motivated by the persistence of involuntary smoking as a public health problem and the need to evaluate the substantial new evidence reported since 1986. This report substantially expands the list of topics that were included in the 1986 report. Additional topics include SIDS, developmental effects, and other reproductive effects; heart disease in adults; and cancer sites beyond the lung. For some associations of involuntary smoking with adverse health effects, only a few studies were reviewed in 1986 (e.g., ear disease in children); now, the relevant literature is substantial. Consequently, this report uses meta-analysis to quantitatively summarize evidence as appropriate. Following the approach used in the 2004 report (*The Health Consequences of Smoking*, USDHHS 2004), this 2006 report also systematically evaluates the evidence for causality, judging the extent of the evidence available and then making an inference as to the nature of the association.

Evidence Evaluation

Following the model of the 1964 report, the Surgeon General's reports on smoking have included comprehensive compilations of the evidence on the health effects of smoking. The evidence is analyzed to identify causal associations between smoking and disease according to enunciated principles, sometimes referred to as the "Surgeon General's criteria" or the "Hill" criteria (after Sir Austin Bradford Hill) for causality (USDHEW 1964; USDHHS 2004). Application of these criteria involves covering all relevant observational and experimental evidence. The criteria, offered in a brief chapter of the 1964 report entitled "Criteria for Judgment," included (1) the consistency of the association, (2) the strength of the association, (3) the specificity of the association, (4) the temporal relationship of the association, and (5) the coherence of the association. Although these criteria have been criticized (e.g., Rothman and Greenland 1998), they have proved useful as a framework for interpreting evidence on smoking and other postulated causes of disease, and for judging whether causality can be inferred.

In the 2004 report of the Surgeon General, *The Health Consequences of Smoking*, the framework for interpreting evidence on smoking and health was

Table 3

Four-Level Hierarchy for Classifying the Strength of Causal Inferences Based on Available Evidence

Level 1   Evidence is sufficient to infer a causal relationship.

Level 2   Evidence is suggestive but not sufficient to infer a causal relationship.

Level 3   Evidence is inadequate to infer the presence or absence of a causal relationship (which encompasses evidence that is sparse, of poor quality, or conflicting).

Level 4   Evidence is suggestive of no causal relationship.

Source: U.S. Department of Health and Human Services 2004.

revisited in depth for the first time since the 1964 report (USDHHS 2004). The 2004 report provided a four-level hierarchy for interpreting evidence (Table 3). The categories acknowledge that evidence can be "suggestive" but not adequate to infer a causal relationship, and also allows for evidence that is "suggestive of no causal relationship." Since the 2004 report, the individual chapter conclusions have consistently used this four-level hierarchy (Table 3), but evidence syntheses and other summary statements may use either the term "increased risk" or "cause" to describe instances in which there is sufficient evidence to conclude that active or involuntary smoking causes a disease or condition. This four-level framework also sharply and completely separates conclusions regarding causality from the implications of such conclusions.

That same framework was used in this report on involuntary smoking and health. The criteria dating back to the 1964 Surgeon General's report remain useful as guidelines for evaluating evidence (USDHEW 1964), but they were not intended to be applied strictly or as a "checklist" that needed to be met before the designation of "causal" could be applied to an association. In fact, for involuntary smoking and health, several of the criteria will not be met for some associations. Specificity, referring to a unique exposure-disease relationship (e.g., the association between thalidomide use during pregnancy and unusual birth defects), can be set aside as not relevant, as all of the health effects considered in this report have causes other than involuntary smoking. Associations are considered more likely to be causal as the strength of an association increases because competing explanations become less plausible alternatives. However, based on knowledge of dosimetry and mechanisms of injury and disease causation, the risk is anticipated to be only slightly or modestly increased for some associations of involuntary smoking with disease, such as lung cancer, particularly when the very strong relative risks found for active smokers are compared with those for lifetime nonsmokers. The finding of only a small elevation in risk, as in the example of spousal smoking and lung cancer risk in lifetime nonsmokers, does not weigh against a causal association; however, alternative explanations for a risk of a small magnitude need full exploration and cannot be so easily set aside as alternative explanations for a stronger association. Consistency, coherence, and the temporal relationship of involuntary smoking with disease are central to the interpretations in this report. To address coherence, the report draws not only on the evidence for involuntary smoking, but on the even more extensive literature on active somking and disease.

Although the evidence reviewed in this report comes largely from investigations of secondhand smoke specifically, the larger body of evidence on active smoking is also relevant to many of the associations that were evaluated. The 1986 report found secondhand smoke to be qualitatively similar to mainstream smoke inhaled by the smoker and concluded that secondhand smoke would be expected to have "a toxic and carcinogenic potential that would not be expected to be qualitatively different from that of MS [mainstream smoke]" (USDHHS 1986, p. 23). The 2004 report of the Surgeon General revisited the health consequences of active smoking (USDHHS 2004), and the conclusions substantially expanded the list of diseases and conditions caused by smoking. Chapters in the present report consider the evidence on active smoking that is relevant to biologic plausibility for causal associations between involuntary smoking and disease. The reviews included in this report cover evidence identified through search strategies set out in each chapter. Of necessity, the evidence on mechanisms was selectively reviewed. However, an attempt was made to cover all health studies through specified target dates. Because of the substantial amount of time involved in preparing this report, lists of new key references published after these cut-off dates are included in an Appendix. Literature reviews were extended when new evidence was sufficient to possibly change the level of a causal conclusion.

Major Conclusions

This report returns to involuntary smoking, the topic of the 1986 Surgeon General's report. Since then, there have been many advances in the research on secondhand smoke, and substantial evidence has been reported over the ensuing 20 years. This report uses the revised language for causal conclusions that was implemented in the 2004 Surgeon General's report (USDHHS 2004). Each chapter provides a comprehensive review of the evidence, a quantitative synthesis of the evidence if appropriate, and a rigorous assessment of sources of bias that may affect interpretations of the findings. The reviews in this report reaffirm and strengthen the findings of the 1986 report. With regard to the involuntary exposure of nonsmokers to tobacco smoke, the scientific evidence now supports the following major conclusions:

1. Secondhand smoke causes premature death and disease in children and in adults who do not smoke.
2. Children exposed to secondhand smoke are at an increased risk for sudden infant death syndrome (SIDS), acute respiratory infections, ear problems, and more severe asthma. Smoking by parents causes respiratory symptoms and slows lung growth in their children.
3. Exposure of adults to secondhand smoke has immediate adverse effects on the cardiovascular system and causes coronary heart disease and lung cancer.

4. The scientific evidence indicates that there is no risk-free level of exposure to secondhand smoke.
5. Many millions of Americans, both children and adults, are still exposed to secondhand smoke in their homes and workplaces despite substantial progress in tobacco control.
6. Eliminating smoking in indoor spaces fully protects nonsmokers from exposure to secondhand smoke. Separating smokers from nonsmokers, cleaning the air, and ventilating buildings cannot eliminate exposures of nonsmokers to secondhand smoke.

J. B. Copas and J. Q. Shi

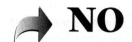

Reanalysis of Epidemiological Evidence on Lung Cancer and Passive Smoking

Objective   To assess the epidemiological evidence for an increase in the risk of lung cancer resulting from exposure to environmental tobacco smoke.

Design   Reanalysis of 37 published epidemiological studies previously included in a meta-analysis allowing for the possibility of publication bias.

Main outcome measure   Relative risk of lung cancer among female lifelong non-smokers, according to whether her partner was a current smoker or a lifelong non-smoker.

Results   If it is assumed that all studies that have ever been carried out are included, or that those selected for review are truly representative of all such studies, then the estimated excess risk of lung cancer is 24%, as previously reported (95% confidence interval 13% to 36%, P < 0.001). However, a significant correlation between study outcome and study size suggests the presence of publication bias. Adjustment for such bias implies that the risk has been overestimated. For example, if only 60% of studies have been included, the estimate of excess risk falls from 24% to 15%.

Conclusion   A modest degree of publication bias leads to a substantial reduction in the relative risk and to a weaker level of significance, suggesting that the published estimate of the increased risk of lung cancer associated with environmental tobacco smoke needs to be interpreted with caution.

Introduction

Exposure to environmental tobacco smoke (passive smoking) is widely accepted to increase the risk of lung cancer, but different epidemiological studies have produced varying estimates of the size of the relative risk. Hackshaw et al. reviewed the results of 37 such studies that estimated the relative risk of lung cancer among female lifelong non-smokers, comparing those whose spouses (or partners) were current smokers with those whose spouses had

From J. B. Copas and J. Q. Shi, "Reanalysis of Epidemiological Evidence on Lung Cancer and Passive Smoking," *British Medical Journal,* vol. 320 (February 12, 2000). Copyright © 2000 by The BMJ Publishing Group. Reprinted by permission. Notes omitted.

never smoked.[1] Of the 37 studies, 31 reported an increase in risk, and the increase was significant in seven studies. The remaining six studies reported negative results, but none of these was significant. Pooling these results using a method which allows for statistical heterogeneity between studies, Hackshaw et al concluded that there is an overall excess risk of 24% (95% confidence interval 13% to 36%).[1] This is strong epidemiological evidence for an association between lung cancer and passive smoking (P < 0.001).

The approach used by Hackshaw et al does not allow for the possibility of publication bias—that is, the possibility that published studies, particularly smaller ones, will be biased in favour of more positive results. We reanalysed the results and looked for evidence of publication bias.

Methods and Results

. . . [T]he relative risks from the 37 epidemiological studies analysed by Hackshaw et al[1] [were] plotted against a measure of the uncertainty in that relative risk. This uncertainty (s) decreases as the size of the study increases so that large studies are on the left of the plot and small studies on the right. The plot shows a trend for smaller studies to give more positive results than the larger studies (correlation = 0.35, P < 0.05, or P = 0.012 by Egger's test[2]). This graph is similar to the funnel plot used in the meta-analysis of clinical trials, when a trend such as this is interpreted as a sign of publication bias.[3] This bias arises when a study is more likely to be written up and submitted to a journal and more likely to be accepted for publication if it reports positive results than if its results are inconclusive or negative. Since it is reasonable to assume that publication is more likely for larger (small s) than smaller (large s) studies, the problem of publication bias will be most evident among the smaller studies, as suggested by the figure. By "publication" we mean the whole process of selecting a study for review.

We reanalysed the results of the 37 epidemiological studies to allow for the trend evident in the figure. Our method describes the apparent relation between relative risk and study size by a curve. This gives a good fit to the observed points. The basic idea of the method is that there is no real relation between study outcome and study size, the relation that we observe is simply an artefact of the process of selecting these studies.

Our method has been published,[4] and further details are available from us on request. The estimated average relative risk depends on a statistical parameter that can be interpreted as the probability that a paper with a certain value of s is published (publication probability). If the publication probability is 1, all papers are published and so there is no possibility of publication bias; the relative risk is then estimated as 1.24 (24% risk excess), agreeing as expected with Hackshaw et al's result.[1] But smaller values of publication probability give smaller estimates of relative risk. We do not know how many unpublished studies have been carried out. Therefore there is no way of estimating the publication probability from any data: all we know is that there is a significant correlation in the funnel plot, so that some degree of publication bias is needed to explain this trend.

Table 1

Estimated Relative Risk and Number of Unpublished Smaller and Larger Studies for Various Values of Publication Probability

Publication probability	Relative risk (95% CI)	P value	No of unpublished studies (*)	
			Small	Large
0.6	1.11 (0.97 to 1.27)	0.110	36	24
0.7	1.13 (1.00 to 1.27)	0.052	23	15
0.8	1.15 (1.03 to 1.28)	0.014	14	9
0.9	1.18 (1.07 to 1.31)	0.002	7	4
n	1.24 (1.13 to 1.36)	<0.001	0	0

(*) Smaller studies s > 0.4; larger studies s [is less than or equal to] 0.4.

Table 1 gives the estimated relative risk for values of publication probability between 0.6 and 1, together with 95% confidence intervals and P values. The P value is less than 5% only when the publication probability is more than about 0.7. The indirect estimate of 19% excess risk derived from studies on biochemical markers (table 5 of Hackshaw et al's paper[1]) agrees with the epidemiological analysis when the publication probability is about 0.9.

For any given value of publication probability it is possible to estimate the number of studies which have been undertaken but not published. This is shown in the final two columns of Table 1. If the publication probability is 0.8 then there are a total of 23 unpublished studies so that the 37 selected ones represent a sample of 37/60 = 62% of all such studies that have been undertaken. If this is the case, then the excess risk is likely to be closer to 15% than 24%. . . .

Conclusions

Although the trend . . . seems clear, Bero et al suggest that the number of unpublished studies is unlikely to be large,[5] and so the problem of publication bias may be less severe here than in systematic reviews of other aspects of medicine. However, the possibility of publication bias cannot be ruled out altogether, and at least some publication bias is needed to explain the trend we found. Our results show that the publication probability does not have to fall much below 1.0 before there is quite a substantial reduction in the estimated risk.

References

1. Hackshaw AK, Law MR, Wald NJ. The accumulated evidence on lung cancer and environmental tobacco smoke. BMJ 1997;315:980–988.
2. Egger M, Smith GD, Schneider M, Minder C. Bias in meta-analysis detected by a simple graphical test. BMJ 1997;315:629–634.

3.   Egger M, Smith GD. Misleading meta-analysis. BMJ 1995;310:752–754.

4.   Copas JB. What works; selectivity models and meta analysis. J R Stat Soc Am 1999; 162:95–109.

5.   Bero LA, Glantz SA, Rennie D. Publication bias and public health policy on environmental tobacco smoke. JAMA 1994;272:133–136.

POSTSCRIPT

Does Secondhand Smoke Endanger the Health of Nonsmokers?

In today's health-conscious society, many people seem to be more aware of what they eat, whether or not they get enough exercise, if they get an adequate amount of sleep, and how much stress they experience. Thus, it is only logical that people also are concerned about possible environmental threats to their health, such as secondhand smoke.

Whether or not secondhand smoke is injurious to nonsmokers is relevant because many businesses have adopted policies and many cities and states have passed laws based on the premise that secondhand smoke is a significant health risk. A number of states restrict smoking in the workplace; most shopping malls prohibit smoking; the military has banned or restricted smoking in many of its facilities; and numerous restaurants forbid smoking in their establishments. New York City and other cities have even banned smoking in bars. Many colleges prohibit smoking in residence halls.

The issue of smoking also has become a point of contention in child custody cases. It has been argued that parents who smoke around their children are unfit parents. Is smoking around children a form of child abuse? Should parental smoking be a consideration in children custody cases? If one thinks that smoking around children is abusive, then would overfeeding children or using television as a babysitter also be considered child abuse?

Increasingly, smokers are being isolated in society; they are almost always pictured as social outcasts. There appears to be a growing contempt and disdain shown toward smokers. The emotionality of this issue often puts smokers on the defensive. This confrontational stance is not conducive to addressing the issue of smokers' rights in a constructive way.

A report released by the Environmental Protection Agency (EPA) links environmental tobacco smoke (ETS) to lung cancer and heart disease in nonsmokers and to respiratory infections in children. The report states that passive smoking is responsible for an estimated 3,000 lung cancer deaths annually in adults, as many as 300,000 childhood cases of bronchitis and pneumonia, and between 8,000 and 26,000 new cases of asthma in children. Although groups in support of restricting environmental tobacco smoke cite the EPA's report as evidence for their position, the report has been criticized for exaggerating and distorting the harmful effects of passive smoke.

The role of the tobacco industry in this issue is discussed in "The Tobacco Industry's Role in the 16 Cities Study of Secondhand Tobacco Smoke: Do the Data Support the Stated Conclusions?" by Richard Barnes, S. Katharine Hammond, and Stanton Glantz in *Environmental Health Perspectives* (December 2006). The effects of secondhand smoke are studied in "Adverse

Health Effects of Prenatal and Postnatal Tobacco Smoke Exposure on Children" by W. Hofhuis, J. C. de Jongste, and P. J. Merkus (*Archives of Disease in Childhood*, December 2003). F. D. Galliland and associates examined the role of secondhand smoke on schoolchildren in "Environmental Tobacco Smoke and Absenteeism Related to Respiratory Illness in Schoolchildren" (*American Journal of Epidemiology*, May 15, 2003). "Second Hand Smoke and Risk Assessment: What Was in It for the Tobacco Industry?" by Norbert Hirschhorn and Stella A. Bialous in *Tobacco Control* (December 2001) addresses how the tobacco industry tries to refute the claims regarding the harms related to secondhand smoke.

ISSUE 15

Is Alcoholism Hereditary?

YES: National Institute on Alcohol Abuse and Alcoholism, from "The Genetics of Alcoholism," *Alcohol Alert* (July 2003)

NO: Grazyna Zajdow, from "Alcoholism's Unnatural History: Alcoholism Is Not a Health Issue, But One of Personal and Existential Pain. Recognising This Would Force Us to Acknowledge One of the Most Successful Methods of Dealing With Alcohol Addiction," *Arena Magazine* (April–May 2004)

ISSUE SUMMARY

YES: The National Institute on Alcohol Abuse and Alcoholism (NIAAA) contends that heredity plays a large role in the development of alcoholism. Family environment may play a role in whether one becomes an alcoholic but individuals inherit characteristics that increase the possibility of developing alcoholism. The NIAAA notes that identical twins are twice as likely to become alcoholic as fraternal twins.

NO: Grazyna Zajdow, a lecturer in sociology at Deakin University, maintains that the concept of alcoholism results from a social construct of what it means to be alcoholic. Because alcoholism is a social stigma, it is viewed as a disease rather than as a condition caused by personal and existential pain. Environmental conditions, especially consumerism, says Zajdow, are the root cause of alcoholism.

Alcoholism is a serious health problem throughout the world. The number of people with an addiction to alcohol surpasses the number of addicts of any other drug. Estimates from the National Institute on Alcohol Abuse and Alcoholism indicate that there are approximately 10 million to 20 million alcoholics in the United States and millions more that are problem drinkers. Yet, it is not fully understood what determines a person's disposition to alcoholism. For years scientists have been reporting that there is a genetic tendency towards alcoholism. Research shows that there may exist specific biochemical and behavioral differences in the way sons and daughters of alcoholics respond to alcohol that may be a key about why these children are more prone to becoming addicted to or abusive of the drug.

Children of alcoholics have been consistently shown to have higher rates of alcoholism than children of nonalcoholics. Children of alcoholics are two to four times more likely to become alcoholic than children of nonalcoholic parents, according to the National Council on Alcoholism. Thus, alcoholism has been called a "family disease" because it tends to run in families.

The degree to which hereditary and biological risk factors make some individuals more likely candidates for addiction once they begin drinking is unknown. Psychological forces and environmental influences may also play a major role in predisposing one to alcoholism. Certainly, there is agreement among experts that a combination and interplay of all three of these factors—biological, psychological, and environmental—are responsible for alcoholic behaviors.

In one of the largest studies ever conducted on females and alcoholism, the *Journal of the American Medical Association* reports that heredity plays a major role in determining whether a woman becomes an alcoholic. Researchers found that genes do not automatically cause alcoholism, but they do account for 50 percent to 61 percent of a woman's risk of becoming an alcoholic. The report mirrors the results for men. Another research group found that college-aged sons of alcoholics tend to have a lower hormonal response to alcohol and feel less drunk when they drink too much when compared to young men whose parents are not alcoholic. And, many adoption and twin studies indicate a genetic predisposition to alcoholism among children of alcoholic parents.

Although many scientists and psychologists believe that there is a genetic component of alcoholism for many people, genetic theories are still inconclusive. Researchers have not identified a single gene that carries a predisposition to alcohol abuse. Some argue that risk factors for alcoholism cannot be translated directly into genetic and biological terms and that factors such as personality traits, values, individual needs, attitudes, family upbringing, peers, and other sociocultural influences in a person's life affect one's use or abuse of alcohol.

Studies of family members show (1) common causal factors that are shared among relatives and (2) risk factors that are unique to an individual family member's life experiences and environment. In addition to sharing genes, many family members share similar environments, customs, culture, diet, and patterns of behavior. The interaction of these factors may be the foundation for a pattern of alcoholism in the family or individual family member. Thus, the conclusion that the sole cause of alcoholism is genetic is viewed skeptically because there are too many other psychological and environmental factors that play a key role in the onset of alcoholism.

The National Institute on Alcohol Abuse and Alcoholism (NIAAA) argues that alcoholism has a genetic component and is not the result of family environment. The NIAAA maintains that there are differences in the brains of alcoholics that may account for their alcoholism. Grazyna Zajdow contends that alcoholism is not based on genetics but on society's view of what constitutes alcoholism. Zajdow argues that addictive drinking choices.

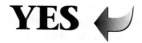

The Genetics of Alcoholism

Research has shown conclusively that familial transmission of alcoholism risk is at least in part genetic and not just the result of family environment.[1] The task of current science is to identify what a person inherits that increases vulnerability to alcoholism and how inherited factors interact with the environment to cause disease. This information will provide the basis for identifying people at risk and for developing behavioral and pharmacologic approaches to prevent and treat alcohol problems. The advances being made now are built on the discovery 50 years ago of the role in inheritance of DNA, the genetic material in cells that serves as a blueprint for the proteins that direct life processes. Alcoholism research, like other fields, is capitalizing on the scientific spinoffs of this milestone, among them the Human Genome Project and related efforts to sequence the genomes, the complete DNA sequences, of selected animals.

A Complex Genetic Disease

Studies in recent years have confirmed that identical twins, who share the same genes, are about twice as likely as fraternal twins, who share on average 50 percent of their genes, to resemble each other in terms of the presence of alcoholism. Recent research also reports that 50 to 60 percent of the risk for alcoholism is genetically determined, for both men and women.[2-5] Genes alone do not preordain that someone will be alcoholic; features in the environment along with gene–environment interactions account for the remainder of the risk.

Research suggests that many genes play a role in shaping alcoholism risk. Like diabetes and heart disease, alcoholism is considered genetically complex, distinguishing it from genetic diseases, such as cystic fibrosis, that result primarily from the action of one or two copies of a single gene and in which the environment plays a much smaller role, if any. The methods used to search for genes in complex diseases have to account for the fact that the effects of any one gene may be subtle and a different array of genes underlies risk in different people.

Scientists have bred lines of mice and rats that manifest specific and separate alcohol-related traits or phenotypes, such as sensitivity to alcohol's

From "Alcohol Alert:, the National Institute on Alcohol Abuse and Alcoholism", no. 60, July 2003.

intoxicating and sedative effects, the development of tolerance, the suscepti-bility to withdrawal symptoms, and alcohol-related organ damage.[6, 7] Risk for alcoholism in humans reflects the mix and magnitude of these and other phenotypes, shaped by underlying genes, in interaction with an environment in which alcohol is available. Genetic research on alcoholism seeks to tease apart the genetic underpinnings of these phenotypes and how they contribute to risk.

One well characterized relationship between genes and alcoholism is the result of variation in the liver enzymes that metabolize (break down) alcohol. By speeding up the metabolism of alcohol to a toxic intermediate, acetaldehyde, or slowing down the conversion of acetaldehyde to acetate, genetic variants in the enzymes alcohol dehydrogenase (ADH) or aldehyde dehydrogenase (ALDH) raise the level of acetaldehyde after drinking, causing symptoms that include flushing, nausea, and rapid heartbeat. The genes for these enzymes and the alle-les, or gene variants, that alter alcohol metabolism have been identified. Genes associated with flushing are more common among Asian populations than other ethnic groups, and the rates of drinking and alcoholism are correspondingly lower among Asian populations.[8, 9]

Genes, Behavior, and the Brain

Addiction is based in the brain. It involves memory, motivation, and emo-tional state. The processes involved in these aspects of brain function have thus been logical targets for the search for genes that underlie risk for alcoholism. Much of the information on potential alcohol-related genes has come from research on animals. Research has demonstrated a similarity in the mechanisms of many brain functions across species as well as an overlap between the genomes of animals—even invertebrates—and humans.

One approach to identifying alcohol-related genes is to start with an aspect of brain chemistry on which alcohol is thought to have an impact, and work forward, identifying and manipulating the underlying genes and ulti-mately determining whether the presence or absence of different forms, or alleles, of a gene influence alcoholism risk. For example, genetic technology now permits scientists to delete or inactivate specific genes, or alternatively, to increase the expression of specific genes, and watch the effects in living animals. Because genes act in the context of many other genes, interpretation of these studies can be difficult. If one gene is disabled, for example, others may compen-sate for the loss of function. Alternatively, the loss of a single gene throughout development may be harmful or lethal. Nonetheless, these techniques can provide important clues to function. These approaches have been used to study how altering the expression of genes encoding the receptors (or their subunits) for neurotransmitters and intracellular messenger molecules alters the response to alcohol.[10]

Scientists also have an increasing array of methods for locating alcohol-related genes and gene locations and only then determining how the genes function, an approach known as reverse genetics. Quantitative trait loci (QTL) analysis seeks to identify stretches of DNA along chromosomes that influence traits, like alcohol sensitivity, that vary along a spectrum (height is another quantitative trait). QTLs have been identified for alcohol sensitivity, alcohol preference, and withdrawal severity.[11] Ultimately, the goal is to identify and determine which candidate genes within the QTLs are responsible for the observed trait. Among the candidate genes already known to lie near alcohol-related QTLs are several that encode neurotransmitter receptors and neurotransmitters themselves. One of these, neuropeptide Y (NPY), lies within a QTL for alcohol preference in rats. NPY is a small protein molecule that is abundant in the brain and has been shown to influence the response to alcohol.[12]

Scientists also can scan the genome to identify genes whose activity differs among animals that respond differently to alcohol. The methods used are designed to measure the amount of messenger RNA which, as the first intermediary in the process by which DNA is translated into protein, is a reflection of gene expression. The advantage of this approach is its power to survey the activities of thousands of genes, some of which might not otherwise have been identified as candidates for involvement in alcohol-related behavior. Recent work in rats identified a gene that is differentially expressed in brain regions of alcohol-preferring rats and nonpreferring rats. The gene is within an already identified QTL for alcohol preference and codes for alpha-synuclein, a protein that has been shown to regulate dopamine transmission.[13]

Genetic Studies in Humans

Knowledge gained from animal studies has assisted scientists in identifying the genes underlying brain chemistry in humans. Much research suggests that genes affecting the activity of the neurotransmitters serotonin and GABA (gamma-aminobutyric acid) are likely candidates for involvement in alcoholism risk. A recent preliminary study looked at five genes related to these two neurotransmitters in a group of men who had been followed over a 15-year period.[14] The men who had particular variants of genes for a serotonin transporter and for one type of GABA receptor showed lower response to alcohol at age 20 and were more likely to have met the criteria for alcoholism. Another study found that college students with a particular variant of the serotonin transporter gene consumed more alcohol per occasion, more often drank expressly to become inebriated, and engaged more frequently in binge drinking than students with another variant of the gene.[15] The relationships between neurotransmitter genes and alcoholism are complex, however; not all studies have shown a connection between alcoholism risk and these genes.

Individual variation in response to stressors such as pain is genetically influenced and helps shape susceptibility to psychiatric diseases, including alcoholism. Scientists recently found that a common genetic variation in an enzyme (catechol-0-methyltransferase) that metabolizes the neurotransmitters dopamine and norepinephrine results in a less efficient form of the enzyme and increased pain susceptibility.[16] Scientists in another study found that the same genetic variant influences anxiety in women. In this study, women who had the enzyme variant scored higher on measures of anxiety and exhibited an electroencephalogram (EEG) pattern associated with anxiety disorders and alcoholism.[17]

The drug naltrexone has been shown to help some, but not all, alcohol-dependent patients reduce their drinking. Preliminary results from a recent study showed that alcoholic patients with different variations in the gene for a receptor on which naltrexone is known to act (the mu-opioid receptor) responded differently to treatment with the drug.[18] This work demonstrates how genetic typing may in the future be helpful in tailoring treatment for alcoholism to each individual.

NIAAA's Collaborative Study on the Genetics of Alcoholism (COGA) is searching for alcohol-related genes through studies of families with multiple generations of alcoholism. Using existing markers—known variations in the DNA sequence that serve as signposts along the length of a chromosome—and observing to what extent specific markers are inherited along with alcoholism risk, they have found "hotspots" for alcoholism risk on five chromosomes and a protective area on one chromosome near the location of genes for alcohol dehydrogenase.[19] They have also examined patterns of brain waves measured by electroencephalogram. EEGs measure differences in electrical potential across the brain caused by synchronized firing of many neurons. Brain wave patterns are characteristic to individuals and are shaped genetically—they are quantitative genetic traits, varying along a spectrum among individuals. COGA researchers have found that reduced amplitude of one wave that characteristically occurs after a stimulus correlates with alcohol dependence, and they have identified chromosomal regions that appear to affect this P300 wave amplitude.[20] Recently, COGA researchers found that the shape of a characteristic brain wave measured in the frequency stretch between 13 and 25 cycles per second (the "beta" wave) reflected gene variations at a specific chromosomal site containing genes for one type of GABA receptor.[21] They suggest that this site is in or near a previously identified QTL for alcoholism risk. Thus, brain wave patterns reflect underlying genetic variation in a receptor for a neurotransmitter known to be involved in the brain's response to alcohol. Findings of this type promise to help researchers identify markers of alcoholism risk and ultimately, suggest ways to reduce the risk or to treat the disease pharmacologically.

Genetics Research—A Commentary by NIAAA Director, Ting-Kai Li, M.D.

Even from the first drink, individuals differ substantially in their response to alcohol. Genetics research is helping us understand how genes shape the metabolic and behavioral response to alcohol and what makes one person more vulnerable to addiction than another. An understanding of the genetic underpinnings of alcoholism can help us identify those at risk and, in the long term, provide the foundation for tailoring prevention and treatment according to the particular physiology of each individual.

References

1. **National Institute on Alcohol Abuse and Alcoholism (NIAAA).** The Genetics of Alcoholism. *Alcohol Alert* No. 18. Rockville, MD: NIAAA, 1992.

2. **Heath, A.C.;** Bucholz, K.K.; Madden, P.A.F.; et al. Genetic and environmental contributions to alcohol dependence risk in a national twin sample: Consistency of findings in women and men. *Psychological Medicine* 27:1381–1396, 1997.

3. **Heath, A.C.,** and Martin, N.G. Genetic influences on alcohol consumption patterns and problem drinking: Results from the Australian NH&MRC twin panel follow-up survey. *Annals of the New York Academy of Sciences* 708:72–85, 1994.

4. **Kendler, K.S.;** Neale, M.C.; Heath, A.C.; et al. A twin-family study of alcoholism in women. *American Journal of Psychiatry* 151:707–715, 1994.

5. **Prescott, C.A.,** and Kendler, K.S. Genetic and environmental contributions to alcohol abuse and dependence in a population-based sample of male twins. *American Journal of Psychiatry* 156: 34–40, 1999.

6. **Crabbe, J.C.** Alcohol and genetics: New models. *American Journal of Medical Genetics (Neuropsychiatric Genetics)* 114:969–974, 2002.

7. **Tabakoff, B.,** and Hoffman, P.L. Animal models in alcohol research. *Alcohol Research & Health* 24(2):77–84, 2000.

8. **Li, T.K.** Pharmacogenetics of responses to alcohol and genes that influence alcohol drinking. *Journal of Studies on Alcohol* 61:5–12, 2000.

9. **Makimoto, K.** Drinking patterns and drinking problems among Asian-Americans and Pacific Islanders. *Alcohol Health & Research World* 22(4):270–275, 1998.

10. **Bowers, B.J.** Applications of transgenic and knockout mice in alcohol research. *Alcohol Research & Health* 24(3):175–184, 2000.

11. **Crabbe, J.C.;** Phillips, T.J.; Buck, K.J.; et al. Identifying genes for alcohol and drug sensitivity: Recent progress and future directions. *Trends in Neurosciences* 22(4):173–179, 1999.

12. **Pandey, S.C.;** Carr, L.G.; Heilig, M.; et al. Neuropeptide Y and alcoholism: Genetic, molecular, and pharmacological evidence. *Alcoholism: Clinical and Experimental Research* 27:149–154, 2003.

13. **Liang, T.;** Spence, J.; Liu, L.; et al. α-Synuclein maps to a quantitative trait locus for alcohol preference and is differentially expressed in alcohol-preferring and nonpreferring rats. *Proceedings of the National Academy of Sciences of the U.S.A.* 100(8): 4690–4695, 2003.

14. **Schuckit, M.A.;** Mazzanti, C.; Smith, T.L.; et al. Selective genotyping for the role of 5-HT_{2A}, 5-HT_{2C}, and $\text{GABA}_{\alpha6}$, receptors and the serotonin transporter in the level of response to alcohol: A pilot study. *Biological Psychiatry* 45:647–651, 1999.

15. **Herman, A.I.;** Philbeck, J.W.; Vasilopoulos, N.L.; and Depetrillo, P.B. Serotonin transporter promoter polymorphism and differences in alcohol consumption behaviour in a college student population. *Alcohol and Alcoholism* 38: 446–449, 2003.

16. **Zubieta, J.-K.;** Heitzeg, M.M.; Smith, Y.R.; et al. COMT val[158]met genotype affects μ-opioid neurotransmitter responses to a pain stressor. *Science* 299: 1240–1243, 2003.

17. **Enoch, M.A.;** Xu, K.; Ferro, E.; et al. Genetic origins of anxiety in women: A role for a functional catechol-O-methyltransferase polymorphism. *Psychiatric Genetics* 13(1):33–41, 2003.

18. **Oslin, D.W.;** Berrettini, W.; Kranzler, H.R.; et al. A functional polymorphism of the μ-opioid receptor gene is associated with naltrexone response in alcohol-dependent patients. *Neuropsychopharmacology* 28:1546–1552, 2003.

19. **Edenberg, H.J.** The collaborative study on the genetics of alcoholism: An update. *Alcohol Research & Health* 26(3):214–217, 2002.

20. **Begleiter, H.;** Porjesz, B.; Reich, T.; et al. Quantitative trait loci analysis of human event-related brain potentials: P3 voltage. *Electroencephalography and Clinical Neurophysiology* 103(3):244–250, 1998.

21. **Porjesz, B.;** Almasy, L.; Edenberg, H.J.; et al. Linkage disequilibrium between the beta frequency of the human EEG and a GABA$_A$ receptor gene locus. *Proceedings of the National Academy of Sciences of the U.S.A.* 99:3729–3733, 2002.

Grazyna Zajdow

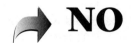 **NO**

Alcoholism's Unnatural History: Alcoholism Is Not a "Health" Issue, But One of Personal and Existential Pain. Recognising This Would Force Us to Acknowledge One of the Most Successful Methods of Dealing With Alcohol Addiction

Watching former Tasmanian premier Jim Bacon on TV, resigning himself to continuing a course of palliative care for lung cancer and urging young Australians not to be "idiots" and smoke, reminds one that there is such a thing as addiction. Bacon prefers to say he was stupid rather than addicted. And this is to a substance that is not mind-altering!

This example gives us an interesting view of how we deal with addictive substances on a social and personal level. Addiction is a problem for the late modern world because it questions the very basis of consumption and choice. In a wider social world, choice is everything; for the addict, choice can be death. Yet the Australian response to addiction is marked by ambivalence, particularly in the case of addiction to alcohol. Despite the widespread acknowledgement of the serious nature of this social problem, the attitude to one of the most successful ways of dealing with alcoholism—through Alcoholics Anonymous—is often one of downright antagonism. As a sociologist who reads the literature on addictions and problematic drug use, I often wonder why—and here I will try to unravel the mystery.

The most prominent narrative of addiction in the last few years in Australia and other places is the narrative of social construction. This narrative presents drug use as an integral part of the social world and cuts it loose from biology and physiology. Addiction only exists if there is a stigmatised role of "addict." Without this deviant category there would not be a notion of addiction. Thomas de Quincey wrote about his seventeen-year addiction to opium and even lengthier time with laudanum. He could write so openly because there was no

From *Arena Magazine*, issue 70, April–May 2004, pp. 41–43. Copyright © 2004 by Arena Magazine.

notion of addiction as a stigmatised social category at the time, but what he described was addiction nonetheless.

There is also the postmodern, discursive view of addiction as an extension of social constructionism. Discourses of addiction, in this view, are part of the Foucauldian notion of disciplinary power and knowledge. The addict is part of the "web of power" that plugs him/her into a network that constrains and limits the individual. This is a particularly abstract notion of addiction that rarely admits to material reality of the individual body, or even the social body. This narrative comes not from the sociological study of the experience of addiction, but cultural studies research on written texts such as the book *What's Wrong with Addiction* by Helen Keane.

These narratives of addiction often merge and become entangled in academic discussions. Combine these with the antagonism-towards-the-disease model of addiction that is sometimes—erroneously in my view—linked to Temperance and Prohibition and we might get an idea of why AA and its models have had such bad press, particularly on the social welfare Left. Take a typical example from a major textbook called *Drug Use in Australia,* in which one chapter refers to the AA model of addiction as the grand narrative of the "alcoholic as sinner." The evidence the authors present is one person's reported statements in an AA meeting from another academic text! Another chapter presents it as a disease model of addiction—but nowhere in the text is any of the large-scale and in-depth studies of AA referred to.

I would argue that the fundamental fact about alcoholism must be that this problem lies in the individual body as much as the social body and it is experienced as a highly individual pain. This pain is materially real and cannot be explained away as a form of discourse, amenable to the linguistic contortions of postmodernity or dismissed as simply a social construction. Alcoholics are different from non-alcoholics. The difference is not easy to distinguish—it only really becomes apparent in its most extreme manifestations—but it is there. I cannot say that my first drink of alcohol changed my life—I cannot even remember it—but I know plenty of alcoholics who say just that. They remember their first drink and how it made them feel. For some who always believed they were different or outsiders, their first drink made them feel part of humanity. For others, their natural shyness disappeared and they became loquacious and humorous. Again others just drank themselves into a stupor from the first moment because they hated the world so much and never seemed to leave this state, at least not until the pain became too great and they permanently left this world.

The sociologist Norman Denzin, in his opus *The Alcoholic Society,* wrote that every alcoholic he talked to drank "to escape an inner emptiness of self." Of course, many of us experience an inner emptiness at many times of our lives, but what Denzin talks about is an emptiness which is a constant. For Denzin, the "alcoholic self" is constantly in search of fulfilment through alcohol, but alcohol just pushes the alcoholic further away from him/herself and all others. No drug or cognitive therapy produces permanent fulfilment—only sobriety through the experience of likeminded others. One could suggest that the divided self produced by alcoholism precedes the first drink, and an existential pain must exist which is married to some physiological and biochemical response to alcohol. There is some genetic component, but what it is and how it works is not understood, and it is unlikely that any pharmaceutical therapy can ever offer a solution—though medical experts, along with pharmaceutical companies are always hinting at the possibility. For Denzin, the answer to the individual alcoholic's pain is the community of others, specifically the community of alcoholics. He is talking, of course, about Alcoholics Anonymous.

A Parallel World

Many years ago, I worked as a youth worker in what was known as the Community Youth Support Scheme. We worked out of an old house, but there was one room that we did not use and which was generally locked. One day I had to go in to do something and I felt that I had stumbled on the meeting room of a secret order, like the Masons. What struck me at first was the terrible odour of tobacco (this was in the days when we could smoke absolutely anywhere) and then I noticed the banners on the wall. They were full of strange language which included the terms God, higher power and surrender. It looked to me as if I had fallen through a hole in the floor and found myself in a parallel world. My stoned friends and I lived off jokes about it for years.

Thus, as a sociologist and a materialist, feminist and atheist, my first AA meeting—which I attended as a non-alcoholic—came as a shock to me. I imagined it had to be a cult, that it produced automatons who were close to born-again Christians. For me, the answer to alcohol and drug problems was to sweep away poverty and inequality; the social and personal body were indistinguishable— what was good for one was equally good for the other. After listening to the unmediated stories of pain, anguish and redemption, I came to believe that I was wrong. Not that poverty and inequality should not be swept away, but that alcoholism would be swept away with them. However, I did meet many stalwarts of the Left in those AA meetings and stalwarts they stayed. I know academics, unionists, politicians, writers, folk singers, musos from the 1970s who regularly maintain their sober conditions through AA. To get to this position and stay in AA, these people had to cross a line that would have been unimaginable, and the only explanation can be the intense, existential pain they experienced when they drank.

Many, whatever the drug of choice had originally been, ended up drinking themselves into oblivion. It may only have been because alcohol was the cheapest and most freely available. There are many paths into addiction and many different categories of addicts. In the end, I never truly understood what they were doing or what they were feeling. I could not understand, ever. I am not like them. I do not feel their pain, I could never cause pain to people the way they did, and nothing I do could ease their suffering. I suspect this is one of the reasons there is such a distrust of AA and its notion of alcoholism—that alcoholism produces a different category of individual, one not amenable to the niceties of living in the world as nonaddicts might do.

But I do know people who are like them. They come together in rooms (no longer smoke-ridden) and recite a prayer at the end of their meetings. Most of them have found some kind of religious understanding; many are still atheists; but all have some form of spiritual fulfilment. Those meetings are more egalitarian than almost any other community they may belong to, although sexism and racism still exist to some extent.

Here people seek to change the way they live in the world and it is a change in morality, as much as in alcohol consumption. We may find the way that television has taken up this public confession distasteful, but the AA meeting is not an episode of Oprah—it is not a mediated televisual experience. To the same extent as any conversation, it is unmediated. It also demands an ethical understanding of individual experience. Obviously some people are better at it than others. An old AA saying is that a sober horse-thief is still a horse-thief.

There are many well-known people who admit to membership of AA. Even in death, however, many people's friends and relatives often refuse to acknowledge the importance of AA in their lives. It is as if acknowledging AA is a recognition that some things (like sobriety) are more important than motherhood or friendship or other social roles.

Why are we so reluctant to recognise this state of addiction that some people find themselves in? There are strong cultural and economic forces that make alcoholism almost impossible to speak about. To recognise it would mean having to do something about it. In Australia at the moment, it would mean having to deal with the availability of help to overcome the problems of drunkenness, and it would mean facing up to the key issue of whether it should be portrayed to any degree as a "health" issue. While it has health consequences, it is not a health issue; it is an issue of personal and existential pain. Even after his public humiliation, Democrats leader Andrew Bartlett would not admit to an alcohol problem. He called it instead a "health" problem. More people are now willing to admit to problems with depression but few mention that they have been compulsively drinking a depressant for most of their adult lives. They are happy to admit to Prozac but not the sobriety (or lack of).

It is more than likely that it is a cultural distrust of AA, its religiosity and its American influence, that keeps many antagonistic to it. Ultimately, one of the most powerful arguments in AA's favour is that it works. A sixty-year follow-up by the writer George Vaillant—carried out fifteen years after the release of his *The Natural History of Alcoholism*, which looked at American men with clear alcohol problems in the 1940s—found that those who were still alive were most likely to be abstinent.

Beyond that, most alcohol-related problems in Australia are not connected to alcoholism or addiction, but to drunkenness and its consequences. Indeed, alcoholics or chronic heavy drinkers make up between 5 and 15 percent of the drinking population. Mixed with aggressive forms of masculinity, drunkenness contributes to all forms of violent crime, from the minor altercation in the pub between drunken bulls, to domestic assault and then to deaths of all sorts. It does not matter whether it is used as a form of excuse or "time-out"—without the intoxicating effects of alcohol, violent crime would be much reduced.

Large and small epidemiological studies show quite clearly that the cheaper and more readily available the alcohol is, and the greater the number of alcohol outlets, the greater the problems that exist. Some cultural factors may ameliorate or enhance its worst effects, but the reality is that humans, especially those in societies which are based on endless consumerism, will endlessly consume alcohol and other intoxicating substances. Attempting to minimise its most harmful effects without dealing with supply is to park an ambulance at the bottom of the cliff. I am not saying we should not provide the ambulance, but we cannot pretend that it is anything more than that. It is here that the abstract nature of academic discussions combines with libertarian constructions of personal choice. Resistance, then, to the restriction of the supply of alcohol means that we are really unable to effectively deal with the worst aspects of alcohol consumption.

POSTSCRIPT

Is Alcoholism Hereditary?

Is there a significant, substantiated relationship between heredity and alcoholism? The National Institute on Alcohol Abuse and Alcoholism (NIAAA) notes that numerous studies demonstrate a high probability of biological vulnerability to alcohol addiction. The NIAAA claims that there are differences in the brains of alcoholics compared to others. Critics agree that alcoholism runs in families, but they argue that there are critical environmental and psychological risk factors for alcoholism that cannot be overlooked. In the final analysis, this issue comes down to which research one chooses to accept.

Some experts have expressed concern for certain people who feel that alcoholism is a family legacy. An individual who believes that he or she is destined to become an alcoholic because his or her mother, father, aunt, uncle, or grandparent has suffered from alcoholism may become alcoholic to satisfy a self-fulfilling prophecy. Some psychologists believe this may have lamentable consequences for such individuals who feel that alcoholism is their destiny anyway.

Whether or not alcoholism is genetic or environmental has serious implications. For example, if a genetic predisposition to alcoholism was conclusively proven, then medical therapies could be designed to help those who had the hereditary risk. Second, if a person was diagnosed as having a genetic predisposition, then he or she could adopt behaviors that would help avoid problem drinking. That is, they would become aware of the hereditary factor and adjust their attitudes and actions accordingly. If alcoholism is environmental, then one's environment could be altered to influence drinking behavior.

Because of the lack of conclusive evidence identifying heredity as the primary cause for alcoholism, it may be wise to err on the side of caution with regard to consigning children of alcoholics to a fate of alcoholism. On the other hand, research that consistently finds higher rates of alcoholism and alcohol abuse among children of alcoholics cannot be dismissed. This link alone provides ample support for additional funding of research studies that may delineate the exact nature of and risk factors of alcoholism. Still, efforts against the perils of alcoholism via progressive alcohol prevention and education programs to meet the needs of children of alcoholics as well as the general public need to be strengthened.

Two interesting publications that provide a different look at the genetic basis of alcoholism are "Recent Progress in the Genetics of Alcoholism," in *10th Special Report to the U.S. Congress on Alcohol and Health and Alcohol: The World's Favorite Drug* by Griffith Edwards (St. Martin's Press, 2001). In "Finding the Future Alcoholic" (*The Futurist*, May/June 2002), Steven Stocker describes attempts to identify children who may become alcoholic. In "Research Finds Alcohol Tolerance Gene" (*The San Francisco Chronicle*, December 12, 2003), Carl Hall examines how come some people can tolerate alcohol's effects better than others.

ISSUE 16

Should Marijuana Be Approved for Medical Use?

YES: Sherwood O. Cole, from "An Update on the Effects of Marijuana and Its Potential Medical Use: Forensic Focus," *The Forensic Examiner* (Fall 2005)

NO: Drug Enforcement Administration, from *The DEA Position on Marijuana* (May 2006)

ISSUE SUMMARY

YES: Sherwood O. Cole, a professor emeritus of psychology at Rutgers University, argues in favor of allowing marijuana for medicinal purposes despite the fact that it has some adverse effects, especially on cognition and mental health and on the respiratory and cardio-vascular systems. Some of the potential medical uses of marijuana include reducing fluid pressure in the eyes of glaucoma patients, reducing nausea associated with cancer treatment, stimulating appetite in AIDS patients, and reducing convulsions of epileptic patients.

NO: The Drug Enforcement Administration (DEA) states that marijuana has not been proven to have medical utility. The DEA cites the positions of the American Medical Association, the American Cancer Society, the American Academy of Pediatrics, and the National Multiple Sclerosis Society to support its position. The DEA feels that any benefits of medicinal marijuana are outweighed by its drawbacks.

Numerous states have passed referenda to legalize marijuana for medical purposes. Despite the position of these voters, however, the federal government does not support the medical use of marijuana, and federal laws take precedence over state laws. A major concern of opponents of these referenda is that legalization of marijuana for medicinal purposes will lead to its use for recreational purposes.

Marijuana's medicinal qualities have been recognized for centuries. Marijuana was utilized medically as far back as 2737 B.C., when Chinese emperor Shen Nung recommended marijuana, or cannabis, for medical use. By the 1890s some medical reports had stated that cannabis was useful as a pain reliever. However, despite its historical significance, the use of marijuana for medical treatment is still a widely debated and controversial topic.

Marijuana has been tested in the treatment of glaucoma, asthma, convulsions, epilepsy, and migraine headaches, and in the reduction of nausea, vomiting, and loss of appetite associated with chemotherapy treatments. Many medical professionals and patients believe that marijuana shows promise in the treatment of these disorders and others, including spasticity in amputees and multiple sclerosis. Yet others argue that there are alternative drugs and treatments available that are more specific and effective in treating these disorders than marijuana and that marijuana cannot be considered a medical replacement.

Because of the conflicting viewpoints and what many people argue is an absence of reliable, scientific research supporting the medicinal value of marijuana, the drug and its plant materials remain in Schedule I of the Controlled Substances Act of 1970. This act established five categories, or schedules, under which drugs are classified according to their potential for abuse and their medical usefulness, which in turn determines their availability. Drugs classified under Schedule I are those that have a high potential for abuse and no scientifically proven medical use. Many marijuana proponents have called for the Drug Enforcement Administration (DEA) to move marijuana from Schedule I to Schedule II, which classifies drugs as having a high potential for abuse but also having an established medical use. A switch to Schedule II would legally allow physicians to utilize marijuana and its components in certain treatment programs. To date, however, the DEA has refused.

Currently, marijuana is used medically but not legally. Most of the controversy surrounds whether marijuana and its plant properties are indeed of medical value and whether the risks associated with its use outweigh its proposed medical benefits. Research reports and scientific studies have been inconclusive. Some physicians and many cancer patients say that marijuana greatly reduces the side effects of chemotherapy. Many glaucoma patients believe that marijuana use has greatly improved their conditions. In view of these reports by patients and the recommendations by some physicians to allow inclusion of marijuana in treatment, expectations have been raised with regard to marijuana's worth as a medical treatment.

Marijuana opponents argue that the evidence in support of marijuana as medically useful suffers from far too many deficiencies. The DEA, for example, believes that studies supporting the medical value of marijuana are scientifically limited, based on biased testimonies of ill individuals who have used marijuana and their families and friends, and grounded in the unscientific opinions of certain physicians, nurses, and other hospital personnel. Furthermore, marijuana opponents feel that the safety of marijuana has not been established by reliable scientific data weighing marijuana's possible therapeutic benefits against its known negative effects.

In the following selections, Sherwood Cole asserts that the federal government should allow marijuana to be used for medical purposes despite the fact that it has some drawbacks. The Drug Enforcement Agency (DEA) argues that marijuana should not be used for legal medical purposes because the current research on marijuana's medicinal benefits is inconclusive. Other drugs are available that preclude the need to use marijuana.

YES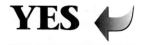

Sherwood O. Cole

An Update on the Effects of Marijuana and Its Potential Medical Use: Forensic Focus

Introduction

Marijuana is the most commonly used illicit drug in the United States (National Institute on Drug Abuse [NIDA], n.d.; Compton, Grant, Colliver, Glantz, & Stinson, 2004). The task of offering expert testimony on the clinical or psychological effects of the drug is particularly difficult. This is due to two primary factors: (1) the controversy related to classifying marijuana compared to other psychoactive drugs and (2) the widespread lack of a balanced perspective on the effects of marijuana.

Regarding the first factor, marijuana is not a simple drug (it contains over 200 compounds) and, unlike most psychoactive drugs, is hard to describe from a single perspective. Also, its effects are phase-dependent and, to a large degree, individualistic. Accordingly, rather than classifying marijuana among other psychoactive drugs, most authors prefer to treat it as a separate topic or issue (Ray & Ksir, 2004). Most certainly, marijuana is not a narcotic, as it is often incorrectly referred to by law-enforcement agencies and the legal system.

Regarding the second factor, the public is bombarded with culturally confusing messages about the risks and benefits of marijuana (Alexander, 2003). The public and some professionals view marijuana from two conflicting perspectives, resulting in a lack of a balanced (moderate) view of its action. Some view marijuana as a very dangerous drug while others see it as a harmless drug. Those viewing marijuana as a dangerous drug are supported by the federal government's prohibition of possession and use of the drug and by outdated and unproven horror stories about marijuana-related criminal acts (Ray & Ksir, 2004). Those viewing marijuana as a harmless drug base their opinions primarily on personal experiences with the drug and on the belief that the federal government has been lying and exaggerating the potential danger of marijuana.

In view of the above issues, there seems to be a specific need to provide updated data on marijuana for scientific accuracy and forensic credibility. Forensic science relies upon facts and scientific findings (not speculation or anecdotal information), and the value of forensic testimony is seriously compromised in those instances where such standards are not implemented.

This article attempts to present an updated picture of the effects, potential dangers, and possible beneficial uses of marijuana in hopes that it will provide a valuable database for scientific reporting in the context of expert forensic testimony. In order to assure that the picture of marijuana presented here is current, only recent studies are reviewed. While no attempt has been made to exhaust all available studies, a genuine attempt has been made to be representative and fair in reviewing such findings.

The Nature of Marijuana and Its Action

Marijuana (also referred to as cannabis in the literature) is a preparation of leafy material from the cannabis plant (Cannabis sativa). While herbal cannabis contains over 400 compounds, including over 60 cannabinoids, its most important and primary active ingredient is delta-9-tetrahydrocannabinol (THC) (Ashton, 2001). Cannabinoids are chemicals that are unique to the cannabis plant and are structurally related to THC. The main recreational purpose of marijuana is its euphoric effect or high, although the drug can also produce dysphoric reactions such as panic and anxiety (Ashton). The potency of marijuana varies depending upon the part of the plant used and the amount of resin present. The flowering top of the plant contains the most resin, with the leaves and fibrous stalk containing progressively less. While marijuana of past years may have been relatively harmless, experimentation and crossbreeding have resulted in an increase in the potency of the drug found on the market today (Compton et al., 2004; ElSohly, et al., 2000). Evidence obtained from confiscated marijuana suggests that its increase in potency nearly doubled during the period from the early 90s to the late 90s (ElSohly, et al.). There is also some suggestion that the increase in the potency of marijuana may contribute to the rising rate in abuse (Compton et al.).

The mechanism of action underlying cannabinoids has only recently been clarified (D'Souza & Kosten, 2001) and involves the identification of two receptor subtypes referred to as CB1 and CB2 (Ledent et al., 1999; Watson, Benson, & Joy, 2000). CB1 receptors are distributed throughout the central nervous system including the cerebral cortex, hippocampus, amygdala, basal ganglia, cerebellum, thalamus, and brainstem (Ashton, 2001) as well as some areas of the peripheral nervous system (Ledent et al.). The newly discovered endogenous cannabinoid anandamide is believed to be a critical pre-synaptic component of neurotransmitter systems related to CB1 subtype systems and involved in the central mediation of marijuana effects (Ashton). This conclusion finds support in studies where pretreatment with the CB1 antagonist SR 141716 blocked the effects of smoked marijuana on self-reports of acute intoxication (Huestis et al., 2001) as well as the effects of peripherally administered anandamide on induced overeating (Williams & Kirkham, 1999). In contrast to CB1 receptors, less is known about CB2 receptor types, although they are found mainly in immune cells. However, the role of cannaboids in the immune system is likely to be multifaceted and, at present, remains vague (Watson et al., 2000).

Marijuana Dependence, Withdrawal, and Treatment

While the latest edition of the American Psychiatric Association's Diagnostic and Statistical Manual of Mental Disorders recognizes marijuana dependence (2000), it is less certain about marijuana withdrawal symptoms and their clinical significance. However, evidence clearly suggests that individuals using marijuana can develop both dependence and withdrawal symptoms, although under a narrower range of conditions than with some other drugs (Watson et al., 2000; Johns, 2001). Such withdrawal symptoms include restlessness, insomnia, anxiety, increased aggression, anorexia, muscle tremors, and autonomic effects (Ashton, 2001). In heavy users of marijuana, these symptoms appear to be more pronounced during the initial 10 days of abstinence, but some symptoms may persist as long as 28 days (Kouri & Pope, 2000). The symptoms are similar in type and magnitude to those observed with nicotine withdrawal and less severe than those observed with alcohol or opiate withdrawal (Budney, Hughes, Moore, & Novy, 2001). While the development of tolerance to the drug may lead some marijuana users to escalate dosage, the presence of withdrawal symptoms encourages continued use of the drug.

While the treatment of marijuana dependence is still in its infancy, there appear to be some interesting prospects on the horizon. For one, there is some optimism about the potential therapeutic use of the CB1 antagonist SR 141716A (and possibly other similar antagonists) in the treatment of marijuana dependence, although caution is advised (D'Souza & Kosten, 2001). In contrast to chemical treatment, brief intervention programs that utilize multi-component therapy (motivational, cognitive, behavioral) appear to be more effective than single component therapy in treating cannabis-dependent adults (Babor, 2004). Additional intervention programs directed at curbing marijuana use/abuse include the use of targeted public service announcements with high-sensation-seeking adolescents (Palmgreen, Donohew, Lorch, Hoyle, & Stevenson, 2001) and family skill training to equip parents with drug information and coping strategies (Spoth, Redmond, & Shin, 2001).

One additional important finding of interest is the evidence from animal studies of an interconnected role of CBI and opiate receptors in brain areas and its potential importance to the mediation of addictive behavior (Ledent et al., 1999). The cross-sensitization observed between delta-9-THC and morphine, which was symmetrical, suggests that common neurobiological substrates may be involved in addiction to marijuana and opiates (Cadoni, Pisanu, Solinas, Acquas, & DiChiara, 2001). These homologies between cannabinoids and opiates, while not providing direct evidence for a causal relationship between cannabis and opiate use, are nonetheless consistent with this possibility (Parolaro & Rubino, 2002). The functional link in the mechanism of addictive action by both types of drugs may be through u-opiate receptor influence on mesolimbic dopamine systems (Manzanares et al., 1999; Rubino, Massi, Vigano, Fuzio, & Parolaro, 2000). While there may also be functional links between cannabinoid properties and other centrally acting drugs, these links are at present less clearly defined (Wiley & Martin, 2003).

Deleterious Effects of Marijuana

The areas reviewed here include (1) the effects of marijuana on cognitive performance; (2) the potential role of marijuana as a stepping-stone to "hard drug" use; and (3) the relationship of marijuana use to the later development of psychotic illness. Following this, comments will be made regarding some additional marijuana effects of continued interest in the literature.

The effects of marijuana on cognitive performance. The impairment of cognitive performance by cannabis is generally well accepted in the literature. In some respects, this impairment is similar to that observed with alcohol and includes slow reaction time, lack of coordination, deficits in concentration, and impairment in performance of complex tasks (Ashton, 2001). However, two specific issues appear to be of primary interest in the context of such impairment: (1) the influence of amount of marijuana on cognitive impairment, and (2) the duration or sustaining power of the cognitive impairment produced by the drug.

Regarding the first of these issues, evidence clearly suggests that there is a direct relationship between the amount of marijuana use and the degree of cognitive impairment. For example, in studies where a large battery of neuropsychological tests were employed, abstaining subjects with a history of heavy marijuana use performed significantly less well than controls or subjects with a history of moderate drug use (Bolla, Brown, Eldreth, Tate, & Cadet, 2002; Solowij et al., 2002). Interestingly, while heavy marijuana users differed from controls on the majority of tests administered in one study, the moderate drug users differed very little from controls (Solowij et al.). In general, while the impairment in cognitive functions resulting from marijuana use is moderate, it would appear to have the potential of impairing driving ability, operation of equipment, task proficiency, and daily functioning.

Regarding the duration or sustaining power of cognitive impairment resulting from marijuana use, results are less consistent. For example, some evidence suggests that the cognitive deficits associated with cannabis use may persist up to only 7 days after subjects last smoked the drug (Pope, Gruber, Hudson, Huestis, & Yurgelun-Todd, 2001), while other evidence suggests that such cognitive deficits may persist up to 28 days after abstinence from marijuana (Bolla et al., 2002). Such a difference in findings raises critical issues related to possible mechanisms by which the drug mediates such discrepancies. In the case of the short-term deficits, the effects may simply be associated with marijuana-induced agitation associated with withdrawal from the drug often lasting this long (Pope et al.). However, in the case of cognitive deficits persisting up to 28 days, such an explanation is inadequate. In this case, the deficits may be due to neurological changes in the previously mentioned cannabinoid receptor systems and the effect of marijuana on such systems over a longer period of time (Solowij et al., 2002). In addition, marijuana-induced hypoactivity in the posterior cerebellum may play an immediate role in such a cognitive deficit, particularly in light of the role of this brain area in the sense of timing (Block et al., 2000a). The effects of marijuana on attention-related regional cerebral blood flow may also play some underlying role in such a cognitive deficit (Block et al., 2000b). However, the relevance of these changes in activity level and blood flow to the issue of duration of cognitive impairment remains unclear.

While the bulk of evidence strongly supports the findings of a cognitive impairment produced by marijuana, one study reported no evidence for cognitive decline between heavy, light, and non-users of cannabis (Lyketsos, Garrett, Liang, & Anthony, 1999). However, the failure to detect cognitive decline in this case may reflect insufficient heavy or chronic use of cannabis or the use of insensitive assessment instruments (Solowij et al., 2002).

The potential role of marijuana as a stepping stone to "hard drugs." Marijuana has long been referred to as a gateway drug, implying that its use serves as a stepping stone to the later use of other "hard drugs" (e.g., heroin, cocaine, hallucinogens, etc.). Such an assumption finds strong support in studies where both national diversity and differences in subsequent "hard drug" use have been investigated.

In one Australian twin study, twin pair members who had used cannabis by age 17 had higher additional drug-use rates than their twin siblings who had not used cannabis by age 17 (Lynskey et al., 2003). It is unlikely such differences were due to environmental factors since the twin pairs were raised in the same household. While the association between early marijuana use and later additional drug use did not differ significantly between monozygotic and dizygotic twins, the age of initiation of cannabis use (before age 17) was influenced by heritable factors (Lynskey et al.).

Additional non-twin studies conducted in New Zealand and the United States generally support the findings of the above study in that early cannabis use preceded the later use of other illicit drugs (Fergusson & Horwood, 2000; Wagner & Anthony, 2002; Merline, O'Malley, Schulenberg, Bachman, & Johnston, 2004). In one of these studies, subjects previously using cannabis on more than 50 occasions per year demonstrated hazards of subsequent illicit drug use that were 59 times higher than non-users (Fergusson & Hotwood). Another one of these studies also points out the persistence of such subsequent drug use; it was still rather prevalent among adults 35 years of age, although influenced by adult role and experiences (Merline et al.). Not only does marijuana use increase the risk of subsequent illicit drug use, it also increases the risk of problems in general, which limits the individual's adjustment and performance (Brook, Balka, & Whiteman, 1999).

While there is little dispute over the influence of early marijuana use on subsequent "hard drug" use, one of the major focal points of recent studies has been on the possible mechanism mediating such a relationship. One author suggests that the relationship is due to the fact that initial cannabis use may encourage later broader experimentation, reduce perceived risk of using other drugs, and bring users into contact with other drugs (Lynskey et al., 2003). A similar view is the suggestion that the interconnection between early marijuana use and subsequent illicit drug use is due to drug exposure opportunities; i.e., marijuana users will increasingly be exposed to greater opportunities to experiment with other drugs (Wilcox, Wagner, & Anthony, 2002). While both of the above mechanisms have a ring of truth about them, one cannot rule out, in light of previous evidence of cross-sensitization of delta-9-tetrahydrocannabinol and morphine (Cadoni et al., 2001), the potential role of neurobiological substrates in such a relationship. Although such a mechanism may not mediate the relationship between early marijuana use and all types of subsequent "hard drug" use, it may serve some role in the subsequent use of opioids. It is also possible that the relationship between early marijuana use and subsequent illicit drug use is non-causal and reflects factors not yet adequately addressed by studies (Fergusson & Horwood, 2000).

The relationship of marijuana use to later development of psychotic illness. One of the most interesting and important areas of marijuana research in recent years is the relationship between early marijuana use and the subsequent development of mental illness. In general, recent evidence obtained from cross-sectional national studies supports the conclusion that the previous use of marijuana significantly increases the subsequent occurrence of schizophrenia (van Os et al., 2002; Arseneault, Cannon, Witton, & Murray, 2004; Veen et al., 2004) and major depression (Brook, Brook, Zhang, Cohen, & Whiteman, 2002). Overall, cannabis use appears to confer a two-fold risk of the later development of schizophrenia compared to that found in the general population (Arseneault et al.). Further evidence also suggests that, while gender and age may further influence the onset of the first psychotic episode, it is the use of cannabis itself that proves to be a much stronger predictor of the onset of the first psychotic episode (Veen et al., 2004). Parenthetically, it is of further interest to note that comorbidity (presence of additional mental illness) is also present in many adolescent substance users (including marijuana users) (Latimer, Stone, Voight, Winters, & August, 2002; Robbins et al., 2002). Such an overlap in adolescent predictors increases, markedly, the difficulty of defining the association between early marijuana use and subsequent mental illness (McGee, Williams, Poulton, & Moffitt, 2000).

While the evidence for the previous use of marijuana increasing the subsequent development of mental illness is relatively strong, the mechanism underlying this linkage is a controversial and highly debated topic. Although it is fairly clear that the linkage between previous marijuana use and mental illness is not simply a fortuitous or temporal association, suggestions as to the causative factors that may contribute to it are diversified. For example, one author suggests that early cannabis use may trigger or exacerbate symptoms of mental illness in subjects who may already be at genetic risk for developing the mental illness (Veen et al., 2004). This view appears to have some credibility in light of the aforementioned evidence for a co-occurrence of drug use and mental illness in adolescents (Latimer et al., 2002; Robbins et al., 2002). However, the majority of evidence suggests that cannabis use demonstrates temporal priority in relationship to mental illness (precedes it) and can produce psychosis in individuals who have no history of mental illness (Johns, 2001; van Os et al., 2002). More realistically, it may be appropriate to suggest that cannabis use is likely to play a causal role with regard to psychosis, but that it is not a necessary or sufficient condition for schizophrenia (Arseneault et al., 2004). That is to say, cannabis use is a component cause, one part of a constellation of causes that leads to subsequent schizophrenia (Arseneault et al.).

Additional evidence suggests that such a "component cause" explanation of the linkage between cannabis use and mental illness may not go far enough (Leweke, Giuffrida, Wurster, Emrich, & Piomelli, 1999). In this case, the level of endogenous cannabinoids in the cerebrospinal fluids of schizophrenics was significantly higher than in controls, suggesting that a type of "hyper-cannabinergic state" in the central nervous system may contribute to the pathogenesis of schizophrenia (Leweke et al.). However, the relatively small sample of subjects in this study (10 schizophrenic patients) somewhat restricts the generalities of the findings. It is quite apparent that the final word on the mechanism underlying the linkage between marijuana use and subsequent mental illness awaits further study.

Additional miscellaneous marijuana effects. The harmful effects of marijuana on the respiratory and cardiovascular systems have long been recognized (National Institute on Drug Abuse, n.d.; Ashton, 2001). Like tobacco, marijuana smoke increases the risk of cancer and lung damage (Watson et al., 2000). This should not be surprising since marijuana contains most of the same chemical components (except nicotine) that are found in tobacco. Also, the smoking of marijuana causes changes in the cardiovascular system that are, in general, characteristic of stress (Ray & Ksir, 2004). Recent studies further emphasize the increased risk of cardiac problems associated with such changes. For example, evidence suggests that chronic abuse of marijuana may increase the risk of stroke in young men aged 18-30 years (Bulletin Board, 2002) and that such an increased risk remains well past the period of withdrawal symptoms caused by abstinence from the drug. Additional evidence suggests that, within 1 hour after smoking marijuana, the risk of myocardial infarction onset was elevated approximately 5 fold (Mittleman, Lewis, Maclure, Sherwood, & Muller, 2001). Fortunately, after 1 hour, the risk of such an effect decreases markedly. While the risk of myocardial infarction significantly increases after smoking marijuana, the risk is much less than that associated with cocaine use (Mittleman et al., 1999).

Another long-standing interest associated with marijuana use is the concept of "amotivational syndrome" (Ray & Ksir, 2004). This syndrome is generally described as a diminished motivation accompanied by a loss of energy and drive to work. Such characteristics can, undoubtedly, have an important impact on one's ability to learn, school performance, and general effectiveness in dealing with everyday problems. However, such a syndrome may represent nothing more than the ongoing intoxication in frequent marijuana users (Johns, 2001). This appears to be particularly plausible in light of the long half-life of marijuana in the body and the fact that daily smokers can be chronically intoxicated (Ray & Ksir, 2004).

Finally, the impairment of short-term memory (ability to easily recall information learned just seconds or minutes before) by marijuana remains one of the most consistent findings in the literature. Since CB 1 receptors are distributed in the hippocampus, interference with their function may play a role in such impairment by marijuana, possibly by disrupting the encoding process (Hampson & Deadwyler, 1999). As to whether such an impairment in short-term memory is more permanent or tends to diminish with the passage of time is debatable (Johns, 2001). In any event, such impairment in short-term memory has the potential for impacting cognitive performance as discussed previously.

The Potential Medical Use of Marijuana

One of the most hotly-debated issues in our society is the legalization of marijuana for medical purposes. In spite of the continued debate, the evidence for the medical benefits of the drug grows and presently includes, by conservative estimate, the following uses (Watson, ct al., 2000; Ray & Ksir, 2004):

1. Reduction of the fluid pressure in the eyes of glaucoma patients.
2. Reduction of severe nausea caused by certain drugs in the treatment of cancer.
3. Stimulation of appetite and reduction of pain associated with wasting syndrome in patients with cancer and AIDS.
4. As a possible anticonvulsant in the treatment of epilepsy.

While the potential medical benefits of marijuana are generally recognized, the legalization of the drug for such purposes has, nevertheless, been hampered by three critical issues:

1. Marijuana is labeled a Schedule I drug under the Controlled Substance Act of 1970, which implies it has no accepted medical use and has high abuse potential. Accordingly, it is not available by prescriptions written by physicians.
2. There is general fear by the public that the legalization of marijuana for medical purposes would open the door to a general increased availability and abuse of the drug in our society.
3. There may not be a necessity for legalizing marijuana for medical purposes since there are presently alternative drugs that are equally effective and available for treatment.

Each of these issues will be briefly discussed in order to disclose the nature and potential fallacy of the position. It is hoped that such a discussion will indicate that medical marijuana may have a future, albeit in a slightly different direction than it is presently going.

Regarding the labeling of marijuana as a Schedule I drug by the federal government (FDA) and its lack of availability by prescription, the issue is not black and white. The National Institute on Drug Abuse did provide medical-grade marijuana cigarettes to a few patients with FDA approval of a "compassionate use" protocol (Ray & Ksir, 2004). The labeling of the drug as Schedule I pertains to the plant (botanical product) or to synthetic equivalents of the plant, not to all drugs containing THC (The Science of Medical Marijuana, n.d.). For example, Marinol (dronabinol) is a synthesized drug in capsule form containing THC in sesame oil and is available by prescription under a Schedule II label (The Science of Medical Marijuana, n.d.). The factor limiting the prescribing of Marinol by physicians may simply be the lack of awareness of the drug's efficacy or the fact that a Schedule II label, while making the drug available, is still a restricted category. In any case, the future of Marinol and other potential cannabinoid medications would appear to be found in pure drugs delivered by some means other than smoking (Watson et al., 2000).

The most promising delivery system to date would appear to be some form of inhalation, owing to the rapid onset and potential for better titration by the patient (The Science of Medical Marijuana, n.d.). Ironically, the federal government's handling of the marijuana issue has been so poor that a growing number of states have passed ballot initiatives (e.g., California's Proposition 215) designed to allow individuals to grow their own marijuana (Nofziger, 1998). This has led to addition al state and federal legal action that has only further delayed a solution to the medical-marijuana issue (Murphy, 2004; Ray & Ksir, 2004).

Regarding the issue of general fear by the public that the legalization of marijuana for medical purposes would encourage a general increase in the illicit use and abuse of the drug in society, the answer is not immediately clear. However, evidence available suggests that this is not the case. For example, a comparison of marijuana use practices in two cities that are very similar demographically but different in legal availability of marijuana for recreational use (San Francisco, California, and Amsterdam, Netherlands) indicated such practices do not differ in the two locations (Reinarman, Cohen, & Kaal, 2004). Since total removal of criminalization restraints (Amsterdam) does not appear to increase the abuse potential over that observed in the context of such restraints (San Francisco), the partial relaxing of drug-control standards in making medical marijuana available would not appear to exacerbate marijuana abuse problems.

Furthermore, a time-series analysis could be undertaken to determine whether society is consuming marijuana at higher rates or in greater quantities than it was prior to medical legalization (Yacoubian, 2001). Such results could be achieved by monitoring the use of marijuana with national data collection systems (e.g., The National House Survey on Drug Abuse, The Drug Abuse Warning Network, etc.). A further benefit of the relaxing of drug control standards in making medical marijuana available might possibly be the control in the spread of disease by clean needle programs and controlled environments for drug use.

Regarding the fact that the legalization of marijuana may not be necessary because there are alternative drugs that are equally effective and available for treatment, the statement may be partially true and partially false. In the case of some treatment contexts, additional available drugs may be better and safer than marijuana. This appears to be true in the case of the treatment of fluid pressure in the eyes of glaucoma patients with available prescription eye drops. The effect of marijuana, in this case, is short-lived and the doses so high that the modest benefits gained are outweighed by the side effects (Watson et al. 2000). Also, in the case of the possible use of marijuana as an anticonvulsant, the available drug Dilantin (phenytoin) may prove to be equally effective.

In other instances, medical marijuana may not necessarily be better than other legal drugs on the market, but simply an alternative choice in the array of available medications. If marijuana is chosen as an alternative medication to those legally available, it is important to keep in mind that smoked marijuana is a complex mixture of active and inactive ingredients (The Science of Medical Marijuana, n.d.). Accordingly, concerns arise about product consistency, potency of active ingredients, and contamination.

While the debate over medical marijuana continues, cannabinoids are being developed for therapeutic application beyond those previously mentioned here. One of the most important new applications of cannabinoids is their potential role in "neuroprotection," a role associated with their antioxidant action (The Science of Medical Marijuana, n.d.). However, the future of such medications would appear to be found in pure drugs (chemically defined), not with the use of the plant or smoked form of marijuana (Watson et al., 2000).

Summary and Concluding Comments

Marijuana is not a completely benign substance but, rather, is a powerful drug with a variety of effects. Accordingly, it is important to examine these effects in a fair and balanced manner. This article attempts to do this by, first of all, presenting a general review on the nature of marijuana, its mechanisms of action, and evidence for dependence. Following this, the adverse effects of the marijuana on cognitive performance, the drug's role as a "stepping stone" to hard drugs, its potential for contributing to the development of mental illness, and other effects are reviewed for the purpose of demonstrating the cost associated with the drug's use. While these adverse effects are real, they are well within the range of effects tolerated by other medications on the market (Watson et al., 2000). A counterbalance to the adverse effects of marijuana is the fact that the drug clearly has some therapeutic value, albeit in a somewhat different form than the smoked one. Undoubtedly, the future of the growing medical use of cannabinoids depends upon the development of pure drugs, where the consistency of content, purity, and potency of the product can be carefully controlled.

Such a balanced and up-to-date view on the effects of marijuana, as presented here, is particularly important in the context of the forensic need to assure the accuracy and reliability of expert testimony. Such accuracy and reliability of testimony would appear to be particularly critical in light of the United States Supreme Court's ruling in the Daubert decision (Daubert v. Merrell Dow, 1993). While previous evidence was admissible on the basis of its "general acceptance" in the scientific community, the Daubert decision established a new set of criteria for courts to determine the admissibility of evidence. An outline and discussion of these criteria are presented elsewhere (Bloomer & Hurwitz, 2002; Cole, 2003). One of these criteria, "the actual or potential rate of error in the expert's methodology," is particularly relevant to the present discussion. For example, any inaccuracy or deficiency in the assessment of marijuana effects can potentially increase the rate of error in the testimony offered by expert witnesses. Protective measures appear to be particularly relevant in the case of marijuana, where anecdotal information and unscientific assumptions about the drug are still prevalent in the public mindset.

While there has been considerable debate as to whether the Daubert decision has made it easier or more difficult to admit expert testimony (Joseph, Atkins, & Flaks, 2000), there is little doubt that the decision has provided useful and standardized rules for such admission. Contrary to the loose criteria for expert testimony in existence prior to the Daubert decision, testimony that is subjective and controversial is now more likely to be excluded as unreliable (Cole, 2003). Experts in the courtroom are expected to employ the same level of intellectual rigor that characterizes their practices.

Expert witnesses need to become more aware of the scientific basis of their evidence, and up-to-date data is critical to this process. The evidence presented here provides a solid and current database for such witnessing related to marijuana effects. Thorough preparation by a potential witness will increase his or her credibility and will allow the witness to speak with authority and effectiveness.

While serving as an expert witness on the effects of marijuana (or any other psychoactive drug) can be an exciting and challenging role, the changes that have taken place in court procedures suggest the need for better and more thorough preparation. In the final analysis, it is important to remember that the legal game is still an adversarial system of justice.

References

Alexander, D. (2003). A marijuana screening inventory (experimental version): Description and preliminary psychometric properties. The American Journal of Drug and Alcohol Abuse, 29, 619–646.

American Psychiatric Association. (2000). Diagnostic and Statistical Manual of Mental Disorders (text revision). Washington, DC: Author.

Arseneault, L., Cannon, M., Witton, J., & Murray, R. M. (2004). Causal association between cannabis and psychosis: Examination of the evidence. The British Journal of Psychiatry, 184, 110–117.

Ashton, C. H. (2001). Pharmacology and effects of cannabis: A brief review. The British Journal of Psychiatry, 178, 101–106.

Babor, T. F. (2004). Brief treatments for cannabis dependence: Findings from a randomized multisite trial. Journal of Consulting and Clinical Psychology, 72, 455–466.

Block, R. I., O'Leary, D. S., Hichwa, R. D., Augustinack, J. C., Ponto, L. L. B., Ghoneim, M. M., Arndt, S., Ehrhardt, J. C., Hurtig, R. R., Watkins, G. L., Hall, J. A., Nathan, P. E., & Andreasen, N. C. (2000a). Cerebellar hypoactivity in frequent marijuana users. Neuro Report, 11, 749–753.

Block, R. I., O'Leary, D. S., Augustinack, J. C., Ponto, L. L. B., Ghoneim, M. M., Hurtig, R. R., Hall, J. A., & Nathan, P. E. (2000b). Effects of frequent marijuana use on attention-related regional cerebral blood flow. Society for Neuroscience Abstract, 26, 2080.

Bloomer, R. H., & Hurwitz, B. (2002, September). So you're going to testify: What every young neuropsychologist should know about tests and the courts. Paper presented at the American College of Forensic Examiners Conference, Orlando, FL.

Bolla, K. I., Brown, K., Eldreth, D., Tate, K., & Cadet, J. L. (2002). Dose-related neurocognitive effects of marijuana use. Neurology, 59, 1337–1343.

Brook, J. S., Balka, E. B., & Whiteman, M. (1999). The risks for late adolescence of early adolescent marijuana use. American Journal of Public Health, 89, 1549–1554.

Brook, D. W., Brook, J. S., Zhang, C., Cohen, E, & Whiteman, M. (2002). Drug use and the risk of major depressive disorder, alcohol dependence, and substance use disorders. Archives of General Psychiatry, 59, 1039–1044.

Budney, A. J., Hughes, J. R., Moore, B. A., & Novy, P. L. (2001). Marijuana abstinence effects in marijuana smokers maintained in their home environment. Archives of General Psychiatry, 58, 917–924.

Bulletin Board (2002). Chronic marijuana abuse may increase risk of stroke. NIDA Notes, 17, 14–15.

Cadoni, C., Pisanu, A., Solinas, M., Acquas, E., & DiChiara, G. (2001). Behavioral sensitization after repeated exposure to A9-tetrahydrocannabinol and cross-sensitization with morphine. Psychopharmacology, 158, 259–266.

Cole, S. O. (2003). Comorbidity of mental illness and drug treatment requirements: Impact on forensic evidence. The Forensic Examiner, 12 (11 & 12), 28–34.

Compton, W. M., Grant, B. F., Colliver, J. D., Glantz, M. D., & Stinson, F. S. (2004). Prevalence of marijuana use disorders in the United States, 1991–1992 and 2001–2002. Journal of the American Medical Association, 291, 2114–2121.

Daubert v. Merrell Dow Pharmaceuticals, Inc. (1993). 113, S. Ct. 2786.

D'Souza, D. C., & Kosten, T. R. (2001). Cannabinoid antagonists: A treatment in search of an illness. Archives of General Psychiatry, 58, 330–331.

ElSohly, M. A., Ross, S. A., Mehmedic, Z., Arafat, R., Yi, B., & Banahan, B. F. (2000). Potency trends of A9-THC and other cannabinoids in confiscated marijuana from 1980-1997. Journal of Forensic Science, 45, 24–30.

Fergusson, D. M., & Horwood, L. J. (2000). Does cannabis use encourage other forms of illicit drug use? Addiction, 95, 505–520.

Hampson, R. E., & Deadwyler, S. A. (1999). Cannabinoids, hippocampal function and memory. Life Sciences, 65, 715–723.

Huestis, M. A., Gorelick, D. A., Heishman, S. J., Preston, K. L., Nelson, R. A., Moolchan, E. T., & Frank, R. A. (2001). Blockade of effects of smoked marijuana by the CB1-selective cannabinoid receptor antagonist SR 141716. Archives of General Psychiatry, 58, 322–328.

Johns, A. (2001). Psychiatric effects of cannabis. The British Journal of Psychiatry, 178, 116–122.

Joseph, G. W., Atkins, E. L., & Flaks, D. K. (2000). Admissibility of expert psychological testimony in the era of Daubert. The case of hedonic damages. American Journal of Forensic Psychology, 1 & 3–34.

Kouri, E. M., & Pope, H. G., Jr. (2000). Abstinence symptoms during withdrawal from chronic marijuana use. Experimental and Clinical Psychopharmacology, 8, 483–492.

Latimer, W. W., Stone, A. L., Voight, A., Winters, K. C., & August, G. J. (2002). Gender differences in psychiatric comorbidity among adolescents with substance use disorders. Experimental and Clinical Psychopharmacology, 10, 310–315.

Ledent, C., Valverde, O., Cossu, G., Petitet, E, Aubert, J-F, Beslot, E, Bohme, G. A., Imperato, A., Pedrazzini, T., Roques, B. E, Vassart, G., Fratta, W., & Parmentier, M. (1999). Unresponsiveness to cannabinoids and reduced addictive effects of opiates in CB1 receptor knockout mice. Science, 283, 401–404.

Leweke, F. M., Giuffrida, A., Wurster, U., Emrich, H. M., & Piomelli, D. (1999). Elevated endogenous cannabinoids in schizophrenia. NeuroReport, 10, 1665–1669.

Lyketsos, C. G., Garrett, E., Liang, K. Y., & Anthony, J. C. (1999). Cannabis use and cognitive decline in persons under 65 years of age. American Journal of Epidemiology, 149, 794–800.

Lynskey, M. T., Heath, A. C., Bucholz, K. K., Slutske, W. S., Madden, P. A. E, Nelson, E. C., Statham, D. J., & Martin, N. G. (2003). Escalation of drug use in early-onset cannabis users vs. co-twin controls. Journal of the American Medical Association, 289, 427–433.

Manzanares, J., Corchero, J., Romero, J., Fernandez-Ruiz, J. J., Ramos, J. A., & Fuentes, J. A. (1999). Pharmacological and biochemical interactions between opioids and cannabinoids. Trends in Pharmacological Science, 20, 287–294.

McGee, R., Williams, S., Poulton, R., & Moffitt, T. (2000). A longitudinal study of cannabis use and mental health from adolescence to early adulthood. Addiction, 95, 491–503.

Merline, A. C., O'Malley, P. M., Schulenberg, J. E., Bachman, J. G., & Johnston, L. D. (2004). Substance use among adults 35 years of age: Prevalence, adulthood predictors, and impact of adolescent substance use. American Journal of Public Health, 94, 96–102.

Mittleman, M. A., Mintzer, D., Maclure, M., Tofler, G. H., Sherwood, J. B., & Muller, J. E. (1999). Triggering of myocardial infarction by cocaine. Circulation, 99, 2737–2741.

Mittleman, M. A., Lewis, R. A., Maclure, M., Sherwood, J. B., & Muller, J. E. (2001). Triggering myocardial infarction by marijuana. Circulation, 103, 2805–2809.

Murphy, D. E. (2004, February 26). Court allows medical use of marijuana. New York Times.

National Institute on Drug Abuse. (n.d.). Info-Facts-marijuana. . . .

Nofziger, L. (1998). Forward in Marijuana Rx: The patients' fight for medicinal pot. New York: Thunder's Mouth Press.

Palmgreen, P., Donohew, L., Lorch, E. P., Hoyle, R.H., & Stevenson, M. T. (2001). Television campaigns and adolescent marijuana use: Tests of sensation seeking targeting. American Journal of Public Health, 91, 292–296.

Parolaro, D., & Rubino, T. (2002). Is cannabinoid transmission involved in rewarding properties of drugs of abuse? British Journal of Pharmacology, 136, 1083–1084.

Pope, H. G., Jr., Gruber, A. J., Hudson, J. I., Huestis, M. A., & Yurgelun-Todd, D. (2001). Neuropsychological performance in long-term cannabis users. Archives of General Psychiatry, 58, 909–915.

Ray, O., & Ksir, C. (2004). Drugs, society, and human behavior (10th ed.). New York: McGraw-Hill.

Reinarman, C., Cohen, P. D. A., & Kaal, H. L. (2004). The limited relevance of drug policy: Cannabis in Amsterdam and in San Francisco. American Journal of Public Health, 94, 836–842.

Robbins, M. S., Kumar, S., Walker-Barnes, C., Feaster, D. J., Briones, E., & Szapocznik, J. (2002). Ethnic differences in comorbidity among substance-abusing adolescents referred to outpatient therapy. Journal of the American Academy of Child and Adolescent Psychiatry, 41, 394–401.

Rubino, T., Massi, P., Vigano, D., Fuzio, D., & Parolaro, D. (2000). Long-term treatment with SR141716A, the CB1 receptor antagonist, influences morphine withdrawal syndrome. Life Sciences, 66, 2213–2219.

Solowij, N., Stephens, R. S., Roffman, R. A., Babor, T., Kadden, R., Miller, M., Christiansen, K., McRee, B., & Vendetti, J. (2002). Cognitive functioning of long-term heavy cannabis users seeking treatment. Journal of the American Medical Association, 287, 1123–1131.

Spoth, R. L., Redmond, C., & Shin, C. (2001). Randomized trial of brief family interventions for general populations: Adolescent substance use outcomes 4 years following baseline. Journal of Consulting and Clinical Psychology, 69, 627–642.

The Science of Medical Marijuana. (n.d.). . . .

van Os, J., Bak, M., Hanssen, M., Bijl, R. V., de Graaf, R., & Verdoux, H. (2002). Cannabis use and psychosis: A longitudinal population-based study. American Journal of Epidemiology, 156, 319–327.

Veen, N. D., Selten, J-P., van der Tweel, 1., Feller, W. G., Hock, H. W., & Kahn, R. S. (2004). Cannabis use and age at onset of schizophrenia. American Journal of Psychiatry, 161, 501–506.

Wagner, F. A., & Anthony, J. C. (2002). Into the world of illegal drug use: Exposure opportunity and other mechanisms linking the use of alcohol, tobacco, marijuana, and cocaine. American Journal of Epidemiology, 155, 918–925.

Watson, S. J., Benson, J. A., Jr., & Joy, J. E. (2000). Marijuana and medicine: Assessing the science base. Archives of General Psychiatry, 57, 547–552.

Wilcox, H. C., Wagner, F. A., & Anthony, J. C. (2002). Exposure opportunity as a mechanism linking youth marijuana use to hallucinogen use. Drug and Alcohol Dependence, 66, 127–135.

Wiley, J. L., & Martin, B. R. (2003). Cannabinoid pharmacological properties common to other centrally acting drugs. European Journal of Pharmacology, 471, 185–193.

Williams, C. M., & Kirkham, T. C. (1999). Anandamide induces overeating: Mediation by central cannabinoid (CB1) receptors. Psychopharmacology, 143, 315–317.

Yacoubian, G. S., Jr. (2001). Beyond the theoretical rhetoric: A proposal to study the consequences of drug legalization. Journal of Drug Education, 31, 319–328.

Sherwood O. Cole, PhD, Diplomate of the American Board Psychological Specialties.

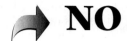 **NO**

The DEA Position on Marijuana

The campaign to legitimize what is called "medical" marijuana is based on two propositions: that science views marijuana as medicine, and that DEA targets sick and dying people using the drug. Neither proposition is true. Smoked marijuana has not withstood the rigors of science—it is not medicine and it is not safe. DEA targets criminals engaged in cultivation and trafficking, not the sick and dying. No state has legalized the trafficking of marijuana, including the twelve states that have decriminalized certain marijuana use.[1]

Smoked Marijuana Is Not Medicine

There is no consensus of medical evidence that smoking marijuana helps patients. Congress enacted laws against marijuana in 1970 based in part on its conclusion that marijuana has no scientifically proven medical value. The Food and Drug Administration (FDA) is the federal agency responsible for approving drugs as safe and effective medicine based on valid scientific data. FDA has not approved smoked marijuana for any condition or disease. The FDA noted that "there is currently sound evidence that smoked marijuana is harmful," and "that no sound scientific studies supported medical use of marijuana for treatment in the United States, and no animal or human data supported the safety or efficacy of marijuana for general medical use."[2]

In 2001, the Supreme Court affirmed Congress's 1970 judgment about marijuana in *United States v. Oakland Cannabis Buyers' Cooperative et al.*, 532 U.S. 438 (2001), which held that, given the absence of medical usefulness, medical necessity is not a defense to marijuana prosecution. Furthermore, in *Gonzales v. Raich*, 125 S.Ct. 2195 (2005), the Supreme Court reaffirmed that the authority of Congress to regulate the use of potentially harmful substances through the federal Controlled Substances Act includes the authority to regulate marijuana of a purely intrastate character, regardless of a state law purporting to authorize "medical" use of marijuana.

The DEA and the federal government are not alone in viewing smoked marijuana as having no documented medical value. Voices in the medical community likewise do not accept smoked marijuana as medicine:

- The American Medical Association has rejected pleas to endorse marijuana as medicine, and instead has urged that marijuana remain a

From the Justice Department, *The DEA Position on Marijuana*, May 2006.

prohibited, Schedule I controlled substance, at least until more research is done.[3]

- The American Cancer Society "does not advocate inhaling smoke, nor the legalization of marijuana," although the organization does support carefully controlled clinical studies for alternative delivery methods, specifically a THC skin patch.[4]
- The American Academy of Pediatrics (AAP) believes that "[a]ny change in the legal status of marijuana, even if limited to adults, could affect the prevalence of use among adolescents." While it supports scientific research on the possible medical use of cannabinoids as opposed to smoked marijuana, it opposes the legalization of marijuana.[5]
- The National Multiple Sclerosis Society (NMSS) states that studies done to date "have not provided convincing evidence that marijuana benefits people with MS," and thus marijuana is not a recommended treatment. Furthermore, the NMSS warns that the "long-term use of marijuana may be associated with significant serious side effects."[6]
- The British Medical Association (BMA) voiced extreme concern that down-grading the criminal status of marijuana would "mislead" the public into believing that the drug is safe. The BMA maintains that marijuana "has been linked to greater risk of heart disease, lung cancer, bronchitis and emphysema."[7] The 2004 Deputy Chairman of the BMA's Board of Science said that "[t]he public must be made aware of the harmful effects we know result from smoking this drug."[8]
- The American Academy of Pediatrics asserted that with regard to marijuana use, "from a public health perspective, even a small increase in use, whether attributable to increased availability or decreased perception of risk, would have significant ramifications."[9]

In 1999, The Institute of Medicine (IOM) released a landmark study reviewing the supposed medical properties of marijuana. The study is frequently cited by "medical" marijuana advocates, but in fact severely undermines their arguments.

- After release of the IOM study, the principal investigators cautioned that the active compounds in marijuana may have medicinal potential and therefore should be researched further. However, the study concluded that "there is little future in smoked marijuana as a medically approved medication."[10]
- For some ailments, the IOM found ". . . potential therapeutic value of cannabinoid drugs, primarily THC, for pain relief, control of nausea and vomiting, and appetite stimulation."[11] However, it pointed out that "[t]he effects of cannabinoids on the symptoms studied are generally modest, and in most cases there are more effective medications [than smoked marijuana]."[12]
- The study concluded that, at best, there is only anecdotal information on the medical benefits of smoked marijuana for some ailments, such as muscle spasticity. For other ailments, such as epilepsy and glaucoma, the study found no evidence of medical value and did not endorse further research.[13]
- The IOM study explained that "smoked marijuana . . . is a crude THC delivery system that also delivers harmful substances." In addition,

"plants contain a variable mixture of biologically active compounds and cannot be expected to provide a precisely defined drug effect." Therefore, the study concluded that "there is little future in smoked marijuana as a medically approved medication."[14]

- The principal investigators explicitly stated that using smoked marijuana in clinical trials "should not be designed to develop it as a licensed drug, but should be a stepping stone to the development of new, safe delivery systems of cannabinoids."[15]

Thus, even scientists and researchers who believe that certain active ingredients in marijuana may have potential medicinal value openly discount the notion that smoked marijuana is or can become "medicine."

DEA has approved and will continue to approve research into whether THC has any medicinal use. As of May 8, 2006, DEA had registered every one of the 163 researchers who requested to use marijuana in studies and who met Department of Health and Human Services standards.[16] One of those researchers, The Center for Medicinal Cannabis Research (CMCR), conducts studies "to ascertain the general medical safety and efficacy of cannabis and cannabis products and examine alternative forms of cannabis administration."[17] The CMCR currently has 11 on-going studies involving marijuana and the efficacy of cannabis and cannabis compounds as they relate to medical conditions such as HIV, cancer pain, MS, and nausea.[18]

At present, however, the clear weight of the evidence is that smoked marijuana is harmful. No matter what medical condition has been studied, other drugs already approved by the FDA, such as Marinol—a pill form of synthetic THC—have been proven to be safer and more effective than smoked marijuana.

Marijuana Is Dangerous to the User and Others

Legalization of marijuana, no matter how it begins, will come at the expense of our children and public safety. It will create dependency and treatment issues, and open the door to use of other drugs, impaired health, delinquent behavior, and drugged drivers.

This is not the marijuana of the 1970's; today's marijuana is far more powerful. Average THC levels of seized marijuana rose from less than one per cent in the mid-1970's to a national average of over eight per cent in 2004.[19] And the potency of "B.C. Bud" is roughly twice the national average—ranging from 15 per cent to as high as 25 per cent THC content.[20]

Dependency and Treatment:

- Adolescents are at highest risk for marijuana addiction, as they are "three times more likely than adults to develop dependency."[21] This is borne out by the fact that treatment admission rates for adolescents reporting marijuana as the primary substance of abuse increased from 32 to 65 per cent between 1993 and 2003.[22] More young people ages

12–17 entered treatment in 2003 for marijuana dependency than for alcohol and all other illegal drugs combined.[23]

- "[R]esearch shows that use of [marijuana] can lead to dependence. Some heavy users of marijuana develop withdrawal symptoms when they have not used the drug for a period of time. Marijuana use, in fact, is often associated with behavior that meets the criteria for substance dependence established by the American Psychiatric Association."[24]

- Of the 19.1 million Americans aged 12 or older who used illicit drugs in the past 30 days in 2004, 14.6 million used marijuana, making it the most commonly used illicit drug in 2004.[25]

- Among all ages, marijuana was the most common illicit drug responsible for treatment admissions in 2003, accounting for 15 per cent of all admissions—outdistancing heroin, the next most prevalent cause.[26]

- In 2003, 20 per cent (185,239) of the 919,833 adults admitted to treatment for illegal drug abuse cited marijuana as their primary drug of abuse.[27]

Marijuana As a Precursor to Abuse of Other Drugs:

- Marijuana is a frequent precursor to the use of more dangerous drugs, and signals a significantly enhanced likelihood of drug problems in adult life. The *Journal of the American Medical Association* reported, based on a study of 300 sets of twins, "that marijuana-using twins were four times more likely than their siblings to use cocaine and crack cocaine, and five times more likely to use hallucinogens such as LSD."[28]

- Long-term studies on patterns of drug usage among young people show that very few of them use other drugs without first starting with marijuana. For example, one study found that among adults (age 26 and older) who had used cocaine, 62 per cent had initiated marijuana use before age 15. By contrast, less than one per cent of adults who never tried marijuana went on to use cocaine.[29]

- Columbia University's National Center on Addiction and Substance Abuse reports that teens who used marijuana at least once in the last month are 13 times likelier than other teens to use another drug like cocaine, heroin, or methamphetamine, and almost 26 times likelier than those teens who have never used marijuana to use another drug.[30]

- Marijuana use in early adolescence is particularly ominous. Adults who were early marijuana users were found to be five times more likely to become dependent on any drug, eight times more likely to use cocaine in the future, and fifteen times more likely to use heroin later in life.[31]

- In 2003, 3.1 million Americans aged 12 or older used marijuana daily or almost daily in the past year. Of those daily marijuana users, nearly two-thirds "used at least one other illicit drug in the past 12 months." More than half (53.3 per cent) of daily marijuana users were also dependent on or abused alcohol or another illicit drug compared to those who were nonusers or used marijuana less than daily.[32]

- Healthcare workers, legal counsel, police and judges indicate that marijuana is a typical precursor to methamphetamine. For instance, Nancy Kneeland, a substance abuse counselor in Idaho, pointed out that "in almost all cases meth users began with alcohol and pot."[33]

Mental and Physical Health Issues
Related to Marijuana:

- John Walters, Director of the Office of National Drug Control Policy, Charles G. Curie, Administrator of the Substance Abuse and Mental Health Services Administration, and experts and scientists from leading mental health organizations joined together in May 2005 to warn parents about the mental health dangers marijuana poses to teens. According to several recent studies, marijuana use has been linked with depression and suicidal thoughts, in addition to schizophrenia. These studies report that weekly marijuana use among teens doubles the risk of developing depression and triples the incidence of suicidal thoughts.[34]
- Dr. Andrew Campbell, a member of the New South Wales (Australia) Mental Health Review Tribunal, published a study in 2005 which revealed that four out of five individuals with schizophrenia were regular cannabis users when they were teenagers. Between 75–80 per cent of the patients involved in the study used cannabis habitually between the ages of 12 and 21.[35] In addition, a laboratory-controlled study by Yale scientists, published in 2004, found that THC "transiently induced a range of schizophrenia-like effects in healthy people."[36]
- Smoked marijuana has also been associated with an increased risk of the same respiratory symptoms as tobacco, including coughing, phlegm production, chronic bronchitis, shortness of breath and wheezing. Because cannabis plants are contaminated with a range of fungal spores, smoking marijuana may also increase the risk of respiratory exposure by infectious organisms (i.e., molds and fungi).[37]
- Marijuana takes the risks of tobacco and raises them: marijuana smoke contains more than 400 chemicals and increases the risk of serious health consequences, including lung damage.[38]
- According to two studies, marijuana use narrows arteries in the brain, "similar to patients with high blood pressure and dementia," and may explain why memory tests are difficult for marijuana users. In addition, "chronic consumers of cannabis lose molecules called CB1 receptors in the brain's arteries," leading to blood flow problems in the brain which can cause memory loss, attention deficits, and impaired learning ability.[39]
- Carleton University researchers published a study in 2005 showing that current marijuana users who smoke at least five "joints" per week did significantly worse than non-users when tested on neurocognition tests such as processing speed, memory, and overall IQ.[40]

Delinquent Behaviors and Drugged Driving:

- In 2002, the percentage of young people engaging in delinquent behaviors "rose with [the] increasing frequency of marijuana use." For example, according to a National Survey on Drug Use and Health (NSDUH) report, 42.2 per cent of youths who smoked marijuana 300 or more days per year and 37.1 per cent of those who did so 50–99 days took part in serious fighting at school or work. Only 18.2 per cent of those who did not use marijuana in the past year engaged in serious fighting.[41]

- A large shock trauma unit conducting an ongoing study found that 17 per cent (one in six) of crash victims tested positive for marijuana. The rates were slightly higher for crash victims under the age of eighteen, 19 per cent of whom tested positive for marijuana.[42]
- In a study of high school classes in 2000 and 2001, about 28,000 seniors each year admitted that they were in at least one accident after using marijuana.[43]
- Approximately 15 per cent of teens reported driving under the influence of marijuana. This is almost equal to the percentage of teens who reported driving under the influence of alcohol (16 per cent).[44]
- A study of motorists pulled over for reckless driving showed that, among those who were not impaired by alcohol, 45 per cent tested positive for marijuana.[45]
- The National Highway Traffic Safety Administration (NHTSA) has found that marijuana significantly impairs one's ability to safely operate a motor vehicle. According to its report, "[e]pidemiology data from road traffic arrests and fatalities indicate that after alcohol, marijuana is the most frequently detected psychoactive substance among driving populations." Problems reported include: decreased car handling performance, inability to maintain headway, impaired time and distance estimation, increased reaction times, sleepiness, lack of motor coordination, and impaired sustained vigilance.[46]

Some of the consequences of marijuana-impaired driving are startling:

- The driver of a charter bus, whose 1999 accident resulted in the death of 22 people, had been fired from bus companies in 1989 and 1996 because he tested positive for marijuana four times. A federal investigator confirmed a report that the driver "tested positive for marijuana when he was hospitalized Sunday after the bus veered off a highway and plunged into an embankment."[47]
- In April 2002, four children and the driver of a van died when the van hit a concrete bridge abutment after veering off the freeway. Investigators reported that the children nicknamed the driver "Smokey" because he regularly smoked marijuana. The driver was found at the crash scene with marijuana in his pocket.[48]
- A former nurse's aide was convicted in 2003 of murder and sentenced to 50 years in prison for hitting a homeless man with her car and driving home with his mangled body "lodged in the windshield." The incident happened after a night of drinking and taking drugs, including marijuana. After arriving home, the woman parked her car, with the man still lodged in the windshield, and left him there until he died.[49]
- In April 2005, an eight year-old boy was killed when he was run over by an unlicensed 16 year-old driver who police believed had been smoking marijuana just before the accident.[50]
- In 2001, George Lynard was convicted of driving with marijuana in his bloodstream, causing a head-on collision that killed a 73 year-old man and a 69 year-old woman. Lynard appealed this conviction because he allegedly had a "valid prescription" for marijuana. A Nevada judge agreed with Lynard and granted him a new trial.[51] The case has been appealed to the Nevada Supreme Court.[52]

- Duane Baehler, 47, of Tulsa, Okalahoma was "involved in a fiery crash that killed his teenage son" in 2003. Police reported that Baehler had methamphetamine, cocaine and marijuana in his system at the time of the accident.[53]

Marijuana also creates hazards that are not always predictable. In August 2004, two Philadelphia firefighters died battling a fire that started because of tangled wires and lamps used to grow marijuana in a basement closet.[54]

Marijuana and Incarceration

Federal marijuana investigations and prosecutions usually involve hundreds of pounds of marijuana. Few defendants are incarcerated in federal prison for simple possession of marijuana.

- In 2001, there were 24,299 offenders sentenced in federal court on drug charges. Of those, only 2.3 per cent (186 people) were sentenced for simple possession.[55] In addition, it is important to recognize that many inmates were initially charged with more serious crimes but negotiated reduced charges to simple possession through plea agreements.[56]
- According to the latest survey data in a 2005 ONDCP study, marijuana accounted for 13 per cent of all state drug offenders in 1997, and of the inmates convicted of marijuana offenses, only 0.7 per cent were incarcerated for marijuana possession alone.[57]

The Foreign Experience

The Netherlands:

- Due to international pressure on permissive Dutch cannabis policy and domestic complaints over the spread of marijuana "coffee shops," the government of the Netherlands has reconsidered its legalization measures. After marijuana became normalized, consumption nearly tripled—from 15 per cent to 44 per cent—among 18 to 20 year-old Dutch youth.[58] As a result of stricter local government policies, the number of cannabis "coffeehouses" in the Netherlands was reduced—from 1,179 in 1997[59] to 737 in 2004, a 37 per cent decrease in 7 years.[60]
- About 70 per cent of Dutch towns have a zero-tolerance policy toward cannabis cafes.[61]
- In August 2004, after local governments began clamping down on cannabis "coffeehouses" seven years earlier, the government of the Netherlands formally announced a shift in its cannabis policy through the United National International Narcotics Control Board (INCB). According to "an inter-ministerial policy paper on cannabis, the government acknowledged that 'cannabis is not harmless'—neither for the abusers, nor for the community." Netherlands intends to reduce the number of coffee shops (especially those near border areas and schools), closely monitor drug tourism, and implement an action plan to discourage cannabis use. This public policy change brings the Netherlands "closer

towards full compliance with the international drug control treaties with regard to cannabis."[62]

- Dr. Ernest Bunning, formerly with Holland's Ministry of Health and a principal proponent of that country's liberal drug philosophy, has acknowledged that, "[t]here are young people who abuse soft drugs . . . particularly those that have [a] high THC [content]. The place that cannabis takes in their lives becomes so dominant they don't have space for the other important things in life. They crawl out of bed in the morning, grab a joint, don't work, smoke another joint. They don't know what to do with their lives."[63]

Switzerland:

- Liberalization of marijuana laws in Switzerland has likewise produced damaging results. After liberalization, Switzerland became a magnet for drug users from many other countries. In 1987, Zurich permitted drug use and sales in a part of the city called Platzpitz, dubbed "Needle Park." By 1992, the number of regular drug users at the park reportedly swelled from a "few hundred at the outset in 1987 to about 20,000." The area around the park became crime-ridden, forcing closure of the park. The experiment has since been terminated.[64]

Canada:

- After a large decline in the 1980s, marijuana use among teens increased during the 1990s as young people became "confused about the state of federal pot law" in the wake of an aggressive decriminalization campaign, according to a special adviser to Health Canada's Director General of drug strategy. Several Canadian drug surveys show that marijuana use among Canadian youth has steadily climbed to surpass its 26-year peak, rising to 29.6 per cent of youth in grades 7-12 in 2003.[65]

United Kingdom:

- In March 2005, British Home Secretary Charles Clarke took the unprecedented step of calling "for a rethink on Labour's legal down-grading of cannabis" from a Class B to a Class C substance. Mr. Clarke requested that the Advisory Council on the Misuse of Drugs complete a new report, taking into account recent studies showing a link between cannabis and psychosis and also considering the more potent cannabis referred to as "skunk."[66]
- In 2005, during a general election speech to concerned parents, British Prime Minister Tony Blair noted that medical evidence increasingly suggests that cannabis is not as harmless as people think and warned parents that young people who smoke cannabis could move on to harder drugs.[67]

The Legalization Lobby

The proposition that smoked marijuana is "medicine" is, in sum, false—trickery used by those promoting wholesale legalization. When a statute dramatically reducing penalties for "medical" marijuana took effect in Maryland in October 2003, a defense attorney noted that "[t]here are a whole bunch of people who like marijuana who can now try to use this defense." The attorney observed that lawyers would be "neglecting their clients if they did not try to find out what 'physical, emotional or psychological'" condition could be enlisted to develop a defense to justify a defendant's using the drug. "Sometimes people are self-medicating without even realizing it,'" he said.[68]

- Ed Rosenthal, senior editor of *High Times*, a pro-drug magazine, once revealed the legalizer strategy behind the "medical" marijuana movement. While addressing an effort to seek public sympathy for glaucoma patients, he said, "I have to tell you that I also use marijuana medically. I have a latent glaucoma which has never been diagnosed. The reason why it's never been diagnosed is because I've been treating it." He continued, "I have to be honest, there is another reason why I do use marijuana . . . and that is because I like to get high. Marijuana is fun."[69]
- A few billionaires—not broad grassroots support—started and sustain the "medical" marijuana and drug legalization movements in the United States. Without their money and influence, the drug legalization movement would shrivel. According to National Families in Action, four individuals—George Soros, Peter Lewis, George Zimmer and John Sperling—contributed $1,510,000 to the effort to pass a "medical" marijuana law in California in 1996, a sum representing nearly 60 per cent of the total contributions.[70]
- In 2000, The New York Times interviewed Ethan Nadelmann, Director of the Lindesmith Center. Responding to criticism that the medical marijuana issue is a stalking horse for drug legalization, Mr. Nadelmann stated: "Will it help lead toward marijuana legalization? . . . I hope so."[71]
- In 2004, Alaska voters faced a ballot initiative that would have made it legal for adults age 21 and older to possess, grow, buy, or give away marijuana. The measure also called for state regulation and taxation of the drug. The campaign was funded almost entirely by the Washington, D.C.-based Marijuana Policy Project, which provided "almost all" the $857,000 taken in by the pro-marijuana campaign. Fortunately, Alaskan voters rejected the initiative.[72]
- In October 2005, Denver voters passed Initiative 100 decriminalizing marijuana based on incomplete and misleading campaign advertisements put forth by the Safer Alternative For Enjoyable Recreation (SAFER). A Denver City Councilman complained that the group used the slogan "Make Denver SAFER" on billboards and campaign signs to mislead the voters into thinking that the initiative supported increased police staffing. Indeed, the Denver voters were never informed of the initiative's true intent to decriminalize marijuana.[73]
- The legalization movement is not simply a harmless academic exercise. The mortal danger of thinking that marijuana is "medicine" was graphically illustrated by a story from California. In the spring of 2004, Irma Perez was "in the throes of her first experience with the drug ecstasy" when, after taking one ecstasy tablet, she became ill and told friends that she felt like she was "going to die." Two teenage acquaintances did not seek medical care and instead tried to get Perez to smoke marijuana. When that failed due to her seizures, the friends tried to

force-feed marijuana leaves to her, "apparently because [they] knew that drug is sometimes used to treat cancer patients." Irma Perez lost consciousness and died a few days later when she was taken off life support. She was 14 years old.[74]

Still, There's Good News

Continued Declines in Marijuana Use among Youth

In 2005, the *Monitoring the Future (MTF)* survey recorded an overall 19.1 per cent decrease in current use of illegal drugs between 2001 and 2005, edging the nation closer to its five-year goal of a 25 per cent reduction in illicit drug use in 2006. Specific to marijuana, the 2005 MTF survey showed:

- Between 2001 and 2005, marijuana use dropped in all three categories: lifetime (13%), past year (15%) and 30-day use (19%). Current marijuana use decreased 28 per cent among 8th graders (from 9.2% to 6.6%), and 23 per cent among 10th graders (from 19.8 per cent to 15.2%).[75]

Increased Eradication

- As of September 20, 2005, DEA's Domestic Cannabis Eradication/ Suppression Program supported the eradication of 3,054,336 plants in the top seven marijuana producing states (California, Hawaii, Kentucky, Oregon, Tennessee, Washington and West Virginia). This is an increase of 315,628 eradicated plants over the previous year.[76]
- For the 2005 eradication season, a total of 5 million marijuana plants have been eradicated across the United States. This is a one million plant increase over last year. The Departments of Agriculture and Interior combined have eradicated an estimated 1.2 million plants during this 2005 eradication season.[77]

Appendix A

Acronyms Used in "The DEA Position on Marijuana"

AAP: American Academy of Pediatrics

ACS: American Cancer Society

AMA: American Medical Association

BBC: British Broadcasting Company

B.C.: Bud British Columbia Bud

BMA: British Medical Association

CB1: Cannabinoid Receptor 1: one of two receptors in the brain's endocannabinoid (EC) system associated with the intake of food and tobacco dependency.

CMCR: Center for Medicinal Cannabis Research

DASIS: Drug and Alcohol Services Information System

DEA: Drug Enforcement Administration

FDA: Food and Drug Administration

HIV: Human Immunodeficiency Virus

INCB: International Narcotics Control Board

IOM: Institute of Medicine

IOP: Intraocular Pressure

LSD: Diethylamide-Lysergic Acid

MS: Multiple Sclerosis

NHTSA: National Highway Traffic Safety Administration

NIDA: National Institute on Drug Abuse

NMSS: National Multiple Sclerosis Society

NORML: National Organization for the Reform of Marijuana Laws

NSDUH: National Survey of Drug Use and Health

ONDCP: Office of National Drug Control Policy

TEDS: Treatment Episode Data Set

THC: Tetrahydrocannabinol

Endnotes

1. As of April 2006, the eleven states that have decriminalized certain marijuana use are Arizona, Alaska, California, Colorado, Hawaii, Maine, Montana, Nevada, Oregon, Rhode Island, Vermont, and Washington. In addition, Maryland has enacted legislation that recognizes a "medical marijuana" defense.

2. "Inter-Agency Advisory Regarding Claims That Smoked Marijuana Is a Medicine." U.S. Food and Drug Administration, April 20, 2006. . . .

3. "Policy H-95.952 'Medical Marijuana.'" *American Medical Association.* See also, American Medical Association, Featured Council on Scientific Affairs. "Medical Marijuana (A-01)." June 2001. In 2001, the AMA updated their policy regarding medical marijuana reflecting the results of this study. It should be noted that a few medical organizations have offered limited support to the concept of "medical" marijuana. For example, the American Academy of Family Physicians has said that it opposes the use of marijuana "except under medical supervision and control, for specific medical indications." Largely at the urging of one activist—a lobbyist and former Board member of NORML—the American Nurses Association has endorsed "medical" marijuana under "appropriate prescriber supervision," and the American Academy of HIV Medicine, a group of about 1,800 members founded in 2000, has taken the view that marijuana should not only be made available for "medical" use, but should be excluded altogether as a Schedule I drug.

4. "Experts: Pot Smoking Is Not Best Choice to Treat Chemo Side-Effects." American Cancer Society. 22 May 2001. . . .

5. Committee on Substance Abuse and Committee on Adolescence. "Legalization of Marijuana: Potential Impact on Youth." *Pediatrics* Vol. 113, No. 6 (6 June 2004): 1825-1826. *See also,* Joffe, Alain, MD, MPH, and Yancy, Samuel, MD. "Legalization of Marijuana: Potential Impact on Youth." *Pediatrics* Vol. 113, No. 6 (6 June 2004): e632-e638h.

6.   National MS Society. "Information Sourcebook." *National MS Society.* December 2004. . . .

7.   "Doctors' Fears at Cannabis Change." BBC News. 21 January 2004.

8.   Manchester Online. "Doctors Support Drive Against Cannabis." *Manchester News.* 21 January 2004. . . .

9.   Joffe, Alain, MD, MPH, Yancy, Samuel W., MD, the Committee on Substance Abuse and the Committee on Adolescence, Technical Report: "Legalization of Marijuana: Potential Impact on Youth", American Academy of Pediatrics, 6 June 2004.

10. Institute of Medicine. "Marijuana and Medicine: Assessing the Science Base." (1999). Summary. (12 April 2005).

11. Id.

12. Institute of Medicine. "Marijuana and Medicine: Assessing the Science Base." (1999). Executive Summary. . . .

13. Institute of Medicine. "Marijuana and Medicine: Assessing the Science Base." (1999). Summary. . . .

14. Institute of Medicine. "Marijuana and Medicine: Assessing the Science Base." (1999). Summary. . . .

15. Benson, John A., Jr. and Watson, Stanley J., Jr. "Strike a Balance in the Marijuana Debate." *The Standard-Times.* 13 April 1999.

16. DEA, Office of Diversion Control. 8 May 2006.

17. "CMCR Mission Statement." *Center for Medicinal Cannabis Research.* . . .

18. DEA, Office of Diversion Control. 6 January 2006.

19. Marijuana Potency Monitoring Project. "Quarterly Report #87." *Marijuana Potency Monitoring Project.* 8 November 2004.

20. "BC Bud: Growth of the Canadian Marijuana Trade." *Drug Enforcement Administration, Intelligence Division.* December 2000.

21. "Teens at High Risk for Pot Addiction." *The Seattle Post-Intelligencer.* 6 January 2004.

22. Department of Health and Human Services, Substance Abuse and Mental Health Services Administration, Office of Applied Studies. *Treatment Episode Data Set (TEDS) 1993-2003: National Admissions to Substance Abuse Treatment Services.* November 2005, Table 5.1b. . . .

23. Id.

24. "Marijuana Myths & Facts: The Truth Behind 10 Popular Misperceptions." *Office of National Drug Control Policy.* . . .

25. Department of Health and Human Services, Substance Abuse and Mental Health Services Administration, Office of Applied Studies. *Overview of Findings from 2004 National Survey on Drug Use and Health.* September 2005.

26. Department of Health and Human Services, Substance Abuse and Mental Health Services Administration, Office of Applied Studies. Treatment Episode Data Set (TEDS) 1993-2003: *National Admissions to Substance Abuse Treatment Services.* November 2005. Page 74; Table 2.1b. . . .

27. Id., Tables 2.1a and 5.1a. There were 284,361 primary marijuana admissions in 2003, with 99,122 of those being juvenile marijuana admissions, meaning that there were 185,239 adult marijuana admissions.

28. "What Americans Need to Know about Marijuana." *Office of National Drug Control Policy.* October 2003.

29. Gfroerer, Joseph C., et al. "Initiation of Marijuana Use: Trends, Patterns and Implications." *Department of Health and Human Services, Substance Abuse and Mental Health Services Administration, Office of Applied Studies.* July 2002. Page 71.

30. "Non-Medical Marijuana II: Rite of Passage or Russian Roulette?" *CASA Reports*. April 2004. Chapter V, Page 15.

31. "What Americans Need to Know about Marijuana," 9.

32. Department of Health and Human Services, Substance Abuse and Mental Health Services Administration, Office of Applied Studies. "Daily Marijuana Users." *The NSDUH Report*. 26 November 2004.

33. Furber, Matt. "Threat of Meth-'the Devil's Drug'—increases." *Idaho Mountain Express and Guide*. 28 December 2005.

34. "Drug Abuse; Drug Czar, Others Warn Parents that Teen Marijuana Use can Lead to Depression." *Life Science Weekly*. 31 May 2005.

35. Kearney, Simon. "Cannabis is Worst Drug for Psychosis." *The Australian*. 21 November 2005.

36. Curtis, John. "Study Suggests Marijuana Induces Temporary Schizophrenia-Like Effects." *Yale Medicine*. Fall/Winter 2004.

37. "Marijuana Associated with Same Respiratory Symptoms as Tobacco," *YALE News Release*. 13 January 2005. . . . *See also*, "Marijuana Causes Same Respiratory Symptoms as Tobacco," January 13, 2005, . . .

38. "What Americans Need to Know about Marijuana," page 9.

39. "Marijuana Affects Brain Long-Term, Study Finds." Reuters. 8 February 2005. *See also*: "Marijuana Affects Blood Vessels." BBC News. 8 February 2005; "Marijuana Affects Blood Flow to Brain." *The Chicago Sun-Times*. 8 February 2005; Querna, Elizabeth. "Pot Head." *US News & World Report*. 8 February 2005.

40. "Neurotoxicology; Neurocognitive Effects of Chronic Marijuana Use Characterized." Health & Medicine Week. 16 May 2005.

41. Department of Health and Human Services, Substance Abuse and Mental Health Services Administration (SAMHSA), Office of Applied Sciences. "Marijuana Use and Delinquent Behaviors Among Youths." *The NSDUH Report*. 9 January 2004.

42. "Drugged Driving Poses Serious Safety Risk to Teens; Campaign to Urge Teens to 'Steer Clear of Pot' During National Drunk and Drugged Driving (3D) Prevention Month." *PR Newswire*. 2 December 2004.

43. O'Malley, Patrick and Johnston, Lloyd. "Unsafe Driving by High School Seniors: National Trends from 1976 to 2001 in Tickets and Accidents After Use of Alcohol, Marijuana and Other Illegal Drugs." *Journal of Studies on Alcohol*. May 2003.

44. Id.

45. "White House Drug Czar Launches Campaign to Stop Drugged Driving." *Office of National Drug Control Policy Press Release*. 19 November 2002.

46. Couper, Fiona, J., Ph.D., page 11.

47. Orange County Register. "Nation: Drug Test Positive for Driver in Deadly Crash." *Orange County Register*. 14 May 1999.

48. Edmondson, Aimee. "Drug Tests Required of Child Care Drivers—Fatal Crash Stirs Change; Many Already Test Positive." *The Commercial Appeal*. 2 July 2003.

49. McDonald, Melody and Boyd, Deanna. "Jury Gives Mallard 50 Years for Murder; Victim's Son Forgives but Says 'Restitution is Still Required.'" *Fort Worth Star Telegram*. 28 June 2003.

50. "Boy, 8, Who Was Struck While Riding Bike Dies." *The Dallas Morning News*. 25 April 2005.

51. "Lastest News in Brief from Northern Nevada." *The Associated Press State & Local Wire*. 30 April 2005.

52. Washoe County District Attorney's Office. 6 January 2006.

53. The Associated Press. "Police: Driver in Fatal Crash had Drugs in System." *The Associated Press.* 1 June 2003.

54. The Associated Press. "Murder Charges Filed in Blaze that Killed Two Fire-fighters." *The Associated Press.* 21 August 2004.

55. Office of National Drug Control Policy. "Who's Really in Prison for Marijuana?" May 2005. Page 22.

56. "Marijuana Myths & Facts." Page 22.

57. "Who's Really in Prison for Marijuana? Page 20.

58. "What Americans Need to Know about Marijuana," ONDCP, Page 10.

59. Dutch Health, Welfare and Sports Ministry Report. 23 April 2004.

60. INTRAVAL Bureau for Research & Consultancy. "Coffeeshops in the Nether-lands 2004." *Dutch Ministry of Justice.* June 2005. . . .

61. Id.

62. International Narcotics Control Board. "INCB Welcomes 'Crucial and Signifi-cant Change in Dutch Cannabis Policy.'" *United Nations Information Service.* 2 March 2005. The action plan to discourage cannabis use includes elements such as drug prevention campaigns, mass-media anti-drugs campaign, increased treatment efforts to cannabis users, and encouragement of administrative and criminal law enforcement efforts. *See also*: "International Narcotics Control Board Annual Report Focuses on Need to Integrate Drug Demand, Supply Strategies." *SOC/NAR/924 Press Release.* 3 February 2005. . . . "Press Briefing by International Narcotics Control Board." 3 January 2005. . . .

63. Collins, Larry. "Holland's Half-Baked Drug Experiment." *Foreign Affairs* Vol. 73, No. 3. May-June 1999: Pages 87–88.

64. Cohen, Roger. "Amid Growing Crime, Zurich Closes a Park it Reserved for Drug Addicts." *The New York Times.* 11 February 1992.

65. Adlaf, Edward M. and Paglia-Boak, Angela, Center for Addiction and Mental Health, *Drug Use Among Ontario Students*, 1977-2005, CAMH Research Docu-ment Series No. 16. The study does not contain data on marijuana use among 12th graders prior to 1999. See also: *Canadian Addiction Survey, Highlights* (November 2004) and *Detailed Report* (March 2005), produced by Health Canada and the Canadian Executive Council on Addictions; *Youth and Marijuana Quantitative Research' 2003 Final Report*, Health Canada; Tibbetts, Janice and Rogers, Dave. "Marijuana Tops Tobacco Among Teens, Survey Says: Youth Cannabis Use Hits 25-Year Peak," *The Ottawa Citizen*, 29 October 2003.

66. Koster, Olinka, Doughty, Steve, and Wright, Stephen. "Cannabis Climbdown." *Daily Mail* (London). 19 March 2005. See also. Revill, Jo, and Bright, Martin. "Cannabis: the Questions that Remain Unanswered." The Observer. 20 March 2005; Steele, John and Helm, Toby. "Clarke Reviews "Too Soft" Law on Cannabis." The Daily Telegraph (London). 19 March 2005; Brown, Colin. "Clarke Orders Review of Blunkett Move to Downgrade Cannabis." *The Inde-pendent (London).* 19 March 2005.

67. "Blair's 'Concern' on Cannabis." The Irish Times. 4 May 2005. See also, Russell, Ben. "Election 2005: Blair Rules Out National Insurance Rise." *The Independent (London).* 4 May 2005.

68. Craig, Tim. "Md. Starts to Allow Marijuana Court Plea; Penalty Can be Cut for Medicinal Use." *The Washington Post.* 1 October 2003, sec B.

69. From a videotape recording of Mr. Rosenthal's speech, as shown in "Medical Marijuana: A Smoke Screen."

70. "A Guide to Drug Related State Ballot Initiatives." *National Families in Action.* 23 April 2002. . . .

71. Wren, Christopher S. "Small But Forceful Coalition Works to Counter U.S. War on Drugs." *The New York Times*, 2 January 2000.

72. Brant, Tataboline. "Marijuana Campaign Draws in $857,000." *The Anchorage Daily News*. 30 October 2004.

73. Gathright, Alan. "Pot Backers Can't Stoke Hickenlooper." *Rocky Mountain News*. 27 October 2005.

74. Stannard, Matthew B. "Ecstasy Victim Told Friends She Felt Like She Was Going to Die." *The San Francisco Chronicle*, 4 May 2004. The Chronicle reported that Ms. Perez was given ibuprofen and "possibly marijuana," but DEA has confirmed that the drug given to her was indeed marijuana.

75. *Monitoring the Future,* 2005. Supplemented by information from the Office of National Drug Control Policy press release on the 2005 MTF Survey, December 19, 2005.)

76. DEA Domestic Cannabis Eradication/Suppression Program, 2005 eradication season.

77. Id.

POSTSCRIPT

Should Marijuana Be Approved for Medical Use?

The delay in the medicalization of marijuana stems from arduous and restrictive procedures of the federal government according to many people who support marijuana's medical use. They argue that the federal government prevents research from being conducted that would validate the medical benefits of marijuana. Thus, they argue that the government blocks people in need from receiving medication that is both therapeutic and benign. The government's objection to marijuana, according to these supporters, is based more on politics than scientific evidence.

From the federal government's perspective, promoting marijuana as a medicinal agent would be a mistake because it has not been proven medically useful or safe. Moreover, it feels that the availability of marijuana should not be predicated on personal accounts of its benefits or whether the public supports its use. Also, the Drug Enforcement Agency (DEA) disputes that although those studies show that marijuana may have medical value, much of that research has been based on bad scientific methodology and other deficiencies. The results of previous research, the DEA contends, do not lend strong credence to marijuana's medicinal value.

Some people have expressed concern about what will happen if marijuana is approved for medicinal use. Would it then become more acceptable for nonmedical, recreational use? Would it not be easy for people to get prescriptions for marijuana even though they may not have a medical need for the drug? There is also a possibility that some people would misinterpret the government's message and think that marijuana cures cancer when, in fact, it would only be used to treat the side effects of the chemotherapy.

A central question is if physicians feel that marijuana use is justified to properly care for seriously ill patients, should they promote this form of medical treatment even though it falls outside the law? Does the relief of pain and suffering for patients warrant going beyond what federal legislation says is acceptable? Also, should physicians be prosecuted if they recommend marijuana to their patients? What about the unknown risks of using an illegal drug? Is it worthwhile to ignore the possibility that marijuana may produce harmful side effects in order to alleviate pain or to treat other ailments?

Many marijuana proponents contend that the effort to prevent the legalization of marijuana for medical use is purely a political battle. Detractors maintain that the issue is purely scientific—that the data supporting marijuana's medical usefulness are inconclusive and scientifically unsubstantiated. And although the chief administrative law judge of the Drug Enforcement Administration (DEA) made a recommendation to change the status of marijuana from

Schedule I to Schedule II, the DEA and other federal agencies are not compelled to do so, and they have resisted any change in the law.

Articles that discuss whether marijuana should be legalized as a medication include "Medical Marijuana, Compassionate Use, and Public Policy: Expert Opinion or Vox Populi?" by Peter Cohen (*The Hastings Center Report,* May–June 2006); "Respectable Reefer," by Gary Greenberg (*Mother Jones,* November 2005); and "Medical Marijuana" (*The Economist,* April 27, 2006). Two additional articles that deal with specific medical uses of marijuana are "Cannabis Has Potential as a Drug to Relieve the Side Effects of Cancer and Its Treatment," by Donald Abrams (*Oncology News International,* March 1, 2006) and "Cannabis and AIDS" by Jule Klotter (*Townsend Letter for Doctors and Patients,* June 2006).

ISSUE 17

Should Schools Drug Test Students?

YES: Office of National Drug Control Policy, from *Strategies for Success: New Pathways to Drug Abuse Prevention* (Fall/Winter 2006)

NO: Jennifer Kern, Fatema Gunja, Alexandra Cox, Marsha Rosenbaum, Judith Appel, and **Anjuli Verma,** from *Making Sense of Student Drug Testing: Why Educators Are Saying No* (January 2006)

ISSUE SUMMARY

YES: The Office of National Drug Control Policy (ONDCP), an agency of the federal government, maintains that it is important to test students for illicit drugs because testing reduces drug use and improves the learning environment in schools. The ONDCP purports that the majority of students support drug testing. In addition, drug testing does not decrease participation in extracurricular activities.

NO: Jennifer Kern and associates maintain that drug testing is ineffective and that the threat of drug testing may dissuade students from participating in extracurricular activities. Moreover, drug testing is costly, it may make schools susceptible to litigation, and it undermines relationships of trust between students and teachers. Drug testing, according to Kern, does not effectively identify students who may have serious drug problems.

$\mathbf{A}$ttempting to reduce drug use by students is a desirable goal. Whether or not drug testing students is a means to achieve this goal is the subject of this debate. If it can be shown that drug testing results in less student drug use, then it is worthwhile. However, people on both sides of this issue do not agree on whether drug use is curtailed by drug testing.

According to the Office of National Drug Control Policy (ONDCP), drug testing acts as a deterrent to drug use. The threat of drug testing, states the ONDCP, has been shown to be extremely effective in reducing drug use by students in schools who participate in extracurricular activities as well as by individuals in the workplace. On the other hand, Jennifer Kern and associates believe that drug testing does not have an impact on drug use. They indicate that drug testing is counterproductive in that the threat of drug testing will cause many students to avoid extracurricular activities. Moreover, drug testing may lead to false positives in which students may be erroneously accused of using drugs.

Should the expense of drug testing be a factor in whether schools test students? Very few students are detected as having used illegal drugs. When school districts are strapped for funds, is drug testing a good use of funds? Critics maintain that a more effective strategy for reducing drug use would be better drug education programs that are geared to having students understand the hazards associated with drugs. Drug testing is geared to preventing drug use, not to reducing the harms that come from drug use.

An important question evolves around the legality of drug testing. Does drug testing unfairly discriminate against student athletes? In June 2002, the Supreme Court, in a 5 to 4 decision, ruled that random drug testing for all middle and high school students participating in extracurricular activities is allowable. Prior to 2002, only student athletes could be tested. Should students who participate in school government, band, plays, or other school-related activities undergo drug testing?

One reason the federal government supports drug testing is that students who use drugs do not perform as well academically as those students who do not use drugs. The point of drug testing, states the federal government, is to help students, not to punish them. One criticism of drug testing is that it focuses on illegal drugs. Teenagers are far more likely to use tobacco and alcohol than illegal drugs. Drug testing does not address the problem of tobacco and alcohol use. Tobacco and alcohol cause far more harm than illegal drugs. Drug testing proponents agree that tobacco and alcohol are not adequately addressed, but that does not mean that students should not be tested for illegal drugs.

In the following selections, the Office of National Drug Control Policy (ONDCP) advocates drug testing as a means of reducing illegal drug use by students. The ONDCP claims that the threat of drug testing is sufficient for stopping drug use or preventing drug use from occurring in the first place. Jennifer Kern and her associates question the effectiveness of drug testing. They maintain that drug testing has the opposite effect in that many students will choose not to participate in extracurricular activities for fear of testing positive for illegal drugs.

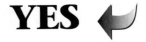

YES

Office of National Drug Control Policy

Strategies for Success: New Pathways to Drug Abuse Prevention

Principals Claim Testing Brings a Wealth of Benefits

Evidence suggesting the efficacy of random student drug testing as a tool to reduce drug use among youth is mounting. Results of a recent survey in Indiana corroborate what some educators and substance-abuse experts have maintained for years: drug testing is a promising drug prevention strategy.

Testing may not only reduce illicit drug use, the report suggests, it may also help improve the learning environment in schools by diminishing the culture of drugs. Principals participating in the survey indicated they believe drug testing has no negative effect on school morale or participation in sports or extracurricular activities, and that costs are minimal.

Published in the February 23 issue of *West's Education Law Reporter,* "The Effectiveness and Legality of Random Student Drug Testing Programs Revisited" presents findings from an April 2005 survey of principals at 65 Indiana high schools. Of the 56 schools that responded to the written survey, 54 used drug testing as part of their substance-abuse prevention programs. Two-thirds of the principals responding to the questionnaire said they based their answers on written student surveys.

The report, written by Joseph R. McKinney, chairman of the Department of Educational Leadership at Ball State University, is a follow-up to a survey conducted at the same high schools in 2002–2003, a time when the schools had either just begun or resumed their drug testing programs. Several years earlier, schools across Indiana had been forced to halt all drug testing because a ruling by a state appeals court had declared them unconstitutional. A landmark decision in June 2002 by the U.S. Supreme Court cleared the way by ruling that middle and high schools can conduct random drug tests of students participating in extracurricular activities.

The 2005 study is an attempt to learn about the effectiveness of drug testing programs by asking survey respondents what changes, if any, occurred in student drug use and other behavior at the target schools after nearly three years with testing programs in place. Its purpose, as stated in the report, is to shed light on two issues facing school districts trying to decide whether to test

From the Office of National Drug Control Policy, *Pathways to Drug Abuse Prevention,* Fall/Winter 2006.

students for drug use: Are drug testing programs effective in reducing and preventing drug use, and are they legal?

McKinney is optimistic on both counts. "The Supreme Court has spoken," he writes, "and so have several state and federal courts. Random student drug testing [RSDT] is legal with some limitations." In McKinney's opinion, "The research on RSDT also speaks volumes on the effectiveness of drug testing programs. RSDT programs are effective in deterring, reducing and detecting illegal drug use among students."

While some indicators remained constant between surveys, almost every reported change in drug-use behavior or related activities was a change for the better. For example, more than half (58 percent) of the principals in the 2005 study who relied on written student surveys for their responses said student drug use had decreased since the previous study. The rest said levels of use remained the same. Additionally, 41 percent of the full group of principals reported that the positive drug-test result rate—the percentage of students testing positive for drug use—had decreased, while 56 percent said the rate had not changed since the previous survey.

Among the encouraging results to emerge from the McKinney survey is that in no case was drug testing seen to have a negative impact on the classroom. Despite critics' concerns that drug testing erodes student morale, 100 percent of the responding Indiana principals whose schools have drug testing programs said their experiences showed these claims to be untrue. (One left the question blank.)

Reporting on data collected from the survey, McKinney also addresses charges that drug testing discourages participation in sports and other extra-curricular activities and is too costly. More than half of the high schools with drug testing programs reported that levels of participation in athletic programs remained the same from 2003 to 2005. The rest said participation increased. None reported that participation levels had gone down. As for the expense, the overwhelming majority (91 percent) of schools with testing programs reported that the per-test cost was only $30 or less. Almost two-thirds said the drug tests cost no more than $20 each.

Although overall youth drug use has decreased by nearly 20 percent Nationwide since 2001, illegal drugs remain a significant threat to young people. A 2005 survey of teens by the National Center on Addiction and Substance Abuse at Columbia University found that 62 percent of high schoolers and 28 percent of middle schoolers report that drugs are used, kept, or sold at their schools. According to the 2005 Youth Risk Behavior Survey, almost half of all students (47.6 percent) have used marijuana by the time they finish high school.

Results of the McKinney survey cannot, of course, be construed as a definitive measure of student drug use or attitudes, nor do they prove a causal relationship between drug testing and reduced levels of use. Still, taken as a whole, the survey data offer compelling evidence that random drug testing can be helpful in the effort to keep students drug free. The report bolsters the notion that random drug testing, used in conjunction with other methods as part of a comprehensive program for preventing and treating substance abuse, can be a useful and potentially effective drug abuse prevention tool.

KEY FINDINGS

Here are key findings of the McKinney report, which compares the results of an April 2005 survey of 65 Indiana high schools with data collected from the same schools in 2002–2003:

Principals Report:

Student Drug Use*
- Decreased: 58 percent
- Remained the same: 42 percent
- Increased: 0 percent

Per-Test Cost
- $30 or less: 91 percent of surveyed schools
- $20 or less: 63 percent of surveyed schools

Positive Drug-Test Result Rate
- Decreased: 41 percent
- Remained the same: 56 percent
- Increased: 3 percent

Effects of Drug Testing on Peer Pressure to Use Drugs
- Testing limits the effects of peer pressure: 91 percent
- Testing does not limit the effects of peer pressure: 9 percent

Participation in Athletic Programs
- Decreased: 0 percent
- Remained the same: 54 percent
- Increased: 46 percent

Participation in Extracurricular Activities
- Decreased: 0 percent
- Remained the same: 55 percent
- Increased: 45 percent

Impact Upon Morale
- Principals reporting that, based on their experiences, random drug testing does not have a negative impact in the classroom: 100 percent

* Responses based on written student surveys

Drugs and Testing: Looking at the Big Picture

Imagine a surgeon turning down the opportunity to use a powerful medical procedure that is government-approved, affordable, available, easy to use, and potentially life-saving.

It makes no sense.

The same could be said about schools that pass up a promising new technique for combating the scourge of substance abuse: random student drug testing. As any good surgeon knows, better methods bring better results.

Parents and educators have a responsibility to keep young people safe from drug use. In recent years we have made solid, measurable progress toward that end. According to the latest national survey in the Monitoring the Future series, the proportion of 8th-, 10th-, and 12th-grade students combined who use illicit drugs continued to fall in 2006, the fifth consecutive year of decline for these age groups. Similarly, results of the 2005 Youth Risk Behavior Survey show that rates of current marijuana use among high school students have dropped from a peak of 26.7 percent in 1999 to 20.2 percent.

This is good news, to be sure, but hardly reason to drop our guard. Consider: In 2006, according to Monitoring the Future, a fifth (21 percent) of today's 8th graders, over a third (36 percent) of 10th graders, and about half (48 percent) of 12th graders in America had tried illegal drugs at some point in their lives. Proportions indicating past-year drug use were 15 percent, 29 percent, and 37 percent, respectively, for the same grade levels.

Marijuana remains the greatest single drug threat facing our young people. Past-year marijuana use among 18- to 25-year-olds (the group with the highest drug-use rates) fell 6 percent from 2002 to 2005, according to the National Survey on Drug Use and Health. And yet, despite reduced rates in this and other user categories, marijuana still ranks as the most commonly used of all illicit drugs, with a rate of 6 percent—14.6 million current users—for the U.S. population age 12 and older. This is particularly disturbing because marijuana use can lead to significant health, safety, social, and learning or behavioral problems, and kids are the most vulnerable to its damaging effects.

Adding more cause for concern is the emergence of new threats, such as prescription-drug abuse. Over the past decade, youth populations have more than tripled their non-medical use of prescription drugs. Nearly one in five teens has taken prescription medications to get "high," according to a recent study by the Partnership for a Drug-Free America.

Our task, then, is to keep forging ahead and working to defeat drug abuse wherever it should arise. And to do this, we need all the help we can get. It is vital that we make use of the best tools at our disposal to protect young people from a behavior that destroys bodies and minds, impedes academic performance, and creates barriers to success.

Drug testing is just such a tool. For decades, drug testing has been used effectively to help reduce drug use in the U.S. Military and the Nation's workforce. Now this strategy is available to any school that understands the devastation of drug use and is determined to push back. Many of our schools urgently need effective ways to reinforce their anti-drug efforts. A random drug testing program can help them.

In June 2002, the U.S. Supreme Court broadened the authority of public schools to test students for illegal drugs. The ruling allows random drug tests not just for student athletes, but for all middle and high school students participating in competitive extracurricular activities. School administrators, however, need to consult with their counsels about any additional state law requirements regarding student drug testing.

Scientists know that drug use can interfere with brain function, learning, and the ability to retain information (see "The Biology of Drug Addiction," page 12). Any drug use at school disrupts the learning environment for all students. It spreads like a contagious disease from peer to peer and is, in this regard, nothing less than a public health threat. Schools routinely test for tuberculosis and other communicable diseases that jeopardize student health. Clearly, there is every reason to test for drugs as well.

It is important to understand that random student drug testing is not a panacea or an end in itself. Nor is it a substitute for other techniques or programs designed to reduce drug use by young people. Testing is only part of the solution and cannot do the job alone. For maximum effectiveness, it should be used in combination with other proven strategies in a comprehensive substance-abuse prevention and treatment program.

Schools considering adding a testing program to their current prevention efforts will find reassurance in knowing drug testing can be done in a way that is compassionate and respectful of students' privacy, pride, and dignity. The purpose of testing, after all, is not to punish or stigmatize kids who use drugs. Rather, it is to prevent drug use in the first place, and to make sure users get the help they need before the disease of addition can spread. Drug testing is also affordable. Discussions with individual schools indicate that, on average, a high school with 1,000 students will spend approximately $1,500 a year to test 70 students, or 10 percent of the pool of eligible students.

As the number of schools with testing programs grows, so does the body of evidence suggesting that random student drug testing can have beneficial effects on school morale. Students feel safer participating in an activity when they know their classmates are drug-free. As former drug users get and stay clean, they make healthier and better choices about how to spend leisure time, and they are more likely to engage in school activities. School pride and spirit increase as students, parents, and the school community become more involved in the school environment.

Our Road to Random

Robert Razzano

On October 2, 2003, a young man made the ultimate decision of his life. It was a decision that would affect his family, friends, and community. That young man's name was Michael Mikkanen.

Michael was a model high school student who had it all. He was an athlete, honor student, popular, and personable. His future was full of promise and opportunities. The pressure of his transition from high school to his first year in college led to severe anxiety, depression, and instability. His inability to cope led to drug use. Heroin was cheap and easy to get. Michael's addiction became so intense that it led to crime to feed his habit. Eventually Michael was arrested and jailed. On his first night behind bars, Michael made the fateful decision to take his own life.

At the funeral home, Michael's mother pleaded with me to do something to help our young people with the drug problem in our city. As I sat there with my eldest son and watched Michael's friends walk up to the casket,

I made a commitment to myself that I would try to fulfill the appeal of Michael's mother. Shortly thereafter I started my research on random and reasonable-suspicion drug testing.

As an administrator for the New Castle Area School District in Pennsylvania, I presented my research at our monthly administrative meetings. Superintendent George Gabriel asked me to select a committee and to present a proposal for drug testing to the school board. My committee included parents, coaches, the district attorney, school board members, the band director, and the athletic director. We spoke with many other school districts that already had a written drug testing policy. The committee spent six months working on the proposal, which Michael's mother and I presented to the school board. The board approved it, and the policy was implemented for the 2004/2005 school year.

The purpose of the random drug testing policy for the New Castle Area School District is to create a drug-free setting for all students and district employees. It is our belief that participation on any interscholastic athletic team or in any extracurricular activity is a privilege and not a right. The students who volunteer to take part in these programs are expected to accept the responsibilities granted to them by this privilege.

We recognized that drug use by school-age children is becoming more prevalent and dangerous in the community and believed the problem had to be addressed to ensure the health, safety, and welfare of all the students within the district. The need for a random drug testing policy is predicated upon the risk of immediate physical harm to drug users and to those with whom the users play sports or participate in extracurricular activities.

Drug use is not only a national problem, but a local problem. The objectives of our district's random drug testing program are to establish a deterrent to drug use and to take a proactive approach toward creating a truly safe and drug-free school. We believe the random drug testing policy undermines the effects of peer pressure by providing students with a legitimate reason to refuse to use illegal drugs. The policy also, we believe, will encourage students who use drugs to participate in drug treatment programs.

Over the past two years, we have administered 2,221 drug tests to our 7th- to 12th-grade students. Less than 1 percent tested positive for illegal drugs. Of the 1,112 students tested during the 2004/2005 school year, there were eight positive tests (five freshman and three seniors). In 2005/2006, we tested 1,109 students. Only two tested positive. The parents of all those students were notified, and each student was obligated to follow the consequence phase of the policy.

The consequences phase includes suspension from extracurricular or athletic activities, assessment from a certified drug and alcohol counselor, five consecutive weeks of drug testing, and an automatic referral to the student assistance program. Also included in our policy is a parental request referral: if parents request that their son or daughter be drug-tested, that student will be added to the random sample list on the next scheduled date.

I am not under the illusion that drug testing is a panacea in the war on drugs. However, I unequivocally believe that a random drug testing policy is a strong deterrent and helps our young people say "no" to drugs. A drug testing

AROUND THE U.S., HOPEFUL SIGNS AT SCHOOLS WITH TESTING

Drug testing programs have shown great promise in reducing student drug use. Here are some encouraging numbers from school districts around the country.

Community High School District #117 Lake Villa, Illinois

Results of the American Drug and Alcohol Survey for 9th through 12th graders in 2005–2006 show a 29 percent decrease in past-year drug use, down from 30 percent in 2002 to 21 percent in 2006; and a 33 percent decrease in past-month drug use, down from 18 percent in 2002 to 12 percent in 2006.

Oceanside Unified School District Oceanside, California

The Oceanside District saw an increase in drug use among student-athletes in 2004 after their drug testing program was eliminated. The school reinstated the program during the 2005–2006 school year. More than half of student athletes surveyed in 2006 said the school's current drug testing program made it easier for them to say no to drugs.

Eagle Mountain-Saginaw Independent School District Fort Worth, Texas

Ninth through 12th graders showed a decline in substance use in 8 of 13 substances from 2004 to 2005, according to a school substance use survey.

Paradise Unified School District Paradise, California

Paradise High School staff noted a decrease in school disciplinary actions for student drug use during the 2005–2006 school year after drug testing began. The California Healthy Kids Survey results for Paradise Valley indicate that past-month drug use by 11th graders decreased 12 percent since 2003.

Pulaski County Board of Education Somerset, Kentucky

The number of disciplinary infractions related to drug use decreased 26 percent from 76 incidents in 2004-05 to 56 incidents in 2005-06 after one year of student drug testing.

program is worth the effort even if it saves only one life. I know Michael Mikkanen's family would agree.

British Educator Calls Testing Program a Success

Peter Walker is not the type to sit idly by and wait for others to find solutions. Beneath that jovial, self-effacing manner and soft English accent lies an iron determination. "In this world," the longtime educator told a group of ONDCP staffers and guests during a recent visit, "if you think there's a problem and you can do something about it—you do it."

Before stepping down last spring as headteacher (headmaster) of the Abbey School in Faversham, Kent County, England, Walker took his own advice to heart. He knew about the problem of drug abuse, about how drugs create barriers to education, burden society, and destroy young lives. So in a bold and historic move, he did something about it.

Early last year, Walker launched the first random student drug testing program at a public school in the United Kingdom. The program is open to all students but is entirely voluntary; both the student and parents must give their consent before testing can occur. And though more research must be done to determine the program's full impact, Walker needs no further convincing. For him, the signs of success are everywhere.

The Numbers

Walker spent nearly a year developing the testing program, consulting with students, parents, teachers, staff, government officials, local police, and others. "I was overwhelmed by the support," he said.

Particularly encouraging was the response of parents: 86 percent gave permission for their children to be tested.

From the time testing began in January 2005 until last spring, 600 of the nearly 1,000 students at the Abbey School had been tested for drug use (using the oral-fluids method). Only four refused when their names were called. And of all the samples tested that first year, just one was positive for drug use.

Academic Achievement

When the testing program began, Walker went on record with his belief that examination results would improve within the first year. It was a risky prediction, he said, "because in the UK, if a school doesn't meet its targets, the headteacher is the first to go." At year's end, however, he was able to report that the exam results were not only the best in the school's history, they beat out the previous record by a remarkable ten percent.

Reduced Crime

Levels of crime, too, have plunged since testing began, Walker said. Last winter, a policeman came to his office and asked why crime rates at Abbey School had dropped below those at the other area schools within the past year. Walker wouldn't go so far as to claim that drug testing alone was responsible for the decline. "But," he said, "I will claim that drug testing might have had an influence."

Improved Morale

And then there are the intangible signs of success. Morale, for instance, has improved noticeably throughout the school since testing began, Walker said.

When the program was announced, more than half of the staff agreed to make themselves eligible for testing—"and they weren't even asked."

As for the students, they not only accept the program, Walker said, "They support it. They want it. They believe in it, and they're proud of it." For one thing, he continued, testing gives them a way to resist what he called the greatest motivation for taking drugs in the first place: peer pressure. Fear of being called up for a drug test gives students a convenient excuse to say no to drugs, he said. "If they can come up with their own reasons that their peer group will accept, you're on a winner."

A drug testing program, Walker explained, also shifts some of the emphasis away from the students who may be using drugs and focuses needed attention on those who strive to avoid them. From the start, he set out to achieve two main goals through drug testing. The first was to prevent drug use before it begins—by far the cheapest and most effective way to combat substance abuse.

The second main goal was to improve the quality of life for kids who choose not to take drugs. Indeed, gaining the cooperation of the non-using majority of students is vital to the program's success. "That's the trick," said Walker. One day last fall, he overheard a student telling a visiting reporter that she welcomed the program. With drug testing, she explained, "the kids now feel that they're being protected. They're feeling valued."

MYTH VS. FACT

Myth
Participation in extracurricular activities decreases when schools implement random student drug testing programs.

Fact
To date, more than 750 schools have implemented random student drug testing programs. A number of these schools indicate that the presence of a testing program does not appear to reduce levels of student participation in extracurricular activities; in fact, the levels have remained stable or actually increased. In Florida's Polk County schools, for example, where athletes are randomly drug-tested, 448 more students tried out for sports in 2005 than in 2004, and 319 more students tried out for sports in 2004 than in 2003.

Published studies support these findings. In Oregon, the Student Athlete Testing Using Random Notification (SATURN) study found that sport-activity participation increased by over 10 percent in schools with a random testing program. In addition, on a recent survey of high school principals in Indiana with 54 principals responding, 45 percent of principals in schools with random student drug testing programs reported increases in student participation, and no principals reported a decrease (see "Principals Claim Testing Brings a Wealth of Benefits,". . .).

Any good drug-prevention program requires what Walker calls a "total package" of student support. "Do it in isolation," as he put it, "and you're on a loser." It is pointless to address substance abuse only occasionally or half-heartedly, such as during "drug awareness month," he said. Instead, it has to be part of a package that encompasses broad aspects of the students' lives, from academics and health education to sexual and financial matters.

Looking Ahead

The Abbey School's drug testing program has become a catalyst for big changes in England. Prompted by its success, the government is rolling out a pilot drug testing program this fall for all schools in Kent. If all goes well, the plan is to extend drug testing to schools throughout the country.

Walker, meanwhile, though retired as headteacher, remains nonetheless an educator, actively spreading the word as a government-appointed ambassador for random drug testing. "I'm not an evangelist," he said, "and I'm not selling anything. But I believe this can make a difference to young people."

Jennifer Kern, Fatema Gunja, Alexandra
Cox, Marsha Rosenbaum, Judith Appel,
and Anjuli Verma

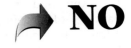 **NO**

Making Sense of Student Drug Testing: Why Educators Are Saying No

Executive Summary

Comprehensive, rigorous and respected research shows there are many reasons why random student drug testing is not good policy:

- Drug testing is not effective in deterring drug use among young people;
- Drug testing is expensive, taking away scarce dollars from other, more effective programs that keep young people out of trouble with drugs;
- Drug testing can be legally risky, exposing schools to potentially costly litigation;
- Drug testing may drive students away from extracurricular activities, which are a proven means of helping students stay out of trouble with drugs;
- Drug testing can undermine trust between students and teachers, and between parents and children;
- Drug testing can result in false positives, leading to the punishment of innocent students;
- Drug testing does not effectively identify students who have serious problems with drugs; and
- Drug testing may lead to unintended consequences, such as students using drugs (like alcohol) that are more dangerous but less detectable by a drug test.

There *are* alternatives to drug testing that emphasize education, discussion, counseling and extracurricular activities, and that build trust between students and adults.

Random Drug Testing Does Not Deter Drug Use

Proponents assert the success of random student drug testing by citing a handful of reports from schools that anecdotally claim drug testing reduced drug use. The only formal study to claim a reduction in drug use was based on a snapshot of two schools and was suspended by the federal government for lack of sound methodology.[1, 2]

In a 2005 report evaluating the available evidence, Professor Neil McKeganey critiqued the methodology and biases of the studies repeatedly presented in support of random student drug testing, saying, "It is a matter of concern that student drug testing has been widely developed within the USA . . . on the basis of the slimmest available research evidence."[3]

Largest National Study Shows Drug Testing Fails

The first large-scale national study on student drug testing found virtually no difference in rates of drug use between schools that have drug testing programs and those that do not.[4] Based on data collected between 1998 and 2001 from 76,000 students nationwide in 8th, 10th and 12th grades, the study found that drug testing did not have an impact on illicit drug use among students, including athletes.

Dr. Lloyd D. Johnston, an author of the study, directs *Monitoring the Future,* the leading survey by the federal government of trends in student drug use and attitudes about drugs. According to Dr. Johnston, "**[The study] suggests that there really isn't an impact from drug testing as practiced . . . I don't think it brings about any constructive changes in their attitudes about drugs or their belief in the dangers associated with using them.**"[5] Published in the April 2003 *Journal of School Health,* the study was conducted by researchers at the University of Michigan and funded in part by the National Institute on Drug Abuse (NIDA).

Follow-Up Study Confirms Results: Drug Testing Fails

The researchers at the University of Michigan conducted a more extensive study later that year with an enlarged sample of schools, an additional year of data and an increased focus on random testing programs.[6] The updated results reinforced their previous conclusions:

> So, does drug testing prevent or inhibit student drug use? Our data suggest that, as practiced in recent years in American secondary schools, it does not . . . The two forms of drug testing that are generally assumed to be most promising for reducing student drug use—random testing applied to all students . . . and testing of athletes—did not produce encouraging results.[7]

The follow-up study was published in 2003 as part of the Youth, Education and Society (YES) Occasional Papers Series sponsored by the Robert Wood Johnson Foundation.

The strongest predictor of student drug use, the studies' authors note, is students' attitudes toward drug use and their perceptions of peer use. The authors recommend policies that address "these key values, attitudes and perceptions" as effective alternatives to drug testing.[8] The results of these national studies are supported by numerous other surveys and studies that examine the effectiveness of various options for the prevention of student drug misuse.[9]

Who Says No to Random Drug Testing?

A groundswell of opposition has emerged to random drug testing among school officials, experts, parents and state legislatures.

School Officials and Parents Say No to Drug Testing

> We stopped testing because "we didn't think it was the deterrent that we thought it would be . . . we didn't think it was as effective with the money we spent on it."
>
> —Scot Dahl. President at school board in Guymon, Oklahoma[10]

> We decided not to drug test because "it really is a parental responsibility . . . it is not our job to actually test [students]."
>
> —Harry M. Ward, Superintendent in Mathews County, Virginia[11]

> "The concerns of parents [in opposing a student drug testing proposal] have ranged from the budgetary issues to losing our focus on education to creating a threatening environment."
>
> —Laura Rowe, President of Band Aids, a parent association of the high school band program in Oconomowoc, Wisconsin[12]

> "We object to the urine-testing policy as an unwarranted invasion of privacy. We want school to teach our children to think critically, not to police them."
>
> —Hans York, parent and Deputy Sheriff in Wahkiakum, Washington[13]

> "I would have liked to see healthy community participation that stimulates thoughtful interaction among us. Instead, this [drug testing] policy was steamrolled into place, powered by mob thinking."
>
> —Jackie Puccetti, parent in El Paso, Texas[14]

Educators and School Officials

The majority of school officials—including administrators, teachers, coaches, school counselors and school board members—have chosen not to implement drug testing programs. With their concerns rooted in knowledge and practical experience, school officials object to drug testing for a variety of reasons, including the cost of testing, the invasion of privacy and the unfair burden that student drug testing places on schools. For many educators and school officials, drug testing simply fails to reflect the reality of what works to establish safe school environments.

Experts

Physicians, social workers, substance abuse treatment providers and child advocates agree that student drug testing cannot replace pragmatic drug prevention measures, such as after-school activities. Many prominent national organizations representing these groups have come forward in court to oppose drug testing programs. These groups include the American Academy of Pediatrics, the National Education Association, the American Public Health Association, the National Association of Social Workers, and the National Council on Alcoholism and Drug Dependence. These experts have stated: **"Our experience—and a broad body of relevant research—convinces us that a policy [of random student drug testing]** *cannot* **work in the way it is hoped to and will, for many adolescents, interfere with more sound prevention and treatment processes."**[15]

Experts Say No to Drug Testing

"Social workers, concerned with a child's well-being, question whether [drug testing] will do more harm than good . . . What is most effective in keeping kids away from drugs and alcohol are substance abuse prevention programs based on scientific research."

—Elizabeth J. Clark, Ph.D., A.C.S.W., M.P.H., Executive Director of the National Association of Social Workers[16]

"Protecting America's youth from alcohol and drugs requires more than a simple drug test. We need a greater commitment to prevention and treatment . . . At-risk and marginal students need the support systems and mentoring relationships that extracurricular activities provide. Excluding students who test positive for drugs will likely exacerbate their problems."

—Bill Burnett, President, the Association for Addiction Professionals[17]

"Let us not rush to accept the illusory view that drug testing in schools is the silver bullet for the prevention of youth substance abuse . . . While [drug tests] are increasing in popularity, their efficacy is unproven and they are associated with significant technical concerns."

—Dr. John R. Knight, Director of the Center for Adolescent Substance Abuse Research at Children's Hospital in Boston and Dr. Sharon Levy, Director of Pediatrics for the Adolescent Substance Abuse Program at Children's Hospital in Boston[18]

The Oklahoma policy "falls short doubly if deterrence is its aim: It invades the privacy of students who need deterrence least, and risks steering students at greatest risk for substance abuse away from extra-curricular involvement that potentially may palliate drug problems."

—U.S. Supreme Court Justice Ruth Bader Ginsburg's Dissenting Opinion in Board of Education of Pottawatomie v. Earls[19]

Parents

Many parents oppose drug testing for the same reasons as school staff and administrators. In addition, some parents believe that schools are misappropriating their roles when they initiate drug testing programs. They believe that it is the role of parents, not schools, to make decisions about their children's health.

State Governments

Since the U.S. Supreme Court's 2002 decision that schools may randomly drug test students participating in competitive extracurricular activities, several state legislatures have opposed student drug testing after hearing community and expert concerns about privacy, confidentiality, potential liability and overall effectiveness. For example, the Hawaii legislature tabled a bill that would have established a drug testing pilot program at several public high schools.[20] In Louisiana, a bill was defeated that would have mandated drug testing state scholarship recipients.[21]

Drug Testing Has a Negative Impact on the Classroom

Drug testing can undermine student-teacher relationships by pitting students against the teachers and coaches who test them, eroding trust and leaving students ashamed and resentful.

As educators know, student-teacher trust is critical to creating an atmosphere in which students can address their fears and concerns about drug use itself, as well as the issues that can lead to drug use, including depression, anxiety, peer pressure and unstable family life.[22] Trust is jeopardized if teachers act as confidants in some circumstances but as police in others.

Drug testing also results in missed classroom instruction. Officials at some schools with testing programs reported that many students would flagrantly ridicule the testing process by stalling for hours to produce a urine sample—during which time they remained absent from class.[23]

THE HUMAN COSTS OF DRUG TESTING:
A CASE IN POINT

Lori Brown of Texas felt her son was wronged by his school's random drug testing program. Seventeen-year-old Mike, an upstanding senior at Shallowater High School near Lubbock, Texas, was taking a number of medications for allergies, as well as some antibiotics, when his school randomly tested him. One of these antibiotics, his doctor later confirmed, can cause a false positive for cocaine. The school failed to properly follow their own policies by neglecting to ask Mike to list the medications he was taking. To make matters worse, South Plains Compliance, the drug testing company hired by the school to administer the tests, maintained that their procedures were 100 percent accurate despite the extenuating circumstances.

After the test came up positive for cocaine, Lori had Mike tested several times by their own physician for her own peace of mind. Each test confirmed what she already knew: Mike was not using cocaine. Lori defended her son, explaining to school authorities what she learned from Mike's doctor. But they refused to listen. Over the next six months, he was "randomly" picked for testing several more times and began to feel harassed and stigmatized as a result.

"In my opinion, schools are using the [drug] testing program as a tool to police students, when they should be concentrating on education," Lori says.

Finally, Lori and Mike had reached their emotional limit when a South Plains Compliance representative yelled at Mike for not producing enough urine for his sixth test. Together they decide to remove him from the drug testing program. As a result, Mike could no longer participate in extracurricular activities.

PROBLEMS WITH DIFFERENT TYPES OF TESTS[24]

School officials lack the expertise to determine which type of testing is more reliable.

Urine	Marijuana Cocaine Opiates Amphetamine PCP	$10–$50 per test	• Tests commonly used in schools often do not detect alcohol or tobacco • Since marijuana stays in the body longer than other drugs, drugs like cocaine, heroin and methamphetamine often go undetected • Test is invasive and embarrassing • Specimen can be adulterated
Hair	Marijuana Cocaine Opiates Amphetamine PCP MDMA/ [Ecstasy]	$60–$75 per test	• Expensive • Cannot detect alcohol use • Will not detect very recent drug use • The test is discriminatory: dark-haired people are more likely to test positive than blondes, and African Americans are more likely to test positive than Caucasians • Passive exposure to drugs in the environment, especially those that are smoked, may lead to false positive results
Sweat Patch	Marijuana Cocaine Opiates Amphetamine PCP	$20–$50 per test	• Limited number of labs able to process results • Passive exposure to drugs may contaminate patch and result in false-positives • People with skin eruptions, excessive hair, or cuts and abrasions cannot wear the patch
Saliva	Marijuana Cocaine Opiates Amphetamine PCP	$10–$50 per test	• Detects only very recent use and limited number of drugs • New technology; accuracy rates and testing guidelines not established

Drug Testing is Expensive and a Waste of School Resources

Drug testing costs schools an average of $42 per student tested, which amounts to $21,000 for a high school testing 500 Students.[25] This figure is for the initial test alone and does not include the costs of other routine components of drug testing, such as additional tests throughout the year or follow-up testing.

The cost of drug testing often exceeds the total a school district spends on existing drug education, prevention and counseling programs combined. In fact, drug testing may actually take scarce resources away from the very health and treatment services needed by students who are misusing drugs.

The process for dealing with a positive test is usually long and involved; not only must a second test be done to rule out a false positive result, but treatment referral and follow-up systems must also be in place. In one school district, the cost of detecting the 11 students who tested positive amounted to $35,000.[26]

Beyond the initial costs, there are long-term operational and administrative expenses associated with student drug testing, including:

- Monitoring students' urination to collect accurate samples;
- Documentation, bookkeeping and compliance with confidentiality requirements; and
- Tort or other insurance to safeguard against potential lawsuits.

COST-BENEFIT ANALYSIS IN DUBLIN, OHIO[27]

In Dublin, Ohio, school administrators ended their drug testing program and hired two full time substance abuse counselors instead, concluding that drug testing reduces resources for more effective drug prevention programs.

	Drug Testing	Substance Abuse Counselor
Cost of program	$35,000 per school year	$32,000 annual starting salary per counselor
Number of students	Out of 1,473 students tested, 11 tested positive	Prevention programs for all 3,581 high school students incorporated in a weekly class curriculum
Cost per student	$24 per student for drug test $3,200 per student who tested positive	$18 per student for drug prevention, education and intervention Intervention programs for all targeted students who need help

Not All Drug Testing is Protected Under the Law

In 2002, by a margin of five to four, the U.S. Supreme Court in *Board of Education of Pottawatomie v. Earls* permitted public school districts to drug test students

U.S. SUPREME COURT DID NOT SAY . . .

- The Court DID NOT say that schools are required to test students involved in competitive extracurricular activities.
- The Court DID NOT say drug testing of all students or specific groups of students outside of those participating in competitive extracurricular activities [i.e. student drivers) is constitutional.
- The court DID NOT say it is constitutional to drug test elementary school children.
- The Court DID NOT say that it is constitutional to test by means other than urinalysis.
- The Court DID NOT say that schools are protected from lawsuits under their respective state laws.

participating in competitive extracurricular activities. In its ruling, however, the Court only interpreted *federal* law. Schools are also subject to *state* law, which may provide greater protections for students' privacy rights. These laws vary greatly from state to state and, in many states, the law may not yet be well-defined by the courts.

Since the 2002 *Earls* decision, lawsuits have been filed in many states, including Indiana, New Jersey, Oregon, Pennsylvania, Texas and Washington, challenging school districts' drug testing policies.[28] Most of these school districts will spend thousands of taxpayer dollars battling these lawsuits with no guarantee of success.

What National Experts Said to the U.S. Supreme Court[29]

A mandatory drug testing policy "injects the school and its personnel, unnecessarily, into a realm where parental and medical judgment should be preeminent."

—American Academy of Pediatrics, et al.

School drug testing policies often operate "in disregard for prevention and treatment principles that doctors and substance abuse experts view as fundamental . . ."

—American Public Health Association, et al.

"There is growing recognition that extracurricular involvement plays a role in *protecting* students from substance abuse and other dangerous health behaviors."

—National Education Association, et al.

The risk that testing students for illicit drugs "will be understood to signal that alcohol and tobacco are of lesser danger is not an idle concern."

—National Council on Alcoholism and Drug Dependence, et al.

Random Drug Testing is a Barrier to Joining Extracurricular Activities

Random drug testing is typically directed at students who want to participate in extracurricular activities, including athletics, which have proven among the most effective pathways to preventing adolescent drug use. However, all too often drug testing policies actually prevent students from engaging in these activities.

Research shows a vastly disproportionate incidence of adolescent drug use and other dangerous behavior occurs during the unsupervised hours between the end of classes and parents' arrival home in the evening.[30]

Research also shows that students who participate in extracurricular activities are:

- Less likely to develop substance abuse problems;
- Less likely to engage in other dangerous behavior such as violent crime; and
- More likely to stay in school, earn higher grades, and set and achieve more ambitious educational goals.[31]

In addition, after-school programs offer students who are experimenting with or misusing drugs productive activities as well as contact with teachers, coaches and peers, who can help them identify and address problematic drug use.

The Tulia Independent School District, one of the many districts facing heightened public concerns about privacy and confidentiality, has seen a dramatic reduction in student participation in extracurricular activities since implementing drug testing.[32] . . .

Drug Testing Results in False Positives That Punish Innocent Students

A positive drug test can be a devastating accusation for an innocent student. The most widely used drug screening method, urinalysis, will falsely identify some students as illicit drug users when they are not actually using illicit drugs, because drug testing does not necessarily distinguish between drug metabolites with similar structures. For example:

- Over-the-counter decongestants may produce a positive result for amphetamine.[33]
- Codeine can produce a positive result for heroin.[34]
- Food products with poppy seeds can produce a positive result for opiates.[35]

VIOLATING CONFIDENTIALITY

When Tecumseh High School in Oklahoma enacted its random drug testing program, the school failed to ensure the protection of private information concerning prescription drug use submitted under the testing policy. The choir teacher, for instance, looked at students, prescription drug lists and inadvertently left them where other students could see them. The result of a positive test, too, were disseminated to as many as 13 faculty members at a time. Other students figured out the results when a student was abruptly suspended from his/her activity shortly after the administration of a drug test.[36] This not only violates students' privacy rights, but can also lead to costly litigation.

Out of a desire to eliminate the possibility for false positives, schools often ask students to identify their prescription medications before taking a drug test. This both compromises students' privacy rights and creates an added burden for schools to ensure that students' private information is safely guarded.

Drug Testing is Not the Best Way to Identify Students With a Drug Problem

Drug testing says very little about who is misusing or abusing drugs. Thousands of students might be tested in order to detect a tiny fraction of those who may have used the drugs covered by the test. Additionally, students misusing other harmful substances not detected by drug tests will not be identified. If schools rely on drug testing, they may undervalue better ways of detecting young people who are having problems with drugs. Most often, problematic drug use is discovered by learning to recognize its common symptoms. Properly trained

FIRST, ASK THESE HARD QUESTIONS

- Has the drug test been proven to identify students likely to have future problems and to clear those who will not?
- Have schools been proven to be more appropriate or cost-effective places to perform these tests than a doctor's office?
- Are resources in place to assist students who fail the test, regardless of health insurance status or parental income?
- Is the financial interest of a proprietary firm behind the test's promotion?
- Is the school staff using precious time to elicit parental permission, explain the test, make the referrals and assure follow-up?

Adapted from the American Association of School Administrators' website[37] teachers, coaches and other school officials can identify symptoms of a potential drug problem by paying attention to such signs as student absences, erratic behavior, changes in grades and withdrawal from peers.

Drug Testing Has Unintended Consequences

Students may turn to more dangerous drugs or binge drinking   Because marijuana is the most detectable drug, with traces of THC remaining in the body for weeks, students may simply take drugs that exit the body quickly, like methamphetamine, MDMA (Ecstasy) or inhalants.[38] Knowing alcohol is less detectable, they may also engage in binge drinking, creating health and safety risks for students and the community as a whole.

Students can outsmart the drug test   Students who fear being caught by a drug test may find ways to cheat the test, often by purchasing products on the Internet. A quick Internet search for "pass drug test" yields nearly four million hits, linking students to websites selling drug-free replacement urine, herbal detoxifiers, hair follicle shampoo and other products designed to beat drug tests. Students may also try dangerous home remedies. The president of the school board for Guymon, Oklahoma, described a frantic parent who had caught her daughter drinking bleach;[39] the district's drug testing program was subsequently abandoned. In one Louisiana school district, students who were facing a hair test shaved their heads and body hair, making a mockery of the drug testing program.[40]

Students learn that they are guilty until proven innocent   Students are taught that under the U.S. Constitution people are presumed innocent until proven guilty and have a reasonable expectation of privacy. Random drug testing undermines both lessons; students are assumed guilty until they can produce a clean urine sample with no regard for their privacy rights.

Alternatives to Student Drug Testing

The current push to increase drug testing comes from the drug testing industry as well as well-intentioned educators and parents frustrated by the lack of success of drug prevention programs such as Drug Abuse Resistance Education (DARE).[41] However, there are more effective ways to keep teens out of trouble with drugs.

Engage Students in After-School Programs

Schools and local communities should help engage students in extracurricular activities and athletics, as these are among the best deterrents to drug misuse.

Incorporate Reality-Based Drug Education into the School Curriculum

Drugs of all sorts abound in our society. We are constantly confronted by a wide variety of substances with recreational and medicinal uses that can be purchased over-the-counter, by prescription and illegally. Since our decisions about drugs of all kinds should be based on complete, accurate information, quality drug education should be incorporated into a broad range of science disciplines, including physiology, chemistry and biology as well as psychology, history and sociology. Drug education should avoid dishonest scare tactics and should also recognize the wide spectrum of drug use and misuse, and the reasons why young people might choose to use (or not use) drugs.

Provide Counseling

Schools should provide counseling for students who are using drugs in a way that is causing harm to themselves or others. An emerging model that stresses relationships between students and counselors is that of a comprehensive Student Assistance Program (SAP).[42] Such a program advocates a mix of prevention, education and intervention. Counselors who teach about drugs can remain an important resource for students after the formal session ends, while trained student counselors can engage those students who feel more comfortable talking about their problems with peers.[43]

Allow Students to Be Assessed and Treated by Healthcare Professionals

Schools can refer students to healthcare professionals who can play a role in screening, intervening and referring adolescents to treatment. Several screening tools other than urinalysis, such as questionnaires, are available to healthcare professionals in diagnosing drug abuse among adolescents.[44]

Encourage Parents to Become Better Informed

Informed parents play a key role in preventing and detecting student drug misuse, so they should learn as much as they can. Schools can encourage parents to open a dialogue when adolescents are first confronted with alcohol and other intoxicating drugs, usually in middle school. At this point, "drug talks" should be two-way conversations. It is important for parents to teach, as well as learn from, their children.[45]

Cultivate Trust and Respect Among Students and Adults

Trust and respect are perhaps the most important elements of relationships with teens. Young people who enjoy the confidence of their parents and teachers, and who are expected to assume responsibility for their actions, are the most likely to act responsibly. They need to practice responsibility while in high school, where they have a crucial parental and school safety net.

The combination of these methods will help ensure that students:

- **Receive comprehensive, science-based information;**
- **Receive help when they need it; and**
- **Stay busy and involved in productive activities when the school day ends.**

Resources

Studies on Students, Drug Testing and/or After-School Activities

Neil McKeganey, *Random Drug Testing of Schoolchildren: A Shot in the Arm or a Shot in the Foot for Drug Prevention?* (York, UK: Joseph Rowntree Foundation, 2005). . . .

Ryoko Yamaguchi, Lloyd D. Johnston, and Patrick M. O'Malley, *Drug Testing in Schools: Policies, Practices, and Association With Student Drug Use,* Youth, Education, and Society (YES) Occasional Papers Series (Ann Arbor, MI: The Robert Wood Johnson Foundation, 2003). . . .

Ryoko Yamaguchi, Lloyd D. Johnston, and Patrick M. O'Malley, "Relationship Between Student Illicit Drug Use and School Drug-Testing Policies," *Journal of School Health* 73, no. 4 (2003): pp. 159–164. . . .

William J. Bailey, "Suspicionless Drug Testing in Schools," Indiana Prevention Resource Center (1998). . . .

Julie Pederson and others, "The Potential of After-School Programs" in *Safe and Smart: Making After-School Hours Work for Kids* (Washington, D.C.: U.S. Department of Education and U.S. Department of Justice, 1998). . . .

Nicholas Zill, Christine Winquist Nord, and Laura Spencer Loomis, "Adolescent Time Use, Risky Behavior and Outcomes: An Analysis of National Data," U.S. Department of Health and Human Services (1995). . . .

Recommended Reading and Viewing

Rodney Skager, Ph.D., *Beyond Zero Tolerance: A Reality-Based Approach to Drug Education and Student Assistance* (San Francisco, CA: Drug Policy Alliance, 2005). This 23-page booklet offers educators an approach to secondary school drug education that is honest, interactive and cost-effective. The booklet also addresses student assistance and restorative practices as an alternative to punitive zero tolerance policies. . . .

Brave New Films, *The ACLU Freedom Files: The Supreme Court* (2005) is a television show featuring the story of Lindsay Earls, the high school sophomore who opposed her school's drug testing policy for violating her privacy. Screen the half-hour program online and see how she stood up for her beliefs in front of the U.S. Supreme Court. Lindsay Earls was a student at Tecumseh High School, a member of the debate team and a performer in the choir, when a mandatory drug testing policy was instituted for anyone participating in extracurricular activities. She opposed the order as an unconstitutional invasion of her privacy in *Board of Education of Pottawatomie v. Earls.* The show traces the Earls' family experience and gives an insider's view of the high court and the justices who serve on it. . . .

Andrew Weil, M.D. and Winifred Rosen, *From Chocolate to Morphine: Everything You Need to Know About Mind-Altering Drugs* (Boston, MA: Houghton Mifflin, 2004).

Marsha Rosenbaum, Ph.D., *Safety First: A Reality-Based Approach to Teens, Drugs and Drug Education* (San Francisco, CA: Drug Policy Alliance, 2004). This 20-page booklet provides parents and educators with pragmatic ways to address teenage drug use. . . . The Safety First website also contains "fact sheets" about drugs, strategies for talking with teens, news about teen drug use and drug education, an "Ask the Experts" column containing questions submitted by parents and educators, links to relevant sites, ordering information and more.

Mark Birnbaum and Jim Schermbeck, *Larry v. Lockney* (Dallas, TX: Independent Television Service, KERA Unlimited and Public Broadcasting Service, 2003). This documentary follows a parent's fight against a student drug testing program in his son's school. The film's website includes lesson plans and other related resources. . . .

Friend-of-the-Court brief of the American Academy of Pediatrics, et al. in Support of Lindsay Earls, in *Earls*, 536 U.S. 822 (2002). . . .

American Bar Association, *Teaching about Drug Testing in Schools* adapted from Street Law, Inc. (1999). This lesson plan educates students about drug testing in schools and allows them to consider and discuss the consequences of a student drug testing policy. . . .

Recommended Websites

"Drug Testing Fails" provides resources for parents, educators, coaches, and other interested and concerned adults, who believe that safe and trusting learning environments are critical to our young people's health and safety, and that student drug testing programs get in the way of creating that kind of environment. . . .

"A Test You Can't Study For" is a special ACLU web feature on student drug testing that includes a guide for students, fact sheets, reports and other materials. . . .

Student for Sensible Drug Policy (SSDP), an organization with more than 115 college and high school chapters nationwide, is committed to providing education on harms caused by the war on drugs, working to involve youth in the political process, and promoting an open, honest and rational discussion of alternative solutions to our nation's drug problems. SSDP offers talking points, background materials and organizational assistance to students and families working to counteract drug testing programs in their school districts. . . .

Endnotes

1. Office for Human Research Protections to Peter O. Kohler, M.D., president, Oregon Health and Science University, determination letter, October 24, 2002; Adil E. Shamoo and Jonathan D. Moreno, "Ethics of Research Involving Mandatory Drug Testing of High School Athletes in Oregon," *The American Journal of Bioethics* 4, no. 1 (2004): pp. 25-31.

2. Linn Goldberg, the author of the study suspended by federal authorities, now agrees that "even his study did not prove that testing limits consumption. 'Schools should not implement a drug testing program until they're proven to work,' he added. 'They're too expensive. It's like having experimental surgery that's never been shown to work.'" Greg Winter, "Study Finds No Sign That Testing Deters Students' Drug Use," *New York Times,* May 17, 2003.

3. Neil McKeganey, *Random Drug Testing of Schoolchildren: A Shot in the Arm or a Shot in the Foot for Drug Prevention?* (York, UK: Joseph Rowntree Foundation, 2005), p. 12. . . .

4. Ryoko Yamaguchi, Lloyd D. Johnston, and Patrick M. O'Malley, "Relationship Between Student Illicit Drug Use and School Drug-Testing Policies," *Journal of School Health* 73, no. 4 (2003): pp. 159-164. . . .

5. Greg Winter, "Study Finds No Sign That Testing Deters Students' Drug Use," *New York Times,* May 17, 2003.

6. Ryoko Yamaguchi, Lloyd D. Johnston, and Patrick M. O'Malley, *Drug Testing in Schools, Policies, Practices, and Association With Student Drug Use,* Youth, Education, and Society (YES) Occasional Papers Series (Ann Arbor, MI: The Robert Wood Johnson Foundation, 2003. . . .

7. Ibid., p. 16.

8. Ryoko Yamaguchi, Lloyd D. Johnston, and Patrick M. O'Malley, "Relationship Between Student Illicit Drug Use and School Drug-Testing Policies," *Journal of School Health* 73, no. 4 (2003): p. 164.

9. See, for example: Nicholas Zill, Christine Winquist Nord, and Laura Spencer Loomis, "Adolescent Time Use, Risky Behavior and Outcomes: An Analysis of National Data," U.S. Department of Health and Human Services (1995). . . . Lee Shilts, "The Relationship of Early Adolescent Substance Use to Extracurricular Activities, Peer Influence, and Personal Attitudes," *Adolescence* 26, no. 103 (1991): pp. 613, 615; William J. Bailey, "Suspicionless Drug Testing in Schools," Indiana Prevention Resource Center (1998). . . . Robert Taylor, "Compensating Behavior and the Drug Testing of High School Athletes," *The Cato Journal* 16, No. 3 (1997). . . . and Rodney Skager, *Beyond Zero Tolerance: A Reality-Based Approach to Drug Education and Student Assistance* (San Francisco, CA: Drug Policy Alliance, 2005).

10. Jessica Raynor, "Guymon to Eliminate Drug Program," *Amarillo Globe-News Online,* August 15, 2002. . . .

11. Andrew Petkofsky, "School Scraps Drug Testing; but Mathews Will Make Kits Available," *Richmond Times Dispatch,* July 27, 2002.

12. Kay Nolan, "District Drops Random Drug Testing Plan; Proposal for Oconomowoc Schools Lacks Parents' Support," *Milwaukee Journal Sentinel,* October 22, 2003.

13. ACLU of Washington, "First Lawsuit Filed Challenging Suspicionless Student Urine-Testing in Washington," press release, December 17, 1999. . . .

14. Jackie Puccetti to Cathedral High School Community, February 28, 2003. . . .

15. Brief of Amici Curiae American Academy of Pediatrics, et al. at 1, *Board of Education of Independent School District No. 92 of Pottawatomie County, et al. v. Lindsay Earls, et al.,* 536 U.S. 822 (2002) (No. 01-332). . . .

16. National Association of Social Workers, "Social Workers Disagree with Supreme Court Decision to Test Students for Drug Use," press release, June 27, 2002. . . .

17. The Association for Addiction Professionals, "Supreme Court Ruling on Student Drug Testing Misguided: NAADAC Speaks Out Against Court's Approval of Random Drug Tests for Public School Students," press release, June 27, 2002. . . .

18. John R. Knight and Sharon Levy, "An F for School Drug Tests," *Boston Globe,* June 13, 2005.

19. *Board of Education of Independent School District No. 92 of Pottawatomie County, et al. v. Lindsay Earls, et al.,* 536 U.S. 822 (2002) (Ginsburg, R., dissenting).

20. Hawaii State Legislature, HB 273 "Relating to Education: Drug Testing Public School Students," Introduced January 21, 2005. . . .

21. Louisiana State Legislature, SB117 "Tuition Opportunity Program for Students," Considered April 24, 2003. . . .

22. See, for example: Clea A. McNeely, James M. Nonnemaker, and Robert W. Blum, "Promoting School Connectedness: Evidence from the National Longitudinal Study of Adolescent Health," *Journal of School Health* 72, no. 4 (2002): pp. 138-46; Rodney Skager, *Beyond Zero Tolerance: A Reality-Based Approach to Drug Education and Student Assistance* (San Francisco: Drug Policy Alliance, 2005).

23. "Proposed Random Drug Testing Plan Expected to Pass with Minor Changes," *Drug Detection Report,* 15 no. 10 (2005): p. 77.

24. "Student Drug Testing: An Investment in Fear," Drug Policy Alliance. . . .

25. Robert L. DuPont. Teresa G. Campbell and Jacqueline *J. Mazza, Report of a Preliminary Study: Elements of a Successful School-Based Student Drug Testing Program* (Rockville, MD: United States Department of Education, 2002), p. 8.

26. Mary Bridgman and Dean Narciso, "Dublin Halts Drug Tests; School District Stops Screening Athletes," *Columbus Dispatch,* June 26, 2002.

27. Mary Bridgman and Dean Narciso, "Dublin Halts Drug Tests; School District Stops Screening Athletes," *Columbus Dispatch,* June 26, 2002; Dublin Coffman High School Guidance Department, personal communication., July 2003; Richard Caster, Executive Director of Administration at the Dublin Schools, personal communication, April 2005; "Student Drug Testing: An Investment in Fear," Drug Policy Alliance. . . .

28. "ACLU Drug Testing Cases Across the Nation," ACLU. . . .

29. Statements come from the Brief of Amici Curiae of the American Academy of Pediatrics, et al., *Board of Education of Independent School District No. 92 of Pottawatomie County. et al. v. Lindsay Earls,* 536 U.S. 822 (2002) (No. 01-332). . . .

30. Julie Pederson and others, "The Potential of After-School Programs" in *Safe and Smart: Making After-School Hours Work for Kids* (Washington, D.C.: U.S. Department of Education and U.S. Department of Justice, 1998). . . .

31. Maureen Glancy, F. K. Willits and Patricia Farrell, "Adolescent Activities and Adult Success and Happiness: Twenty-four years later," *Sociology and Social Research* 70, no. 3 (1986): p. 242.

32. Plaintiffs in the lawsuit *Bean v. Tulia Independent School District,* claim that, "In 1990-1991 participation of black seniors was 100% in extracurricular clubs and activities and 100% in sports; while the 2000-2001 participation rates [after student drug testing] of black seniors fell to 0% within both." Affidavit of Nancy Cozette Bean, p. 3, *Bean v. Tulia Independent School District,* 2003 WL 22004511 (N.D. Tex. Feb. 18, 2003).

33. American Civil Liberties Union, *Drug Testing: A Bad Investment* (New York: ACLU, 1999), p. 18. . . .

34. Ibid.

35. C. Meadway, S. George, and R. Braithwaite, "Opiate Concentrations Following the Ingestion of Poppy Seed Product: Evidence for 'The Poppy Seed Defense,'" *Forensic Science International* 96, no. 1 (1998): pp. 29-38; American Civil Liberties Union, *Drug Testing: A Bad Investment* (New York: ACLU, 1999), p. 18. . . .

36. Respondents' Brief at 3, *Board of Education of Independent School District No. 92 of Pottawatomie County, et al. v. Lindsay Earls. et al.,* 536 U.S. 822 (2002) (No. 01-332).

37. Howard Taras, "Maximizing Student Health Resources," American Association of School Administrators (2003). . . .

38. American Civil Liberties Union, *Drug Testing: A Bad Investment* (New York: ACLU, 1999), p. 13. . . .

39. Annette Fuentes, "Student Drug Tests Aren't the Answer" *USA Today,* June 10, 2005.

40. Rob Nelson, "Jeff Schools Trim Drug Test Loophole; Hair Samples Will be Required by Policy," *Times Picayune,* July 11, 2003.

41. U.S. General Accounting Office, *Youth Illicit Drug Use Prevention: DARE Long-Term Evaluations and Federal Efforts to Identify Effective Programs* (Washington, D.C.: January 15, 2003).

42. Student Assistance Programs (SAPs) are comprehensive models for the delivery of K-12 prevention, intervention and support services. SAPs are designed to reduce student risk factors, promote protective factors, and increase personal development and decision-making skills by students. For information about developing SAPs, see the National Student Assistance Association. . . .

43. See: Rodney Skager, *Beyond Zero Tolerance: A Reality-Based Approach to Drug Education and Student Assistance* (San Francisco, CA: Drug Policy Alliance, 2005). . . .

44. Physician Leadership on National Drug Policy, *Adolescent Substance Abuse: A Public Health Priority; An Evidence-Based. Comprehensive and Integrative Approach* (Providence, RI: Physician Leadership on National Drug Policy, 2002), pp. 23-31. . . . These tools include the Personal Experience Inventory (PEI), Drug Abuse Screening Test for Adolescents (DAST-A), and Adolescent Drug Involvement Scale (ADIS), among others.

45. See: Marsha Rosenbaum, *Safety First: A Reality-Based Approach to Teen, Drugs, and Drug Education* (San Francisco, CA: Drug Policy Alliance, 2004). . . .

POSTSCRIPT

Should Schools Drug Test Students?

Advocates for random drug testing and people opposed to drug testing do not agree on whether such programs reduce illegal drug use. Regardless of whether drug testing curtails the use of drugs, some critics are concerned that drug testing programs undermine relationships of trust between students and teachers. Teachers are often put in the position of enforcers.

An important question evolves around the role of parents regarding their children. Is it the responsibility of schools to test students for drug use? Should parents be responsible for their children's behavior? In addition, if students test positive for drugs, is it the school's or the parents' responsibility to deal with this problem?

Another concern regarding drug testing is that some schools may be susceptible to litigation. What is the school's role if a student is falsely identified as having used drugs? The federal government recognizes this risk and strongly supports that school districts who randomly drug test students have safeguards in the event that students test positive. Moreover, what actions should schools take if students test positive for drugs? Is the purpose to punish or help students who test positive? Lastly, which school personnel should have access to the results of drug tests? Generally, it is recommended that only school administrators and parents have access to this confidential information.

Some school administrators oppose drug testing on the grounds that such programs create a threatening environment. In addition, some administrators feel that drug testing represents an unwarranted invasion of privacy. Others maintain that whether or not students use drugs is the responsibility of parents, not schools. Proponents of drug testing point out that many parents abdicate their parental responsibilities. They claim that schools are the logical place to implement drug testing.

One concern is that students will try to outsmart the drug test. Whether or not one can fool a drug test is not the point. The point is that students may engage in unhealthy practices to avoid detection. One only has to surf the Internet to find hundreds of advertisements discussing ways to beat drug tests. One can purchase herbal detoxifiers, hair follicle shampoo, or drug-free replacement urine.

According to Supreme Court Justice Ruth Bader Ginsburg, drug testing "risks steering students at greater risk for substance abuse away from extracurricular involvement that potentially may palliate drug problems." At the present time, the vast majority of schools do not randomly drug test student athletes.

The Office of National Drug Control Policy (ONDCP) does not support that all schools drug test students. Its position is that schools should drug test if it or the community feels that there is a drug problem among its students. Without community support, drug testing is not advocated. Because the ONDCP recognizes that some students may test falsely positive, it recommends that reputable drug testing laboratories be used.

The legality of random drug testing is reviewed in "Respect Versus Surveillance: Drug Testing Our Students," by Larry Brendtro and Gordon Martin in *Reclaiming Children and Youth* (Summer 2006). Two articles that point to the effectiveness of drug testing programs to reduce drug use are "High School Drug Testing Program Dramatically Reduces Drug Use" in *Medical Letter on the CDC and FDA* (February 2, 2003) and Norm Brodsky's article "Street Smarts" in *INC Magazine* (November 2004). In their article "Relationship Between Student Illicit Drug Use and School-testing Policies" (*Journal of School Health*, April 2003), Ryoko Yamaguchi, Lloyd D. Johnston, and Patrick O'Malley argue that drug testing had no impact on whether high school students used illegal drugs.

ISSUE 18

Does Drug Abuse Treatment Work?

YES: Susan L. Ettner, David Huang, Elizabeth Evans, Danielle Rose Ash, Mary Hardy, Mickel Jourabchi, and Yih-Ing Hser, from "Benefit-Cost in the California Treatment Outcome Project: Does Substance Abuse Treatment 'Pay for Itself'?" *Health Services Research* (February 2006)

NO: United Nations, from *Investing in Drug Abuse Treatment* (2003)

ISSUE SUMMARY

YES: Author Susan L. Ettner and associates maintain that not only do people in substance abuse treatment benefit, but that taxpayers also benefit. They estimate that about seven dollars is saved for every dollar spent on treatment. Individuals in treatment are less likely to engage in criminal activity and they are more likely to be employed.

NO: The report from the United Nations Office on Drugs and Crime argues that drug abuse treatment does not cure drug abuse. Most people who go through drug treatment relapse. Drug abuse treatment does not get at the root causes of drug abuse: crime, family disruption, loss of economic productivity, and social decay. At best, treatment may minimize drug abuse.

Numerous drug experts feel that more funding should go toward preventing drug use from starting or escalating and toward treating individuals who are dependent on drugs. Today, when taxpayers dispute how their tax monies are spent, the question of whether government funds should be used to treat people who abuse drugs is especially relevant. Questions surrounding this debate include: Does drug abuse treatment reduce criminal activity associated with drugs? Will drug addicts stop their abusive behavior if they enter treatment? Will more drug addicts receive treatment than currently do if services are expanded? Will the availability and demand for illegal drugs decline?

The research on the effectiveness of drug treatment is mixed. In *The Effectiveness of Treatment for Drug Abusers Under Criminal Justice Supervision* (National Institute of Justice, 1995), Douglas S. Lipton states that drug abuse treatment not only reduces the rate of arrests but also reduces crime and lowers the cost to taxpayers over the long run. Also, it has been shown that illicit drug use is curtailed by drug abuse treatment and that treated drug addicts are better able to function in society and to maintain employment. Perhaps most important, drug treatment may prove beneficial in curbing the escalation of HIV (human immunodeficiency virus), the virus that causes AIDS.

Some experts contend that reports regarding the effectiveness of drug treatment are not always accurate and that research on drug abuse has not been subjected to rigorous standards. Some question how effectiveness should be determined. If a person relapses after one year, should the treatment be considered ineffective? Would a reduction in an individual's illegal drug use indicate that the treatment was effective, or would an addict have to maintain complete abstinence? Also, if illegal drug use and criminal activity decline after treatment, it is possible that these results would have occurred anyway, regardless of whether the individual had been treated.

There are a variety of drug treatment programs. One type of treatment program developed in the 1960s is *therapeutic communities*. Therapeutic communities are usually residential facilities staffed by former drug addicts. Although there is no standard definition of what constitutes a therapeutic community, the program generally involves task assignments for addicts, group intervention techniques, vocational and educational counseling, and personal skill development. Inpatient treatment facilities are the most expensive type of treatment and are often based on a hospital model. These programs are very structured and include highly regimented schedules, demanding rules of conduct, and individual and group counseling.

Outpatient treatment, the most common drug treatment, is less expensive, less stigmatizing, and less disruptive to the abuser's family than other forms of treatment. Vocational, educational, and social counseling is provided. Outpatient treatment is often used after an addict leaves an inpatient program. One type of treatment that has proliferated in recent years is the self-help group. Members of self-help groups are bound by a common denominator, whether it is alcohol, cocaine, or narcotics. Due to the anonymous and confidential nature of self-help groups, however, it is difficult to conduct follow-up research to determine their effectiveness.

Individuals addicted to narcotics are often referred to methadone maintenance programs. Methadone is a synthetic narcotic that prevents narcotic addicts from getting high and eliminates withdrawal symptoms. Because methadone's effects last about 24 hours, addicts need to receive treatment frequently. Unfortunately, the relapse rate is high once addicts stop treatment. Because there is much demand for methadone maintenance in some areas, there are lengthy waiting lists. A newer, more effective drug for treating narcotic addiction is buprenorphine.

In the following selections, Susan Ettner and associates maintain that drug abuse treatment is beneficial and cost effective. The United Nations International Drug Control Program argues that drug abuse treatment is ineffective because treatment programs do not get at the root cause of addiction.

YES ⬅

Susan L. Ettner, David Huang, Elizabeth Evans, Danielle Rose Ash, Mary Hardy, Mickel Jourabchi, and Yih-Ing Hser

Benefit-Cost in the California Treatment Outcome Project: Does Substance Abuse Treatment "Pay for Itself"?

Objective. To examine costs and monetary benefits associated with substance abuse treatment.

Data Sources. Primary and administrative data on client outcomes and agency costs from 43 substance abuse treatment providers in 13 counties in California during 2000–2001.

Study Design. Using a social planner perspective, the estimated direct cost of treatment was compared with the associated monetary benefits, including the client's costs of medical care, mental health services, criminal activity, earnings, and (from the government's perspective) transfer program payments. The cost of the client's substance abuse treatment episode was estimated by multiplying the number of days that the client spent in each treatment modality by the estimated average per diem cost of that modality. Monetary benefits associated with treatment were estimated using a pre–post treatment admission study design, i.e., each client served as his or her own control.

Data Collection. Treatment cost data were collected from providers using the Drug Abuse Treatment Cost Analysis Program instrument. For the main sample of 2,567 clients, information on medical hospitalizations, emergency room visits, earnings, and transfer payments was obtained from baseline and 9-month follow-up interviews, and linked to information on inpatient and outpatient mental health services use and criminal activity from administrative databases. Sensitivity analyses examined administrative data outcomes for a larger cohort ($N = 6,545$) and longer time period (1 year).

Principal Findings. On average, substance abuse treatment costs $1,583 and is associated with a monetary benefit to society of $11,487, representing a greater than 7:1 ratio of benefits to costs. These benefits were primarily because of reduced costs of crime and increased employment earnings.

From *Health Services Research*, February 2006, pp. 192–213. Copyright © 2006 by Blackwell Publishing, Ltd. Reprinted by permission. www.blackwell-synergy.com

Conclusions. Even without considering the direct value to clients of improved health and quality of life, allocating taxpayer dollars to substance abuse treatment may be a wise investment. . . .

In spite of advances in treatment and technology, successfully treating those addicted to alcohol and drugs and helping them maintain abstinence remains a challenge. Traditional health services research on these topics has focused on the effectiveness of treatments and access to treatment. In recent years, however, there has been greater focus on assessing the societal impact of addiction and substance abuse treatment. A substantial body of empirical evidence suggests that in addition to the cost of substance abuse treatment itself, drug and alcohol abuse are associated with increases in a wide range of costs (Harwood et al. 1998; Holder 1998a; French, Salome, and Carney 2002; McCollister and French 2003; Salome et al. 2003; Sindelar et al. 2004), including those associated with crime and the criminal justice system (Wall et al. 2000; Vencill and Sadjadi 2001); medical care, especially hospital and emergency room (ER) (French, Salome, Krupski et al. 2000; Wall et al. 2000; Hunkeler et al. 2001; Office of National Drug Control Policy 2001; Palepu et al. 2001; Sturm 2001, 2002); infectious diseases such as HIV/AIDS, hepatitis, and tuberculosis (Daley et al. 2000; Mark et al. 2001); pre- and postnatal care (Mark et al. 2001); mental disorders (Harwood et al. 1998); and government and private transfer payments and other social programs (Gresenz et al. 1998; Merrill and Fox 1998; Cook and Moore 2000; Mark et al. 2001), including unemployment benefits, welfare payments, disability benefits, and food stamps. Evidence on the effects of substance abuse on unemployment and impaired work productivity is somewhat more mixed, with some suggestion that drinking may not have the same adverse effects as alcohol or drug abuse (Mullahy and Sindelar 1998; Cook and Moore 2000; Wall et al. 2000; Feng et al. 2001; Mark et al. 2001; Vencill and Sadjadi 2001).

Successful substance abuse treatment can have an extraordinarily important impact on lives; yet, in many instances, these programs are needed by those who are indigent and hence dependent on services that are publicly financed. In a cost-cutting environment, public funding for substance abuse treatment competes more broadly with other uses of limited societal resources for improving population health. Given the stigma associated with substance abuse and perhaps an underlying skepticism about the value of rehabilitation, financing for substance abuse treatment may not be readily provided in the current policy climate. Pressure therefore exists for advocates to demonstrate that the benefits of substance abuse treatment can be explained not only in human terms but also in monetary terms. Policymakers are generally more inclined to support treatment programs if they "pay for themselves" through reductions in other types of costs, e.g., health care, criminal justice costs, etc. With one notable exception (Alexandre et al. 2002), the literature in this area has consistently suggested that substance abuse treatment is associated with net benefits.

Previous studies were, however, subject to certain limitations, including the inability to compare the benefits with the cost of the treatment; small sample sizes; potential lack of generalizability beyond randomized-controlled trial settings, populations, and interventions; inability to measure a comprehensive array of costs, including both health care and crime; and age of the data. For example, Holder's (1998a, b) reviews of the older literature identify the cost savings resulting from substance abuse treatment, but did not provide information on the cost of the treatment itself, so estimates of the benefit:cost ratio were not available. In the more recent literature, several studies looked at reductions in health care costs or use only (Zywiak et al. 1999; Goodman et al. 2000; Parthasarathy et al. 2001); conversely, other studies looked only at reductions in crime (Flynn et al. 1999; Daley et al. 2000; Aos et al. 2001). One study (Mauser et al. 1994) adopted a more comprehensive approach in exploring the monetary benefits associated with substance abuse treatment, including savings related to both health care and crime, but had a relatively small sample size that made detection of statistically significant differences challenging. Other studies incorporated multiple outcome measures like criminal activity, health services utilization, and employment status but were performed with narrowly defined populations (Daley et al. 2000; French et al. 2002b, 2003; Logan et al. 2004) or were focused on particular treatment modalities (Barnett and Hui 2000; French, Salome, and Carney 2002), or insured populations (French, Salome, Krupski et al. 2000; Goodman et al. 2000; Humphreys and Moos 2001; Parthasarathy et al. 2001).

A number of the other studies assessed the cost–benefit of one treatment modality only relative to another modality. For example, Flynn et al. (1999) compared long-term residential and outpatient drug-free treatment, while Salome et al. (2003) compared the results of one outpatient modality that initiated with inpatient treatment with another that did not. Weisner et al. (2000) compared outcomes from day hospital treatment to traditional outpatient regimens, and Holder et al. (2000) compared outcomes of cognitive behavior therapy, motivational enhancement therapy, or a Twelve-Step facilitation treatment. Still other studies compare enhanced interventions with standard ones. Hartz et al. (1998) evaluated the value of contingency contracting, while Avants et al. (1999) compared outcomes from a standard versus an enhanced treatment. Koenig et al. (2000a, b) looked at the marginal costs and benefits associated with increased treatment duration and intensity; French, McCollister et al. (2002a) compared a modified therapeutic community to treatment-as-usual for homeless mentally ill substance abusers; and Fleming et al. (2002) examined the benefit–cost of a brief intervention for problem drinkers.

In the present study, we address the benefit–cost question using data from the California Treatment Outcome Project (CalTOP), a large demonstration project that collected outcomes data on clients admitted to 43 substance abuse treatment providers in 13 counties in California. CalTOP was the successor to the California Drug and Alcohol Treatment Assessment Program (CalDATA), a large-scale study of the effects of alcohol and drug treatment on participant behavior, treatment costs, and economic benefits to society (Gerstein et al. 1994) that suggested that substance abuse treatment was associated with a 7:1 ratio of benefits to costs. CalDATA was conducted 10 years earlier than CalTOP, prior to a number of changes in the California substance abuse treatment system and treatment population, such as increased methamphetamine users, decreases in the average length of treatment, and concomitant increases in the number of prior treatment episodes (Urada 2000). CalTOP also improved upon other aspects of CalDATA, including its reliance on a discharge sample and 50 percent response rate; its lack of a baseline survey, which meant that analyses were based on self-reports of events occurring up to 3 years earlier; its reliance on self-reported crime; and its comparison of benefits with the cost of the initial treatment episode only (35 percent of clients reentered treatment during follow-up).

Methods

Study Design

As detailed in the CalTOP Final Report (Hser et al. 2002, 2003), the 43 CalTOP providers administered the ASI-Lite (McLellan et al. 1980, 1992) to all of their clients at intake. CalTOP subjects were comparable at intake to those entering treatment statewide, except that CalTOP had slightly fewer criminal justice clients, slightly more patients with a secondary drug problem, and fewer methadone programs. A consecutive census of intake clients was then asked to participate in follow-up surveys at 3 and 9 months, using the same instrument. At intake and 9 months post-intake, self-reported information was collected from clients on ER visits and hospital nights for medical problems during the past 30 days and 6 months, as well as money received from employment, unemployment, disability/retirement, and welfare during the past 30 days. Of the 3,314 clients targeted for the 3-month follow-up, 86 percent were interviewed, 8 percent were not found, 3 percent were incarcerated, 2 percent refused the interview, less than 1 percent were deceased, and less than 1 percent were not interviewed for other reasons. Of the 3,715 clients targeted for the 9-month follow-up, 73 percent were interviewed, 20 percent were not found, 5 percent were incarcerated, less than 1 percent refused the interview when contacted, less than 1 percent were deceased, and less than 1 percent were not interviewed for other reasons. An attrition analysis showed that clients who did and did not complete each follow-up interview were not statistically different in terms of age, ethnicity, marital and educational status, employment, primary drug, treatment history, and legal status at admission. The only significant difference was that 50 percent of the clients who completed the follow-up interviews were female, compared with 43 percent of those who did not.

To determine the ratio of costs to monetary benefits associated with substance abuse treatment, the estimated average direct cost of substance abuse treatment ("treatment cost") was compared with the average change in nontreatment costs associated with treatment (hereinafter referred to as the "monetary benefits"). Substance abuse treatment costs were calculated using a combination of cost data collected from providers and administrative data on days in treatment. Monetary benefit measures were derived from survey and administrative data, and depending on the study perspective taken, included medical care, mental health services, criminal activity, earnings, and government transfer payments. To estimate the monetary benefits, we compared nontreatment costs before and after admission with treatment, i.e., each client served as his or her own "control." All costs and benefits were adjusted to

2001 using the appropriate Consumer Price Index component. To the extent possible, the analyses follow the benefit–cost guidelines outlined in French, Salome, Sindelar et al. (2002). The main perspective adopted was that of the "social planner," in which all costs and benefits are included, regardless of the party to whom they accrue.

Study Cohort and Follow-up Period

The main analyses were based on the cohort of clients entering substance abuse treatment between January 4, 2000 and May 31, 2001, who also completed a 9-month follow-up survey ($N = 2,567$). These analyses utilized 3- and 9-month follow-up ASI data and administrative data. Because the follow-up period was only 9 months, the "look-back" period for the preadmission data was also 9 months. Sensitivity analyses were conducted using all clients entering substance abuse treatment between January 4, 2000 and May 31, 2001 ($N = 6,545$), using only administrative data and a 1-year follow-up period. The second cohort was larger and had a longer follow-up period, but the first cohort had more complete data on the benefits of substance abuse treatment. . . .

Discussion

Our best estimate is that on average, substance abuse treatment costs $1,583 and is associated with a societal benefit of $11,487, representing a 7:1 ratio of benefits to costs (9:1 when arrest data are "inflated" to proxy for actual crimes committed). This ratio is based on weighted average treatment costs, which reflect expected costs of treatment; 9-month follow-up of clients in all modalities with follow-up survey data, so that as many sources of benefit as possible could be included in the analysis; and benefit measures that demonstrate significant change, so that the estimates are robust to rare events. Sixty-five percent of the total benefit was attributable to reductions in crime costs, including incarceration. Twenty-nine percent was because of increased employment earnings, with the remaining 6 percent because of reduced medical and behavioral health care costs.

A review of 11 studies (McCollister and French 2003) found that the benefit–cost ratios associated with substance abuse treatment ranged from 1.33 to 23.33 and that benefits were overwhelmingly because of reductions in criminal activity, with smaller contributions of earnings, and averted health care. Our conclusion is similar, especially when inflating the arrest data. Our benefit–cost ratio is also similar to the CalDATA estimate, despite differences in study design and methodology. However, our estimates of substance abuse treatment costs tend to be lower than those in previous studies. An earlier literature review by Roebuck, French, and McLellan (2003) suggested that the average cost per treatment episode was $7,358 for MM, $1,944 for standard outpatient, and $9,426 for residential. Our estimates were $2,737, $838, and $2,791, respectively, based on weighted per diem estimates. The lower episode costs in CalTOP were because of shorter lengths of treatment for MM and residential, as the weekly cost of treatment was actually higher ($99 and $235, respectively, in CalTOP, compared with $91 and $194 in Roebuck et al.). For outpatient, lower episode costs were also attributable to lower weekly costs, around $48 versus $121 in Roebuck et al. These discrepancies might reflect geographic differences in the intensity and duration of treatment.

Our findings should be interpreted with caution, given a number of study limitations. The results may not generalize to non-CalTOP providers, especially those in other states. Attrition may have biased the estimated cost–benefit ratio among the "intake+follow-up" cohort if the clients who were women, incarcerated, or could not be located were more costly on average than the clients who were successfully tracked. Compared with the statewide data, the CalTOP sample slightly underrepresented methadone clients, although statewide methadone clients only account for 10 percent of the total treatment population. We may have slightly overestimated benefit–cost ratios if they were based on the average across CalTOP programs of all modalities. Reductions in nontreatment costs may be overstated because of regression to the mean, i.e., persons entering substance abuse treatment often have hit the bottom and "have nowhere to go but up." A related issue is whether clients who were court-mandated to enter treatment were deterred in the short run from committing further criminal activities. Unfortunately, randomization to treatment is neither logistically nor ethically possible in a large-scale, "realworld" study of this type, plus randomized-controlled studies lack the external validity of observational studies. The pre–post study design has strong advantages over observational studies comparing substance abusers who do and do not enter treatment, because of the selection bias inherent in the latter. The high ratio of benefits to costs makes it less plausible that the cost of substance abuse treatment would have outweighed its benefits if regression to the mean and deterrence effects could have been taken into account. Although it was not possible to study these effects using CalTOP data, we analyzed studies including a "no-treatment" control group from a published meta-analysis of drug abuse treatment outcomes (Prendergast et al. 2002). These analyses suggested that the controls had pre–post differences in outcomes that were about half as large as those in the treatment group. Applying this ratio to CalTOP, the $1,583 in treatment costs would be compared with a benefit of $5,744 ($11,487/2).

The relatively short 9-month follow-up period may understate the monetary benefits associated with treatment if its effects persist over the longer run; alternatively, the additional benefits accrued beyond the 9-month window might be offset by additional costs if the patients relapse and require further treatment. Most of the other study limitations are likely to lead to conservative biases, e.g., the inability to cost out certain crimes (especially those related to drug manufacture and sales, which showed the largest reductions following treatment) and to measure probation and parole costs and costs imposed on family members and friends. Systematic underreporting of hospitalizations, ER use, days incarcerated, and employment income would tend to understate the benefits of treatment as long as the under-reporting was similar for a given client before and after treatment. The lack of comprehensive outpatient medical care data could have induced either a conservative or liberal bias, depending on whether engagement in substance abuse treatment increased referrals to medical providers or primarily improved physical health so that less medical care was needed. Treatment costs may have been slightly underestimated because providers estimated the depreciated costs of their furniture to be zero.

The CalTOP study provided a number of important lessons for conducting future analyses of the cost–benefit of substance abuse treatment. Given concerns about respondent burden, use of a shorter version of the DATCAP is desirable and we do not believe much critical information would be lost. A brief version of the DATCAP has been pilot tested (French, Roebuck, and McLellan 2004). . . . Similarly, the ASI-6 will be better suited for economic evaluation studies than the older version used for CalTOP. The most important sources of monetary benefits (crime, hospitalizations, and earnings) occurred in domains that can be measured using administrative data. As omission of many other sources of monetary benefit induces only a conservative bias, a reasonable cost–benefit analysis might be conducted without the time and expense of primary data collection from clients. Use of administrative data only has the added advantage of allowing the entire client population to be included in the analysis. Long administrative data lags suggest that cost–benefit analyses may need to be based on older data, but lags pose less of a threat to the validity of the findings if treatment systems or client populations do not change rapidly over time. If primary data collection is used as the primary or a supplementary source of information, an instrument designed specifically for cost–benefit analyses should be administered. For example, the most recent version of the Addiction Severity Index (the forthcoming ASI-6) has been redesigned to permit economic evaluation.

Nontrivial differences by treatment modality were observed. Although the benefits associated with outpatient treatment were lower than for residential treatment, the costs were also lower, so the net return on investment was actually higher for outpatient than for residential treatment. No statistically significant monetary benefits were identified among the MM clients, likely because of the small sample size and low power. Alternatively, benefits may be smaller for the MM clients, because of the long-term nature of methadone treatment. The strongest effects of treatment are likely to occur soon after the client becomes drug-free. The overwhelming majority of MM clients had prior treatment admissions, suggesting that many may have been on methadone for a long time and hence already realized any reductions in crime in past years. The baseline level of crime costs was much lower for MM clients than for either outpatient or residential clients, suggesting little room for additional improvement. In other words, our "pre" admission measurement period may not actually precede the receipt of treatment for these clients, but rather, reflect a phase in ongoing treatment. Again, however, the lack of precision in the estimates when looking separately at MM clients precludes us from drawing firm conclusions about the relative magnitudes of the effects for methadone versus outpatient or residential clients. In general, caution must be exercised in making comparisons across modalities, because substance abusers tend to move in and out of treatment and across treatment modalities during their life course. Furthermore, the modality comparisons were based on initial treatment modality, so attribution of benefits to a single modality may be misleading.

Taken as a whole, our findings suggest that even without considering the health and quality-of-life benefits to the clients themselves, spending taxpayer dollars on substance abuse treatment may be a wise investment. Further research is needed to establish a link between the monetary benefits of treatment and the duration and intensity of treatment. Challenges in identifying this relationship include collecting reliable data on the services received by clients and addressing selection bias (i.e., more acute clients probably receive more intensive services, at least to begin with, but more motivated clients are likely to have higher retention rates). Despite these challenges, such an analysis would seem to be the logical next step in building on the CalTOP findings. . . .

References

Alexandre, P., H. Salome, M. French, J. Rivers, and C. McCoy. 2002. "Consequences and Costs of Closing a Publicly Funded Methadone Maintenance Clinic." *Social Science Quarterly* 83 (2): 519–36.

Aos, S., P. Phipps, R. Barnoski, and R. Lieb. 2001. *The Comparative Costs and Benefits of Programs to Reduce Crime, Version 4.0 (Document No. 01-05-1201).* Olympia, WA: Washington State Institute for Public Policy.

Avants, S., M. Kelly, S. Arther, L. Jody, B. Rounsaville, R. Schottenfeld, S. Stine, N. Cooney, R. Rosencheck, S. Li, and T. Kosten. 1999. "Day Treatment versus Enhanced Standard Methadone Services for Opioid-Dependence Patients: A Comparison of Clinical Efficacy and Cost." *American Journal of Psychiatry* 156 (1): 27–33.

Barnett, P., and S. Hui. 2000. "The Cost-Effectiveness of Methadone Maintenance." *Mount Sinai Journal of Medicine* 67 (5 & 6): 365–74.

Beck, A., and B. Shipley. 1997. Bureau of Justice Statistics Special Report: Recidivism of Prisoners Released in 1983. U.S. Department of Justice, Office of Justice Programs.

California State Auditor. 1998. *California Department of Corrections: The Cost of Incarcerating Inmates in State-Run Prisons is Higher Than the Department's Published Cost.* Sacramento, CA: Bureau of State Audits.

Cohen, M. 2001. "Calculations for Cost of Gang-Related Crime" [accessed on September 17, 2003]. . . .

Cook, P., and M. Moore. 2000. "The Economics of Alcohol Abuse and Alcohol-Control Policies." *Health Affairs* 21 (2): 120–33.

Daley, M., M. Argeriou, D. McCarty, J. Callahan, D. Shephard, and C. Williams. 2000. "The Costs of Crime and the Benefits of Substance Abuse Treatment for Pregnant Women." *Journal of Substance Abuse Treatment* 19 (4): 445–58.

Feng, W., W. Zhou, J. Beutler, B. Booth, and M. French. 2001. "The Impact of Problem Drinking on Employment." *Health Economics* 10 (6): 509–21.

Fleming, M. F., M. P. Mundt, M. T. French, L. B. Manwell, E. A. Stauffacher, and K. L. Barry. 2002. "Brief Physician Advice for Problem Drinkers: Long-Term Efficacy and Benefit–Cost Analysis." *Alcoholism: Clinical and Experimental Research* 26 (1): 36–43.

Flynn, P., P. Kristiansen, J. Porto, and R. Hubbard. 1999. "Costs and Benefits of Treatment for Cocaine Addiction in DATOS." *Drug and Alcohol Dependence* 57 (2): 167–74.

French, M., and R. Martin. 1996. "The Costs of Drug Abuse Consequences: A Summary of Research Findings." *Journal of Substance Abuse Treatment* 13 (6): 453–66.

French, M. T., K. A. McCollister, S. Sacks, K. McKendrick, and G. DeLeon. 2002a. "Benefit Cost Analysis of a Modified Therapeutic Community for Mentally Ill Chemical Abusers." *Evaluation and Program Planning* 25 (2): 137–48.

——. 2002b. "Benefit–Cost Analysis of Addiction Treatment in Arkansas: Specialty and Standard Residential Programs for Pregnant and Parenting Women." *Substance Abuse* 23 (1): 31–51.

French, M. T., M. C. Roebuck, M. L. Dennis, S.H. Godley, H. Liddle, and F. M. Tims. 2003. "Outpatient Marijuana Treatment for Adolescents: Economic Evaluation of a Multisite Field Experiment." *Evaluation Review* 27 (4): 421–59.

French, M. T., M. C. Roebuck, and A. T. McLellan. 2004. "Cost Estimation When Time and Resources Are Limited: The Brief DATCAP." *Journal of Substance Abuse Treatment* 27 (3): 187–93.

French, M. T., H. J. Salome, and M. Carney. 2002. "Using the DATCAP and ASI to Estimate the Costs and Benefits of Residential Addiction Treatment in the State of Washington." *Social Science and Medicine* 55 (12): 2267–82.

French, M., H. Salome, A. Krupski, J. McKay, D. Donovan, A. McLellan, and J. Durell. 2000. "Benefit–Cost Analysis of Residential and Outpatient Addiction of Treatment in the State of Washington." *Evaluation Review* 24 (6): 609–34.

French, M. T., H. J. Salome, J. L. Sindelar, and A. T. McLellan. 2002. "Benefit–Cost Analysis of Addiction Treatment: Methodological Guidelines and Application Using the DATCAP and ASI." *Health Services Research* 37 (2): 433–55.

Gerstein, D., R. Dean, R. Johnson, M. Foote, N. Suter, K. Jack, G. Merker, S. Turner, R. Bailey, K. Malloy, E. Williams, H. Harwood, and D. Fountain. 1994. Evaluating Recovery Services: The California Drug And Alcohol Treatment Assessment (CalDATA), Methodology Report (Control No. 92-00110). Department of Alcohol and Drug Programs, State of California.

Goodman, A., J. Tilford, J. Hankin, H. Holder, and E. Nishiura. 2000. "Alcoholism Treatment Offset Effects: An Insurance Perspective." *Medical Care Research and Review* 57 (1): 51–75.

Gresenz, C., K. Watkins, and D. Podus. 1998. "Supplemental Security Income (SSI), Disability Insurance (DI), and Substance Abusers." *Community Mental Health Journal* 34 (4): 337–50.

Hartz, D., P. Meek, N. Piotrowski, D. Tusel, C. Henke, K. Delucchi, K. Sees, and S. Hall. 1998. "A Cost-Effectiveness and Cost–Benefit Analysis of Contingency Contracting-Enhanced Methadone Detoxification Treatment." *American Journal of Drug and Alcohol Abuse* 25 (2): 207–18.

Harwood, H., D. Fountain, and G. Livermore. 1998. *The Economic Costs of Alcohol and Drug Abuse in the United States, 1992*. Rockville, MD: National Institute on Drug Abuse.

Holder, H. D. 1998a. "Cost Benefits of Substance Abuse Treatment: An Overview of Results from Alcohol and Drug Abuse." *Journal of Mental Health Policy and Economics* 1: 23–9.

——. 1998b. "The Cost Offsets of Alcoholism Treatment." *Recent Developments in Alcoholism* 14: 361–74.

Holder, H. D., R. A. Cisler, R. Longabaugh, R. L. Stout, A. J. Treno, and A. Zweben. 2000. "Alcoholism Treatment and Medical Care Costs from Project MATCH." *Addiction* 95: 999–1013.

Hser, Y., E. Evans, S. Ettner, D. Huang, and R. Picazo. 2003. *The California Treatment Outcome Project Supplement to the Final Report. Submitted to the California Department of Alcohol and Drug Programs*. Los Angeles, CA: UCLA Integrated Substance Abuse Programs.

Hser, Y., E. Evans, C. Teruya, M. Hardy, D. Urada, Y. Huang, R. Picazo, H. Shen, J. Hsieh, and D. Anglin. 2002. *The California Treatment Outcome Project (CalTOP) Final Report Submitted to the California Department of Alcohol and Drug Programs*. Los Angeles, CA: UCLA Integrated Substance Abuse Programs.

Humphreys, K., and R. Moos. 2001. "Can Encouraging Substance Abuse Patients to Participate in Self-Help Groups Reduce Demand for Health Care? A Quasi-Experimental Study." *Alcoholism Clinical and Experimental Research* 25 (5): 711–6.

Hunkeler, E., Y. Hung, D. Rice, C. Weisner, and T. Hu. 2001. "Alcohol Consumption Patterns and Health Care Costs in an HMO." *Drug and Alcohol Dependence* 64: 181–90.

Koenig, L., H. Harwood, J. Henrick, K. Sullivan, and N. Sen. 2000a. *Do the Benefits of More Intensive Substance Abuse Treatment Offset the Costs? (Caliber/NEDS Contract No. 270-97-7016).* Rockville, MD: Center for Substance Abuse Treatment, Substance Abuse and Mental Health Services Administration, Department of Health and Human Services.

Koenig, L., H. Harwood, K. Sullivan, and N. Sen. 2000b. "The Economic Benefits of Increased Treatment Duration and Intensity in Residential and Outpatient Substance Abuse Treatment Settings." *Journal of Psychopathology and Behavioral Assessment* 22 (4): 399–417.

Logan, T. K.,W. Hoyt, K. E. McCollister, M. T. French, C. Leukefeld, and L. Minton. 2004. "Economic Evaluation of Drug Court: Methodology, Results, and Policy Implications." *Evaluation and Program Planning* 27: 381–96.

Mark, T., G. Woody, T. Juday, and H. Kleber. 2001. "The Economic Costs of Heroin Addiction." *Drug and Alcohol Dependence* 61: 195–206.

Mauser, E., K. VanStelle, and D. Moberg. 1994. "The Economic Impact of Diverting Substance-Abusing Offenders into Treatment." *Crime and Delinquency* 40 (4): 568–88.

McCollister, K. E., and M. T. French. 2003. "The Relative Contribution of Outcome Domains in the Total Economic Benefit of Addiction Interventions: A Review of First Findings." *Addiction* 98: 1647–59.

McLellan, A., H. Kushner, D. Metzger, R. Peters, I. Smith, G. Grissom, H. Pettinati, and M. Argeriou. 1992. "The Fifth Edition of the Addiction Severity Index." *Journal of Substance Abuse Treatment* 9: 199–213.

McLellan, A., L. Luborsky, G. Woody, and C. O'brien. 1980. "An Improved Diagnostic Evaluation Instrument for Substance Abuse Patients: The Addiction Severity Index." *Journal of Nervous and Mental Disease* 168: 26–33.

Merrill, J., and K. Fox. 1998. *The Impact of Substance Abuse on Federal Spending. Cost–Benefit/Cost-Effectiveness Research of Drug Abuse Prevention: Implications for Programming and Policy (Report No. 76).* Rockville, MD: National Institute on Drug Abuse.

Miller, T., M. Cohen, and B. Wiersama. 1996. *Victim Costs and Consequences: A New Look. Final Summary Report Presented to the National Institute of Justice, January, 1996.* Rockville, MD: National Institute of Justice.

Mullahy, J., and J. L. Sindelar. 1998. "Drinking, Problem Drinking, and Productivity." *Canadian Medical Association Journal* 165 (4): 415–20.

Office of National Drug Control Policy. 2001. *The Economic Costs of Drug Abuse in the United States, 1992–1998. (Publication No. NCJ-190636.)* Washington, DC: The Executive Office of the President.

Palepu, A., M. Tyndall, H. Leon, J. Muller, M. O'Shaughnessy, M. Schechter, and A. Anis. 2001. "Hospital Utilization and Costs in a Cohort of Injection Drug Users." *Canadian Medical Association Journal* 165 (4): 415–20.

Parthasarathy, S., C. Weisner, T. Hu, and C. Moore. 2001. "Association of Outpatient Alcohol and Drug Treatment with Health Care Utilization and Costs: Revisiting the Offset Hypothesis." *Journal of Studies on Alcohol* 62 (1): 89–97.

Prendergast, M. L., D. Podus, E. Chang, and D. Urada. 2002. "The Effectiveness of Drug Abuse Treatment: A Meta-Analysis of Comparison Group Studies." *Drug and Alcohol Dependence* 67 (1): 53–72.

Roebuck, M. C., M. T. French, and A. T. McLellan. 2003. "DATStats: Results from 85 Studies Using the Drug Abuse Treatment Cost Analysis Program (DATCAP)." *Journal of Substance Abuse Treatment* 25: 51–7.

Salome, H. J., M. T. French, C. Scott, M. Foss, and M. L. Dennis. 2003. "Investigating the Economic Costs and Benefits of Addiction Treatment: Econometric Analysis of the Chicago Target Cities Project." *Evaluation and Programming Planning* 26 (3): 325–38.

Sindelar, J. L., M. Jofre-Bonet, M. T. French, and A. T. McLellan. 2004. "Cost-Effectiveness Analysis of Addiction Treatment: Paradoxes of Multiple Outcomes." *Drug and Alcohol Dependence* 73: 41–50.

Sturm, R. 2001. *The Costs of Covering Mental Health and Substance Abuse as Medical Care in Private Insurance Plans (RAND Health Publication No. CT-180)*. Chicago: RAND.

———. 2002. "The Effects of Obesity, Smoking and Drinking on Medical Problems and Costs." *Health Affairs* 21 (2): 245–53.

Urada, D. 2000. *California State Treatment Needs Assessment Program Existing Service Utilization, and Outcomes: Interim Report (Under Contract No. 270-98-7052)*. Los Angeles, CA: California Department of Alcohol and Drug Programs.

Vencill, C., and Z. Sadjadi. 2001. "Allocation of the California War Costs: Direct Expenses, Externalities, Opportunity Costs, and Fiscal Losses." *Justice Policy Journal* 1 (1): 1–40.

Wall, R., J. Rehm, B. Fischer, B. Brands, L. Gliksman, J. Stweard, W. Medved, and J. Blacke. 2000. "Social Costs of Untreated Opioid Dependence." *Journal of Urban Health: Bulletin of the New York Academy of Medicine* 77 (4): 688–722.

Weisner, C., J. Mertens, S. Parthasarathy, C. Moore, E. Hunkleler, T. Hu, and J. Selby. 2000. "The Outcome and Cost of Alcohol and Drug Treatment in an HMO: Day Hospital versus Traditional Outpatient Regimens." *Health Services Research* 35 (4): 791–812.

Zywiak, W., N. Hoffman, R. Stout, S. Hagberg, A. Floyd, and S. DeHart. 1999. "Substance Abuse Treatment Cost-Offsets Vary with Gender, Age, and Abstinence Likelihood." *Journal of Health Care Financing* 26 (1): 33–9.

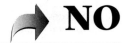
Investing in Drug Abuse Treatment

Summary

Drug addiction produces serious, pervasive and expensive social problems. Regardless of whether substance abuse is a sin, a crime, a bad habit or an illness, society has a right to expect that an effective public policy or approach to the "drug abuse problem" will reduce drug-related crime, unemployment, family dysfunction and disproportionate use of medical care.

Science has made great progress over the past several years, but it is still not possible to account fully for the physiological and psychological processes that transform controlled, voluntary "use" of alcohol and/or other drugs into uncontrolled, involuntary "dependence" on those substances, and there is still no cure. What can be done is to treat use "effectively" and to provide an attractive return on societal investment in treatment. . . .

Importantly, the research shows that while motivation for treatment plays an important role in maintaining treatment participation, most substance-abusing patients enter treatment with combinations of internal motivation and family, employment or legal pressure. Those pressures can be combined with treatment interventions for the benefit of the patient and society.

The evidence is compelling that, at the present state of knowledge, addiction is best considered a chronic relapsing condition. It is true that not all cases of addiction are chronic and some who meet diagnostic criteria for substance dependence recover completely without treatment. However, many of those who develop addiction disorders suffer multiple relapses following treatments and are thought to retain a continuing vulnerability to relapse for years or perhaps a lifetime. Like so many other illnesses, it is impossible to predict whether or when an acute care strategy is likely to achieve complete remission. For example, while change in diet, exercise and lifestyle can reduce high blood pressure in some patients without medication or continuing treatment, many others require sustained management with medications as well as regular monitoring of diet, stress and exercise. In considering addiction a chronic condition, it is no longer surprising that incarcerations or brief stabilizations are not effective.

From "Investing in Drug Abuse Treatment," United Nations International Drug Control Programme, 2003.

The available research is quite clear on these points:

- Education does not correct drug dependence: it is not simply a problem of lack of knowledge.
- Consequences of drug use (e.g. hangovers, loss of job, arrest, etc.) appear to be important stimuli leading to entry into drug abuse treatment.
- Very few addicted individuals are able to profit from a corrections-oriented approach by itself. Relapse rates are over 70 per cent from all forms of criminal justice interventions.
- Addiction is not simply a matter of becoming stabilized and getting the drugs out of one's system. Relapse rates following detoxifications are approximately the same as those following incarceration. . . .

Introduction

Problems of substance dependence produce dramatic costs to all societies in terms of lost productivity, transmission of infectious diseases, family and social disorder, crime and, of course, excessive utilization of health care. These alcohol and drug-related problems not only reduce the safety and quality of daily life, they are also a source of substantial expense. For example, it has been estimated that, in the United States of America, the total cost of alcohol abuse in 1990 was 99 billion United States dollars and drug abuse cost approximately US\$ 67 billion, while the total cost of illicit drug abuse in Australia was estimated to be 1,684 million Australian dollars (or US\$ 1,237 million) in 1992. In Canada, the total cost of alcohol abuse in 1992 was estimated to be 7,522 million Canadian dollars (US\$ 6,223 million) and the total cost of illicit drug abuse Can\$ 1,371 million (US\$ 1,134).

Understandably, such problems also produce heated debates regarding what a family, a school, an employer, a Government and/or a society should do to reduce the costs and the threats of substance abuse to the public health and safety of citizens.

There are few countries—regardless of their economic development—with a well developed public treatment system designed to address different substances of abuse and different levels or manifestations of the addiction spectrum. Why have treatment options not been more favourably considered and better developed and disseminated to address the problems of substance dependence? Perhaps the first reason for this is the relative prominence of the social problems caused by drug and alcohol abuse. Crime, family disruption, loss of economic productivity and social decay are the most observable, potentially dangerous and expensive effects of drugs on the social systems of most countries. This is a powerful factor in shaping the general view that the "drug issue" is primarily a criminal problem requiring a social-judicial remedy rather than a health problem requiring prevention and treatment.

A second reason for a diminished role of treatment in most public policies regarding drug abuse is that most societies are sceptical about the effectiveness of substance abuse treatments and most Governments question whether treatment is "worth it." Moreover, recent surveys show that even a majority of general practice physicians and nurses feel that the currently available medical or health-care interventions are not appropriate or effective in treating addiction.

A third reason why treatment options may not have received more attention in public policies regarding drug abuse is the pervasive view that a treatment approach to substance abuse conveys an implicit message that the addiction—and the addiction-related problems—are not the fault of the addicted person; that they "can't help themselves" and that they have no responsibility for the actions that led to—or resulted from—the addiction. In that regard, the view exists that treatments are designed exclusively to help the drug user but not society. Why should a society expend resources to help an individual who may have produced social harms? These are messages that many people find offensive and unfair.

Thus, treatment interventions that admittedly cannot cure addiction and that may be seen as focused only on helping socially stigmatized addicted individuals are not popular in many segments of society. Are those perceptions correct? Is there a role for addiction treatment in public policy aimed at reducing drug-related problems? In the text that follows the issue is considered from several perspectives. The first part of the paper considers the perspective of a Government or public agency questioning the value of any intervention aimed at "drug problems": What would an "effective" intervention do, regardless of whether the intervention were a punitive, criminal justice intervention, an educational intervention, a new social policy or a treatment intervention? Here the paper examines the characteristics of patients who enter addiction treatments—asking where they have come from, who or what agency has referred them to treatment and what goals are expected by those agencies and organizations. This examination is used to develop a set of outcome expectations that would make treatment "worth it" to a society that might be asked to support such an intervention or policy. . . .

Why Are Addiction Treatments Not as Effective as Treatments for Other Illnesses?

Implications for the Delivery and Evaluation of Addiction Treatment

The previous sections of this paper have examined the addiction treatment field from the perspective of its value to society. It would seem that this review would provide a relatively simple answer to what appears to be a direct question of cost and value. Yet it is not a direct question at all. This paper has tried to show that the reasonable expectations of a society regarding any form of intervention designed to "take care of the drug problem" must address many different issues, all typically related to the "addiction-related" problems that are so frightening and costly to society. Multiple perspectives on outcome are not typical in evaluations of medical illnesses. In the treatment of most chronic illnesses "effective" treatments are expected to reduce symptoms, increase function and prevent relapse, especially costly relapse. Thus, as a final perspective on the issue of the effectiveness and worth of addiction treatments, this section now considers an evaluation of the effectiveness of addiction treatments using the criteria typical for evaluations of other chronic illnesses.

Compliance, Symptom Remission and Relapse in Addiction Treatment

It is important to note that addiction does not need to be considered chronic. Many who meet diagnostic criteria for substance dependence recover completely even without treatment. Others have long remissions following treatment. However, many of those who develop addiction disorders suffer multiple relapses following treatments and are thought to retain a continuing vulnerability to relapse for years or perhaps a lifetime. It is possible to argue that as yet there is no reliable "cure" for drug dependence. For the reasons outlined above, those dependent upon alcohol and/or other drugs who attempt to continue but reduce their use are likely to have problems in maintaining "controlled use." Among those who become addicted, patients who comply with the recommended regimen of education, counselling and medication have favourable outcomes during and for at least 6–12 months following treatment. However, most of those who start any type of treatment drop out prior to completion or they ignore their physician's advice to remain on medication and to continue participation in aftercare or self-help groups. It is also well known that problems of low socio-economic status, co-morbid psychiatric conditions and lack of family or social supports are among the most important variables associated with lack of compliance in addiction treatment and with relapse following treatment. Because of multiple co-morbid medical and social conditions and because of poor compliance with the medical and behavioural components of the treatment regimen, one-year follow-up studies have typically shown that only about 40–60 per cent of treated patients are abstinent, although an additional 15–30 per cent have not resumed dependent use during that period.

It is quite discouraging to many in the addiction treatment field that so many drug- and alcohol-dependent patients fail to comply with the recommended course of treatment and that so many subsequently resume substance use. As indicated above, there are now several medications that have demonstrated effectiveness in the treatment of alcohol and opiate dependence. However, for those medications to be effective, they must be taken on a regular basis and lack of patient compliance has severely limited their impact. Ongoing clinical research in this area is focused upon the development of longer-acting or "depot" forms of these medications, as well as behavioural strategies to increase patient compliance.

Compliance, Symptom Remission and Relapse in the Treatment of Chronic Illnesses

Hypertension, diabetes and asthma are well-studied, chronic disorders, requiring continuing care for most if not all of a patient's life. At the same time, these disorders are not necessarily unremitting or unalterably lethal, as long as the treatment regimen of medication, diet and behavioural change are followed. This last point requires elaboration. Treatments for these medical disorders are heavily dependent upon behavioural change and medication compliance to achieve their potential effectiveness. In a recently published review of treatment outcome studies of these disorders, patient compliance with the recommended medical regimen was the most significant determinant of treatment outcome. However, studies have shown that less than 60 per cent of type-1, insulin-dependent, adult diabetics fully comply with their medication schedule and less than 40 per cent of hypertensive or asthmatic patients comply fully with their medication regimens. The problem is even worse for the behavioural and diet changes that are so important for the maintenance of short-term gains in these chronic illnesses. Again, a review of recent studies in the fields of adult-onset diabetes, hypertension and asthma indicates that less than 30 per cent of patients in treatment for these disorders comply with prescribed diet and/or behavioural changes that are designed to increase functional status and to reduce risk factors for reoccurrence of the disorders. Across all three of these chronic medical illnesses, compliance, and ultimately outcome, is poorest among patients with low socio-economic status, low family and social supports or significant psychiatric co-morbidity, as summarized in Table 1.

This review of medication and behavioural compliance in the treatment of other chronic medical illnesses suggests important parallels with the treatment of drug dependence. In all these disorders, lack of patient compliance with the treatment regimen is a major contributor to the reoccurrence of symptoms; and in all these disorders compliance is poorest among those with co-morbid medical, psychiatric, family and social problems. Perhaps because of these similarities in treatment compliance there is also similarity in relapse or reoccurrence rates across all these disorders. In fact, outcome studies indicate that 30–50 per cent of insulin-dependent adult diabetic patients and approximately 50–70 per cent of adult hypertensive and asthmatic patients suffer reoccurrences of their symptoms each year to the point that they require, at least, re-stabilization of their medication and/or additional medical care to re-establish symptom remission. Many of these reoccurrences result in serious health complications. For example, limb amputations and blindness are common results of treatment non-compliance among diabetics. Stroke and cardiac disease are common problems associated with exacerbation of hypertension.

Table 1

Factors Associated with Relapse in Hypertension, Diabetes and Asthma

- Lack of adherence to prescribed medication, diet or behavioural change regimens
- Low socio-economic status
- Low family supports
- Psychiatric co-morbidity

A Chronic Illness Perspective on Treatment and Evaluation Designs

This section focuses on the question of whether the assumptions underlying interventions for acute conditions or those for chronic conditions are more appropriate for the treatment of addiction.

There are no definitive "cures" for any of the chronic medical illnesses reviewed here. Yet it is interesting that despite rather comparable rates of compliance and relapse across all of the disorders examined, there is no serious argument as to whether the treatments for diabetes, hypertension or asthma are "effective" or whether they should be supported by contemporary health insurance. However, this issue is very much in question with regard to treatments for drug dependence. In this regard, it is interesting that the relatively high relapse rates among diabetic, hypertensive and asthmatic patients following cessation of their medications have been considered evidence of the effectiveness of those medications and of the need for compliance enhancement strategies. In contrast, relapses to drug and alcohol use following cessation of addiction treatments has often been considered evidence of treatment failure.

Drug dependence treatments are not provided and especially are not evaluated under the same assumptions that pertain to other chronic illnesses. Particularly important in this regard is that drug dependence treatments are rarely delivered under a continuing care model that would be appropriate for a chronic illness. Indeed, with the exception of methadone maintenance and self-help groups most contemporary treatments for drug dependence are acute-care episodes. For example, it is common for a drug-dependent individual to be admitted to an outpatient rehabilitation programme lasting 30–90 days, rarely accompanied by medical monitoring or medication. This period of treatment is typically followed by discharge with referral to "community sources." While addiction treatment might be conceptualized as ongoing by those in the treatment field, from an operational perspective addiction treatments are delivered in much the same way as one might treat a surgical patient following a joint replacement. Outcome evaluations are typically conducted 6–12 months following treatment discharge, because addiction treatments have been expected to produce lasting reduction in symptoms following termination of treatment. Unlike the treatments for other chronic conditions, the reduction of symptoms during treatment has not been considered adequate to the expectations underlying addiction treatment.

This argument has nothing to do with whether addiction is fundamentally a disease, a bad habit, a social problem or all of the above. Moreover, it does not matter whether the essence of the intervention is the correction of some biological abnormality, the resolution of a psychological process, the teaching of some new behaviour or the development of some improved social support system. The expectations have been that some finite combination of medications, counselling and therapy, social services and/or social support systems should effect essential change in the root causes of addiction, remove those causal factors and result in lasting benefits.

A more realistic expectation is that the interventions currently available will not permanently correct the essence of the problem, only reduce the number and severity of the symptoms and improve personal function, as long as the patient participates in the intervention. This is precisely the same expectation that currently prevails in the treatment of chronic illnesses. Further, an "acute-care" expectation placed upon those types of treatment produces some perverse and even absurd results. For example, consider contemporary goals and the prevailing evaluation strategy for addiction treatments—applied to a hypertension treatment regimen. Patients who meet diagnostic criteria for hypertension would be admitted to an outpatient "hypertension rehabilitation" programme lasting 30–90 days in which they might receive medication, behavioural change therapy, dietary education and an exercise regimen. At the end of that period, the medication would be tapered during the last days of the treatment and the patients would be referred to community sources. The evaluation team would recontact the patient six months later and determine whether the patient had been continuously normotensive throughout that post-treatment period. Only those patients who met that criterion would be considered "successfully treated." Obviously, this hypothetical treatment management strategy and its associated evaluation approach are absurd for any chronic illness, including drug dependence.

POSTSCRIPT

Does Drug Abuse Treatment Work?

Much of the research on drug abuse treatment effectiveness is inconclusive; furthermore, researchers do not agree on what the best way is to measure effectiveness. Determining the effectiveness of drug abuse treatment is extremely important because the federal government and a number of state governments debate how much drug treatment should be funded. Many experts in the drug field agree that much of the money that has been used to deal with problems related to drugs has not been wisely spent. To prevent further waste of taxpayer funds, it is essential to find out if drug abuse treatment works before funding for it is increased.

Another concern related to this issue is that addicts who wish to receive treatment often face many barriers. One of the most serious barriers is that there is a lack of available treatment facilities. Compounding the problem is the fact that many communities resist the idea of having a drug treatment center in the neighborhoods, even though there is little research on the effects of treatment facilities on property values and neighborhood crime rates. Another barrier to treatment is cost, which, with the exception of self-help groups, is expensive. Furthermore, some addicts avoid organized treatment altogether for fear that if they go for treatment, they will be identified as drug abusers by law enforcement agencies. Likewise, many female drug addicts avoid drug treatment because they fear they will lose custody of their children. Among adolescents in drug treatment, 31 percent were female.

Many addicts in treatment are there because they are given a choice of entering either prison or treatment. Are people who are required to enter treatment more or less likely to succeed than people who enter treatment voluntarily? Early studies showed that treatment was more effective for voluntary clients. However, a study conducted by the U.S. federal government of 12,000 clients enrolled in 41 publicly funded treatment centers found that clients referred by the criminal justice system fared as well as if not better than voluntary clients in terms of reduced criminal activity and drug use. People who enter treatment voluntarily have an easier time walking away from treatment. Typically, the longer one stays in treatment, the more likely the treatment will be effective.

One emerging trend is to provide drug treatment to people in prison. Prison-based drug treatment has increased in recent years. Drug abuse treatment to prison inmates has been shown to reduce recidivism.

The publication *Services Research Outcomes Study* by the Office of Applied Studies (U.S. Department of Health and Human Services, January 28, 2004) describes the benefits of drug abuse treatment. Two articles that support drug abuse treatment are "Drug Treatment: The Willard Option" in *Corrections*

Today (April 2004) and "Coming Clean; Drug Treatment" in *The Economist* (October 16, 2004). Donna Lyons examines whether drug addicts should be sent to prison or to treatment in "Conviction for Addiction: States Are Considering No-nonsense Drug Policy Should Mean Prison or Treatment" in *State Legislatures* (June 2002). The advantages of providing drug abuse treatment to addicts in prison are discussed in Peter Anderson's article "Treatment With Teeth: A Judge Explains Why Drug Courts That Mandate and Supervise Treatment Are an Effective Middle Ground to Help Addicts Stay Clean and Reduce Crime" in *The American Prospect* (December 2003).

ISSUE 19

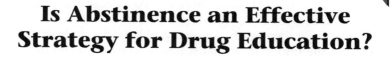

Is Abstinence an Effective Strategy for Drug Education?

YES: Tracy J. Evans-Whipp, Lyndal Bond, John W. Toumbourou, and Richard F. Catalano, from "School, Parent, and Student Perspectives of School Drug Policies," *Journal of School Health* (March 2007)

NO: Marsha Rosenbaum, from *Safety First: A Reality-Based Approach to Teens, Drugs, and Drug Education* (Drug Policy Alliance, 2004)

ISSUE SUMMARY

YES: Tracy J. Evans-Whipp, of the Murdoch Children's Research Institute in Melbourne, Australia, and her colleagues maintain that an abstinence message coupled with harsh penalties is more effective at reducing drug use than a message aimed at minimizing the harms of drugs. They contend that an abstinence message is clear and that a harm reduction message may give a mixed message.

NO: Drug researcher Marsha Rosenbaum states that because many teens experiment with drugs, a message to reduce the harms associated with drugs is necessary. Rosenbaum believes that scare tactics and misinformation about drugs increases the likelihood that teens may have problems if or when they experiment with drugs. Also, a problem with the abstinence-only message is that teens have no one to turn to if they experience problems with drugs.

Drug education is arguably one of the most logical ways of dealing with the problems of drugs in American society. Drug-taking behavior has not been significantly affected by attempts to reduce the demand for drugs, and drug prohibition has not been successful either. One remaining option to explore is drug education. Drug education is not a panacea for eliminating drug problems. Rates of cigarette smoking are much lower today than they were thirty and forty years ago, but it took several decades of public health efforts to achieve this decline. If drug education is to ultimately prove successful, it too will take years.

Many early drug education programs were misguided. One emphasis was on scare tactics. Experts erroneously believed that if young people saw the horrible consequences of drug use, then they would certainly abstain from drugs. Another faulty assumption was that drug use would be affected by knowledge about drugs, but knowledge is not enough. Over 400,000 people die each year from tobacco use, but many adults and teenagers continue to smoke even though most know the grim statistics about tobacco. Young people have a hard time relating to the potential problems like cancer and cirrhosis of the liver (which is caused by long-term alcohol abuse) because these problems take years to manifest themselves. Another problem with early drug education is that much of the information that teachers relayed concerning drugs was either incorrect or exaggerated. Teachers were therefore not seen as credible.

There is a lack of consensus about what a drug education program should encompass. However, there is general agreement among drug prevention experts that drug awareness programs are counterproductive. Many schools conduct drug awareness programs in which, over the course of a week, former drug abusers talk to students about how their lives and families were ruined by drugs, pharmacologists demonstrate the physical effects of drugs, and videos are shown depicting the horrors of drugs. These sensationalized programs stimulate curiosity, and it is not unusual for drug use to increase after one of these presentations.

Many drug prevention programs in the 1970s focused on self-esteem and values clarification. If low self-esteem is a factor in drug use, as many believed, then it would make sense to improve self-esteem to reduce drug use. However, self-esteem is not always a good indicator of drug use. Many young people who have good feelings about themselves use drugs. In addition, many believed that if students clarified their values, they would see the folly of using drugs. This approach overlooked the possibility that young people may turn to drugs because they want to be accepted by their peers, because drugs are forbidden, or simply because they enjoy the high that comes from drug use.

The current emphasis in drug education is on primary prevention. It is easier to have young people not use drugs in the first place than to get them to stop after they have already started using drugs. One popular drug prevention program, Drug Abuse Resistance Education (DARE), attempts to get upper-elementary students to pledge not to use drugs. The rationale is that putting energy into teaching elementary students about drugs rather than high school students will be more likely to reduce drug use because the latter are more likely to have already begun using drugs. The program focuses mainly on tobacco, alcohol, and marijuana. These are considered gateway drugs, which means that students who use other drugs are most likely to have used these first. The longer students delay using tobacco, alcohol, and marijuana, the less likely they will be to use other drugs.

In the following selections, Tracy J. Evans-Whipp and her colleagues feel that the most effective message for reducing drug use is abstinence coupled with harsh punishment. Marsha Rosenbaum believes that an abstinence-only message is ineffective and that a more effective strategy is to reduce the harms associated with drug use.

YES

Tracy J. Evans-Whipp, Lyndal Bond, John W. Toumbourou, and Richard F. Catalano

School, Parent, and Student Perspectives of School Drug Policies

Introduction

Schools are now recognized as much more than centers for academic instruction, with their role in contributing to the health and social well-being of students and staff now widely accepted.(1–5) Schools acknowledge their important influence on preventing youth tobacco, alcohol, and illicit-drug use (and their associated harms) and implement a range of education programs and policy directives to this end.

School drug policies form an important component of school-wide drug prevention, acting to set normative values and expectancies for student behavior as well as documenting procedures for dealing with drug-related incidents. (6) However, it is not clear to what degree, if any, school drug policies influence student behavior and the mechanism by which any such influence occurs. (7,8) Thus, policy makers are provided with little empirical guidance for developing and implementing effective school drug policy. It is likely that schools develop drug policies that reflect the values of the community, state, and country in which they reside, and a recent cross-country comparison of school policies in the United States and Australia(9) indeed found this to be the case.

In working toward an understanding of what constitutes effective school policy, it is important to establish an effective method for collecting information about schools' current policies. Most descriptive accounts of school policies have used school personnel and/or higher level bodies (such as school districts or local education authorities) as informants.(10,11) However, implementation of school drug policy is likely to be a key determinant of policy impact, and investigation of student and parent perspectives of policy provides a broader insight into how policy is carried out in practice. Few studies of school drug policies and student substance-use behaviors have collected information from multiple school policy stakeholders. Where data have been collected from students, the focus has mostly been on student substance-use behaviors rather than on students' understanding of policy content and implementation.(7,12–14) One notable exception is a study by Griesbach et al (15) in which the impact

From *Journal of School Health*, vol. 77, issue 3, March 2007, pp. 138–146. Copyright © 2007 by Blackwell Publishing, Ltd. Reprinted by permission. www.blackwell-synergy.com

of school drug policy components on student smoking at school was measured. This study found that student perceptions of smoking at school were significantly lower in schools where pupil smoking restrictions were consistently enforced, thereby highlighting the importance of measuring policy implementation in addition to documentation. It appears that no other studies have collected information on school drug policy from parents.

We have recently developed and tested a school drug policy survey questionnaire on schools in Victoria, Australia, and Washington State, USA.(9) These 2 states share many sociodemographic characteristics(16) but differ in their approach to drugs, alcohol, and illicit drugs. US drug policies tend to reflect an abstinence-only orientation,(17) whereas Australian policies are based on a combination of abstinence and harm-minimization principles.(17,18) In measuring school policies in states in 2 countries with contrasting policy approaches, a wide variety of policy descriptions and implementation procedures were observed. The survey collected responses from school personnel, usually school principals, who are considered to be knowledgeable about the policy content. The current paper extends the observations collected from school administrators by examining parent and student reports of school drug policy gathered in parallel surveys. Thus, it is possible to compare responses between the 3 groups of respondents to gain a more comprehensive picture of how school policy operates. In particular, cross-comparison of responses will enable us to (1) determine how effectively schools are communicating school drug policy information to parents and students, (2) gain insight into how school policies are implemented, and (3) investigate what policy variables impact students' drug use at school and their perceptions of other students' drug use at school.

Methods

Participants and Procedures

The surveys were conducted in 2003 as part of the International Youth Development Study (IYDS), a longitudinal research study of adolescent substance use and its predictors in Washington State and Victoria. Samples of public and private schools in both states were drawn to constitute representative samples of students at seventh and ninth grade. Procedures for the IYDS sampling, school administrator survey, and student survey have been described previously.(9,19)

This study used data collected from secondary schools and the grade 7 and 9 students (and their parents) attending them.

School administrator survey. The 205 schools (104 from Washington and 101 from Victoria) represent 97.6% of participating secondary (grade 7 through to highest) and mixed (combination of pre-and postgrade 7) schools. The majority of respondents were principals or heads of school (72.1% in Washington and 46% in Victoria), or assistant/vice principals (13.5% in Washington and 22% in Victoria).

Student survey.   Students in grade 7 and grade 9 classes yielded a total of 5085 eligible students, of whom 3899 (76.7%) consented to and participated in the survey (1942 in Washington and 1957 in Victoria). Honesty criteria, which included student reports of being "not honest at all" when completing the survey, using a fictional drug, or using illicit drugs more than 120 times in the past 30 days, were used to remove surveys of 23 students from the sample (8 from Washington and 15 from Victoria).

Parent survey.   Concurrent with the student survey, a 15-minute telephone interview was administered to a parent/guardian of each participating student, using computer-assisted telephone interviewing technology. A total of 1886 Washington parents, representing 98% of the valid student sample, and 1858 Victorian parents (95% of the student sample) were successfully contacted and interviewed. The survey was administered in English for most respondents but also conducted in Vietnamese and Cantonese in Victoria and in Spanish, Korean, Vietnamese, and Russian in Washington. The majority of parents interviewed were biological parents (94% in Washington and 98% in Victoria) and female (74% in Washington and 81% in Victoria).

Measures

Parent awareness of policy and involvement.   School administrators were asked to report how aware they thought parents were of existing substance-use policies and how involved parents were in making decisions and setting substance-use policies at their school.

Awareness of school drug policies was assessed in the parent interview by asking to what degree parents were aware of what happened to a student caught smoking, drinking alcohol, or possessing or using illicit drugs at their child's school. A single construct for parental awareness of school drug policy was generated from the mean of the responses to all 3 items.

Communication methods.   School administrators were asked to indicate which of the following methods they use to communicate policy to parents: parent handbook, structured meetings with school staff (conferences), newsletters/bulletins, letters home to parents, orientation/parent night, or other.

Parents were asked in the interview whether or not details of school drug policies were communicated by their child's school via newsletters or bulletins, parent/teacher meetings, parent handbooks, or student diaries/handbooks, indirectly through their child, or through verbal communication with school staff.

Policy philosophy/orientation.   To index policy orientation toward abstinence-only and harm-minimization principles, administrators were asked to indicate the degree to which the following 2 statements described their school: "School policies emphasize total abstinence from drug use" and "School policies are based on the assumption that most youth will experiment with drugs." For school drug education orientation, administrators were asked to what degree they agreed with these statements: "Drug education programs emphasize total abstinence from drug use" and "Drug education programs emphasize safe drug use rather than no drug use."

To index policy and drug education orientation toward abstinence and harm minimization, respectively, students were asked to indicate the degree to which they agreed with the following two statements: "We are taught to say no to alcohol" and "We are taught to use alcohol safely."

Policy enforcement. Policy enforcement was measured in the school administrator survey by a series of items asking the likelihood of specific consequences for students caught using tobacco, alcohol, and illicit drugs on school grounds or at school events. These included referral to a school counselor or nurse, in-school or out-of-school suspension, expulsion from school, and referral to legal authorities (police).

In the student survey, policy enforcement was assessed by a series of items asking which consequences are used for students caught using tobacco, alcohol, and illicit drugs at school. The consequences given were: he or she would be talked to by a teacher about the dangers of smoking cigarettes/drinking alcohol/using drugs, he or she would be suspended, he or she would be expelled, or the police would be called.

Student drug use on school grounds. Two items in the student survey measured students' perceptions about tobacco and alcohol use at school: "Many students smoke on school grounds without getting caught" and "Many students drink alcohol on school grounds without getting caught."

Students were asked to report their own drug taking on school grounds with the following item: "How many times in the past year (12 months) have you been drunk or high at school?" Responses were dichotomized into "never" and "one or more times" categories.

Results

Parental Awareness of Policy

The percentage of parents aware of specific drug policies at their child's school was higher in Washington than in Victoria (81.6% aware of smoking policies, 86.7% aware of alcohol policies, and 88.8% aware of illicit-drug policies vs 72.1%, 70.3%, and 71.9%, respectively, for Victoria. . . . There was no significant difference between the 2 states in terms of school perceptions of parent awareness (82.5% in Washington vs 80.2% in Victoria, . . . but Victorian schools perceived greater parent awareness than was actually reported by parents.

It was hypothesized that schools that involved their parent body in the policy setting process would report higher levels of parental policy awareness. Less than 10% of schools in both states reported that parents were "very involved" in the policy setting process, and there was no significant difference in the levels of parental policy awareness between schools that did or did not involve parents in policy setting (89% vs 80%). . . .

Methods Used to Communicate Policy

. . . Schools in both states reported that the most commonly used method for communicating school drug policy information to parents was via newsletters/ bulletins and then orientation/parent night. Parents also rated newsletters/ bulletins as the most commonly used method, but in both states, it was reported that parent handbooks and student diaries/handbooks were other commonly used methods. Parent/teacher meetings were not as frequently used.

Washington parents reported the use of each of the communication methods more frequently than Victorian parents, whereas school administrators reported that only one of the communication methods (parent handbook) was used more frequently by Washington schools. . . .

Abstinence and Harm-Minimization Messages

Washington school administrators reported that their school policies placed more emphasis on total abstinence from drug use than policies of Victorian school administrators. . . . Washington school drug education programs also emphasized total abstinence from drug use, whereas Victorian administrators reported that school policies had a stronger abstinence message than did drug education curricula.

More Victorian than Washington school administrators (18% vs 5%) reported that their school drug policies were based on the assumption that most youth will experiment with drugs. Similarly, the harm-minimization concept was adopted within drug education curricula to a much greater extent by Victorian schools than by Washington schools (33% vs 2%) (table not shown). . . .

As with school administrator reports, an emphasis on abstinence was reported by more Washington students and an emphasis on harm minimization by Victorian students. . . .

Policy Enforcement

The most common consequences for all drug policy violations reported by school administrators in both states were referral of the student to a counselor/ nurse or suspension. . . . Highly punitive measures such as expulsion and contacting the police were more commonly used for illicit-drug offences than for tobacco and alcohol policy violations. Washington school administrators were more likely than Victorian administrators to use highly punitive measures.

More Washington than Victorian students reported that highly punitive measures were used for all drug-type violations. Students in both states agreed with school administrators that highly punitive measures were used for illicit-drug offences than for tobacco and alcohol policy violations. Students did not report that referral to a teacher was a common consequence, with only around 50% or less of students reporting use of this method. Victorian students were more likely than Washington students to report this consequence for all drug-type violations.

Policy and Student Drug Use on School Grounds

Students in Victoria were twice as likely to report that students smoke on school grounds without getting caught as students in Washington (61% vs 30%). . . . Perceptions of alcohol use on school grounds were lower than for smoking and similar in both states (12% in Victoria and 14% in Washington) . . . , as was student self-reported drug and/or alcohol use at school in the past year (5% in Victoria and 7% in Washington,). . . .

Characteristics of students, including their being in ninth grade and recent use in the past month, increased their perceptions of smoking on school grounds, and living in Washington reduced the likelihood of perceptions of smoking on school grounds. Student perceptions of smoking on school grounds were lower where students reported having received a strong abstinence drug education message . . . or perceiving harsh penalties if caught smoking at school . . . , parents reported awareness of school drug policy . . . , and if the school reported using an abstinence-based policy . . . or strict policy enforcement. . . . Monitoring of school grounds and bathrooms was significantly associated with higher student perceptions of smoking on school grounds. . . .

Characteristics of students, including being in ninth grade and smoking in the last 30 days, increased the perceptions of drinking on school grounds. Student perceptions of drinking on school grounds were lower when students perceived harsh penalties if caught drinking at school . . . , and were higher if the school reported monitoring of bathrooms. . . .

Ninth grade students and those who used tobacco in the last 30 days reported more drinking or drug taking on school grounds. Student self-reported drinking or drug taking on school grounds was lower where students reported having received a strong abstinence drug education message or a strong harm-minimization drug education message. . . .

Adjusting for state, cohort, and recent (past 30 days) self-reported tobacco use, student perception of harsh penalties for drug policy violations continued to be statistically significantly associated with lower student perceptions of smoking . . . and drinking . . . at school. . . . Student perceptions of a strong abstinence drug education message continued to be statistically significantly associated with lower drug use at school. . . . Harm-minimization drug education continued to be statistically significantly associated with lower perceptions of smoking at school . . . , and marginally significant with self-report of being drunk or high at school. . . . The relationship between school report of monitoring bathrooms and school grounds and high levels of drinking at school also continued to be significant after adjusting for state, cohort, and recent tobacco use. . . . School reports for expulsion for alcohol violations continued to be associated with lower numbers of students reporting being drunk or high at school. . . .

Discussion

This study collected information on school drug policy from 3 different sources and provides detailed insight into policy implementation in schools from 2 countries that have different drug policy environments. Collecting parent reports on policy was important since schools are encouraged to involve their parent body in policy development and ensure that all relevant parties, including parents, are aware of the policy. The considerable investment on the part of schools to achieve this is considered acceptable, as parent involvement is expected to facilitate the school's ability to handle drug incidents in a manner consistent with community expectations, and parental involvement enables parents to enforce similar restrictions outside of school.(22–24) Parents' self-reported awareness of school drug policy in this study indicated that schools in Victoria tend to overestimate slightly how well they are communicating school drug policy information to parents. Interestingly, about 30% fewer Victorian parents reported receiving drug policy information via school news-letters, the most commonly used method, than schools reported using them. It is possible that schools are producing these materials, but that parents do not always receive or remember receiving them. In Washington, about 10% more parents recall receiving drug policy information via school newsletters than schools reported using them.

It is difficult to determine from this study any potential benefits from parent involvement in policy setting since less than 10% of schools reported high levels of parental involvement. This finding is in accordance with other studies in the United States and England that also found low levels of parent involvement in policy setting.(25,26)

How and if student drug use is influenced by school drug policy will be related to students' understanding of policy and their perceptions of its enforcement. This study assessed how well schools communicate their drug policy messages to their students. It appears that schools in both states are successfully communicating their stance on at least alcohol use since the observed differences in policy orientation between schools in the 2 states was also reported by students. By adopting an abstinence-based policy stance to drug issues, Washington schools are able to provide a more consistent message to their students with strong abstinence messages in both drug policy and drug education messages. The harm-minimization concept adopted by most Victorian schools takes a broader view, encouraging abstinence as a key method of reducing harms, but accepting some degree of experimentation and attempting to equip students with knowledge on safe levels of use. As a consequence, Victorian schools report that their policies place strong emphasis on abstinence (the use of drugs being inappropriate at school), while their drug education programs have a greater harm-minimization focus.

Students in both states were generally knowledgeable about the likely consequences for drug policy violations in their school. Students confirmed school reports that Washington schools were more likely than Victorian schools to use highly punitive measures such as expulsion and referral to the police. Students in both states believed that remedial consequences such as counseling were less likely to be used, especially for illicit-drug use, than was indicated by the schools. This disparity in responses might reflect a genuine difference between policy documentation and implementation (ie, schools overreport the use of counseling) or might result from students not being well informed about the remedial consequences of policy violations. It is possible that when communicating school drug policy, schools place more emphasis on the highly punitive consequences to enhance the deterrent effect. The impact of the perception of punitive measures for smoking and drinking is also associated with lower perceptions of smoking and drinking at school, but interestingly, it is less strongly associated with student reports of being drunk or high at school. This area warrants further investigation as there is emerging evidence that the use of education and counseling along with disciplinary sanctions is associated with lower student smoking rates than the use of punitive measures alone.(14,27) The finding that students are generally well aware of their school's policy implementation is an important one as there is strong evidence that school drug policy will only impact student behavior if it is perceived to be well enforced.(15,28,29)

Measuring the impact of school drug policies on student behaviors is a difficult task given the number of known influences on students' decisions to use tobacco, alcohol, and other drugs.(30) It was hypothesized that school policy would be expected to have the greatest effect on student drug use on school grounds. In this study, self-reported drug use on school grounds was measured as well as perceptions of smoking and drinking by other students at school without getting caught. Importantly, reductions in the ORs for these behaviors were observed in schools where students reported receiving an abstinence drug education message and perceived harsh penalties if caught using drugs at school, even when controlling for known influences (cohort, state, and recent tobacco use). Strong harm-minimization messages were also associated with lower levels of self-reported use, indicating that clearly delivered policy messages of either orientation can be effective in lowering levels of drug use at school.

Interestingly, monitoring drug use on school grounds or in bathrooms was associated with increases in perceptions of student smoking and alcohol use but not self-reports of being drunk or high at school. This suggests that monitoring may increase perceptions of student drug use whilst not serving to reduce actual use levels. This may be worrisome since perceptions of drug use are associated with higher levels of drug initiation.(31)

The current study has a number of limitations that should be noted. Only one school informant completed the School Administrator Survey, and it is possible that the responses might more accurately depict school policy if additional school respondents were surveyed. The wording of questions was not always consistent across student, parent, or administrator surveys. For example, when asking about the consequences for policy violations, schools were asked about student referral to a counselor or nurse, whereas students were asked about referral to a teacher. However, there are a number of key strengths to the study, namely its very large representative sample from 2 states with different national drug policy backgrounds, collection of data from 3 key school groups, and measures of actual and perceived student drug use on school grounds.

The implications of this study for school policy makers are preliminary but encouraging. Schools in the 2 study states generally have some impact in educating their students about drug policy. When delivered effectively, policy messages are associated with reduced student drug use at school. Abstinence messages and harsh penalties convey a coherent message to students associated with reduced student drug use at school. Strong harm-minimization messages delivered within a "no drugs at school" context are also associated with reduced drug use at school, but effects are weaker than those for abstinence messages. It is possible that the smaller impact of harm-minimization messages is a result of conflicting messages between policy (abstinence) and drug education (acceptance of experimentation). Harm-minimization advocates would argue that this smaller effect is acceptable given the anticipated reduction in the levels of current and future harmful use and school drop out within the student population. Given that nearly all schools invest substantial time and money developing and implementing policies for tobacco, alcohol, and illicit drugs and drug education, it is imperative that further research is conducted to evaluate which aspects of policy are important in reducing student drug use.

References

1. Commonwealth Department of Health and Family Services. A National Framework for Health Promoting Schools (2000–2003). Canberra Australia: Commonwealth Department of Health and Family Services and Australian Health Promoting Schools Association; 2001.

2. Rutter M, Maughan B, Mortimore P, Ouston J, Smith A. Fifteen Thousand Hours: Secondary Schools and Their Effects on Children. London: Open Books; 1979.

3. Resnick MD, Bearman PS, Blum RW, et al. Protecting adolescents from harm: findings from the National Longitudinal Study on Adolescent Health. JAMA. 1997;278(10):823–832.

4. Bond L, Patton G, Glover S, et al. The Gatehouse Project: can a multilevel school intervention affect emotional well-being and health risk behaviours? J Epidemiol Community Health. 2004;58(12):997–1003.

5. Patton G, Bond L, Butler H, Glover S. Changing schools, changing health? Design and implementation of the Gatehouse Project. J Adolesc Health. 2003;33(4):231–239.

6. Goodstadt MS. Substance abuse curricula vs. school drug policies. J Sch Health. 1989;59(6):246–250.

7. Evans-Whipp T, Beyers JM, Lloyd S, et al. A review of school drug policies and their impact on youth substance use. Health Promot Int. 2004;19(2):227–234.

8. Flay BR. Approaches to substance use prevention utilizing school curriculum plus social environment change. Addict Behav. 2000;25(6):861–885.

9. Beyers JM, Evans-Whipp T, Mathers M, Toumbourou JW, Catalano RF. A cross-national comparison of school drug policies in Washington State, United States, and Victoria, Australia. J Sch Health. 2005;75(4):134–140.

10. Small ML, Jones SE, Barrios LC, et al. School policy and environment: results from the School Health Policies and Programs Study 2000. J Sch Health. 2001;71(7):325–334.

11. Ross JG, Einhaus KB, Hohenemser LK, Greene BZ, Kann L, Gold RS. School health policies prohibiting tobacco use, alcohol and other drug use, and violence. J Sch Health. 1995;65(8):333–338.

12. Pentz MA, Brannon BR, Charlin VL, Barrett EJ, MacKinnon DP, Flay BR. The power of policy: the relationship of smoking policy to adolescent smoking. Am J Public Health. 1989;79(7):857–862.

13. Charlton A, While D. Smoking prevalence among 16–19 year-olds related to staff and student smoking policies in sixth forms and further education. Health Educ J. 1994;53:28–39.

14. Hamilton G, Cross D, Lower T, Resnicow K, Williams P. School policy: what helps to reduce teenage smoking? Nicotine Tob Res. 2003;5(4):507–513.

15. Griesbach D, Inchley J, Currie C. More than words? The status and impact of smoking policies in Scottish schools. Health Promot Int. 2002;17(l):31–41.

16. McMorris BJ, Hemphill SA, Toumbourou JW, Catalano RF, Patton GC. Prevalence of substance use and delinquent behavior in adolescents from Victoria, Australia and Washington State, USA. Health EducBehav. 2006.

17. Caulkins JP, Reuter P. Setting goals for drug policy: harm reduction or use reduction? Addiction. 1997;92(9):1143–1150.

18. Munro G, Midford R. "Zero tolerance" and drug education in Australian schools. Drug Alcohol Rev. 2001;20(1):105–109.

19. Patton GC, McMorris BJ, Toumbourou JW, Hemphill SA, Donath S, Catalano RF. Puberty and the onset of substance use and abuse. Pediatrics. 2004; 114(3):e300–e306.

20. Stata statistical software: Release 8. College Station, TX: StataCorp; 2001.

21. Carlin JB, Wolfe R, Coffey C, Patton GC. Tutorial in biostatistics: analysis of binary outcomes in longitudinal studies using weighted estimating equations and discrete-time survival methods: prevalence and incidence of smoking in an adolescent cohort. Stat Med. 1999;18(19):2655–2679.

22. Peck DD, Acott C, Richard P, Hill S, Schuster C. The Colorado Tobacco-Free Schools and Communities Project. J Sch Health. 1993;63(5):214–217.

23. Commonwealth Department of Education Training and Youth Affairs. National School Drug Education Strategy, May 1999. . . .

24. Commonwealth Department of Education Science and Training. Innovation and Good Practice in Drug Education. Effective Communication. Canberra: Commonwealth of Australia; 2003: 10.

25. Brener ND, Dittus PJ, Hayes G. Family and community involvement in schools: results from the School Health Policies and Programs Study 2000. J Sch Health. 2001;71(7):340–344.

26. Denman S, Pearson J, Hopkins D, Wallbanks C, Skuriat V. The management and organisation of health promotion: a survey of school policies in Nottinghamshire. Health Educ J. 1999; 58:165–176.

27. Hamilton G, Cross D, Resnicow K, Hall M. A school-based harm minimization smoking intervention trial: outcome results. Addiction. 2005;100(5):689–700.

28. Moore L, Roberts C, Tudor-Smith C. School smoking policies and smoking prevalence among adolescents: multilevel analysis of cross-sectional data from Wales. Tob Control. 2001;10(2):117–123.

29. Wakefield MA, Chaloupka FJ, Kaufman NJ, Orleans CT, Barker DC, Ruel BE. Effect of restrictions on smoking at home, at school, and in public places on teenage smoking: cross sectional study. BMJ. 2000;321(7257):333–337.

30. Hawkins JD, Catalano RF, Miller JY. Risk and protective factors for alcohol and other drug problems in adolescence and early adulthood: implications for substance abuse prevention. Psychol Bull. 1992;112(1):64–105.

31. Hansen WB, Graham JW. Preventing alcohol, marijuana, and cigarette use among adolescents: peer pressure resistance training versus establishing conservative norms. Prey Med. 1991;20(3):414–430.

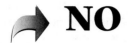 **NO**

Safety First: A Reality-Based Approach to Teens, Drugs, and Drug Education

Drug Education Strategies

Education to prevent drug use has existed in America for over a century. A variety of methods—from scare tactics to resistance techniques—have been used with the intention of encouraging young people to refrain from drug use altogether. Despite the expansion of these abstinence-only programs, it is difficult to know which, if any, are actually successful.

More than half of all high school students in America experiment with illegal drugs, and even more use alcohol. They see for themselves that America is hardly "drug-free." They know there are differences between experimentation, abuse, and addiction; and that the use of one drug does not inevitably lead to the use of others. Adolescence is also a time for trying new things and taking risks.

Yet, conventional drug education programs focus predominantly on abstinence-only messages and are shaped by problematic myths:

Myth #1: Experimentation with drugs is not a common part of teenage culture;

Myth #2: Drug use is the same as drug abuse;

Myth #3: Marijuana is the gateway to drugs such as heroin and cocaine; and

Myth #4: Exaggerating risks will deter young people from experimentation.

Teenagers make their own choices about drugs and alcohol, just as we did. Like us, they sometimes make foolish mistakes. However, since we cannot be there to protect them 100 percent of the time, we have to find ways to trust them when they are not under our watch. It is our responsibility as parents and teachers to engage young people in dialogue, listen to them, and provide a sounding board and resources when they need our help.

Abstinence may be what we'd all prefer for our youth, but this simplistic goal may not be attainable. Our current efforts lack harm reduction education for those students that won't "just say no." In order to prevent drug abuse and drug problems among teenagers who do experiment, we need a fallback strategy that puts safety first.

Educational efforts should acknowledge teens' ability to sort through complex issues and make decisions that will ensure their own safety. The programs should offer credible information, differentiate between use and abuse, and stress the importance of moderation and context. Curricula should be age-specific, stress student participation, and provide objective, science-based materials.

Today's Curricula: Are They Effective?

Existing drug education programs vary tremendously in content, as well as in quality and price. A school typically adopts a particular program and then either uses its own faculty or outside "experts" to teach the program's curriculum. Some programs offer video presentations; others stickers, posters, and activity books. Some are designed to stand alone; others to be integrated into health or science curricula. Some educators hand out T-shirts and certificates when students complete the program; others have graduation ceremonies where students are encouraged to take a pledge to remain drug free.

All programs provide information about the negative consequences of drug use. Most teach resistance or refusal skills. The majority teach students that most people do not use drugs, that abstinence is the societal norm, and that it is socially acceptable not to try drugs.[3]

Increased government funding for "just say no" programs in the 80s resulted in the development and implementation of many new programs promoting an abstinence-only message. While it is very difficult to know which, if any, are effective in preventing drug use, we do know that a majority of students continue to experiment with drugs and alcohol by the time they reach their senior year of high school. Why is there such a disconnect?

Some researchers argue that it is impossible to know whether drug education programs are effective, because the evaluations themselves are too superficial. They tend to measure student attitudes about drugs rather than drug use itself. Unfortunately, attitudes formed about drugs during childhood or early adolescence seem to have little bearing on later decisions, and high school students may offer reasons they've been taught for avoiding drugs, yet use them anyway.[4] Furthermore, some evaluations tend to overly emphasize positive results, while ignoring those that show no effectiveness.[5]

Perhaps most shocking are the consistently negative evaluations of DARE, America's most popular program. DARE reaches 36 million students annually, in nearly 80 percent of school districts in the U.S. In study after study, DARE failed to prevent or reduce drug use among its graduates.[6] These evaluations have troubled educators and parents so much that cities including New York, Salt Lake City, Minneapolis, Oakland, Boulder, and Houston, as well as states, such as Massachusetts, have abandoned the program, forcing DARE to take a close, hard look at its curriculum.

WHAT DO TEENS THINK?

Rarely, if ever, are students themselves asked to evaluate prevention efforts. Listening to the opinions of young people is an important place to begin. Students are hungry for accurate information, but believe that the programs currently in place are not meeting their needs. Here's what some say:

> *"It's like nobody cares what we think . . . The DARE cops just wanted us to do what they told us and our teachers never talked about DARE . . . It seems like a lot of adults and teachers can't bring themselves down to talk to students . . . so you don't care what they think either."*[7]
>
> *"It's just a really unrealistic way of teaching kids how to deal with drugs. It shouldn't be 'just say no,' but 'think about it,' or something like that. Like, 'use your brain.'"*[8]
>
> *"I think they need to make a distinction between drug use and abuse; that people can use drugs and still lead a healthy, productive life. You know, your parents can come home and drink a glass of wine with their dinner. They're not alcoholics."*[9]
>
> *"I think honesty is the core of drug education and the only thing that's going to help people not use drugs. When they're not being bombarded with propaganda for or against drug use, then it's more likely that kids are going to make more informed decisions."*[10]

What's Wrong With Abstinence-Only Education?

Existing programs seem to send mixed messages; blur the lines between use and abuse; use scare tactics; promote misinformation; and undermine the credibility of parents and teachers who provide this false information. Too often, abstinence-only programs ignore young people's exposure to drug use and fail to engage them in a meaningful way.

Mixed Messages

Despite proclamations about the value of being "drug-free," the American people and their children are perpetually bombarded with messages that encourage them to imbibe and medicate with a variety of substances such as alcohol, tobacco, caffeine and over-the-counter and prescription drugs.

The *Journal of the American Medical Association* recently reported that 8 out of 10 adults in the U.S. used at least one medication every week, and half took a prescription drug.[11] More than one in two American adults use alcohol regularly; and 40% have tried marijuana at some time in their lives—a fact not lost on their children.[12]

Today's teenagers have also witnessed the increasing "Ritalinization" of their fellow difficult-to-manage students.[13] And as they watch prime-time commercials for drugs to manage "Generalized Anxiety Disorder," they see more of their parents turning to anti-depressants to cope.

Teenage drug use seems to mirror modern American drug-taking tendencies.[14] Therefore, some psychologists argue, given the nature of our culture, teenage experimentation with legal and illegal mind-altering substances is not deviant.[15]

Use and Abuse

Adults routinely make distinctions between use and abuse. While growing up, young people rapidly learn the difference, too. Most observe their parents and other adults using alcohol (itself a drug) without abusing it. Many also know that their parents, at some point in their lives, used an illegal drug (usually marijuana) without becoming abusers.

In an effort to prevent teenage experimentation, too often programs pretend there is no difference between use and abuse. Some use the terms interchangeably; others emphasize an exaggerated definition of use that categorizes any use of illegal drugs or anything other than one-time experimentation as abuse.

Programs that blur the distinctions undermine educational efforts because students' own experiences tell them the information presented is not believable.[16] As one 17-year-old girl, an 11th-grader in Fort Worth, Texas, put it, *"They told my little sister that you'd get addicted to marijuana the first time, and it's not like that. You hear that, and then you do it, and you say, 'Ah, they lied to me.'"*[17]

Although there is nothing more frightening than a teenager whose use of alcohol and/or other drugs gets out of hand and becomes a problem, virtually all studies have found that the vast majority of students who try drugs do not become abusers.[18] As parents, we can be more effective in dealing with problem use if we are clear and fair about the distinctions.

Scare Tactics and Misinformation

A common belief among many educators, policy makers, and parents is that if teenagers simply believe that drug experimentation is dangerous, they will abstain.[19] As a result, many prevention programs include exaggerated risk and danger messages. Although the old *Reefer Madness*-style messages have been replaced by assertions that we now have scientific evidence of the dangers of drugs, the evidence, particularly about marijuana, just isn't there. When these studies are critically evaluated, few of the most common assertions hold up.

I first realized the dangers of using scare tactics 27 years ago, while working on my doctoral dissertation about heroin addiction. One of my first interviews was with a "nice Jewish girl," like myself, from an affluent suburb in a large metropolitan area. Genuinely intrigued by the different turns our lives had taken, I asked how she had ended up addicted to heroin and in jail. I will never forget what she told me:

> *"When I was in high school they had these so-called drug education classes. They told us if we used marijuana, we would become addicted. They told us if we used heroin, we would become addicted. Well, we all tried marijuana and found we did not become addicted. We figured the entire message must be B.S. So I tried heroin, used it again and again, got strung out, and here I am."*

Marijuana, the most popular illegal drug among teens, is routinely demonized in abstinence-only messages. Many Web sites, including those managed by the federal government, include misinformation about marijuana's potency, its relationship to cancer, memory, the immune system, personality alteration, addiction, and sexual dysfunction.

In *Marijuana Myths, Marijuana Facts: A Review of the Scientific Evidence,* Professor Lynn Zimmer and Dr. John P. Morgan carefully examined the scientific evidence relevant to each of these alleged dangers. They found, in essentially every case, that the claims of marijuana's dangerousness did not hold up.[20] Their findings are not uncommon. Over the years, the same conclusions have been reached by numerous official commissions, including the La Guardia Commission in 1944, the National Commission on Marijuana and Drug Abuse in 1972, the National Academy of Sciences in 1982, and, in 1999, the Institute of Medicine.

A frightening ramification of imparting misinformation is that like the heroin addict I interviewed 27 years ago, teenagers will ignore our warnings completely and put themselves in real danger. The increased purity and availability of "hard" drugs, coupled with teenagers' refusal to heed warnings they don't trust, have resulted in increased risk of fatal overdose such as those we've witnessed among the children of celebrities and in affluent communities.[21]

Another case in point is Ecstasy. Despite a $5 million media campaign to alert young people to its dangers, year after year, government surveys indicate continued use.[22] When I ask teenage users why they have not heeded government warnings, they express deep cynicism. Said one 18-year-old regarding problematic brain changes attributed to Ecstasy, *"Oh yes, they told us about that with marijuana, too. But none of us believes we have holes in our brains, so we just laugh at those messages."*[23]

The Gateway Theory

The gateway theory, a mainstay of drug education, suggests that marijuana use leads to the use of harder drugs such as cocaine and heroin.[24] There is no credible research evidence demonstrating that using one drug causes the use of another.

For example, a large survey conducted by the federal government shows that the vast majority of marijuana users do not progress to the use of more dangerous drugs.[25] Based on the *National Survey on Drug Use and Health,* Zimmer and Morgan calculated that for every 100 people who have tried marijuana, only one is a current user of cocaine.[26] A recent analysis based on the same survey and published in the prestigious *American Journal of Public Health* and a report issued by the Institute of Medicine, also refuted the gateway theory.[27]

Teenagers know from their own experience and observation that marijuana use does not inevitably, or even usually, lead to the use of harder drugs. In fact, the majority of teens who try marijuana do not even use marijuana itself on a regular basis.[28] Therefore, when such information is presented, students discount both the message and the messenger.

The consistent mischaracterization of marijuana may be the Achilles heel of current approaches to prevention, because such misinformation is inconsistent with students' own observations and experience. As a result, teenagers lose confidence in what we, as parents and teachers, tell them. In turn, they are less likely to consider us credible sources of information.

Nowhere to Turn

Most mandated drug education programs are aimed solely at preventing all drug use. After instructions to abstain, the lessons end. There is no information on how to avoid problems or prevent abuse among those who do experiment. Abstinence is seen as the sole measure of success and the only acceptable teaching option.

While the abstinence-only mandate is well meaning, it is clear that this approach is failing. It is unrealistic to believe that teenagers, at a time in their lives when they are most prone to risk-taking, will completely avoid experimentation with alcohol and other drugs.[29] The mandate leaves teachers and parents with nothing to say to the 51 percent of students who say "maybe" or "sometimes" or "yes" to drug use—the very teens we most need to reach.[30]

Teenage Ecstasy use highlight the need for honest drug education and for providing a place to go for information. While there is troubling preliminary research on possible changes in brain chemistry, federally-funded researchers also know that the context of Ecstasy use (high doses, over-exertion, over-heating, and mixing drugs) is responsible for the vast majority of adverse reactions. While claims of brain damage dominate the government's message to young people, no mention is made of how persistent users might avoid short-term problems (drinking water, cooling off, avoiding other drugs, and practicing moderation). It's "just say no" or nothing at all.[31]

Safety First: A Reality-Based Approach

We know that despite our admonitions and advice to abstain, a majority of teenagers will experiment with drugs. Some will use drugs more regularly. This does not mean that they are bad kids or that we are negligent parents. The reality is that drug use is part of teenage culture in America today. In all likelihood, young people will pass through this phase unharmed.

Keeping teenagers free from harm should be our goal. To do this, our challenge is to figure out how to best ensure their safety. To protect youth, a reality-based approach

Provides drug education for life;

Enables teenagers to make responsible decisions by providing honest, science-based information;

Distinguishes between the use and abuse of mindaltering substances;

Emphasizes the legal consequences of drug use; and

Puts safety first.

Drug Education for Life

A range of both legal and illegal substances is available and used by Americans every day. Each of us has to make decisions about prescription drugs, over-the-counter medications, alcohol, tobacco, caffeine, and the like. How much is enough? How much is too much? How does one drug combine with another?

Rather than a stand-alone course designed solely to prevent teenagers from using illegal drugs, real education would be comprehensive and ongoing. Such quality drug education will prepare young people for what lies ahead throughout their lives.

Honest, Science-Based Education

Although their decision-making skills are not perfect, teenagers are learning responsibility, and few young people are interested in destroying their lives or their health. In fact, studies conducted to discover why students quit using drugs found that concerns about health and their own negative experiences with drugs, motivated their decisions. Their choices had little to do with formal drug-education programs.[32]

Q: How much was your decision to use or not use tobacco, alcohol or other drugs due to the classes and activities in your school?

A: Not at all-43%, A little-17%, Somewhat-12%, A lot-7%, Completely-8%, Don't know-13%."[33]

While teens are still growing intellectually, they are capable of rational thinking.[34] The majority of teenagers actually do make careful decisions about drug use. According to the 2002 *National Survey on Drug Use and Health,* although experimentation is widespread, 88 percent of 12–17-year-olds refrained from regular use.[35] Effective drug education programs should be based on sound science and acknowledge teenagers' ability to understand, analyze, and evaluate their options.

Distinguish Between Use and Abuse

The majority of drug use (with the possible exception of nicotine) does not lead to addiction or abuse. Instead, 80–90 percent of users control their use of psychoactive substances.[36]

Context is crucial. Students who use alcohol, marijuana, or other drugs need to understand there is a huge difference between use and abuse, between occasional and daily use. If they persist, students need to know that they can and must control their use by practicing moderation and limiting use. For example, it is never appropriate to use intoxicants at school, at work, while participating in sports, or while driving.

Legal Consequences

All drugs, including alcohol and tobacco, are illegal for teenagers. Young people need to understand the consequences of violating laws against the use, possession, and sale of drugs. With increasing methods of detection, such as school drug testing and escalating zero-tolerance efforts, illegality is a risk in and of itself, extending well beyond the physical effects of drug use. There are real, lasting consequences of using drugs and being caught, including expulsion from school, a criminal record, and lasting stigma. The Higher Education Act, now being challenged by many student groups, denies college loans for students convicted of any drug offense.

Young people need to know that if they are caught in possession of drugs, they will find themselves at the mercy of the criminal justice system. Half a million Americans are behind bars today for violating drug laws. As soon as teenagers turn 18, they can be prosecuted as adults, and run the risk of serving long mandatory sentences, even for what they see as a minor offense. In Illinois, for example, an individual caught with 15 doses of Ecstasy will serve a minimum of four years in state prison.

Putting Safety First

We must not write off teens who use alcohol and other drugs. While stressing the value of abstinence, we should have a fallback strategy that provides young people with credible information and resources so they do the least possible harm to themselves and those around them.

Instead of banning automobiles, which kill far more teenagers than drugs do, we enforce traffic laws, prohibit driving while intoxicated, and insist that drivers wear seat belts. When attention was drawn to the increased numbers of teenagers dying in drunk-driving accidents, responsible-drinking programs promoted the concept of "designated drivers," which is credited with saving thousands of lives.

Sexuality education shifted away from abstinence-only messages in the mid-80s when we learned that the use of condoms could prevent the spread of HIV and other sexually transmitted diseases. At that time, parents, teachers, and policy makers made the choice to put safety first. Safe sex and reality-based sexuality education was introduced into curricula throughout the country. This approach, according to the CDC, has resulted not just in increased use of condoms among those who were sexually active, but also in decreasing the overall rates of sexual activity among teenagers.[37]

These comprehensive prevention strategies provide strong models for restructuring our drug education efforts.

Making Safety First Drug Education Work

As teachers, parents, and role models for young people, we have a responsibility to fill the gaps left by today's incomplete school-based drug prevention. Here are some suggestions on how we can make a difference.

Put Drug Education into Education

The subject of drugs can be integrated into a variety of high school courses and curricula, including physiology and biology (how drugs affect the body), psychology (how drugs affect the mind), chemistry (what's contained in drugs), history and civics (how drugs have been handled by the government), and social studies (who uses which drugs, and why).

Course textbooks should be revised, updated, and expanded. School boards should rethink their approach: replacing or enhancing stand-alone prevention programs with modules devoted to the study of drugs in hard and social science classes.

Ideally, students will be included in the development of new drug education programs and classes will have more interaction and less lecturing. Through experience, family and peer exposure, and the media, teenagers often know more than we think they do. If we want drug education to be credible, formal curricula should incorporate the observations and experiences of young people, themselves.[38]

After School Programs

Not surprisingly, most teenage drug use occurs between 3 p.m. and 6 p.m. Structured activities for youth during these hours can be an important step toward true prevention.

A voluntary, after-school drop-in program for middle and high school students who want to talk freely, openly, and anonymously about drugs could also be a valuable resource. A drug and alcohol expert can be available for one to three hours in the same room each week. The room should be comfortable, quiet, and equipped with a computer with Internet access, since a primary function of such a program is to help students research their own questions.

If a student's drug use becomes a problem, the after-school dropin program enables her to make informal contact with a professional, even if she is not ready for formal treatment. If problems escalate, a referral to the appropriate agency can be made.

Just Say Know

Everyone involved—teenagers, parents, teachers, counselors—needs to take responsibility for learning about the physiological and sociological effects of drugs. This involves reading, using the Internet for research, and asking questions.

There are no easy answers when it comes to drugs. However, parents can find creative ways to open a dialogue, and listen, listen, listen. If we use natural openings, such as drug use in movies, television, and music to talk and if we remain as non-judgmental as possible, teenagers will seek our guidance. If we become indignant and punitive, teenagers will stop talking to us. It's that simple.

When it comes to "the drug talk," many parents are uneasy about revealing their own experiences, perhaps fearing such admissions might open the door to their teens' experimentation. There is no one resolution to this difficult dilemma. But keep in mind that teenagers generally have a knack for seeing through evasions and half-truths, so honesty is usually the best policy in the long run.

Perhaps most important, teenagers need to trust that the important adults in their lives will provide help, if they need it. They need to know we will pick them up if they need transportation; that they can talk to us if they're frightened, depressed, or ambivalent. Our greatest challenge is to listen and help without excessive admonishment, which will certainly drive our teenagers away.

POSTSCRIPT

Is Abstinence an Effective Strategy for Drug Education?

Before the effectiveness of drug education programs can be determined, it is necessary to define the goals of drug education. Are the goals of drug education to prevent drug use from starting? To prevent drug abuse? To prevent drug dependency? Perhaps the goal of drug education is to teach young people how to protect themselves and others from harm *if* they are going to use drugs. Should the messages about drugs be tailored to different audiences? Without a clear understanding of the goals one wants to achieve in teaching about drugs, it is impossible to determine the effectiveness of drug education.

Before a drug education program can be designed, questions regarding what to include in the drug education curriculum needs to be addressed. Should the primary focus be on teaching abstinence or responsible use? Is it feasible to teach abstinence from some drugs and responsible use of other drugs? The vast majority of high school students have drunk alcohol; should they be taught that they should not drink at all, or should they be taught how to use alcohol responsibly? Is it ethical to teach responsible use of a substance that is illegal? Does the age of the children make a difference in what is taught? Do elementary students have the reasoning skills of high school students? Should the goal be for students to engage in a decision-making process or simply to adopt certain behaviors.

Surveys of drug use by secondary students over the past thirty years show that the rate of drug use is cyclical. Periods of high drug use are followed by periods of lower drug use. This fact could lead one to conclude that drug education has little bearing on whether drugs are used and that other factors contribute to the use, or nonuse, of drugs. It is possible that the availability of drugs is a factor in their use as well as stories in the media.

If drug prevention programs are going to be effective in reducing drug use, schools and other institutions will need to work together. Many young people drop out of school or simply do not attend, so community agencies and faith-based institutions need to become involved. The media have a large impact on young people. What is the best way to incorporate the media in the effort to reduce drug use? Are antidrug commercial spots shown during programs aimed at teenage audiences effective? Do movies and music videos in which drug use is depicted contribute to whether drugs are used?

A number of articles examine factors that influence whether young people engage in drug use. The impact of different messages is reviewed in "Youths' Exposure to Substance Use Prevention Messages:2003" in *The NSDUH (National Survey on Drug Use and Health) Report* (July 29, 2005). Factors such as peers, family, psychological functioning, and stressful life events are discussed in "Risk Factors for Serious Alcohol and Drug Use: The Role of Psychosocial Variables in Predicting the Frequency of Substance Use Among Adolescents," by Maury Nation and Craig Anne Heflinger (*American Journal of Drug and Alcohol Abuse*, August 2006). Lastly, Jeremy Arkes looks at the role of the economy in "Does the Economy Affect Teenage Substance Use?" in *Health Economics* (September 7, 2006).

Contributors to This Volume

EDITOR

RAYMOND GOLDBERG is the associate dean for the School of Professional Studies for the State University of New York at Cortland. Previously, he served as the graduate coordinator for its graduate programs and has been a professor in its health department since 1977. He received his Ph.D. in health education from the University of Toledo, his master's degree from the University of South Carolina, and his bachelor's degree from the University of North Carolina at Pembroke. He is the author of *Drugs Across the Spectrum*, 5th edition (Wadsworth Publishing). He has received over $750,000 in grants for his research in health and drug education.

AUTHORS

JUDITH APPEL is the executive director of Our Family Coalition. Appel has more than 15 years of experience as a public-interest lawyer involved in policy-based work. Appel previously was director of legal affairs for the Drug Policy Alliance, a national, nonprofit organization dedicated to reducing the harm caused by drugs and drug policies. She serves on the Boards of Directors of the Ella Baker Center for Human Rights, Oakland Civil Liberties Alliance, and Coalition on Homelessness.

LYNDAL BOND is the research director for the Adolescent Health and Social Environments Program, Centre for Adolescent Health, Murdoch Children's Research Institute, Melbourne, Australia.

JOSEPH A. CALIFANO, JR., is the chairman of the National Center on Addiction and Substance Abuse at Columbia University. Califano has written several books, including *High Society—How Substance Abuse Ravages America and What to Do About It.*

CAROLYN S. CARTER is a social work professor at Howard University.

RICHARD F. CATALANO is professor and the associate director of the Social Development Research Group at the University of Washington's School of Social Work in Seattle, Washington. For over 25 years, he has led research and program development to promote positive youth development and prevent problem behavior. His work has focused on discovering risk and protective factors for positive and problem behavior, and designing and evaluating programs to address these factors.

THE CENTERS FOR DISEASE CONTROL AND PREVENTION (CDC) is one of the 13 major operating components of the Department of Health and Human Services (HHS), which is the principal agency in the U.S. government for protecting the health and safety of all Americans and for providing essential human services, especially for those people who are least able to help themselves.

BRUCE M. COHEN is a clinical instructor of psychiatry and behavioral sciences at the University of Arkansas for Medical Sciences. He is director of the Child Study Center Clinic and Community Outreach Program in the Division of Pediatric Psychiatry as well as clinical director of Arkansas CARES. His clinical work has focused on children and adolescents with ADHD, learning problems, and depression, and he has extensive experience in school consultation. He earned his B.S. in psychology and his M.S. in clinical psychology (child clinical specialty) from Memphis State University.

SHERWOOD O. COLE is a professor emeritus in the psychology department at Rutgers University.

ALEXANDRA COX works for the Office of Legal Affairs for Drug Policy Alliance, which promotes alternatives to the war on drugs.

LAWRENCE DILLER practices behavioral-developmental pediatrics and family therapy in Walnut Creek, California. He is the author of *Running on Ritalin: A Physician Reflects on Children, Society, and Performance in a Pill.*

DRUG ENFORCEMENT ADMINISTRATION (DEA) has a mission to enforce the controlled substances laws and regulations of the United States and bring to the criminal and civil justice systems of the United States, or any other competent jurisdiction, those organizations and principal members of organizations, involved in the growing, manufacture, or distribution of controlled substances appearing in or destined for illicit traffic in the United States; and to recommend and support nonenforcement programs aimed at reducing the availability of illicit controlled substances on the domestic and international markets.

SUSAN L. ETTNER is professor in the Division of General Internal Medicine and Health Services Research in the UCLA Department of Medicine and in the Department of Health Services in the UCLA School of Public Health. Dr. Ettner obtained her Ph.D. in economics at the Massachusetts Institute of Technology in 1991. She was on the faculty of Harvard Medical School in the Department of Health Care Policy prior to joining UCLA as a tenured associate professor in 1999.

ELIZABETH EVANS is affiliated with the UCLA Integrated Substance Abuse Programs in Los Angeles.

TRACY J. EVANS-WHIPP is a research manager for the Centre for Adolescent Health, Murdoch Children's Research Institute, Melbourne, Australia.

MICHAEL FUMENTO is an author, journalist, and attorney specializing in science and health issues. He is a science columnist for Scripps-Howard and a senior fellow of the Hudson Institute in Washington, D.C. He has also been a legal writer for the *Washington Times* and an editorial writer for the *Rocky Mountain News* in Denver, and he was the first "National Issues" reporter for *Investor's Business Daily*. Fumento has lectured on science and health issues throughout the world, including Great Britain, France, the Czech Republic, Greece, Austria, China, and South America. His publications include *BioEvolution: How Biotechnology Is Changing Our World* (Encounter Books, 2003).

PETER GORMAN is an investigative journalist and former editor-in-chief of High Times magazine. He spends at least 3 months of every year living in Peru, where he works with Ayahuasca and other plant-based medicines, as well as doing political work. Much of his writing, both in Peru and the United States, has focused on the on-going War on Drugs.

FATEMA GUNJA attended Cornell University. After graduating, she worked on drug policy issues, first as a communications coordinator at the American Civil Liberties Union and then as the first director of the Drug Policy Forum of Massachusetts. During her drug policy days, she became a passionate spokesperson and writer on racial justice and students' rights in the context of the War on Drugs.

MARY HARDY is affiliated with the UCLA Integrated Substance Abuse Programs in Los Angeles.

MATTHEW HERPER is a staff writer for Forbes Magazine and has written extensively on health-related matters.

YIH-ING HSER is affiliated with the UCLA Integrated Substance Abuse Programs in Los Angeles.

DAVID HUANG is affiliated with the UCLA Integrated Substance Abuse Programs in Los Angeles.

WILLIAM G. IACONO is a Distinguished McNight University Professor. He also is the director of the Clinical Science and Psychopathology Research Training Program in the Psychology Department and an adjunct professor for the Institute of Child Development.

CATHY INOUYE lives in Guatemala City and volunteers for the human rights NGO SEDEM (Seguridad en Democracia). SEDEM monitors the continuing role of the military, police, and intelligence forces in Guatemala.

MICKEL JOURABCHI is a resident of Encino, California.

JENNIFER KERN is a research associate at the Drug Policy Alliance's Office of Legal Affairs in Berkeley. Ms. Kern serves as the national campaign coordinator for DPA's "Drug Testing Fails Our Youth," a public education project. She has been interviewed by a wide range of national print and broadcast media, including *Newsweek, Reuters, The Associated Press, Washington Post, Christian Science Monitor, Houston Chronicle,* and *Milwaukee Journal Sentinel,* among others.

HERBERT KLEBER founded at Columbia University the Division on Substance Abuse, now one of the leading centers in the country. Dr. Kleber is the author of more than 200 papers, and the coeditor of the *American Psychiatric Press Textbook of Substance Abuse Treatment.*

ROBERT LANGRETH is a reporter, who joined *Forbes Magazine* as senior editor. His articles cover the pharmaceutical industry, medicine, and science.

LISA N. LEGRAND received her Ph.D. in behavioral genetics and clinical psychology from the University of Minnesota in 2003 and is currently a research associate at the Minnesota Center for Twin and Family Research (MCTFR).

ROBERT A. LEVY, a senior fellow in constitutional studies, joined Cato in 1997 after 25 years in business. He is a director of the Institute for Justice and a member of the board of visitors of the Federalist Society. Levy received his Ph.D. in business from the American University in 1966.

PAUL A. LOGLI is state's attorney for Winnebago County, Illinois, and a lecturer at the National College of District Attorneys. A member of the Illinois State Bar since 1974, he is a nationally recognized advocate for prosecutorial involvement in the issue of substance-abused infants. He earned his J.D. from the University of Illinois.

ROSALIND B. MARIMONT is a retired mathematician and scientist, having done research and development for the National Institute of Standards and Technology (formerly the Bureau of Standards) for 18 years and for the National Institute of Health (NIH) for another 19. She started in electronics defense work during World War II, then went into the logical design of the early digital computers during the 1950s. At the NIH she studied and published papers on human vision, speech, and other biomathematical subjects. Since her retirement she has been active in health policy issues, particularly the war on smoking.

MERRILL MATTHEWS, JR., is a public policy analyst specializing in health care, Social Security, welfare, and Internet issues, and the author of numerous studies in health policy, as well as other public policy issues. Currently a visiting scholar with the Institute for Policy Innovation, he is former president of the Health Economics Roundtable for the National Association for Business Economics and former health policy adviser for the American Legislative Exchange Council. Matthews also serves as the medical ethicist for the University of Texas Southwestern Medical Center's Institutional Review Board for Human Experimentation. He earned his Ph.D. in philosophy and humanities from the University of Texas at Dallas.

MATT McGUE is a professor of psychology at the University of Minnesota and a past president of the Behavior Genetics Association. He has co-directed the Minnesota Center for Twin and Family Research for the last dozen years.

LEEMON McHENRY is a professor in the Philosophy Department at the California State University at Northridge.

JUDITH McMULLEN is a graduate of Yale Law School, who joined the faculty in 1987 and teaches in the areas of Family Law, Trusts & Estates, and Property. Her articles on family and children's issues have appeared in the *University of Michigan Journal of Law Reform*, the *Indiana Law Review*, and other publications.

MATTHEW J. MITTEN is the director of the National Sports Law Institute and the LL.M. in sports law program for foreign lawyers at Marquette University Law School in Milwaukee, Wisconsin. He currently teaches courses in Amateur Sports Law, Professional Sports Law and Torts and has also taught Antitrust Law, Comparative Sports Law, International Sports Law, Legal Ethics and Professional Responsibility, and a Sports Law seminar.

ETHAN NADELMANN is the founder and executive director of the Drug Policy Alliance, the leading organization in the United States promoting alternatives to the war on drugs. Nadelmann received his BA, JD, and PhD from Harvard, and a master's degree in international relations from the London School of Economics. In 1994, Nadelmann founded the Lindesmith Center, a drug policy institute created with the philanthropic support of George Soros. In 2000, the growing Center merged with another organization to form the Drug Policy Alliance, which advocates for drug policies grounded in science, compassion, health, and human rights.

THE NATIONAL INSTITUTE ON ALCOHOL ABUSE AND ALCOHOLISM (NIAAA) provides leadership in the national effort to reduce alcohol-related problems by conducting and supporting research in a wide range of scientific areas including genetics, neuroscience, epidemiology, health risks and benefits of alcohol consumption, prevention, and treatment. The NIAAA coordinates and collaborates with other research institutes and federal programs on alcohol-related issues. It also collaborates with international, national, state, and local institutions, organizations, agencies, and programs engaged in alcohol-related work. The NIAAA translates and disseminates research findings to health care providers, researchers, policymakers, and the public.

NATIONAL INSTITUTE ON DRUG ABUSE (NIDA) has as its mission to lead our nation in bringing the power of science to bear on drug abuse and addiction.

THE OFFICE OF NATIONAL DRUG CONTROL POLICY establishes policies, priorities, and objectives for the nation's drug control program. The goals of the program are to reduce illicit drug use, manufacturing, and trafficking; drug-related crime and violence; and drug-related health consequences.

MARSHA ROSENBAUM is director of the Safety First project and director of the San Francisco office of the Drug Policy Alliance. She received her doctorate in medical sociology from the University of California at San Francisco in 1979. From 1977 to 1995, Rosenbaum was the principal investigator on National Institute on Drug Abuse-funded studies of heroin addiction, methadone maintenance treatment, MDMA (Ecstasy), cocaine, and drug use during pregnancy. She is author of three books: *Women on Heroin, Pursuit of Ecstasy: The MDMA Experience* (with Jerome E. Beck), and *Pregnant Women on Drugs: Combating Stereotypes and Stigma* (with Sheigla Murphy).

DANIELLE ROSE ASH is a doctoral student who is associated with the Division of General Internal Medicine and Health Services Research at the David Geffen School of Medicine at UCLA.

SALLY SATEL is the staff psychiatrist at the Oasis Clinic in Washington, D.C. She serves on the advisory committee of the Center for Mental Health Services of the Substance Abuse and Mental Health Services Administration. She has written widely in academic journals on topics in psychiatry and medicine, and has published articles on cultural aspects of medicine and science in numerous magazines and journals. Dr. Satel is author of *Drug Treatment: The Case for Coercion* (AEI Press, 1999) and *PC, M.D.: How Political Correctness Is Corrupting Medicine* (Basic Books, 2001), and is coauthor, with Christina Hoff Sommers, of *One Nation under Therapy* (St. Martin's Press, 2005).

JACOB SULLUM is a senior editor at *Reason*, a monthly magazine that covers politics and culture from a libertarian perspective.

JAMES THORNTON is a writer for *Men's Health, Field & Stream, National Geographic Adventure*, and other magazines. His health writing has been nominated three times for the National Magazine Awards, and he won this so-called "Oscars of the magazine business" once (in 1998, for three articles on different aspects of male health).

JOHN W. TOUMBOUROU is associate professor at the Department of Paediatrics, University of Melbourne, and a senior researcher at the Center for Adolescent Health. He is a founding member and outgoing chair of the College of Health Psychologists within the Australian Psychological Society. Professor Toumbourou is a principal investigator on a number of studies investigating healthy youth development including the Australian Temperament Project (investigating the role of childhood temperament and behavior in the prediction of adolescent substance use, delinquency, and depression), and the International Youth Development study (a collaborative longitudinal study with the University of Washington).

UNITED NATIONS INTERNATIONAL DRUG CONTROL PROGRAMME (UNDCP) AND THE UNITED NATIONS CENTRE FOR INTERNATIONAL CRIME PREVENTION (CICP) are part of the United Nations Office on Drugs and Crime (UNODC), which was formerly called the United Nations Office for Drug Control & Crime Prevention (ODCCP). UNDCP cooperates with governmental and nongovernmental organisations as well as with the business community. Its experts help requesting states to become party to and give effect to the United Nations drug control conventions. UNDCP also performs laboratory services, provides training materials, and can refer those in need to the appropriate medical advice. In the area of demand reduction, a multiphase regional programme designed to train professionals in the treatment of drug abuse has been successfully completed, creating a core cadre of over 600 professionals and sustainable national training programmes in training professionals in the treatment of drug abuse.

U.S. DEPARTMENT OF HEALTH AND HUMAN SERVICES is the United States government's principal agency for protecting the health of all Americans and providing essential human services, especially for those who are least able to help themselves.

ANJULI VERMA is the public education coordinator at the ACLU Drug Law Reform Project (DLRP), located in Santa Cruz, California. She creates and executes public education campaigns around the DLRP's litigation and is active in national ACLU campaigns to defend and disband regional narcotics task forces, expose drug laws' disproportionate impact on women and families, especially in communities of color, and educate the rave and other music communities about their rights.